MEDICAL RADIOLOGY
Diagnostic Imaging

Editors:
A. L. Baert, Leuven
K. Sartor, Heidelberg

M. Filippi · N. De Stefano · V. Dousset
J.C. McGowan (Eds.)

MR Imaging in White Matter Diseases of the Brain and Spinal Cord

With Contributions by

R. Bammer · A. Bertolino · A. Bizzi · L. R. Caplan · M. Castillo · N. De Stefano · V. Dousset
B. J. Emmer · F. Fazekas · M. Filippi · K. W. Fishbein · G. B. Frisoni · J. L. Go · J. A. Gomes
S. J. Hickman · M. A. Horsfield · T. W. J. Huizinga · P. Jezzard · A. Kangarlu · P. E. Kim
B. K. Kleinschmidt-DeMasters · M. Knauth · I. Kovanlikaya · D. L. Kraitchman · R. Lenkinski
D. K. B. Li · C. Marras · M. Maya · M. Mascalchi · J. C. McGowan · D. H. Miller · S. Mori
M. Mortilla · L. Nagae-Poetscher · D. T. Okuda · D. W. Paty · B. Pollo · C. Raybaud · M. A. Rocca
M. Rovaris · F. Salvi · F. Sambataro · S. Schwarz · J. H. Simon · R. G. Spencer · S. Strasser-Fuchs
S. D. Swanson · A. Toosy · A. Traboulsee · M. A. van Buchem · P. C. M. van Zijl · T. L. Vollmer
G. Zhao · C-S. Zee

Foreword by

K. Sartor

With 247 Figures in 601 Separate Illustrations, 41 in Color and 23 Tables

Springer

Massimo Filippi, MD
Director, Neuroimaging Research Unit
Department of Neurology
Scientific Institute and
University Ospedale San Raffaele
Via Olgettina, 60
20132 Milan
Italy

Vincent Dousset, MD, PhD
Professor, Service de Neuroradiologie
Diagnostique et Thérapeutique
CHU Bordeaux Pellegrin and Laboratoire de
Neurobiologie des Affections de la Myéline
Université Victor Segalen Bourdeaux 2
33076 Bordeaux
France

Nicola De Stefano, MD, PhD
Associate Professor
Department of Neurology & Behavioral Sciences
University of Siena
Viale Bracci 2
53100 Siena
Italy

Joseph C. McGowan, PhD
Associate Professor of Electrical Engineering
Department of Electrical Engineering
Maury Hall 227
United States Naval Academy
Annapolis, MD 21402-5025
USA

Medical Radiology · Diagnostic Imaging and Radiation Oncology
Series Editors: A. L. Baert · L. W. Brady · H.-P. Heilmann · M. Molls · K. Sartor

Continuation of Handbuch der medizinischen Radiologie
Encyclopedia of Medical Radiology

ISBN 978-3-642-07298-7 e-ISBN 978-3-540-27644-9

Springer is a part of Springer Science+Business Media

http//www.springeronline.com

Printed in Germany

Medical Editor: Dr. Ute Heilmann, Heidelberg
Desk Editor: Ursula N. Davis, Heidelberg
Production Editor: Kurt Teichmann, Mauer

Printed on acid-free paper 21/3150xq – 5 4 3 2 1 0

Foreword

When magnetic resonance imaging (MRI) started to be used clinically in the early 1980s it rapidly became clear how little information had been provided hitherto by computed tomography (CT) on the various diseases that involve the cerebral (and spinal) white matter. For the first time many white matter abnormalities with too little effect on tissue electron density to render them visible on CT could be shown in vivo. Also, as there was no ionizing radiation involved, these abnormalities could be studied over time ("monitored") with essentially no risk to the patient. Along with the evolution of the new imaging modality, such as the steady improvement of MRI hard- and software and the increasing usage of paramagnetic agents to enhance tissue contrast, radiologists and their clinical colleagues gained insight into both the natural history and the course under therapy of many white matter diseases. It was soon recognized, though, that some white matter diseases had a fairly characteristic or even diagnostic pattern on MRI, while others did not; morphologically there was much overlap between diseases differing in etiology and pathogenesis. Despite this limitation of standard structural (conventional) imaging techniques, MRI eventually gained a decisive role in clinical diagnosis and research of the most important white matter disease, multiple sclerosis (MS).

As the quest for advanced MRI methods to obtain more fundamental information on the various disease processes and to improve differential diagnosis continued, any promising new imaging or measuring technique was tested for its usefulness to study normal and abnormal white matter. Some of the presently available techniques allow us to study crucial aspects of neurometabolism in a quantitative way (magnetization transfer MRI, diffusion-weighted MRI, proton MR spectroscopy), while others provide insight into neurovascular physiology and brain and spinal cord function (perfusion-weighted MRI, functional MRI). The ultimate aim, however, is to develop methods suitable to study white matter structure, metabolism, physiology and function at the cellular and even molecular level, an endeavor likely to be successful only at field strengths above 1.5 T.

In this book, conceived and edited by M. Filippi, N. De Stefano, V. Dousset and J. C. McGowan, an impressive number of world-renowned experts have set new standards of compact information regarding white matter disease. The book deals first with the principles of pertinent modern MRI techniques and then covers in depth the disorders of myelination, including normal brain development, demyelinating diseases, immune-mediated disorders of white matter including vasculitides, white matter disorders related to aging, and white matter disorders secondary to other pathologic conditions.

In this state-of-the-art compendium, I am quite sure, interested (neuro)radiologists, neuroclinicians, and neuroresearchers can find practically everything worthwhile knowing on the in vivo imaging of white matter diseases of the brain and spinal cord. Convinced that the book will be a success, I wish to laud the editors and authors for their joint effort and timely work.

Heidelberg K. Sartor

Preface

The application of magnetic resonance imaging (MRI) to the study of the central nervous system (CNS) has greatly improved our ability to diagnose numerous pathological conditions affecting the brain and the spinal cord, as well as to monitor their evolution. This is particularly true for multiple sclerosis (MS), where the sensitivity of T2-weighted MRI in the detection of white matter lesions, together with the ability of post-contrast T1-weighted images to reflect the presence of acute inflammatory activity, may allow us to demonstrate the dissemination of MS pathology in space and time earlier than the clinical assessment, thus leading to an earlier and more confident diagnosis. However, the whole spectrum of white matter diseases, ranging from inherited and acquired disorders of myelination to neurodegenerative conditions related to aging, has been the focus of many MRI studies since the earliest clinical application of this technology.

In the past few years, in parallel with the advancement of MRI technology, the many limitations of conventional MRI have become evident, both in the diagnostic work-up and in the research setting. Conventional MRI patterns of white matter pathology may, on the one hand, overlap among different CNS diseases, while, on the other, they provide only limited pieces of information on the underlying pathological changes in terms of both accuracy and specificity. As regards this latter issue, conventional MRI has three major limitations. First, T2-weighted signal abnormalities just reflect the presence of increased water content, which may range from transient edema to irreversible demyelination and axonal loss. Secondly, the presence of contrast enhancement indicates that blood-brain barrier permeability is increased and associated with ongoing inflammation, but it does not provide any information about the nature and extent of associated tissue damage. Thirdly, conventional MRI is unable to detect and quantify the presence of damage occurring in the normal-appearing CNS tissues, which have been shown to be diffusely and sometimes severely damaged in many white matter disorders.

Structural and metabolic quantitative MRI techniques, such as magnetization transfer (MT) MRI, diffusion-weighted (DW) MRI and proton MR spectroscopy (1H-MRS), are increasingly being applied to the study of white matter diseases. Other non-conventional MRI techniques, such as functional MRI (fMRI), cell-specific MRI, perfusion MRI, molecular MRI and microscopic imaging with ultra-high-field MRI, are emerging as additional promising tools for improving our understanding of many of these conditions. These MRI techniques represent an extraordinary set of powerful instruments to gain in vivo fundamental insights into the pathogenesis and evolution of white matter damage. MT MRI and DW MRI enable us to quantify the extent of structural changes occurring in T2-visible lesions and in the white matter that appears normal on conventional MR images. 1H-MRS can add information on the biochemical nature of white matter changes, with the potential to improve significantly our ability to monitor inflammatory demyelination and axonal injury. Structural and metabolic MR-based quantitative techniques are also contributing to the understanding of the reparative mechanisms occurring after injury to the CNS. This latter aspect is likely to have a central role in determining the final clinical outcome of all neurological conditions. In this context, fMRI holds substantial promise to elucidate the mechanisms of cortical adaptive reorganization following brain injury, and eventually to achieve a more accurate picture of the balance between tissue damage and repair in various CNS conditions. Cellular MRI, molecular MRI and perfusion MRI have the potential to provide additional pieces of information on the heterogeneous aspects of white matter damage, which might be central for the understanding of the pathogenesis of new lesion formation and evolution. High-field MRI will affect dramatically anatomical visualization, proton and nonproton MRS, fMRI and nonproton imaging and, as a consequence, our ability to image the critical components of white matter diseases. This aspect of MRI technology is progressing rapidly, and the time for a more extensive clinical application of high-field MRI will probably come soon.

The present book aims at providing a complete and updated review of the "state of the art" of the application of conventional, quantitative and functional MRI techniques to the study of white matter disorders of the brain and spinal cord. In the first, extensive section, each chapter examines in details the basic principles, advantages and disadvantages of all the aforementioned MRI techniques. The subsequent sections are clinically driven and focused on the various disorders that can affect the human CNS white matter. The role of MRI in the diagnosis and in monitoring the efficacy of experimental treatment is reviewed extensively, as well as the novel insights provided by quantitative MR techniques into the pathophysiology of all these conditions. We hope that this book will represent a valuable tool for clinicians and researchers who wish to gain a deeper understanding of the complex issues related to diagnosis, work-up and treatment of patients with diseased white matter, as well as a reservoir for new ideas and a stimulus for further investigations.

Milan
Siena
Bordeaux
Annapolis

Massimo Filippi
Nicola De Stefano
Vincent Dousset
Joseph C. McGowan

Contents

MR Techniques: Principles

1 Basis of MRI Contrast

Mark A. Horsfield

CONTENTS

1.1 The Magnetic Resonance Signal

1.1.1 Nuclear Magnetism

In the materials that we traditionally think of as being magnetic (such as iron and steel), the magnetism arises from two properties of electrons: charge (all electrons are negatively charged) and motion (electrons rotate or *spin* about their axis). A moving charge will always generate a magnetic field, and in this way an electrical current flowing through a wire generates a magnetic field around the wire. While a single rotating electron generates a magnetic field, electrons tend to form themselves into pairs, with one electron rotating in one direction and the other electron rotating in the opposite direction. The magnetic field of one electron cancels out the field from the second, and the net magnetism of the pair is zero. In materials with unpaired electron spin, the magnetic field from individual electrons may be randomly aligned, so that under these circumstances the net field from the material will be zero. However, if such a material is brought into a magnetic field (the *applied* magnetic field), this causes a partial alignment of the electrons' magnetic fields and the material becomes slightly, and temporarily magnetized. These types of material are called *paramagnetic*.

We do not usually think of people as being magnetic, and indeed some of the principal constituents of the human body (e.g., water, lipids, proteins) do not show any magnetic effects from their electronic structure. However, another, weaker form of magnetism (nuclear paramagnetism) arises from the charge and spin of nuclear particles in just a few types of nuclei, where the spin of individual protons and neutrons is not canceled out within a nucleus. Table 1.1 shows a list of some of the most interesting nuclei (from a biological point of view) that exhibit nuclear magnetism.

Table 1.1. Biologically interesting nuclei that give an MRI signal

Nucleus	Atomic number	Gyromagnetic ratio (MHz/Tesla)	Relative sensitivity[a]
Hydrogen	1	42.58	1.0
Carbon	13	10.71	0.016
Nitrogen	15	4.31	0.001
Oxygen	17	5.77	0.003
Fluorine	19	40.05	0.83
Sodium	23	11.26	0.093
Phosphorus	31	17.23	0.066

[a] Relative sensitivity indicates the amount of signal (compared to hydrogen) and is for equal numbers of atoms per unit volume of tissue. The relative sensitivity takes into account both the Larmor frequency and the natural abundance of the given isotope.

The hydrogen atom is most commonly used when performing MRI scanning, since the hydrogen nucleus gives the strongest signal, and there is plenty of hydrogen around in the human body in molecules of water, fat and proteins. Potentially, other nuclei could be used, but the poor sensitivity would make for very poor quality images, and excessively long scan times.

M. A. Horsfield, PhD
Department of Cardiovascular Sciences, University of Leicester, Leicester, LE1 5WW, UK

1.1.2 Precession

The hydrogen nucleus spins about its axis, generating the nuclear magnetism, but when the nucleus is placed in a magnetic field, it undergoes another form of rotary motion called precession. This type of motion can also be seen with a child's spinning top if it is tilted at an angle to the gravitational field.

The frequency of this precessional motion is called the *Larmor* frequency, and is proportional to the applied magnetic field strength:

$$f = \gamma B0. \tag{1}$$

In the Larmor equation, above, γ is the gyromagnetic ratio and is constant for all nuclei of the same type, but varies between different types, as shown in Table 1.1.

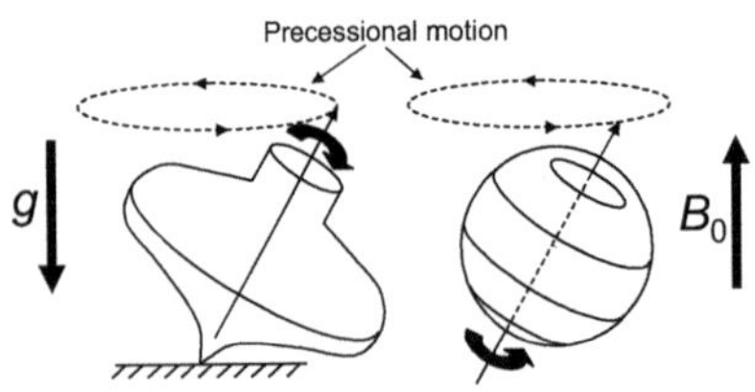

Fig. 1.1. The angular momentum of a spinning top (*left*) interacts with the gravitational field to produce a rotary "precessional" motion. In a similar way, the magnetism of the nucleus (*right*) interacts with the applied *B*0 field to cause precession about the field

1.1.3 Polarization and Coherence

Since nuclear magnetism is a form of paramagnetism, the individual nuclear spins do not have any preferred alignment until they are placed in the applied field (the *B*0 field). A large component of any MRI scanner is the magnet in which the patient lies, which causes the nuclear spins to become aligned, or polarized, such that some spins point in the general direction of the applied field, and some point in a direction opposed to the applied field.

There are slightly more spins aligned with the applied magnetic field than there are opposed to it, although the difference in the numbers is very small. This difference is the *excess population* of spins. Now, when the magnetism of the individual spins is added together, the net result is a small amount of magnetization in the same direction as the applied field that arises within the patient. The amount of this *net magnetization* is proportional to the strength of the applied field, hence the need for a powerful magnet at the heart of the MRI scanner. However, because the net magnetization points in the same direction as the applied field and is much, much smaller than it, it is very difficult to measure directly. We need to tilt the patient's magnetization away from the applied field in order to make it measurable.

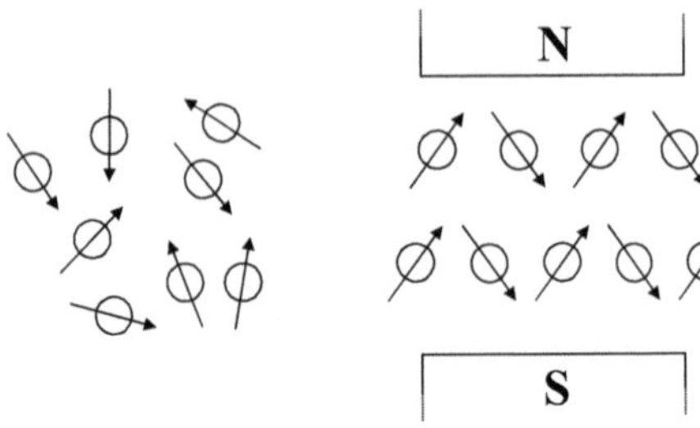

Fig. 1.2. When no magnetic field is applied (*left*), nuclear spins have no preferred alignment so that the net magnetization within the patient is zero. When a magnetic field is applied (*right*), polarization occurs with some spins being aligned with the field, and some opposed to it. There are slightly more spins aligned with the field than opposed, giving rise to magnetism within the patient – the "net magnetization"

1.1.3.1 Radio Frequency Pulses

The patient's net magnetization is made measurable by applying a burst (pulse) of electromagnetic energy. The transfer of energy from the electromagnetic wave to the nuclear magnetization is a *resonance* phenomenon, meaning that the frequency of the pulse must be close the spins' natural frequency (the Larmor frequency) in order to have the desired effect. Since the Larmor frequency is in the radio frequency range (MHz), then the pulse is called a radio frequency (RF) pulse.

Before the RF pulse is applied, the patient's net magnetization is usually shown schematically as in Fig. 1.3. Note that: (a) only the excess population of spins is shown, and (b) although no individual spin is aligned with the *B*0 field, the net result of adding all these spins together is a net magnetization that points in the direction of that field. Since the patient's magnetization has a direction as well as a magnitude, it is a vector quantity called the net magnetization vector, and given the symbol *M*. The magnitude of *M* when the patient has become fully magnetized is given the symbol M_0, and depends on the strength of the *B*0 field and the number of hydrogen atoms per unit volume of tissue that contribute to the magnetization vector. An RF pulse tilts this vector out of alignment with the *B*0 field, and the angle of tilt (or

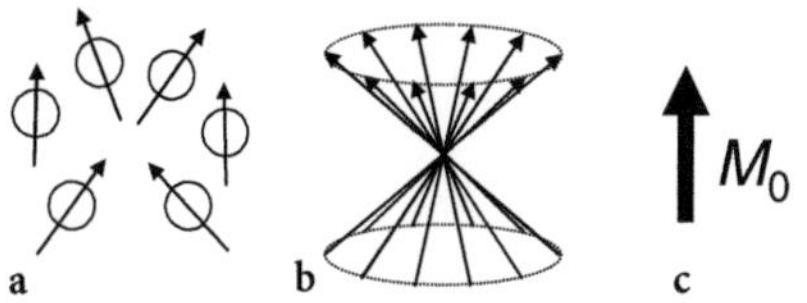

Fig. 1.3a–c. Three different ways of representing the patient's magnetization. **a** The excess population of spins that (by definition) tend to be aligned with the applied field. **b** A schematic representation of these spins, indicating that the component of magnetization perpendicular to *B0* is random, such that any transverse components of magnetization cancel to zero. **c** The resultant magnetization vector after adding the individual nuclear magnets together. This net magnetization vector also points in the same direction as the applied field, and is therefore difficult to detect directly

the *flip angle*) depends on the strength and duration of the RF pulse. When one or more RF pulses is applied, and the MRI signal is measured (see below), then this is called a pulse sequence.

1.1.3.2 90° Pulse – Excitation and FID

A 90° pulse will tilt the net magnetization vector by 90°. If *M* starts off aligned with the *B0* field (by definition, the *z* direction), then a 90° pulse flips the magnetization into the *x-y* plane (see Fig. 1.4).

M then precesses in the *x-y* plane so that, in effect, we now have the patient's magnetization rotating in a plane perpendicular to the applied field. The method of detecting *M* is analogous to a motor car's alternator which generates electricity to power the ignition, lights etc. An alternator consists of a magnet inside some coils of wire, with the magnet being driven by the motor to that it rotates inside the coils. This generates an electromotive force (voltage) within the coils. Similarly, we wrap a coil of wire around the patient (the receiver coil) and can measure an oscillating voltage across the coil, with the frequency of oscillation being equal to the Larmor frequency, and the size of the voltage being dependent on the number of hydrogen nuclei that are within the coil.

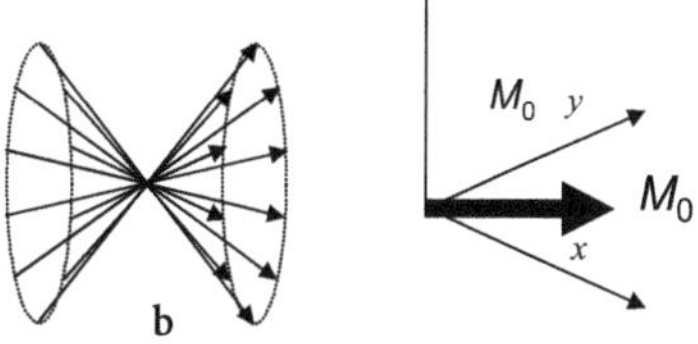

Fig. 1.4a,b. Individual spins (*left*) and the net magnetization vector (*right*) (**a**) before (**a**) and just after (**b**) a 90° RF pulse. The vector has been tilted out of alignment with the *B0* field and into the *x-y* plane

While the magnetization remains in the *x-y* plane, and the individual nuclear spins are oriented in the same direction as shown in Fig. 1.4 (i.e., they are coherent), a voltage will be measured in the coil. However, there are slight, natural variations in the Larmor frequency due to the interactions between magnetic particles (such as the nuclei) within the patient, and these variations in frequency cause the signal to die away (the magnetization loses coherence) normally within the course of a few hundred milliseconds or so. The initial voltage and its subsequent decay are known as the free induction decay (FID), since the voltage is produced by electromagnetic induction, and once *M* is in the *x-y* plane it can rotate freely without further influence from RF pulses.

After application of the 90° RF pulse, the voltage measured in the receiver coil that is wrapped around the patient takes the form of a sinusoidal oscillation with decaying amplitude. The "envelope" that encloses the FID, shown as a dotted line in Fig. 1.6, indicates the rate at which the sinusoid decays, and the time constant that characterizes the decay is called $T2^*$ ("T2 star"). $T2^*$ depends on both the physico-chemical properties of the tissue and on the uniformity, or homogeneity, of the applied magnetic field. Tissues that have a high free water content tend to have longer $T2^*$ values than tissues with a dense matrix of cell membranes and cellular structures. Thus, $T2^*$ can be used as the basis for imaging many pathological tissues such as MS lesions, since the density of these cell membranes and structures is reduced by processes such as demyelination and axonal loss, leading to in-

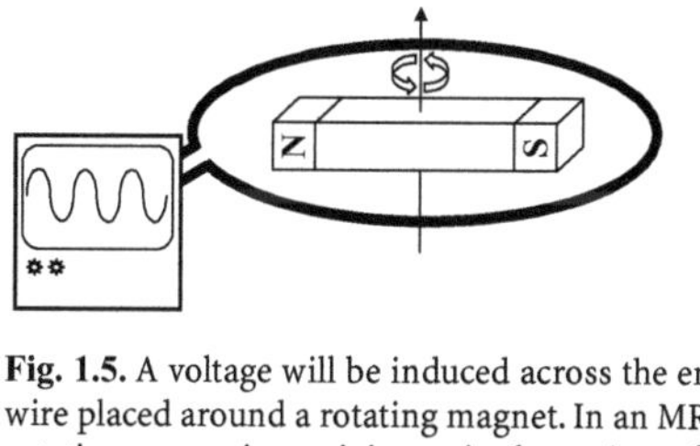

Fig. 1.5. A voltage will be induced across the ends of a coil of wire placed around a rotating magnet. In an MRI scanner, this rotating magnetism originates in the patient after a 90° pulse has been applied. An oscilloscope connected to the coil would show a sinusoidally oscillating voltage, with the frequency of oscillation equal to the Larmor frequency, and the peak-to-peak voltage being proportional to the number of spins within the sensitive region of the coil

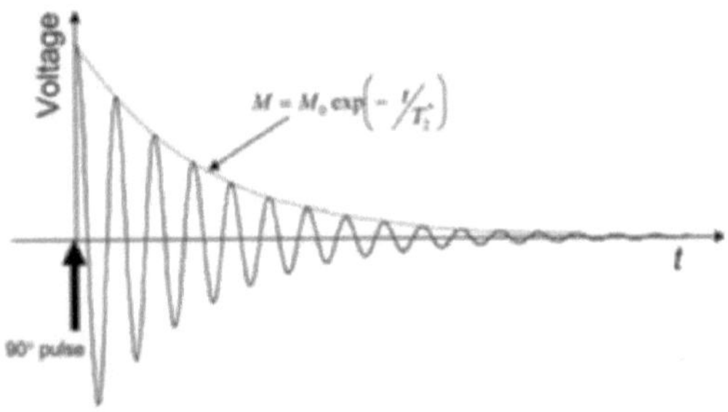

Fig. 1.6. A 90° pulse of RF energy tilts the magnetization vector into the *x-y* plane where it generates an oscillating voltage in the receiver coil. The amplitude of this voltage decays with a time constant T2*

creased T2*. The process of generating image contrast will be described more fully later in this chapter.

As mentioned above, T2* decay contains contributions from both the physico-chemical properties of the tissue, and magnetic field inhomogeneities within the patient. These inhomogeneities may result either from imperfections in the design and manufacture of the magnet, or from the magnetic properties of the patient. Any variations in the tissue's magnetic properties within the patient will result in small but important perturbations in the magnetic field uniformity; these sorts of variation occur, for example, around the interface between the brain tissue and frontal sinuses. It can be seen from the Larmor equation that any variation in *B0* field strength will lead to different precessional frequencies throughout the patient, so that the initial magnetization vector, being composed of magnetization from different parts of the patient, will begin to spread out (or 'dephase') in the *x-y* plane. This is mechanism by which the FID signal decays after it is initially generated by the 90° pulse (Fig. 1.7).

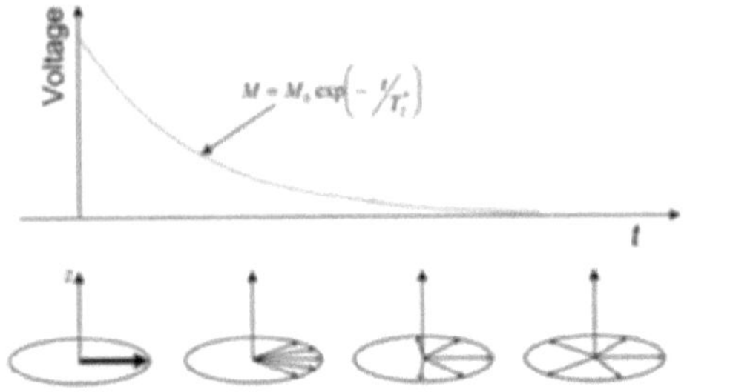

Fig. 1.7. After the 90° pulse creates magnetization in the *x-y* plane, variations in the Larmor frequency within the patient will cause a spreading out, since some magnetization precesses slower, and some faster than the average. This spreading out in the *x-y* plane results in a reduction in the size of the net magnetization vector and is the cause of the decay in the voltage measured in the receiver coil. Deviations from the average motion are shown, so that superimposed on this spreading out is a precession at the average Larmor frequency

1.1.3.3 180° Pulse – Refocusing

The initial 90° pulse rotates the magnetization which is initially along the *z*-axis (longitudinal magnetization) down into the *x-y* plane and generates the measurable or transverse magnetization. Similarly, a 180° pulse rotates the magnetization vectors by 180°, and one use of these pulses is to reverse the dephasing that occurs after a 90° pulse because of the variations in the *B0* field.

Shown in Fig. 1.8 are two packets of magnetization, labeled *a* and *b*, with *a* rotating clockwise (relative to the average) because it experiences a higher *B0* field than average (and hence has a higher precession frequency), and *b* rotating anticlockwise because it experiences a lower *B0* field than average. Deviations from the average motion are shown, so that superimposed on this dephasing is a precession at the average

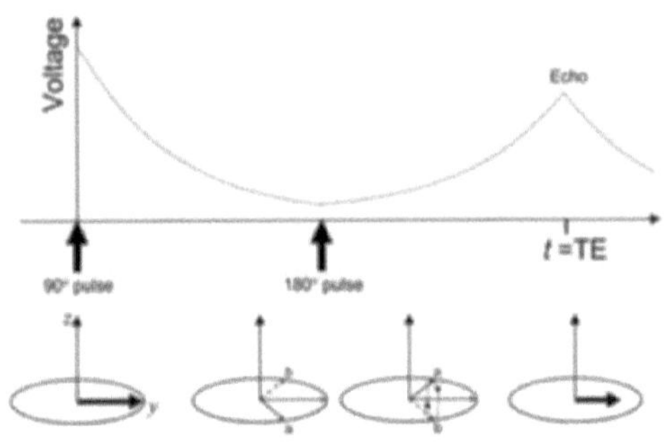

Fig. 1.8. After the initial 90° pulse, dephasing of transverse magnetization occurs, with the magnetization from two locations within the patient, labeled *a* and *b*, being shown. A 180° pulse is applied and rotates the magnetization about the *y*-axis so that the magnetization is flipped over, reversing the phase of *a* and *b*. The magnetization continues to precess and comes back into phase at a time TE called the echo time. Deviations from the average motion are shown, so that superimposed on this is a precession at the average Larmor frequency

Larmor frequency. A 180° pulse will rotate the magnetization about the *y*-axis, which has the effect of reversing the phase that accumulated before this pulse. After the 180° pulse, *a* continues to rotate clockwise and *b* anticlockwise and eventually at a time called the *echo time*, or TE, the individual magnetization vectors come back into phase generating again a high voltage in the receiver coil. This *spin-echo* is what is commonly measured during an MRI scanning sequence.

Notice that the voltage in the receiver coil is somewhat reduced in amplitude compared to the initial amplitude after the 90° pulse. That is because the loss of signal due to T2* relaxation has two causes, and only one of these (the magnetic field inhomogeneities) can be reversed by the 180° pulse. A second cause of signal dephasing is the interactions that occur on a microscopic scale between magnetic entities such as unpaired electrons and other nuclear magnetism within the patient.

Notice also that the echo forms at a time exactly twice that between the 90° pulse and the 180° pulse. If the time between the 90° and 180° pulses is varied, then TE will also vary and the amplitude of the echo will change, as shown in Fig. 1.9. Because the effects of magnetic field inhomogeneity are removed in the process of forming the echo, then the decrease in echo amplitude as TE increases is due only to the microscopic interactions between magnetic particles within the tissue. These interactions are fundamentally related to the physico-chemical properties of the tissue, and not to the vagaries of the uniformity of the magnetic field. The decay of the echo amplitude shown in Fig. 1.9 is exponential with TE and has a time constant called T2, the transverse relaxation time. T2 is also called the spin--spin relaxation time, since the loss of transverse magnetization in this way results largely from interactions between the magnetism of individual spins.

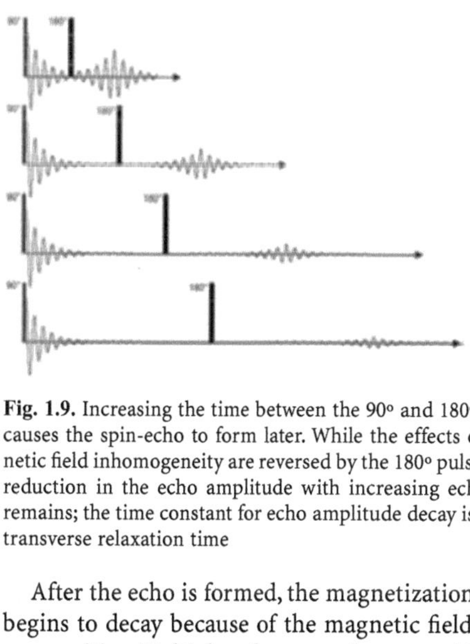

Fig. 1.9. Increasing the time between the 90° and 180° pulses causes the spin-echo to form later. While the effects of magnetic field inhomogeneity are reversed by the 180° pulse, some reduction in the echo amplitude with increasing echo time remains; the time constant for echo amplitude decay is T_2, the transverse relaxation time

After the echo is formed, the magnetization again begins to decay because of the magnetic field inhomogeneities. Multiple echoes can be created by applying a series of 180° pulses. The echoes form between the pulses, and these multiple echoes are called the echo train. In this way, the MRI signal can be measured more than once, since each echo gives us a measurement. The envelope that encloses the peaks of the echoes in the train is also an exponential decay with time constant T2 (Fig. 1.10).

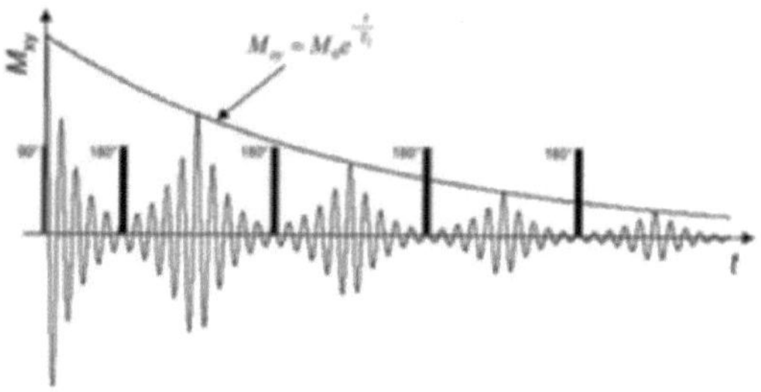

Fig. 1.10. Multiple spin-echoes are formed by applying 180° pulses in succession. The echoes form in the spaces between the pulses, and the amplitude of echoes in the "train" decreases exponentially with a time constant T2

1.2 Relaxation and Image Contrast

1.2.1 Overview

The above has provided the background needed to understand the nature of the MRI signal, how that signal is generated and how it decays due to transverse relaxation (T2*). The following will give more detail about how these processes can be used to create MR images with contrast that helps in the diagnosis and characterization of disease. The brightness of any tissue in an MR image is fundamentally related to the number of hydrogen atoms (or nuclear spins) per unit volume of that tissue since this determines the voltage that is generated in the receiver coil by magnetic induction. However, we can exploit the relaxation characteristics to modulate that brightness according to the physico-chemical properties of the tissue; these properties are different for different tissue types, and for tissue affected by disease.

1.2.2 The Bloch Equations

The nuclear spins exist in equilibrium with their surroundings. At equilibrium, the magnetization within the patient is aligned with *B*0 field (defined as the longitudinal direction, or *z* direction) as illustrated in Fig. 1.3. An RF pulse disturbs the spins from this equilibrium, for example by tilting the net magnetization vector into the *x-y*, or transverse, plane as shown in Fig. 1.4. The Bloch equations, formulated by Felix Bloch in 1946, describe the return of magnetization to equilibrium after such a disturbance.

1.2.2.1 Longitudinal Bloch Equation

This is a differential equation that describes the return of the longitudinal component of magnetization (M_z) to equilibrium:

$$\frac{dM_z}{dt} = -\frac{(M_z - M_0)}{T_1}. \quad (2)$$

The solution to this equation depends on the nature of the disturbance from equilibrium. For example, if a 90° pulse is applied at time t=0, then this tilts the longitudinal magnetization completely into the x-y plane so that M_z = 0. Then the solution, illustrated in Fig. 1.11a, is:

$$M_z = M_0\left(1 - e^{-\frac{t}{T_1}}\right). \quad (3)$$

If, instead, a 180° pulse is applied at time t=0, the longitudinal magnetization is inverted (tilted upside down), so that M_z= -M_0. Then the solution, as shown in Fig. 1.11b, is:

$$M_z = M_0\left(1 - 2e^{-\frac{t}{T_1}}\right). \quad (4)$$

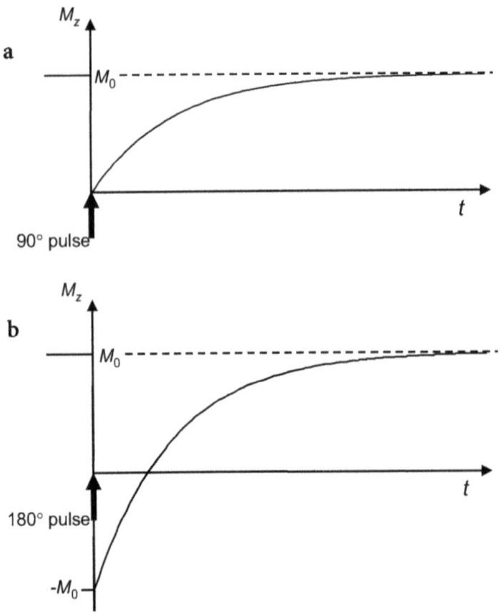

Fig. 1.11a,b. Two particular solutions to the longitudinal Bloch equation. Before an RF pulse is applied, M_z is at its equilibrium value M_0. **a** A 90° pulse tilts the z magnetization into the x-y plane so that M_z=0 at t=0 before it recovers exponentially back to equilibrium. **(b)** A 180° pulse inverts the z magnetization so that M_z=−M_0 at t=0 before again it recovers exponentially to equilibrium

Each of these particular forms is of interest in MRI, since both 90° and 180° pulses are commonly applied, and contrast is affected via the longitudinal magnetization.

1.2.2.2 Transverse Bloch Equation

This is a differential equation that describes the return of the transverse component of magnetization (M_{xy}) to equilibrium:

$$\frac{dM_{xy}}{dt} = -\frac{M_{xy}}{T_2} \quad (5)$$

Of course, at equilibrium, the transverse component of magnetization is zero (see Fig. 1.4a), so this differential equation simply describes how the transverse magnetization returns to zero after it has been disturbed. Again, the solution depends on the nature of the disturbance but if a 90° pulse is applied at time t=0, then this tilts the longitudinal magnetization completely into the x-y plane so that M_{xy} = M_0. Then the solution, illustrated in Fig. 1.12, is:

$$M_{xy} = M_0 e^{-\frac{t}{T_2}}. \quad (6)$$

We have seen in Sect. 1.1.3 that in the real world the magnetic field inhomogeneities cause more rapid decay of transverse magnetization, so that the decay constant should really be T2* in Eq. (6). However, if we measure the transverse magnetization in a spin-echo, as shown in Fig. 1.9, then the decay constant T2 applies.

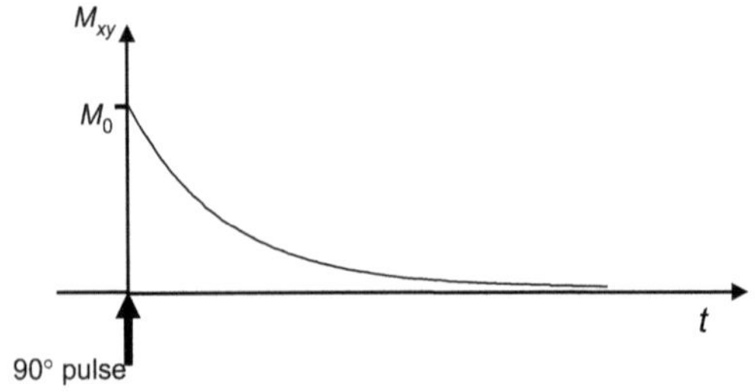

Fig. 1.12. The solution to the transverse Bloch equation when a 90° pulse is applied, converting all z magnetization to transverse magnetization so that M_{xy}=M_0 at t=0. M_{xy} decays exponentially to its equilibrium value of zero

1.2.3 T2-Weighted Imaging

T2-weighted imaging creates image contrast (differences in tissue brightness) that depends on variations in T2. T2-weighted imaging is simpler to understand than T1-weighting, and is therefore discussed first.

After a 90° pulse, the magnetization lies in the *x*-*y* plane and generates the maximum voltage in the receiver coil. This voltage first dies away and then, if a 180° pulse is applied, reforms as an echo at a time TE (Fig. 1.8). The amplitude of the echo depends only on the T2 of the tissue, which in turn reflects the physico-chemical properties of that tissue.

Figure 1.13 shows transverse relaxation curves for two tissues with different T2 values: tissue 'a' has the longer T2 and could represent an MS lesion, while tissue 'b' could represent normal tissue. An echo time can be chosen so that the difference in signal generated by the two tissues, and therefore the difference in brightness, is maximized. When TE is chosen in this way to give contrast, this is known as T2-weighted imaging.

Figure 1.14 shows an axial section of a normal brain, cutting through the lateral ventricles. The same section is shown with three different echo times: 15 ms, 50 ms and 100 ms. Notice that in the top row of images, where the display brightness settings have been kept fixed, the brightness of all tissues decreases with increasing TE, as expected from Fig. 1.12. In the bottom row of images, adjustments have been made to the display brightness setting, as would normally be done, giving the illusion that the signal from some tissues increases with increasing TE.

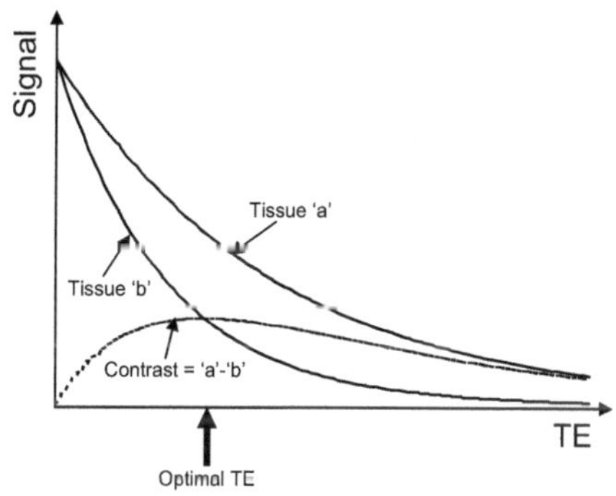

Fig. 1.13. Transverse relaxation curves for two tissues *'a'* and *'b'*, with the difference between *'a'* and *'b'* shown as the *lower dotted curve*. This difference is the contrast between the two tissues, and is maximized by judicious choice of TE in T2-weighted imaging

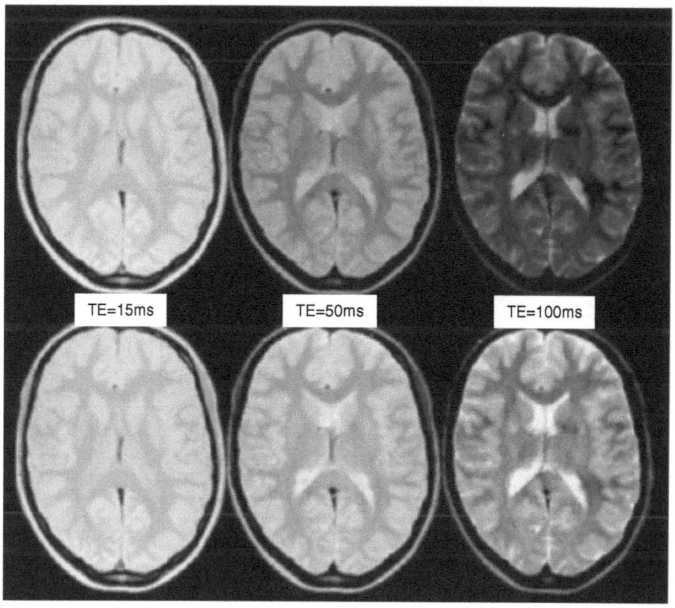

Fig. 1.14. Axial section of a normal brain with increasing echo time (TE) from *left* to *right*. In the *top row* of images, the display brightness settings have been kept fixed, showing that all tissues decline in brightness, with some declining more quickly than others. CSF has the longest T2 and declines most slowly, while gray matter has a slightly longer T2 than white matter and appears brighter in all images largely because of increased proton density. In the *bottom row*, the image display brightness has been adjusted as would be done for filming

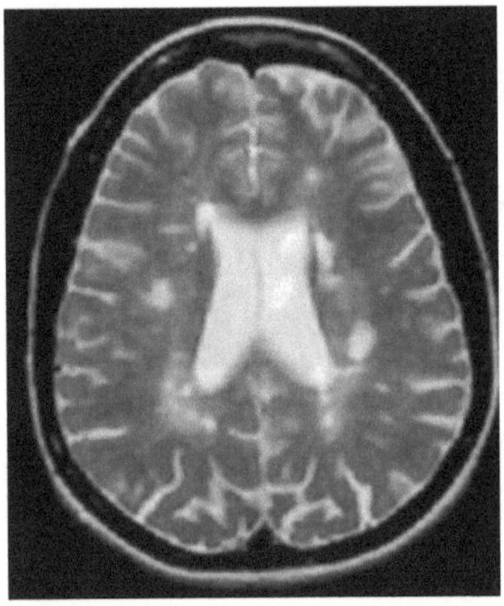

Fig. 1.15. Axial T2-weighted spin-echo image (TE=90 ms) of a patient with multiple sclerosis. Multiple lesions can be seen, particularly around the lateral ventricles, and they are hyperintense because of both their longer T2 and increased proton density

Figure 1.15 shows a typical application of T2-weighted imaging in multiple sclerosis. The echo time has been chosen to give good contrast between normal white matter and the MS lesions, which have an elevated T2 and therefore appear hyperintense on this image.

1.2.4
T2*-Weighted Imaging

T2*-weighted imaging employs the same concept as T2 weighting in that there is a delay between the generation of transverse magnetization and its measurement. The difference is that in a T2*-weighted sequence, no 180° refocusing pulse is used, so that the signal decays partly because of magnetic field inhomogeneities with a time constant T2*. This type of scan is sometimes known as a gradient-echo sequence, or sometimes as a FLASH sequence (an acronym for fast low-angle shot).

1.2.5
T1-Weighted Imaging

Longitudinal magnetization is not directly measured by MRI: to generate a voltage in the receiver coil, this longitudinal magnetization must first be tilted into the *x-y* plane. However, if multiple RF pulses are to be applied, then longitudinal relaxation affects the amount of longitudinal magnetization that is available for tilting when the next pulse is applied.

Consider a sequence of 90° pulses applied in succession, with a time between pulses of TR (the repetition time) as shown in Fig. 1.16. Each pulse tilts the *z*-magnetization down into the *x-y* plane, generating a measurable signal. Between the pulses, M_z recovers according to the curve described by Eq. (3), so at a given TR, different degrees of recovery of the longitudinal magnetization in different tissues produce contrast according to the T1 of these tissues, as illustrated in Fig. 1.17. Remember that the next 90° pulse converts this recovered longitudinal magnetization into measurable signal, so the T1 indirectly affects the amplitude of the signal and therefore the brightness of that tissue in the MR image. Notice that this is only true for signal generated by the second and subsequent pulses, since the amplitude of the signal after the first pulse is independent of the T1; this first signal is usually discarded.

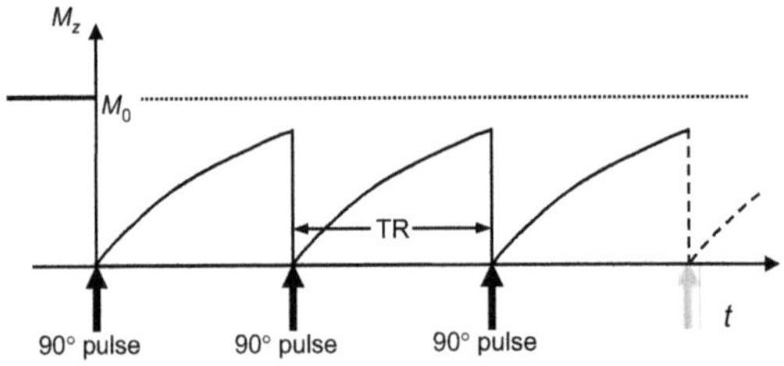

Fig. 1.16. To collect data for an MR image, a series of 90° RF pulses must be applied, with a separation between each pulse of TR. The amount of longitudinal magnetization before each pulse determines how much signal that pulse will generate. Hence, T1 influences the signal intensity in the image as TR is shortened

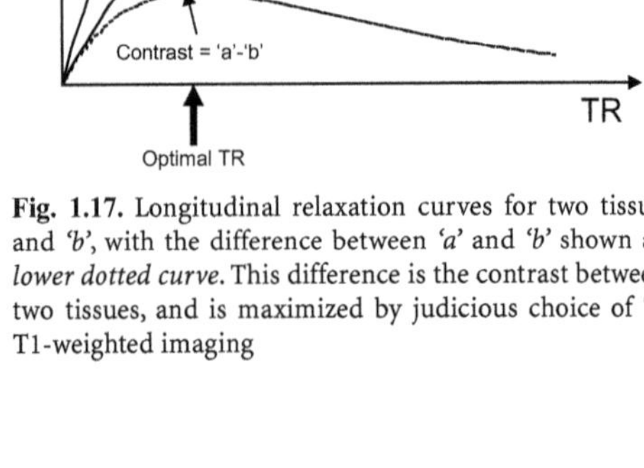

Fig. 1.17. Longitudinal relaxation curves for two tissues *'a'* and *'b'*, with the difference between *'a'* and *'b'* shown as the *lower dotted curve*. This difference is the contrast between the two tissues, and is maximized by judicious choice of TR in T1-weighted imaging

A repetition time can be chosen so that the difference in signal generated by the two tissues, and therefore the difference in brightness, is maximized (see Fig. 1.17). When TR is chosen in this way to give contrast, this is known as T1-weighted imaging.

Figure 1.18 shows a normal brain, with three different repetition times: 600 ms, 1500 ms and 4000 ms. In the top row of images, where the display brightness settings have been kept fixed, the brightness of all tissues decreases as TR is reduced, in line with Fig. 1.11. In the bottom row of images, where adjustments have been made to the display brightness settings, there is the illusion that the signal from some tissues increases with decreasing TR.

T1-weighted imaging is typically used in the head to delineate parenchyma from CSF, and is most frequently used to show tissue hypoplasia or atrophy. Figure 1.19 shows a routine T1-weighted scan typical of those used to answer many clinical questions. The TR on this type of scan is chosen to give high contrast between gray matter and CSF, giving good definition of the outline of the brain structures.

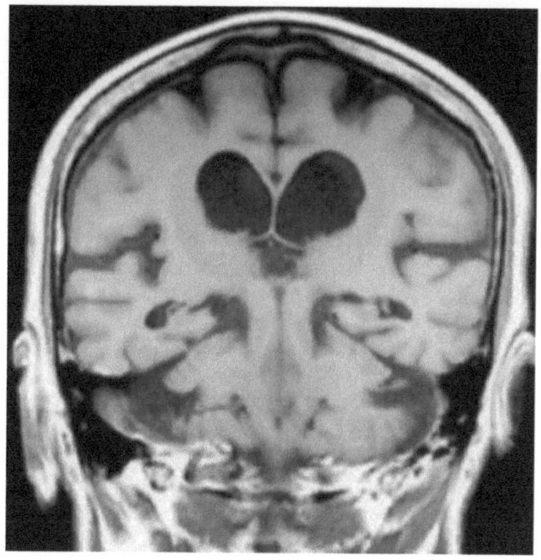

Fig. 1.19. A T1-weighted coronal section through the temporal lobes and lateral ventricles of a female (age 79 years) presenting to memory clinic, showing general atrophy of the brain

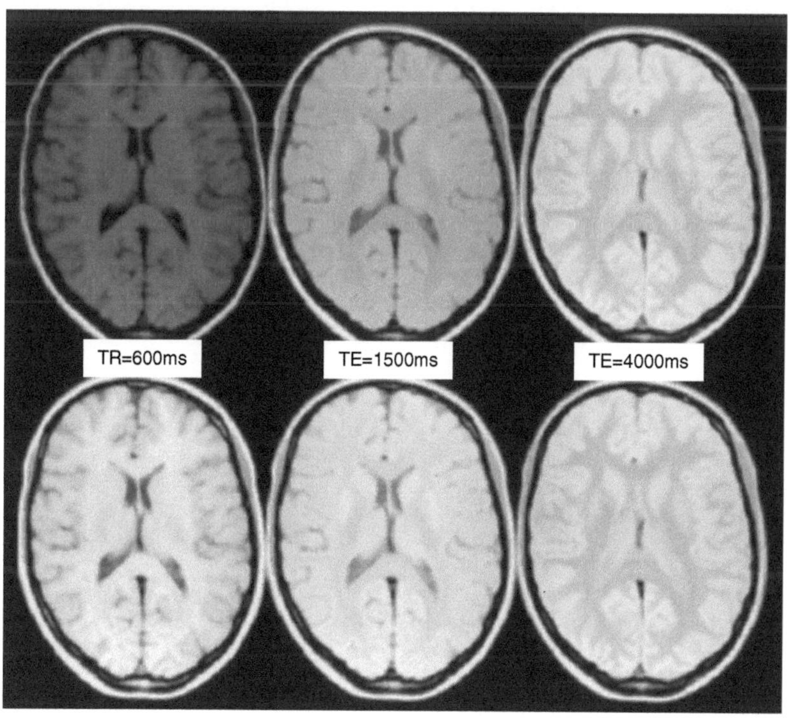

Fig. 1.18. Axial section of a normal brain with increasing repetition time (TR) from *left* to *right*. In the *top row* of images, the display brightness settings have been kept fixed, showing that all tissues increase in brightness as TR is increased, with some increasing more quickly than others. CSF has the longest T1 and increases most slowly, while white matter has a slightly shorter T1 than gray and recovers more quickly. In the *bottom row*, the image display brightness has been adjusted as would be done for filming

1.2.6 Summary of Simple MRI Contrast

The basic factor determining the brightness of a tissue is the number of hydrogen atoms, or protons, per unit volume of tissue, since the signal intensity after an RF pulse is proportional to the proton density in a scan with a long TR and a short TE. Weighting by the relaxation times can be introduced either by shorter repetition time (TR) to give T1 weighting, or by longer echo time (TE) to give T2 weighting. This is summarized and illustrated in Fig. 1.20.

Using a combination of short TR and long TE is not generally useful, since the short TR serves to darken tissues with long relaxation times, while long TE darkens tissues with short relaxation times. Thus, the brightness of all tissues is generally depressed and the resulting image has low intensity and poor contrast (Fig. 1.20).

In biological tissues, it is a general rule that T1 and T2 vary in concert: if T1 is long for a particular tissue, then T2 will also be long, and vice versa. However, there is no strict relationship between them, and the only approximate rule is that the more solid a tissue, or the higher the content of large molecules such as proteins, and lipids in cell membranes then the lower will be both T1 and T2.

An MRI examination will normally comprise more than one imaging pulse sequence. In the CNS, T1-weighted sequences are typically used to show gross anatomy, since the nervous system tissue is shown in relief against a background of dark CSF. Because of this, T1-weighted imaging is sometimes referred to as "anatomical scanning." T2-weighted sequences are normally used to show changes in tissue that are brought about by disease, since the relaxation times are invariably lengthened in damaged tissue and this shows as a bright region. T2-weighted scanning is sometimes referred to as "imaging pathology."

This chapter has aimed to provide a basic understanding of MRI. As with many complex subjects, it is necessary in an introduction to gloss over some important issues and leave questions unanswered. For example, the MR image has been mentioned in very abstract terms, with no detail about how we convert the voltage measured in the receiver coil into an image that is shown on the radiographic film or computer display. More in-depth treatment of specific techniques and pulse sequences is given in later chapters.

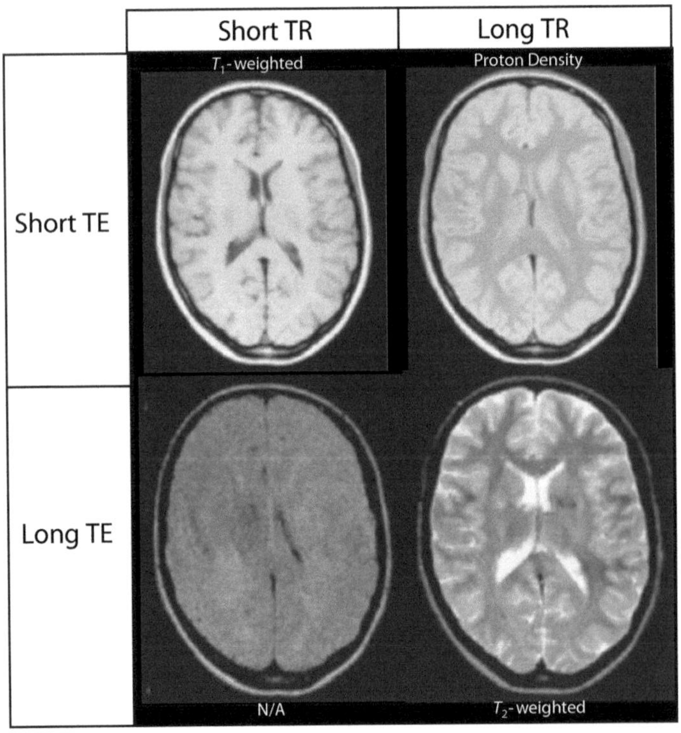

Fig. 1.20. Summary of relaxation time weighting of MR images. The fundamental brightness is determined by the number of hydrogen atoms per unit volume of tissue (proton density). Decreasing the TR introduces T1 weighting, and increasing the TE introduces T2 weighting. A combination of short TR and long TE causes a decrease in intensity for all tissues, giving low signal intensity and little contrast

2 Hardware for Magnetic Resonance Imaging

Kenneth W. Fishbein, Joseph C. McGowan, and Richard G. Spencer

CONTENTS

K. W. Fishbein, PhD
Facility Manager, Nuclear Magnetic Resonance Unit, National Institutes of Health, National Institute on Aging, Intramural Research Program, GRC 4D-08, 5600 Nathan Shock Drive, Baltimore, MD 21224, USA
J. C. McGowan, PhD
Associate Professor of Electrical Engineering, Department of Electrical Engineering, Murray Hall 227, United States Naval Academy, Annapolis, MD 21402-5025, USA
R. G. Spencer, MD, PhD
Chief, Nuclear Magnetic Resonance Unit, National Institutes of Health, National Institute on Aging, Intramural Research Program, GRC 4D-08, 5600 Nathan Shock Drive, Baltimore, MD 21224, USA

2.1 Introduction

While modern magnetic resonance imaging (MRI) instruments vary considerably in design and specifications, all MRI scanners include several essential components. First, in order to create net nuclear spin magnetization in the subject to be scanned, a polarizing magnetic field is required. This main magnetic field is generally constant in time and space and may be provided by a variety of magnets. Once net nuclear spin magnetization is present, this magnetization may be manipulated by applying a variety of secondary magnetic fields with specific time and/or spatial dependence. These may generally be classified into gradients, which introduce defined spatial variations in the polarizing magnetic field, B0, and radio frequency (RF) irradiation, which provides the B1 magnetic field needed to generate observable, transverse nuclear spin magnetization. B0 gradients are generally created by applying an electric current supplied by gradient amplifiers to a set of electromagnetic coil windings within the main magnetic field. Similarly, RF irradiation is applied to the subject by one or more antennas or transmitter coils connected to a set of synthesizers, attenuators and amplifiers known collectively as a transmitter. Under the influence of the main magnetic field, the field gradients and RF irradiation, the nuclear spins within the subject induce a weak RF signal in one or more receiver coils which is then amplified, filtered and digitized by the receiver. Finally, the digitized signal is displayed and processed by the scanner's host computer. In this chapter, we will discuss the various technologies currently in use for these components with an emphasis on critical specifications and the impact that these have on the instrument's performance in specific MRI experiments. While the focus of the current work is imaging, the hardware components described below are also applicable to magnetic resonance spectroscopy (MRS) and this text will include specific information related to spectroscopy where appropriate.

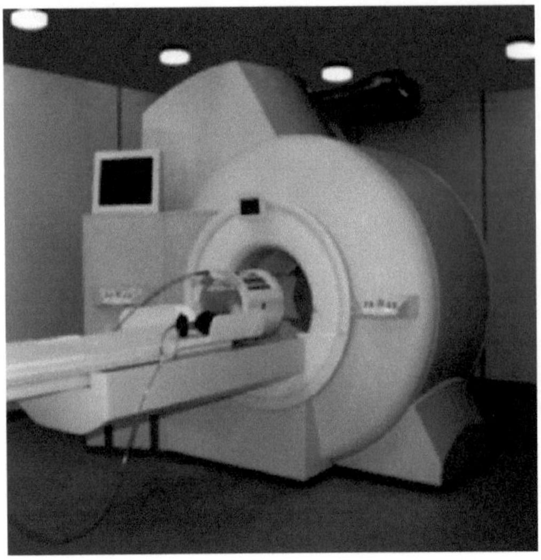

Fig. 2.1. A superconducting clinical magnet system. (Courtesy of Siemens)

2.2 Magnets

The function of a MRI scanner's magnet is to generate a strong, stable, spatially uniform polarizing magnetic field within a defined working volume. Accordingly, the most important specifications for a MRI magnet are field strength, field stability, spatial homogeneity and the dimensions and orientation of the working volume. In addition to these, specifications such as weight, stray field dimensions, overall bore length and startup and operating costs play an important role in selecting and installing a MRI magnet. Magnet types used in MRI may be classified into three categories: permanent, resistive and superconducting. As we shall see, the available magnet technologies generally offer a compromise between various specifications so that the optimum choice of magnet design will depend upon the demands of the clinical applications anticipated and the MRI experiments to be performed.

2.2.1 Permanent Magnets

Permanent magnets for MRI are composed of one or more pieces of iron or magnetizable alloy carefully formed into a shape designed to establish a homogeneous magnetic field over the region to be scanned. These magnets may provide open access to the patient or may be constructed in the traditional, "closed" cylindrical geometry. With care, permanent magnets can be constructed with good spatial homogeneity, but they are susceptible to temporal changes in field strength and homogeneity caused by changes in magnet temperature. The maximum field strength possible for a permanent magnet depends upon the ferromagnetic alloy used to build it, but is generally limited to approximately 0.3 T. The weight of a permanent MRI magnet also depends upon the choice of magnetic material but is generally very high. As an example, a 0.2-T whole-body magnet constructed from iron might weigh 25 tons while the weight of a similar magnet built from a neodymium alloy could be 5 tons. While the field strength of permanent magnets is limited and their weight is high, they consume no electric power, dissipate no heat, and are very stable. Consequently, once installed, permanent magnets are inexpensive to maintain.

2.2.2 Resistive Electromagnets

Other than permanent magnets, all MRI magnets are electromagnets, generating their field by the conduction of electricity through loops of wire. Electromagnets, in turn, are classified as resistive or superconducting depending upon whether the wire loops have finite or zero electrical resistance. Unlike permanent magnets, resistive electromagnets are not limited in field strength by any fundamental property of a magnetic material. Indeed, an electromagnet can produce an arbitrarily strong magnetic field provided that sufficient current can flow through the wire loops without excessive heating or power consumption. Specifically, for a simple cylindrical coil known as a solenoid, the magnetic field generated is directly proportional to the coil current. However, the power requirements and heat generation of the electromagnet increase as the square of the current. Because the stability of the field of a resistive magnet depends both upon coil temperature and the stability of the current source used to energize the magnet coil, these magnets require a power source that simultaneously provides very high current (typically hundreds of amperes) and excellent current stability (less than one part per million per hour). These requirements are technically difficult to achieve and further restrict the performance of resistive magnets. While resistive magnets have been built which generate very high fields over a small volume in the research setting, resistive magnets suitable for human MRI are limited to about 0.2 T. Resistive magnets are generally lighter in weight than permanent magnets of comparable strength, although the power supply and cooling equipment required for their operation add weight and floor space requirements.

2.2.3 Superconducting Electromagnets

Superconducting magnets achieve high fields without prohibitive power consumption and cooling requirements, and are the most common clinical design. In the superconducting state, no external power is required to maintain current flow and field strength and no heat is dissipated from the wire. The ability of the wire to conduct current without resistance depends upon its composition, the temperature of the wire, and the magnitude of the current and local magnetic field. Below a certain critical temperature (T_C) and critical field strength, current less than or equal to the critical current is conducted with no resistance and thus no heat dissipation. As the wire is cooled below T_C, it remains superconducting but the critical current and field generally increase, permitting the generation of a stronger magnetic field. While so-called high-T_C superconductors such as yttrium barium copper oxide can be superconductive when cooled by a bath of liquid nitrogen (77 K or −196°C at 1 bar pressure), limitations to their critical current and field make them thus far impractical for use in main magnet coil construction.

Superconducting MRI magnets are currently manufactured using wire composed of NbTi or NbSn alloys, which must be cooled to below 10 K (−263°C) to be superconducting at the desired field. Therefore, the coil of a superconducting MRI magnet must be constantly cooled by a bath of liquid helium in order to maintain its current and thus its field. As long as the critical temperature, field and current are not exceeded, current will flow through the magnet solenoid indefinitely, yielding an extremely stable magnetic field. However, if the magnet wire exceeds the critical temperature associated with the existing current, the wire will suddenly become resistive. The energy stored in the magnetic field will then dissipate, causing rapid heating and possibly damage to the magnet coil, accompanied by rapid vaporization of any remaining liquid helium in the cooling bath. This undesirable phenomenon is known as a quench.

Because of the need to maintain sufficient liquid helium within the magnet to cool the superconducting wire, the liquid helium is maintained within a vacuum-insulated cryostat or Dewar vessel. In addition, the liquid helium vessel is usually surrounded by several concentric metal radiation shields cooled by cold gas boiling off the liquid helium bath, a separate liquid nitrogen bath or by a cold head attached to an external closed-cycle refrigerator. These shields protect the liquid helium bath from radiative heating and thus reduce liquid helium boil-off losses, thus reducing refill frequency and cost. Magnets incorporating liquid nitrogen cooling require regular liquid nitrogen refills, but liquid nitrogen is less costly than liquid helium and provides cooling with no electrical consumption. Conversely, refrigerator-cooled (refrigerated) magnets need no liquid nitrogen refills but require periodic mechanical service and a very reliable electrical supply. Regardless of design, the cryogenic efficiency of a superconducting magnet is summarized by specifying the magnet's hold time, which is the maximum interval between liquid helium refills. Modern refrigerated magnets typically require liquid helium refilling and maintenance at most once a year while smaller-bore magnets may have a hold time of 2 years or longer. Clearly, the operating costs of a superconducting magnet are inversely related to the magnet's hold time.

Superconducting magnets require periodic cryogen refilling for continued safe operation but little maintenance otherwise. Due to their ability to achieve stable, high magnetic fields with little or no electrical power consumption, superconducting magnets now greatly outnumber other magnet types among both research and clinical MRI facilities. Accordingly, the following discussion of magnet specifications and performance will concentrate on superconducting electromagnet technology.

2.2.4 Magnetic Field Strength

Magnets for MRI are frequently specified by two numbers: field strength in Tesla and bore size in centimeters. The magnetic field strength is the nominal field strength measured at the center of the working volume, where the field is strongest. The nominal Larmor frequency for a given nucleus is directly proportional to the magnetic field strength and thus the strength of a magnet can also be specified in terms of the nominal proton NMR frequency. For example, a MRI scanner equipped with a 4.7-T magnet may also be referred to as a 200-MHz system. There are many advantages and a few disadvantages to performing MRI at the highest magnetic field strength available. Most importantly, with all other conditions held constant, the signal-to-noise ratio (SNR) in an NMR spectrum or a MRI image is directly dependent on the strength of the main magnetic field, B0. The exact relation between SNR and B0 depends upon B0 itself as well as several other factors, but when biological samples are imaged at the typical field strengths used in modern MRI, SNR is approximately linearly dependent upon field strength. Thus, for a voxel of fixed size containing a certain number of water molecules, doubling the magnetic field strength will yield approximately a twofold improvement in SNR. Equivalently, operating at higher magnetic field strength allows one to obtain images with acceptable SNR but greater in-plane resolution and/or thinner slices (Fig. 2.2). While acceptable SNR can be achieved at lower magnetic field strength by signal averaging, SNR increases only as the square root of the number of scans averaged. Consequently, to double SNR at constant B0 field strength, it is necessary to average four times as many scans, quadrupling the total scanning time. This becomes prohibitive in many studies, given the finite stability of biological samples and constraints on magnet time. It can become a particular problem in a variety of applications where high time resolution is essential, including functional MRI.

2.2.4.1 Field Strength and Chemical Shift Effects

In addition to considerations involving imaging resolution, SNR and scan time, the strength of the main magnetic field has important implications for spectral resolution, that is, the spacing in frequency units between resonance lines of different chemical shifts (Fig. 2.3). In addition, in imaging studies the frequency difference between protons in fat and water must be taken into consideration. In these studies, the effect of chemical shift differences on resonance frequency is assumed to be negligible compared with resonance frequency changes due to application of the imaging gradients. If this is a valid assumption, then spatial localization of spins will be independent of chemical shift, as desired. However, at sufficiently high magnetic field strength, the difference in resonance frequency between fat and water protons will become non-negligible due to differing chemical

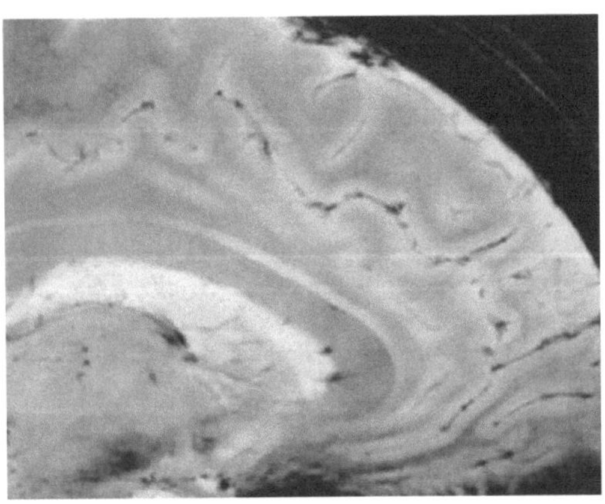

Fig. 2.2. High resolution magnetic resonance image using gradient echo acquisition at 8 T (Ohio State University)

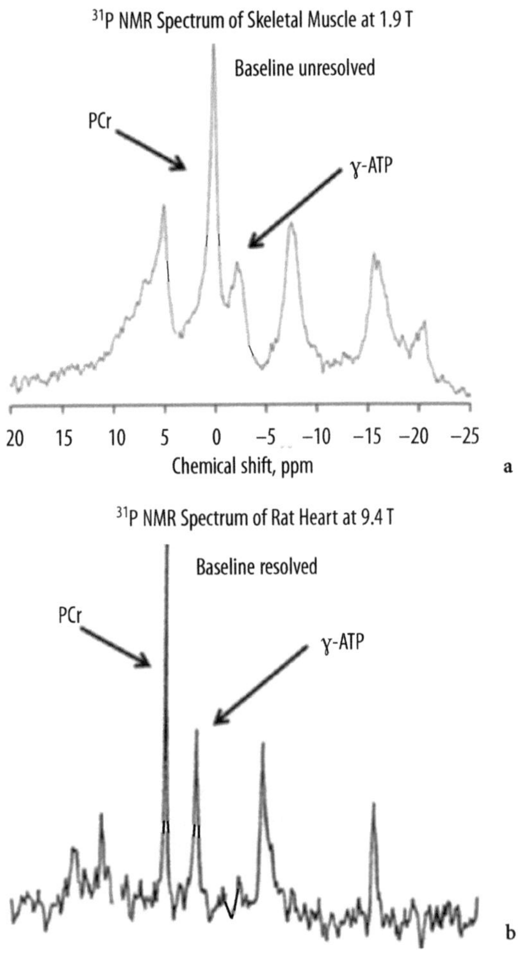

Fig. 2.3a,b. Magnetic resonance phosphorus spectroscopy at 1.9 (a) and 9.4 T (b). The high field spectrum demonstrates improved resolution

shifts. This will be observed as an anomalous shift in position of the fat signal along the read direction in the MRI image, the chemical shift artifact. An example of this effect is shown in Fig. 2.4. The apparent shift in position of the fat signal increases with field strength and similar chemical shift artifacts can be observed for any species with a chemical shift substantially different from water. Chemical shift artifacts can, however, often be attenuated by off-resonance presaturation of the nonaqueous species. In fact, on higher-field instruments, these species can often be saturated with less concomitant saturation of water as a consequence of improved spectral resolution. Other techniques for fat suppression, based on, for example, T1 relaxation time difference, are also available.

2.2.4.2
Magnetic Field Strength and Susceptibility Effects

Magnetic susceptibility, χ, refers to the relative difference between the strength of the magnetic field measured inside and outside an object composed of a specific material. In the most common case, electron shielding results in a reduction of the magnetic field within a substance so that χ is negative. These substances can be thought of as slightly repelling or excluding the external field, and are called diamagnetic. Diamagnetism is a weak effect, resulting in a reduction of the magnetic field within a diamagnetic object of at most a few parts per million (ppm). If the sample to be scanned does not have constant susceptibility, there will be variations in the actual field strength inside the sample. In general, significant B0 inhomogeneity arising from susceptibility differences will be encountered wherever there is a sudden transition in tissue composition or voids in the tissue. For example, a large difference in χ is encountered between brain tissue and pockets of air in the nasal sinuses. In this region of the brain, large distortions in B0 field strength and resulting MRI artifacts are frequently observed at air-tissue interfaces. The presence of metal prostheses or fragments in the body also results in large susceptibility differences. Even if these metal objects are not ferromagnetic, they possess a magnetic susceptibility very different from that of tissue or water and thus may cause pronounced artifacts in their immediate vicinity. An example of a typical artifact caused by variations in susceptibility is shown in Fig. 2.5. Clearly, these variations will change whenever a new sample is inserted into the magnet. Some experimental protocols, particularly in spectroscopy, require corrections for these distortions each time a new sample is inserted for scanning.

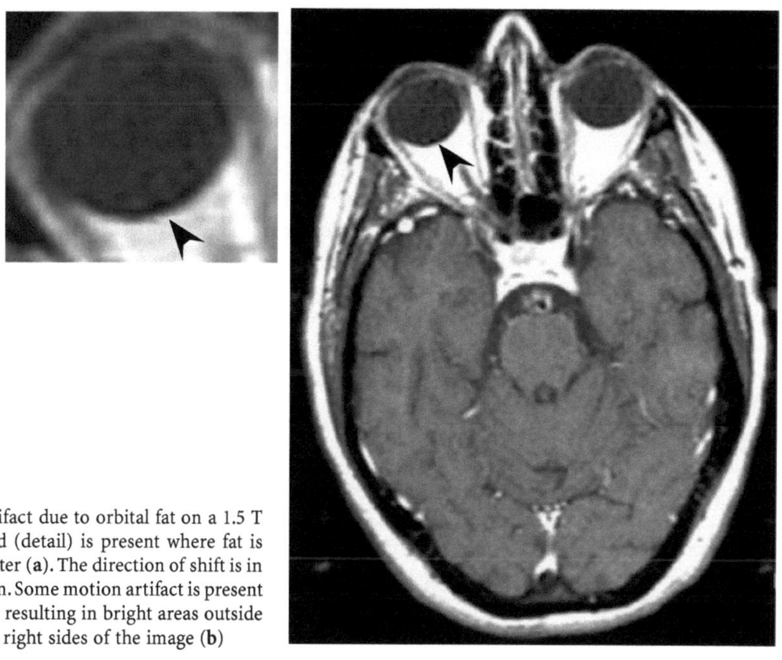

a

b

Fig. 2.4a,b. Chemical shift artifact due to orbital fat on a 1.5 T clinical scanner. A signal void (detail) is present where fat is shifted away from adjacent water (**a**). The direction of shift is in the frequency encode direction. Some motion artifact is present in the phase encode direction resulting in bright areas outside the skull in the lower left and right sides of the image (**b**)

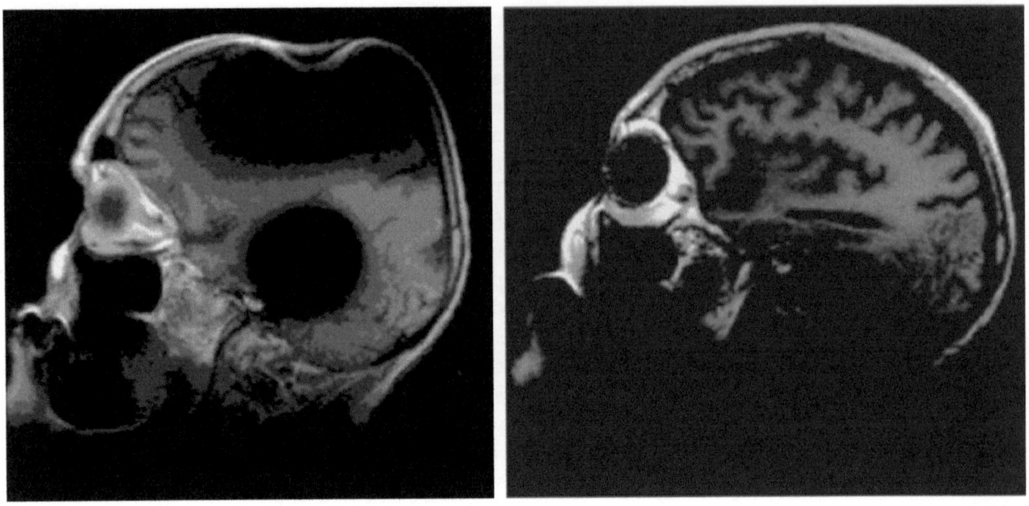

a b

Fig. 2.5a,b. Susceptibility artifact on a 1.5-T clinical scanner. Image (a) was obtained when the patient was wearing a hearing aid. Image (b) followed removal of the hearing aid

Just as the effects of chemical shift differences are magnified at higher magnetic field strength, the effects of differences in susceptibility are similarly amplified. As with chemical shift, susceptibility effects on resonance frequency scale linearly with main magnetic field strength and can result in apparent shifts in position along the read direction in MRI images. More importantly, however, differences in susceptibility within a sample cause inhomogeneities in B0 field strength which result in decreased T2*, broader linewidths and poorer resolution in spectroscopic experiments, and often pronounced imaging artifacts due to signal loss. In practice, particularly large susceptibility differences are found in regions of the body where pockets of air are present, since air has a very different susceptibility than typical tissue. Where susceptibility is exploited for image contrast, for example in some fMRI studies as well as in studies employing exogenous contrast agents, the increase in this effect at higher field may be advantageous.

2.2.4.3 Cost and Siting Considerations

For a given bore size, the higher the magnetic field strength, the greater the size, weight and cost of the magnet become. For superconducting magnets, this is largely the result of the increased number of turns of superconducting wire needed to produce a stronger field in a given working volume. Both the wire itself and the fabrication of the magnet coils are expensive and this cost scales at least linearly with the length of wire required to build the magnet. Moreover, a larger magnet coil demands a larger, heavier cryostat to maintain the coil below its critical temperature. Lastly, as magnetic field strength increases, the internal forces felt by the coil windings increase, necessitating heavier supports and reinforcement within the magnet. The greater size and weight of high field magnets impose demands upon the design of the buildings where they are located. Not only must additional floor space be allocated for the magnet itself, but consideration must also be given to the increased volume of the fringe field (also called stray field) surrounding the magnet in all directions. The fringe field is that portion of the magnetic field that extends outside the bore of the magnet. It is desirable to minimize the dimensions of this field in order to minimize both the effects that the magnet has on objects in its surroundings (e.g., pacemakers, steel tools, magnetic cards) and also the disturbance of the main magnetic field by objects outside the magnet (e.g., passing motor vehicles, rail lines, elevators). While the extent of the fringe field can be reduced by various shielding techniques, the large fringe field of high-field magnets contributes to a need for more space when compared to lower field scanners of comparable bore size.

2.2.5 Magnet Bore Size, Orientation, and Length

In addition to field strength, a traditional, closed, cylindrical MRI magnet is characterized by its bore size. Analogously, magnets for open MRI are described by their gap size, i.e., the distance between their pole pieces. We will refer to either of these dimensions as the magnet's bore size. It is important to note that the magnet bore size does not represent the diameter of the largest object that can be imaged in that magnet. This is due to the fact that the shim coil, gradient coil and radio-frequency probe take up space within the magnet bore, reducing the space available for the subject to be imaged. However, the magnet bore size does place constraints on the maximum inner diameters of each of these components and thus is the primary factor determining the usable diameter available for the patient. For example, a magnet bore diameter of 100 cm is common for whole-body clinical applications, while an 80 cm bore magnet typically only allows insertion of the patient's head once the shim, gradient and radio-frequency coils are installed.

In open MRI magnets, the magnetic field direction is usually vertical and thus perpendicular to the head–foot axis of the patient. An open magnet is depicted in Fig. 2.6. This is to be contrasted with traditional MRI magnets, in which the magnetic field direction is oriented along the long axis of the subject. This difference has consequences for the design of shim, gradient and radio-frequency coils in open MRI. Note that in any magnet, the direction parallel to the B0 magnetic field is always referred to as the Z axis or axial direction while the radial direction is always perpendicular to B0.

In the design of horizontal bore magnets for clinical use, there is an emphasis on minimizing the distance from the front of the magnet cryostat to the center of the magnetic field. Shortening this distance facilitates insertion of the patient and minimizes patient discomfort. However, shortening the magnet coil length may lead to decreased B0 homogeneity, while shortening the magnet cryostat may compromise the insulation of the liquid helium bath and lead to decreased hold time.

2.2.6 Field Stability

The term field stability refers to temporal variation of the magnetic field. Instability in the B0 field from any source directly results in instability in resonance frequency and may thus cause image or spectral artifacts and poor spectral resolution. When these variations are due to intrinsic changes within the magnet (and, for resistive electromagnets, the magnet's power supply), the change in magnetic field strength with time is called drift. A typical specification for the maximum drift rate of a modern superconducting magnet is 0.01–0.1 ppm per hour. Superconducting magnets can also experience field instability associated with changes in the temperature of the liquid helium bath that cools the magnet coils.

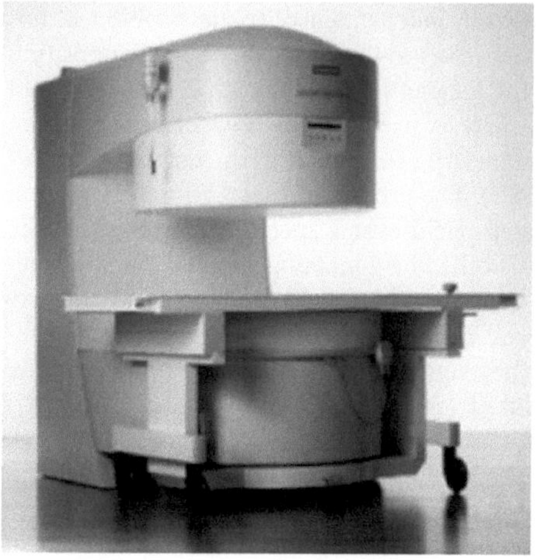

Fig. 2.6. An open clinical magnet system. (Courtesy of Siemens)

Conversely, temporal changes in the magnetic field due to external disturbances, such as moving elevators or trains nearby, are called magnetic interference effects. Magnetic interference can also result from the presence of magnetic fields external to the MRI magnet, such as from large transformers, power lines and motors. External forces may also indirectly affect the magnetic field by causing vibration of the magnet coil and cryostat. For this reason as well as to support the weight of the magnet and magnetic shielding, it is common practice to locate MRI magnets on the lowest floor possible and far away from vibration-generating equipment. Clearly, elimination of external effects on the magnetic field requires careful site planning prior to system installation.

2.2.7 Magnetic Field Homogeneity

While the stability of an MRI magnet refers to the relative variation in the main magnetic field with time, typically independent of spatial position, B0 homogeneity refers to the variation in B0 over position within the magnet's working volume. Magnetic field homogeneity is usually expressed in units of ppm over the surface of a specific diameter spherical volume (DSV). The process of measuring the variation in magnetic field over a specified region inside the magnet is called field mapping. Spatial inhomogeneities in the B0 magnetic field can arise from a variety of sources including imperfections in the construction of the magnet itself. As noted, B0 inhomogeneity also results from variations in the magnetic susceptibility of materials within the magnet coil.

Because homogeneity of the main magnetic field over the imaging or spectroscopic volume is essential, dedicated electromagnetic coils (shim coils) are provided to optimize the B0 field homogeneity within the design of the main magnet. In a superconducting electromagnet, superconducting shims are additional coils of superconducting wire wound coaxially with the main coil in such a way as to generate specific field gradients. For each principal direction, there is typically a dedicated shim coil with an independent electrical circuit. During magnet installation, current may be independently adjusted in the main coil and each of the superconducting shim coils in order to optimize B0 homogeneity within the magnet's working volume. Since, like the main magnet coil, these shim coils are superconducting, large currents may flow through them with no resistance and no external power supply once energized. Thus, superconducting shim coils can generate strong field gradients with high temporal stability. Readjusting the current in these coils is an infrequent operation requiring special apparatus and addition of liquid helium to the magnet.

Unlike superconducting shims, passive shims do not rely upon the flow of electrical current through a coil to generate a field gradient. Instead, they are pieces of ferromagnetic metal of a size and shape designed to improve B0 homogeneity when they are inserted into the magnet.

Magnets are also provided with room temperature shims that can be adjusted on a regular basis as needed. These can be adjusted manually or automatically to compensate for differeces in susceptibility between different patients or patient positions. Since these are resistive electromagnets, they require a stable power supply and their magnitude is limited.

Specifications for magnetic field homogeneity generally distinguish between values achieved by the unshimmed magnet and those obtained after adjusting current in the room-temperature shims. Moreover, homogeneity will be specified over smaller DSVs for smaller bore magnets, as is appropriate for the smaller working volume of the magnet. Usually, homogeneity will be specified for two or more specific DSVs since there is no simple, reliable equation relating field homogeneity to spherical diameter about the field center. A typical field homogeneity specification for a whole-body MRI magnet with optimized room-temperature shims might be 0.06 ppm over a 20-cm DSV and 2 ppm over a 50-cm DSV, while a small-bore research magnet might achieve 2.5 ppm over a 10-cm DSV. In evaluating these specifications, it is important to consider the size of the typical sample to be imaged and the field of view that will be employed.

2.2.8 Magnetic Field Shielding

Because high-field, large bore MRI magnets generate an extensive fringe field, they are capable of both adversely affecting nearby objects as well as experiencing interference from these objects. Since 5 G (0.5 mT) is generally regarded as the maximum safe field for public exposure, the extent of the fringe field is typically described by the dimensions of the 5-G isosurface centered about the magnet. In an unshielded cylindrical magnet, this isosurface is roughly ellipsoidal with a longer dimension along the B0 axis and a shorter radial dimension. The fringe field can be characterized by the radial and axial dimensions of the "5-G line" surrounding the magnet. In order to reduce the magnitude and extent of the fringe field and thus minimize interaction between the magnet and its environment, both passive and active shielding techniques are commonly used. Passive shielding consists of ferromagnetic material placed outside the magnet. Passive shields are generally constructed from thick plates of soft iron, an inexpensive material with relatively high magnetic permeability. In order to shield a magnet with ferromagnetic plates, the substantial attractive force between the magnet and the shielding material must be considered in the design of the magnet. Active shielding consists of one or more electromagnetic coils wound on the outside of the main magnet coil but with opposite field orientation. Typically, in a superconducting magnet, the shield coils are superconducting as well and are energized simultaneously with the main coil during installation. The field generated by the shield coils partially cancels the fringe field of the main coil, thereby reducing the fringe field dimensions. As a rule, both active and passive shielding can reduce the dimensions of the 5-G fringe field by roughly a factor of two in each direction. This often makes it possible to site a magnet in a space too small or too close to a magnetically-sensitive object to accommodate an unshielded magnet of similar size and field strength. New MRI magnets are increasingly designed with built-in active shielding.

2.3 Pulsed Field Gradients

The function of the pulsed field gradient system in an MRI instrument is to generate linear, stable, reproducible B0 field gradients along specific directions with the shortest possible rise and fall times. While the primary use of pulsed field gradients in MRI is to establish a correspondence between spatial position and resonance frequency, gradients are also used for other purposes, such as to irreversibly dephase transverse magnetization. Gradient fields are produced by passing current through a set of wire coils located inside the magnet bore. The need for rapid switching of gradients during pulse sequences makes the design and construction of pulsed field gradient systems quite technologically demanding. The performance of a pulsed field gradient system is specified by parameters including gradient strength, linearity, stability and switching times. In addition, gradient systems are characterized by their bore size, shielding and cooling design.

2.3.1 Uses of Pulsed Field Gradients

Gradient sets are designed to introduce field variation in the X, Y, and Z directions within the magnet. Thus, an X gradient is designed to produce a change in B0 directly proportional to distance along the X direction: $\Delta B0=G_x x$, where x is the distance from the isocenter of the X gradient coil, and similarly for Y and Z. The isocenters for X, Y and Z coils should coincide exactly. Also, the gradient coil set is generally placed so that its isocenter coincides with the B0 field center. The value G_x is the X gradient strength and is typically stated in mT/m or in G/cm (1 G/cm=10 mT/m). By causing the B0 field strength to vary linearly with X position, applying a pulsed field gradient causes the resonance frequency of each nuclear spin to depend linearly upon its X position. If we define the resonance frequency offset $\Delta\nu$ to be zero for a nuclear spin at the isocenter, $\Delta\nu=\nu-\nu_{x=0}$ then we have $\Delta\nu=-\gamma G_x x/2\pi$ whenever the X gradient is switched on. For a particular nucleus, if G_x is known accurately, we can then determine the x position of that nucleus simply by measuring its frequency offset $\Delta\nu$. Similarly, by applying a frequency-selective excitation pulse in conjunction with an X gradient, we can excite nuclear spins located in a specific region along the X axis. This correspondence between B0, frequency and spatial position under the influence of field gradients forms the basis for all magnetic resonance imaging experiments and is illustrated in Fig. 2.7.

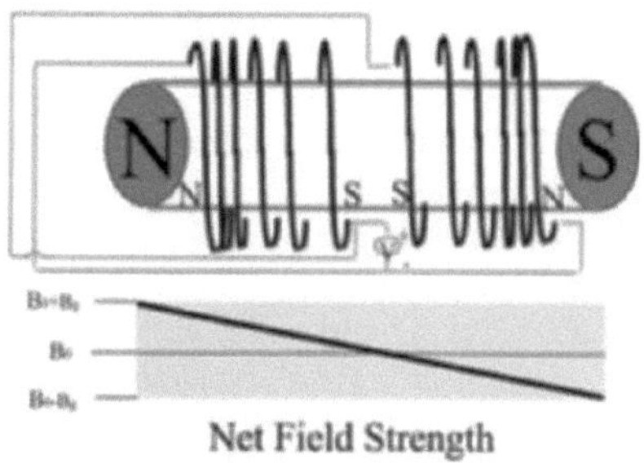

Fig. 2.7. Diagram of a solenoidal gradient coil and the effect on net magnetic field

2.3.1.1 Slice and Volume Selection Gradients

In MRI experiments, slice selection refers to the selective excitation of nuclear spins within a slab with a specific orientation, thickness, and position. This is accomplished by simultaneously applying a pulsed field gradient, called the slice gradient, and a frequency-selective radio-frequency pulse. While the slice gradient is on, the resonance frequency of each nucleus within the gradient coil depends upon its position along the slice gradient direction. The frequency offset and excitation bandwidth of the RF pulse are then set to excite nuclei with a specific range of resonance frequencies, which has the effect of exciting all nuclei located between specific positions along the slice axis. For example, the simultaneous application of a Z slice gradient and a frequency-selective RF pulse will excite all nuclei within a slab perpendicular to the Z axis. To a first approximation, all nuclei in the slab will be excited uniformly, regardless of their positions along the X and Y directions. The thickness of the slab excited by this gradient-RF pulse combination depends upon both the strength of the slice gradient and the excitation bandwidth of the RF pulse. The actual flip angle delivered to a group of spins with a particular resonance frequency depends upon the shape (amplitude and phase modulation), duration, and frequency offset of the RF pulse. If all these parameters are fixed, then the excitation bandwidth is fixed and the slice thickness depends only on the inverse of slice gradient strength:

Slice thickness = 2π (Excitation Bandwidth) / γG_{slice}

Thus, thinner slices can be imaged by increasing the slice gradient strength at a constant excitation bandwidth. While thinner slices can also be achieved by modifying the RF pulse length and shape in order to decrease the excitation bandwidth, this has several practical disadvantages, including longer minimum echo time (TE). Thus, for optimum resolution in the slice direction, it is desirable to have high slice gradient strength. Finally, note that it is possible in an MRI experiment to selectively excite a slice oriented in any direction in three-dimensional space. Slices parallel to the XY, YZ or XZ planes are termed axial (or transverse), sagittal or coronal depending upon the placement of the subject in the scanner. Slices not parallel to any of these planes are called oblique slices. Regardless of slice orientation, the slice gradient is always applied perpendicular to the desired slice plane. Gradients to select oblique slices are created by simultaneously passing current through two or three of the electromagnetic gradient coils X, Y and Z.

Applying three slice-selective gradient and RF pulse pairs in sequence selectively excites nuclei within a defined volume. Once these nuclei have been excited, sampling the resulting NMR signal yields a spectrum reflecting the chemical composition of the selected volume. Just as increased slice gradient strength permits the selection of thinner slices at fixed RF bandwidth, volume-selective NMR spectroscopy experiments gain better spatial resolution with stronger slice gradients. Alternatively, smaller volumes can be selectively excited by decreasing the bandwidth of the RF pulses, but this results in longer minimum echo time TE, and carries other disadvantages.

2.3.1.2
Read Gradients

As we have seen, when a B0 field gradient is applied along a specific axis, the resonance frequency of each nuclear spin becomes dependent on its position along that axis. Picturing each nuclear spin as giving rise to a single, sharp NMR spectral peak at a position-dependent frequency, a large ensemble of spins spread over a range of positions along the gradient axis will give rise to a broad NMR spectrum called a profile. If the peaks from each nucleus are identical except for their center frequency, then the profile represents a histogram displaying the number of nuclei resonating at each frequency and thus located at each position along the gradient axis. Just as in a purely spectroscopic NMR experiment, during the application of the read gradient in a MRI scan, we must digitize the time-domain signal at a sufficiently fast rate to accurately measure the highest frequencies in the spectrum. Mathematically, the minimum digitization rate required to accurately sample the NMR signal for a given spectrum is given by the Nyquist condition: $BW=1/DW \geq 2\nu_{max}$ where ν_{max} is the highest frequency in the spectrum, DW is the dwell time or time increment between successive sample points and BW is the sampling, or acquisition, bandwidth. As long as the read gradient is on, the relative resonance frequency $\Delta\nu$ of any spin is given by $\Delta\nu=-\gamma G_{read}x/2\pi$, where x is the distance from the read gradient isocenter and G_{read} is the strength of the read gradient. Combining these two relations we find that in order to accurately measure a nuclear spin's position along the read direction, that spin must have a distance to isocenter no greater than $\pi \cdot BW/(\gamma G_{read})$. In other words, digitizing the time-domain NMR data with a sweep width of BW, we can only measure positions lying in a region of width $FOV_{read}=2\pi \cdot BW/(\gamma G_{read})$ centered at the read gradient isocenter, where FOV_{read} is the field of view in the read gradient direction.

In digitizing the time-domain NMR signal, we select not only DW, but also the number of samples to collect in the time domain, which is equal to the number of data points in the frequency domain after Fourier transformation, and thus equal to the number of pixels in the MRI image along the read gradient direction. This number of pixels, MTX_{read}, is called the matrix size in the read dimension of the image. The total time over which the NMR signal is digitized is called the acquisition time: $AQ = DW \cdot MTX_{read}$. The spatial resolution, Δx_{read}, of the MRI image along the read direction is simply given by FOV_{read}/MTX_{read}. Recalling that FOV_{read} is given by $2\pi \cdot BW/(\gamma G_{read})$, we observe that spatial resolution in the read direction can be minimized, for constant MTX_{read}, by either minimizing BW or maximizing G_{read}. Minimizing BW has the additional benefit of improving SNR, as we shall discuss in Sect. 2.6, but this also implies longer DW=1/BW, and hence longer AQ and a larger minimum echo time. This may not be acceptable in fast imaging experiments or in the imaging of short T2 or short T2* samples. In contrast, optimizing spatial resolution along the read direction by maximizing G_{read}

with fixed bandwidth has no penalties, but is limited by gradient performance. Thus, in the specification of an MRI scanner, it is relatively advantageous to have a larger maximum G_{read} and a larger maximum BW.

2.3.1.3 Phase Encoding Gradients

A phase encoding gradient in the pulse sequence permits spatial localization in the direction perpendicular to the read gradient direction within the slice plane. This requires multiple acquisitions with a phase encoding gradient inserted between the slice selection and read gradients. During the constant duration phase-encoding period, the nuclear spins undergo a net phase change that depends upon their position along the direction of the phase encoding gradient. This phase change is reflected in a change in the overall intensity of the NMR signal acquired during the read period. With the read and slice gradients operating as discussed above, one can construct a two-dimensional slice-selected MRI image from a sequence of acquisitions performed with incremented phase encoding gradient strength. Likewise, a three-dimensional image can be obtained by simultaneously incrementing phase encoding gradients on two different axes, both perpendicular to the read axis.

2.3.2 Gradient Linearity

As we have mentioned, both shim and pulsed field gradients are typically created by passing electrical current through wire windings. The geometry of the gradient desired determines the shape of the coil windings.

In order to be useful for spatial encoding, either in the read, phase or slice directions, a pulsed field gradient must at a minimum produce a monotonic variation of B0 with X, Y or Z position over the volume of the sample being imaged; this is needed to ensure a one-to-one mapping of B0 field strength to position. In addition, it is highly desirable that the variation of B0 with position be perfectly linear over the sample volume. If this is satisfied, then position and B0 field strength (or resonance frequency) are related by a simple linear transformation, making gradient calibration a simple matter. The term gradient linearity refers to the degree to which a gradient coil generates a perfectly linear variation of B0 with position over a certain range of distances from its isocenter.

2.3.3 Gradient Switching and Eddy Currents

While shim gradients are typically applied continuously and at constant strength, pulsed field gradients must be switched on and off rapidly and frequently during a MRI pulse sequence. This requirement, along with the need for excellent linearity and much higher gradient strength makes pulsed field gradient systems much more challenging to design and build than shim systems. Ideally, we would like to expose the nuclear spins to gradient pulses which turn on and off instantly. In practice, this is not possible due to both inductive and eddy current effects. The finite inductance of the gradient coil affects the dynamics of current and thus gradient amplitude, $\partial B0/\partial x$, on a time scale of hundreds of microseconds. In contrast, eddy current effects influence the B0 field distribution directly on a time scale from milliseconds to seconds. Eddy currents are electrical currents induced in any conductive materials, such as the magnet bore tube, located in close proximity to the gradient coil. These induced currents are proportional to the gradient slew rate, that is, $\partial B0/\partial t = dG/dt$ and thus can be large when the gradient current rises or falls rapidly. Eddy currents flowing through these conductive materials generate a magnetic field oriented opposite in direction to $\partial B0/\partial t$. The nuclear spins experience the sum of the magnetic fields generated by the gradient coil and eddy currents. The net effect is to lengthen both the time required to achieve a stable, usable field gradient as well as the time needed to stabilize the B0 field after the pulse ends. Depending upon the gradient slew rate and the configuration of conductive material inside and outside the gradient coil, eddy current-induced fields may cause the actual B0 distribution felt by the spins to be quite different from the intended distribution. These effects manifest themselves in both broadening and frequency shifts in NMR spectra acquired immediately after a gradient pulse, and contribute to imaging artifacts. One longstanding method of reducing eddy currents is to use gradient preemphasis, in which the input to the gradient amplifiers is calculated to produce the desired gradient in the sample, accounting for coil inductance and eddy current effects. In addition, modern gradient coils are actively shielded. Just as in the design of actively-shielded magnets, these gradient coils are equipped with shield windings which largely cancel the stray field outside the bore of the gradient set. Using a combination of the above techniques, it is possible to achieve a stable B0 field within a few hundred microseconds of the rising or falling edge of a gradient pulse. The actual gradient switching performance of a MRI scanner is often specified by the time required after the beginning of a pulse to reach 90% or 99% of the desired gradient strength. Small microimaging gradient coils can achieve rise and fall times of 100 µs or less while gradient coils for clinical imaging typically require 200–300 µs to achieve 99% stability after gradient switching. Faster gradient switching permits shorter echo times and more rapid acquisitions, and reduces image distortions resulting from undesired time-varying contributions to the spatial distribution of B0. While these effects are noticeable in many MRI experiments, they are particularly pronounced in fast imaging sequences such as echo planar imaging (EPI). In EPI, the read and phase encoding gradients are switched on and off rapidly many times in each scan in order to sample a large number of phase-encoded steps using a train of gradient echoes. Ideally, this gradient switching can be achieved very quickly, permitting an entire two-dimensional image to be acquired in tens of milliseconds. For this to be possible, inductive and eddy current effects must be minimized so that the B0 field achieves the desired magnitude and spatial distribution quickly after each switch. When this is not the case, distortions in the B0 field result in signal loss and distortions in the images. In general, any experiment which requires frequent, rapid gradient switching will produce undistorted images only if considerable care is exercised to minimize gradient stabilization times. Thus, the gradient rise and fall times are critical specifications in the evaluation of any MRI scanner.

2.3.4 Gradient Strength

From the discussion in Sect. 2.3.1, it is clear that strong gradients permit improved in-plane spatial resolution and thinner slices. The gradient strength which is achievable in an actual MRI scanner depends upon several factors. First, just as an electromagnet can be made stronger by increasing the number of turns in the magnet coil, gradient strength can be increased by adding turns to a gradient coil. Unfortunately, this also increases the electrical resistance of the coil and thus the heat dissipated by the coil, I^2R, for a given current, I. This heat must be dissipated by air or water cooling. A larger number of turns also increases the inductance of the coil, which impedes rapid gradient switching. In order to accurately set the field of view and slice thickness and to faithfully depict the sizes and positions of features within a sample, it is necessary that the actual strength of each gradient coil be carefully calibrated. This is typically achieved by imaging an object with known dimensions. With a particular choice of field of view and slice thickness, the pulse amplitude applied to each gradient amplifier is calibrated to give the correct dimensions of the object in MRI slices taken in three orthogonal directions. It is then assumed that the required gradient current will scale linearly with the field of view or slice thickness desired in all other experiments. In other words, we assume that the gradient strength is a linear function of the gradient amplifier input voltage over the operating range of the gradient system. Since all modern gradient amplifiers are linear amplifiers, this is generally an excellent assumption.

2.3.5 Gradient Stability and Duty Cycle

In any imaging experiment, it is important that the amplitude of a gradient pulse be stable following the initial ramp-up period and be reproducible from scan to scan. Failure to meet these conditions results in image distortions for poor gradient stability and ghosting artifacts when gradient reproducibility is inadequate.

The duty cycle of any pulse-generating device is defined as the fraction of time during which the device is active, i.e., producing an output signal, and is expressed as a percentage. A particularly high gradient duty cycle occurs in experiments requiring long echo trains, such as EPI, and when the repetition time TR is very short. In some situations, a burst of strong gradient pulses with a high short-term duty cycle is tolerable to the amplifiers provided that TR is long, so that the long-term duty cycle is low. Both the maximum duty cycle and the tendency of long gradient pulses to droop in amplitude are functions of the capacity of the gradient amplifier power supply to sustain large loads, and the gradient coil's ability to dissipate heat.

2.4 Radio-Frequency Coils

In MRI scanners, radio-frequency transmit coils are used to transmit electromagnetic waves into a sample, creating the oscillating B1 magnetic field needed to excite the nuclear spins. In contrast, receive coils detect the weak signal emitted by the spins as they precess in the B0 field. For typical values of the magnetic field strength B0 encountered in NMR and MRI instruments, these signals lie in the radio-frequency region of the electromagnetic spectrum. Thus, RF coils can be thought of as radio antennas. The same coil may be used for both exciting the spins and receiving the resulting NMR signal, or transmission and reception may be performed by separate coils which are carefully constructed to minimize inductive coupling between them. RF coils are characterized by the volume over which they can generate a uniform B1 field or, equivalently, receive a NMR signal with uniform gain. The most important property of a RF coil, however, is the efficiency with which it converts electromagnetic waves at the specified frequency into electric current, and vice versa. There is a reciprocity relation between the performance of the coil as a transmitter of excitation pulses and as a receiver of faint NMR signals, meaning that both can be optimized simultaneously. A variety of RF coil designs have been developed which attempt to optimize one or both of these specifications over a given volume.

2.4.1 Common RF Coil Designs

2.4.1.1 Solenoidal RF Coils

The solenoidal configuration used for magnet and shim coils is also useful for RF antennas. Driving a solenoidal coil with an alternating current generates a spatially homogeneous time varying B1 magnetic field with the same frequency as the driving current. This produces a torque on nuclear spins which are within the coil and which have a component of their orientation perpendicular to the coil axis. Thus, it is necessary that the coil produce a B1 field which is not parallel to the B0 field. Similarly, a receive coil must be able to detect a time-varying magnetic field perpendicular to B0 in order to detect a NMR signal. Since the B1 field generated by a solenoidal coil is parallel to the bore axis of the solenoid, the coil should be oriented with this axis perpendicular to B0. Consequently, solenoidal coils are primarily used for imaging in vitro samples. Solenoidal RF coils generate very homogeneous fields, especially over samples which are small in diameter and length compared to the dimensions of the solenoid. This enables them to excite and detect a NMR signal from any nuclear spins within the bore of the solenoid. Solenoids are highly efficient as both transmitter and receiver coils and are very simple to construct.

2.4.1.2 Surface Coils and Phased Arrays

A surface coil is a loop of wire which generates or detects B1 fields along a direction perpendicular to the plane of the loop. Like solenoidal coils, surface coils are highly efficient and are easy to build. Since they have a B1 axis perpendicular to the loop plane, surface coils offer convenient access for application to a wide variety of anatomical sites while maintaining B1 perpendicular to B0. However, the RF field generated by a surface coil is very inhomogeneous, with maximum B1 magnitude in the plane of the coil and a rapid falloff in B1 with distance from this plane. Likewise, when used for detecting an NMR signal, a surface coil can only detect nuclei within a short distance from the coil plane. Specifically, when a surface coil is placed against the surface of a sample, nuclei may be excited and detected to a depth approximately equal to the diameter of the coil and over an area approximately equal to the dimensions of the coil. The small, well-defined volume over which a surface coil transmits or receives a signal makes these coils ideal for spatial localization in certain circumstances without requiring the use of field gradients. Surface coils have long been used to obtain in vivo NMR spectra of peripheral muscle, brain, heart, liver and other relatively superficial tissues with simple purely spectroscopic pulse sequences. In MRI scanners, where spatial localization can be achieved by gradients, surface coils are less often used for excitation and are instead primarily employed as high-sensitivity receive-only coils in conjunction with a large, homogeneous transmit-only resonator. The limited area over which a single surface coil can detect a NMR signal can be overcome by combining two or more surface coils to form a phased array coil. These coils must be coupled with electronic components which combine the signals from each coil into a single signal or to multiple, independent receivers. The phased array covers the surface area which a much larger surface coil would observe, but exhibits the higher sensitivity of the small coils which make up the array. Phased array coils are commonly used in clinical imaging of the spine, where an extensive field of view is required but the tissue of interest is relatively superficial. Both individual surface coils and phased arrays can be constructed with curvature to ensure close placement to a given anatomical site, thereby optimizing both sensitivity and depth of view.

2.4.1.3
RF Volume Resonators

When a NMR signal must be excited and detected from deep tissue or where homogeneous excitation is required and a solenoidal coil does not provide convenient patient access, a variety of RF volume resonators is available. These may be defined as cylindrical, multi-loop coils which generate a B1 field perpendicular to the bore axis. A birdcage resonator is very commonly used as a head or body coil in both clinical and animal MRI scanners (see coil in Fig. 2.1). Birdcage resonators can be used in both transmit-receive and transmit-only configurations. In the latter arrangement, a birdcage coil is used to achieve homogeneous excitation over a subject while a surface coil is used for high-sensitivity detection of the signal from a superficial region of the subject. Unlike simpler resonator designs, the birdcage resonator can be operated in quadrature mode in order to achieve an increase in B1 field strength (or, equivalently, detection sensitivity) of a factor of $\sqrt{2}$. In transmission mode, the driving current is split into two separate signals which are simultaneously applied to the birdcage resonator in order to create circularly polarized fields of equal magnitude but 90° out of phase. The vector sum of these fields is a B1 field oriented perpendicular to the resonator's bore axis with a magnitude $\sqrt{2}$ times as great as each component. In reception mode, a quadrature birdcage coil simultaneously detects components of B1 along two orthogonal directions, yielding two separate electrical signals which can be combined with an appropriate electronic circuit external to the resonator. The transverse electromagnetic resonator (TEM), a design relatively new to MRI, has become popular due to its excellent efficiency at very high frequencies, where other resonator designs offer poorer performance. TEM resonators are especially useful for brain imaging on high-field research MRI scanners.

2.4.2
Coil Characteristics and Optimization

For a coil to transmit or receive RF signals at the nuclear magnetic resonance frequency, the coil must be a component of a transmitter or receiver circuit tuned to this frequency. In addition, for efficient transfer of RF power to and from the coil, the electrical impedance of the coil must be matched to the impedance of the transmitter or receiver electronics. Tuning and matching may be achieved by manual or automatic adjustment of variable components located preferably within the coil housing itself or alternatively in a remote enclosure.

The quality factor (Q) measures the efficiency with which the coil converts an electrical signal into radio-frequency radiation or vice versa. Consequently, a coil with high Q is efficient at detecting weak radio frequency NMR signals, creating an electrical signal that may be amplified and digitized by the spectrometer's receiver electronics. A transmitter coil having a high Q indicates that it creates a relatively strong B1 field from an alternating current of a certain amplitude. Because the pulse length τ_{90} needed to achieve a 90° flip angle is simply related to the magnitude of B1 by the equation $\gamma B1\tau_{90}=\pi/2$, the coil efficiency is often specified by stating the 90° pulse length achievable for a specific amount of transmitter power applied to the coil containing a specific sample. Equivalently, coil efficiency can be stated in terms of the transmitter power needed to achieve a 90° flip angle in a given sample with an RF pulse of given duration and shape.

The term filling factor indicates the fraction of a coil's sensitive volume that is occupied by sample. For fixed coil dimensions, quality factor Q and incident transmitter power, the filling factor has minimal effect on the 90° pulse length and the coil's efficiency for exciting the nuclear spins. However, filling factor has a strong effect on sensitivity when detecting a NMR signal, with higher filling factor corresponding to higher sensitivity. For a sample of fixed dimensions, it is advantageous to use the smallest coil that will accommodate the region of the sample to be imaged while providing acceptable RF homogeneity over that region. Using the smallest possible receive coil size also minimizes the amount of sample noise which will be detected along with the NMR signal and thus maximizes signal-to-noise ratio. Because, in practice, it is not possible to achieve both high filling factor and high RF homogeneity with a single transmit/receive coil, it is not uncommon to use a large resonator for homogeneous excitation of the nuclei and a much smaller surface or phased array coil to detect the NMR signal with optimum filling factor, minimum noise pickup and thus maximum SNR. As we described earlier, this crossed coil configuration requires careful adjustment of geometry and synchronization of tuning and detuning to prevent crosstalk between the transmit-only resonator and the receive-only surface coil or coils.

In principle, it is possible to make τ_{90} as short as desired by simply increasing the transmitter power delivered to the coil, even if the transmit coil has low Q. MRI instruments are typically equipped with radio frequency amplifiers delivering kilowatts of power at the NMR frequency and it is very desirable for transmitter coils to be able to operate safely at high power. The ability of a coil to withstand high power pulses depends both on the amplitude of these pulses and their duty cycle. When a coil is exposed to high incident transmitter power, even for a relatively short duration, very large voltages may be created across components such as capacitors and closely-spaced conductors, leading to dielectric breakdown and arcing. Conversely, exposure to long pulses at high power may lead to excessive resistive heating and subsequent failure of inductors and resistive conductors. Just as dissipation of heat within the transmitter coil and associated components imposes a limit on RF power levels and duty cycle in a MRI experiment, care must be taken not to produce excessive heating of the sample, typically an animal or human subject. When exposed to RF radiation, tissue undergoes heating depending upon its dielectric constant. This heat is dissipated largely by blood circulation, which carries heat from deep within the body to the skin and extremities for radiative cooling. When the RF power level and duty cycle are sufficiently low, this cooling mechanism prevents tissue temperatures from rising excessively. Common safety practice is based upon limiting any temperature rise in tissue to one degree Celsius during a MRI examination. In order to satisfy regulatory guidance, MRI experiments performed on living subjects must not exceed certain limits on specific absorption rate (SAR). Power deposition is in general a greater problem at higher field strengths.

2.5 Transmitters

The term transmitter refers to the assembly of electronic components in an MRI scanner which provides an electrical signal to the transmitter coil to excite the nuclear spins. The transmitter system can be divided into low-power components, which create pulsed alternating current signals with defined timing, phase and amplitude modulation, and high-power components, which faithfully amplify this low-level signal and couple it to the transmitter coil. In modern instruments, the low-level RF electronics consist mostly or entirely of digital components while the high-power section of the transmitter is largely analog in design due to the power limitations of available digital components. Accordingly, specifications for the low-power section of an MRI transmitter are based on clock rates and digital resolution of digital-to-analog converters (DACs). In contrast, high-power transmitter subsystems are characterized by the standard amplification specifications of gain, linearity and stability as well as by their power and duty cycle limits. Additional considerations essential for MRI include slew rate, a measure of the speed with which the output of the amplifier can change, and blanking performance, the ability of the amplifier to provide zero output during signal acquisition.

The frequency range of the transmitter must be broad. In proton MRI, for example, the ability to access a wide frequency range about the nominal proton NMR frequency is desirable for several reasons. As we have discussed, it is often desirable to minimize slice thickness by maximizing slice gradient strength rather than by decreasing RF excitation bandwidth, since the latter results in increased echo time and signal losses due to relaxation. Greater slice gradient strength implies a larger dispersion of NMR frequencies along the slice direction. In addition, in order to excite slices anywhere along this direction, the transmitter must be able to generate a wide range of radio frequencies to correspond to different slabs along the slice gradient. For both proton NMR and heteronuclear (i.e., non-proton) experiments, it is desirable to have the capability to study nuclei across their entire chemical shift range. In addition, it is important to be able to excite a variety of nuclei with different gyromagnetic ratios, and hence widely different frequencies.

In addition to setting the frequency, duration and amplitude of an RF pulse, the low-power transmitter system of an MRI scanner must be capable of adjusting the phase of the pulse. By altering the phase relationship between the RF excitation pulse and the receiver reference signal, it is possible to reduce certain artifacts associated with imperfect flip angles, unwanted spin echoes, receiver imbalances and other effects. This technique, called phase cycling, causes the desired signal components to add with each scan while undesired components are subtracted from the accumulated signal.

Once the transmitter's low-power electronics have synthesized a pulsed, amplitude modulated RF signal with the appropriate frequencies and phases, this signal must be amplified to provide sufficient power for spin excitation. High power pulses are needed in NMR and MRI in order to achieve desired flip angles with short pulse durations. In clinical MRI scanners, amplifiers up to 15–25 kW are commonly used. In each case, the RF power required to achieve the desired flip angles with adequately short pulse lengths depends upon the efficiency of the coil at the NMR frequency.

The linearity of the high-power RF amplifier refers to its ability to amplify a signal by a constant factor, that is, with constant gain, over a wide range of input amplitudes. This permits the low-power waveform which is input into the transmitter amplifier system to be faithfully reproduced as a high-power RF excitation pulse. Therefore, it is desirable to have a high-power RF amplifier with minimum variation in gain over the widest possible input amplitude range.

2.6 Radio-Frequency Receiver

After nuclear spins in a sample have been excited by RF pulses, they precess in the main magnetic field as they relax back to equilibrium. This precession induces very small voltages in the receiver coil; this signal can be on the order of microvolts. It is the function of the MRI scanner's receiver train to greatly amplify this signal, filter out unwanted frequency components, separate real and imaginary components and digitize these components for storage and processing by the host computer. The initial amplification occurs at the natural precession frequency of the nuclei using one or more preamplifier stages. In order to help protect these very sensitive preamplifiers from overload and damage by the high-power transmitter pulses as well as to isolate the weak NMR signal from the transmitter pulse ringdown signal, MRI scanners contain a transmit-receive switch. When a single transmit-receive coil is used, the transmit-receive switch alternately connects the coil circuit to the transmitter for spin excitation and to the receiver train for signal detection, amplification, and digitization.

Together, the real and imaginary parts of the NMR signal can be thought of as a complex function with a magnitude and phase at each instant of time. Upon Fourier transformation, this phase-sensitive data yields a spectrum with both positive and negative frequencies centered about the reference frequency. This technique of obtaining a complex, phase-sensitive audio frequency signal by splitting and mixing with phase-shifted reference signals is known as quadrature detection.

Once quadrature detection has been performed, the real and imaginary signals are further amplified and passed through low-pass filters. These filters are set to remove any components with frequencies greater than the spectral width to be digitally sampled. This step is necessary to eliminate any signal components at frequencies too high to be properly digitized with the selected digitization rate, thus preventing high-frequency noise or unwanted resonances from being folded into the digitized signal. Ideally, the low-pass filters should present no attenuation to signal components below the cutoff frequency while totally eliminating any component above this frequency. For any real analog filter, there will always be some attenuation and phase shift as one approaches the cutoff frequency. Thus, the filters are set to a frequency somewhat higher than the full spectral width. This ensures that any resonance occurring within the selected spectral width will receive no significant attenuation from the filters.

Once the NMR signal has been amplified, mixed down to audio frequency and separated into real and imaginary components, it is digitized for computer processing. The ability to digitize rapidly allows one to achieve short echo times in fast imaging and studies of samples with rapid T2 relaxation. Consequently, maximum sampling rate is an important specification for any analog-to-digital converter (ADC), or "digitizer". Just as important is the digital resolution of the ADC. This is the number of bits with which the digitizer represents the amplitude of the signal. It is desirable to amplify the analog signal to be digitized so that it fills as much as possible of the dynamic range, or maximum input amplitude, of the digitizer without exceeding this range. There is a tradeoff in digitizer design between speed and digital resolution. For example, a common 16-bit digitizer can sample the NMR signal at a rate of up to 2 MHz, or 0.5 μs per point, while a 10 MHz digitizer may have a digital resolution of only 12 bits. High digital resolution is advantageous in detecting small spectroscopic peaks in the presence of a much larger peak, as in NMR spectroscopy of metabolites in dilute aqueous solution. A typical MRI scanner is equipped with a 16-bit digitizer with a maximum sampling rate of at least 1 MHz.

Once the NMR signal has been digitized, it may be subjected to a variety of digital signal conditioning procedures. Digital signal processing (DSP) is generally performed by a dedicated microprocessor rather than by the scanner's host computer and the processed signal is accumulated in a dedicated buffer memory. This greatly increases the rate at which data may be accumulated and prevents data loss due to interruptions in data transmission or host computer CPU availability.

3 Spin- and Gradient-Echo Imaging

Dara L. Kraitchman

CONTENTS

3.1 Introduction

In Chap. 1 the fundamental behaviors of a single spin, or of a group of spins, were discussed. In brief summary, after the spins are aligned in a polarizing magnetic field, it is possible to add energy and to cause them to acquire transverse magnetization while giving up longitudinal magnetization. The recovery of longitudinal magnetization and the decay of transverse magnetization are characterized by relaxation times. Signal arises from the transverse component of magnetization and the interaction of that transverse magnetization with the conductors of the radiofrequency (RF) coil, due to Faraday induction. Certain types of signal loss (dephasing) can be reversed by a refocusing pulse to form a spin echo, which is advantageous in that its signal is relatively strong. In this chapter we begin with the MR signal and the spin echo, and develop the construction of images using combinations of RF pulses and application of gradients.

D. L. Kraitchman, VMD, PhD
Associate Professor, Johns Hopkins University, School of Medicine, Department of Radiology, Division of MR Research, 601 N. Caroline Street, Office 4231, Baltimore, MD 21287-0845, USA

3.2 The Spin-Echo Pulse Sequence

3.2.1 Image Encoding

3.2.1.1 Slice Selection

In order to examine only a specific slice in the body rather than exciting the entire body with an RF pulse, a gradient magnetic field is superimposed on the external field, B0, during the application of the RF pulse. This external and additional magnetic field is applied with variable intensity as a function of location. Specifically, the gradient field, as well as the total field that is the sum of the B0 and the gradient, increases from the center of the magnet outward in the positive direction, and decreases in the opposite direction. This establishes a characteristic field strength, and thus, resonance frequency, for each position along the gradient axis.

The thickness of the slice can be selected in two ways. One method is by changing the range of RF pulse frequencies or bandwidth. A smaller range of RF frequencies, such as 64–64.5 mHz, will resonate protons in a thinner slice than a larger range of frequencies, such as 64–65 mHz.

Another method of changing the slice thickness is by modifying the slope or the gradient field. A steeper gradient, i.e., one that has a larger variation in field strength, will cause frequency precession to vary to a larger degree and enable a thinner slice selection.

3.2.1.2
Frequency Encoding

By applying a gradient during the RF pulse, one can select a slice or position in the body as well as the thickness of this slice. If we apply another gradient field during the acquisition of the signal, each position along the gradient direction will be associated by the Larmor relationship with a unique resonance frequency, and the spins at that position will precess according to that frequency. For example, if the gradient pulse is applied along x and increases from the left to right side of the body, then the precession frequency will also increase from left to right (Fig. 3.1). Thus, a one-to-one correspondence between frequency and spatial position is created by using an externally applied magnetic field gradient. Because this gradient creates a relationship between spatial location and frequency, it is called the frequency encoding gradient. A one-dimensional (1D) Fourier transform (FT) of the recorded signal will yield signal amplitudes at different frequencies which correspond to the spatial location in 1D. Note that frequency encoding is not sufficient to uniquely determine the two-dimensional (2D) location within the slice since all protons in one column will have the same frequency. The frequency encoding gradient is often referred to as the read or readout gradient since it is applied during data acquisition or read-out.

3.2.1.3
Phase encoding

In order to discriminate between points within the same column after frequency encoding, we apply another gradient at 90° (or orthogonal) to the frequency encoding gradient. This gradient is called the phase encoding gradient. The phase encoding gradient is applied for a brief period of time, typically prior to the frequency encoding gradient, and causes a change in the frequency of precession for a brief period of time. During the gradient operation, proton spins precess in accordance with the altered magnetic field, and acquire phase angles that are specifically attributable to that field. When the gradient is turned off, the frequency of precession returns to the equilibrium value, but the phase of rotation of the protons is locked in. Thus, when the gradient is turned off, each column (from the previous example) will have a different phase. This is known as phase encoding. Clearly, the magnitude of the phase change is proportional to the magnitude of the phase encoding gradient. By using both frequency and phase encoding gradients, the protons are labeled with both a frequency and phase so that 2D spatial localization can be performed.

Typically, one spin echo is acquired for each gradient magnitude of phase encoding. This simple but powerful form of MR imaging is called the spin-warp pulse sequence and is diagrammed in Fig. 3.2.

3.2.2
Single Spin-Echo

The spin-echo pulse sequence is widely used in clinical practice due to the ease of implementation and the ease of varying parameters that will alter MR contrast based on differences in tissue T1, T2, or proton density. The spin-echo pulse sequence (Fig. 3.3)

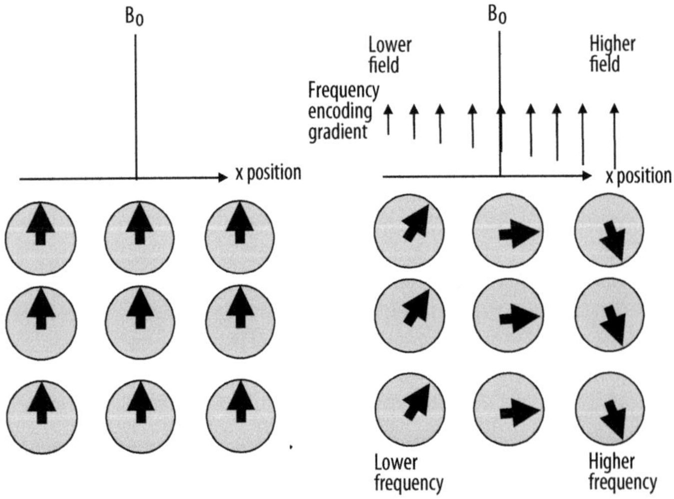

Fig. 3.1. Initially the net magnetization at each pixel is aligned with the magnetic field gradient, B0, as shown for nine representative pixels. Application of the frequency encoding gradient, a linearly varying magnetic field gradient, causes an increased or decreased frequency at each pixel in proportion to the increased or decreased applied field. One dimensional localization can be performed. However, no distinction between pixels in the same column can be made because they are at the same frequency

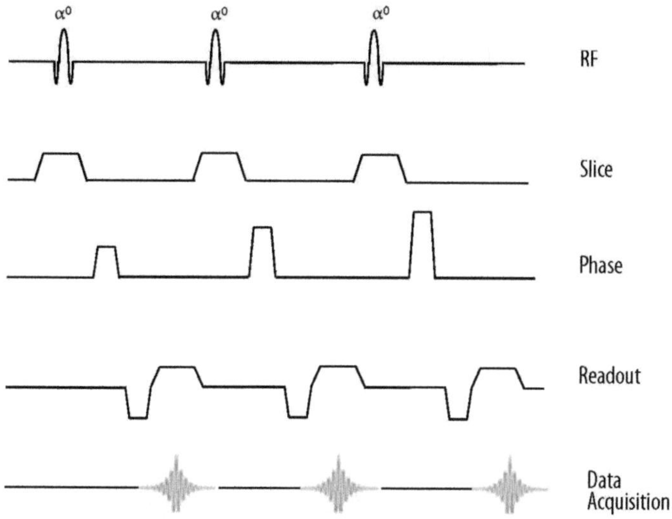

Fig. 3.2. Schematic diagram of the spin warp pulse sequence. A slice selection gradient (*Slice*) is applied during the radiofrequency pulse (*RF*) to excite protons in the slice. Next, a phase encoding gradient (*Phase*) is applied followed by a frequency encoding gradient (*Readout*) during data acquisition for 2D localization. Each line of k-space is obtained with a different magnitude of phase encoding gradient. In this example, three different phase encoding steps are shown

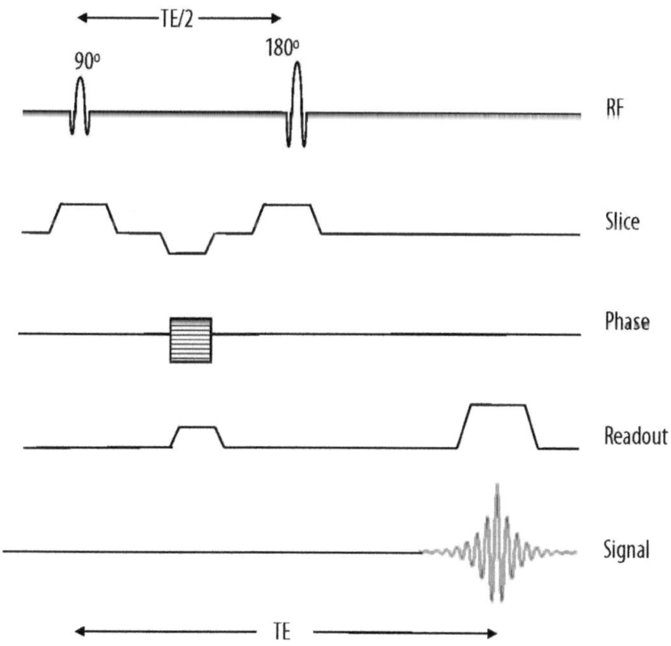

Fig. 3.3. Spin-echo pulse sequence timing diagram where a pair of 90° and 180° radiofrequency (*RF*) pulses are used to create spin echo at echo time (*TE*)

in its simplest form consists of a series of alternating 90° and 180° RF pulses. The 90° RF pulse tips the magnetization such that all the individual spins are in phase (Fig. 3.4). However, because of inhomogeneities in the magnetic field ($T2^*$ effects) dephasing of the spins will occur in addition to the dephasing caused by spin–spin interactions (true T2). The application of a 180° rephasing pulse at some time delay after application of the initial 90° RF pulse nutates the spins such that spins that were precessing more rapidly are now rotating behind the spins that were precessing more slowly (Fig. 3.4). Thus, after an identical time delay, the slower spins have caught up with the faster spins such that the spins are rephased and the spin echo is created (Fig. 3.4). This time between the initial 90° RF pulse and the moment of rephasing when read-out is performed is called the echo time (TE). The time between the application of the 90°

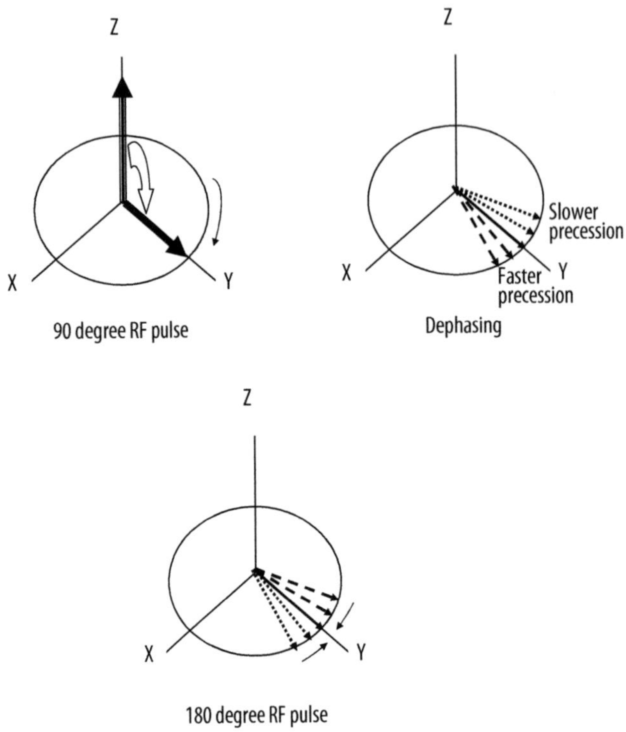

Fig. 3.4. The 90° RF pulse of the spin-echo pulse sequence tips the bulk magnetization to the x-axis with all the spins initially in phase. Due to inhomogeneities in the magnetic field and spin–spin interactions, the spins will dephase with time. The application of a 180° RF refocusing pulse reverses the slower spins *(dotted lines)* and faster spins (*dashed lines*) such that a spin echo is created at the echo time with all the spins rephased

pulse and the 180° pulse is TE/2 (Fig. 3.4). The entire sequence is repeated at a repetition time (TR) that is chosen much longer than TE.

To achieve T1 weighting in a spin-echo pulse sequence, a short repetition time is chosen. Similarly, T2 weighting is achieved by choosing a short TE and a longer TR. Proton density images are obtained with a TR longer than used for T1-weighted imaging and a TE shorter than used for T2-weighted imaging. Typical T1 and T2 values at 1.5 T (and 37°C) are given in Table 3.1.

Table 3.1. Typical T1 and T_2 values at 1.5 T and 37°C

Tissue	T1 (ms)	T2 (ms)
White matter	600–790	90
Gray matter	920–950	100
Cerebrospinal fluid	4500	2000
Fat	250	60
Blood	1200	100–200[a]

[a] Variation in T2 times in blood are due to differences between oxygenated arterial blood and deoxygenated venous blood.

3.2.3 Multi-Echo Spin-Echo

Multi-echo spin-echo sequences are based on the single-echo spin-echo pulse sequence, but use additional 180° refocusing pulse(s) to create additional spin echo(s) (Fig. 3.5). Each spin echo occurs at a different TE and echoes from the same TEs are combined or reconstructed to form a single image. Thus, many images with different degrees of T2-weighting or T2-weighted and proton density images can easily be simultaneously created without extending the imaging time.

3.3 Gradient-Echo Imaging

The main difference between gradient-echo imaging and spin-echo imaging is that in spin-echo imaging the dephasing of spins due to magnet inhomogeneity is refocused. This results in a profound advantage of sensitivity, as the signal is much stronger, all else equal. The cost of this quality advantage is time. The

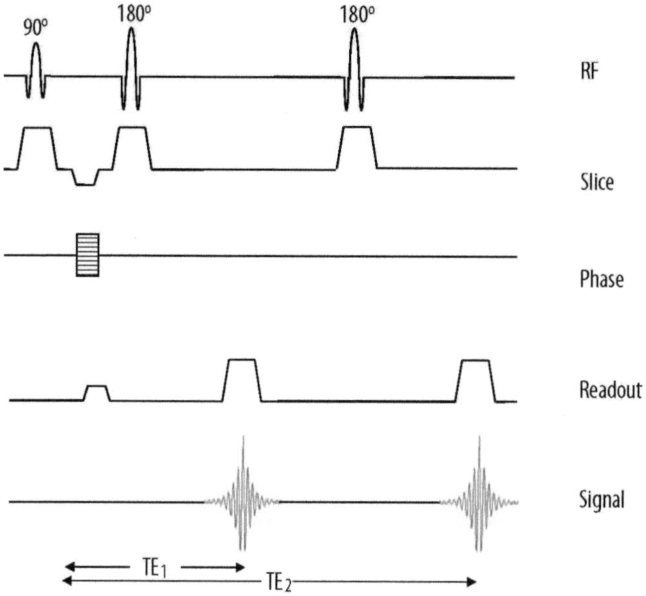

Fig. 3.5. Multi-echo spin-echo pulse sequence timing diagram using multiple refocusing RF pulses to produce several spin echoes each at a different TE (e.g., TE_1 and TE_2)

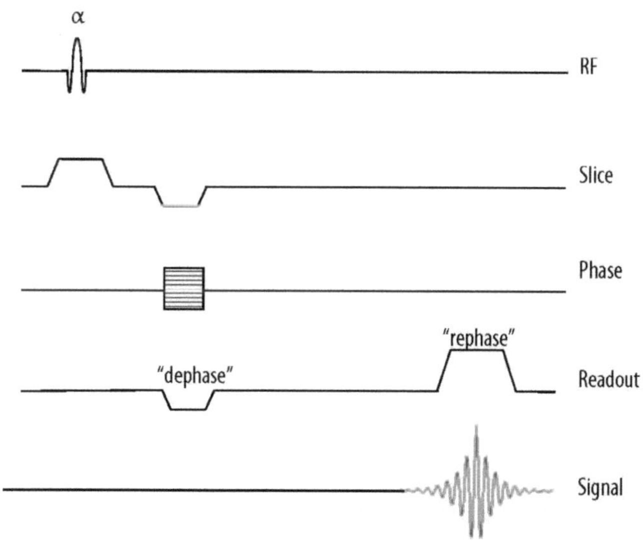

Fig. 3.6. Gradient-echo pulse sequence timing diagram where frequency encoded gradient pulses (i.e., readout) are used to first "dephase" and then "rephase" the spins to create the echo. The flip angle (α), repetition time, and echo time help to determine the degree of T1 and T2 weighting of the image

advent of better constructed, more homogeneous magnets made it possible to obtain imaging data without refocusing the spin-dephasing referred to above. Thus, a new method of imaging was created that did not employ refocusing pulses.

In gradient-echo imaging, paired gradient applications are used to dephase and subsequently rephase the spins. Here, the only rephasing that takes place is a reversal of the intentional dephasing provided by the gradients under control of the pulse sequence. This is in contrast to spin-echo imaging, where dephasing due to magnet imperfections is "corrected" for a sizable advantage in signal-to-noise ratio (SNR).

In gradient-echo imaging, after the phase-encoding gradient is switched off, the frequency encoding gradient is reversed (Fig. 3.6). Spins that initially experienced an increased field due to the phase encoding will precess at a higher frequency. With the reversal of the magnitude of the gradient, the spins that were precessing faster are slowed down and the slower spins precess faster thereby resulting in rephasing of the spins in a manner similar to the 180° refocusing pulse in spin-echo imaging. Thus, while the 180° RF pulse of spin echo refocuses the dephased spins, a negative gradient lobe in gradient-echo imaging initially causes a phase dispersion of spins that are refocused by reversing the gradient.

Gradient-echo imaging techniques are preferred in many applications where the most rapid imaging is required. The use of a gradient reversal to dephase and then rephase spins has several additional positive consequences. Because only a single RF pulse is applied, the echo can be acquired more quickly thereby significantly reducing echo time. In addition, if low flip angles are used, the repetition time can be reduced. These reductions in TR and TE are what enable gradient-echo techniques to acquire images more rapidly than spin-echo techniques. Moreover, since lower flip angles are frequently used with gradient-echo imaging, less energy is deposited than using the 90/180° RF pulses of spin-echo imaging. Therefore, specific absorption rates (SAR), which is defined as the RF power absorbed per unit mass of an object, can be reduced using gradient-echo imaging relative to spin echo.

T2 decay occurs between the dephasing and rephasing gradient pulses. Thus, unlike the 180° RF pulse of spin-echo imaging, rephasing in gradient echo does not completely recover the signal. Because of this loss of signal that cannot be rephased, gradient-echo techniques do not remove the effects of magnetic field inhomogeneities, differences in magnetic susceptibility, or the effects of chemical shift. Thus, gradient-echo techniques are sensitive to $T2^*$ effects. However, the ability to acquire images rapidly with gradient-echo pulse sequences has led to their inclusion in many MR imaging protocols. Moreover, the sensitivity to $T2^*$ changes can be exploited rather than viewed as a hindrance to demonstrate pathologies such as hemorrhage due to a breakdown in the blood–brain barrier or new techniques such as magnetic cell labeling (Bulte et al. 1999). Because the repetition time can be greatly reduced in gradient-echo techniques, often the longitudinal magnetization does not have the time to recover completely. Thus, the next 90° pulse would tip the net magnetization past the transverse plane resulting in reduced signal intensity. In order to not sacrifice the SNR in short TR gradient-echo sequences, a flip angle less than 90° is often used or a steady state of magnetization is achieved by repeated pulsing. In general, gradient-echo techniques are grouped into three major classes: spoiled gradient-echo, refocused gradient-echo, and magnetization-prepared gradient-echo.

3.3.1 Spoiled Gradient-Echo

In spoiled gradient-echo techniques, only longitudinal magnetization is allowed to reach a steady state. Spoiling to minimize the residual transverse magnetization (Frahm et al. 1986) is accomplished either by applying gradient pulses to crush the transverse magnetization or by varying the phase of the RF excitation pulse. Spoiled gradient-echo techniques are often used for short breath-hold acquisitions or contrast-enhanced imaging.

3.3.2 Refocused Gradient-Echo

Refocused gradient-echo techniques are also referred to as fast imaging with steady state precession (FISP), fast field echo (FFE), or gradient acquisition in the steady state (GRASS). Both longitudinal and transverse magnetization are allowed to approach a steady state. Thus, these techniques are based on the steady-state free precession (SSFP) methods. For long TRs and low flip angles, the transverse magnetization decays and the contrast of refocused gradient echo is comparable to spoiled gradient echo. For short TRs and large flip angles, a significant amount of transverse magnetization remains resulting in substantial T2-weighting or an image with mixed T1/T2-weighting. Refocused gradient echo is often used for breath-hold and perfusion imaging.

3.3.3 Magnetization-Prepared Gradient-Echo

In order to provide increased contrast compared to that available by varying TR, TE, and flip angle, additional RF preparation pulses can be applied to "prepare" the net magnetization (Fig. 3.7). Unlike the situation found in refocused gradient echo, the spins do not achieve a steady state condition. Image contrast is very sensitive to the time between the prep pulse and the acquisition of the center of k-space. Thus, changes in the ordering of phase encoding as well as the prep pulse can greatly change image contrast. A 180° RF prep pulse or inversion pulse is commonly used to provide T1-weighting. A 90-180-90° pulse or driven equilibrium approach can be used to provide T2-weighting. Collectively, these magnetization prepared gradient-echo sequences are often referred to as turboFLASH, MP-RAGE (magnetization-prepared rapid-acquisition gradient-echo), and TFE (turbo field-echo).

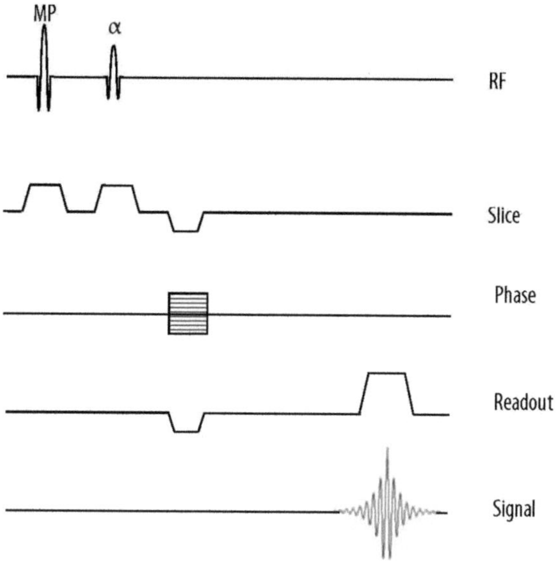

Fig. 3.7. Magnetization prepared gradient-echo pulse sequence timing diagram where a preparation pulse (*MP*) is applied prior to data collection. A 180° prepulse is a special case of magnetization preparation termed "inversion recovery"

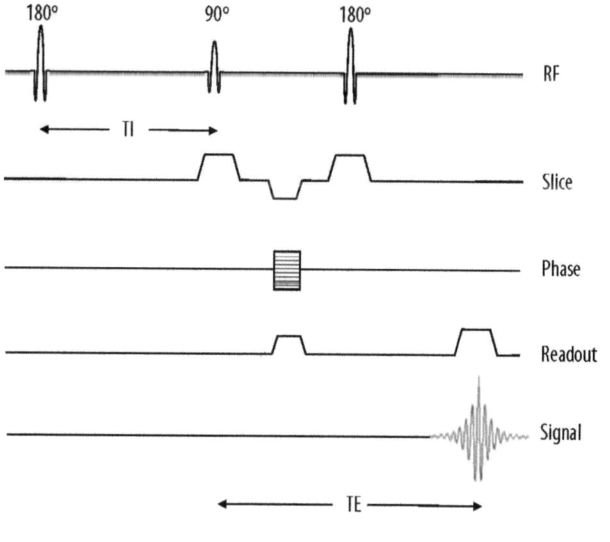

Fig. 3.8. Inversion recovery spin-echo pulse sequence timing diagram where a 180° RF inversion pulse is added prior to the normal spin-echo image acquisition. The inversion time (*TI*) is chosen such that a specific tissue is crossing the null point to obtain maximal tissue contrast

3.4 Inversion Recovery

As mentioned in magnetization-prepared gradient-echo, inversion recovery uses a 180° RF preparation pulse to invert the spins. Inversion recovery (IR) can also be performed with 180° pre-pulse using a spin-echo or fast spin-echo pulse sequence (Fig. 3.8). T1 relaxation of each tissue occurs with each tissue magnetization passing through a null point as it recovers to equilibrium, with a rate depending upon tissue T1 (Fig. 3.9). The time between read-out and the inversion pulse is called the inversion time (TI). By adjusting the TI, such that certain tissues are at the null point during image acquisition, T1 contrast can be maximized (Wehrli et al. 1984). The null point for any individual tissue is determined by: ~ln(2) * T1. For example, by choosing a TI at which cerebrospinal fluid (CSF) is passing thru zero during readout, CSF in the IR image will appear hypointense or black or hence is nulled. Care must be taken when TI is very short. In this case some tissue will still have inverted magnetization,

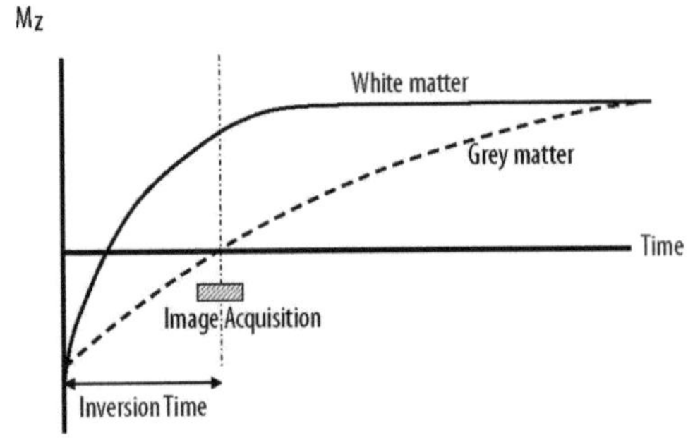

Fig. 3.9. Graphic representation of the recovery of longitudinal magnetization as a function of time for different tissues after an inversion pulse. If the image acquisition (*shaded area*) is placed at the zero crossing (i.e., null point) for a tissue, then maximum contrast between different tissues can be obtained

which will be flipped into the transverse plane and interpreted as positive signal in the images, leading to potential confusion (Young et al. 1985).

3.4.1 Short Inversion Time Recovery

Short tau inversion recovery or STIR is used to enhance contrast between gray and white matter while maintaining a high SNR and suppressing fat. By using a short TI, the signal from fat, which has the shortest T1, can be nulled while preserving soft tissue contrast. At short TI, all other tissue signals are negative which leads to positive values on magnitude reconstructed images (Fig. 3.10). Using STIR, better visualization of structures such as the optic nerve can be obtained (Atlas et al. 1988). STIR is not compatible with intravenous contrast.

3.4.2 Fluid-Attenuated Inversion Recovery

Fluid-attenuated inversion recovery (FLAIR) is a heavily T2-weighted sequence with suppression of the signal from CSF (i.e., fluid) leading to increased conspicuity of brain lesions (Frahm et al. 1986; De Coene et al. 1992). Suppression of the CSF is performed by choosing a null point of ~2200 ms (i.e., 70% of T1 of CSF) combined with a long echo time for T2-weighting (Fig. 3.11). The suppression of the CSF signal leads to decreased artifacts from CSF flow thereby enhancing the conspicuity of small lesions (Hajnal et al. 1992) especially those that are close to the ventricles or sulci.

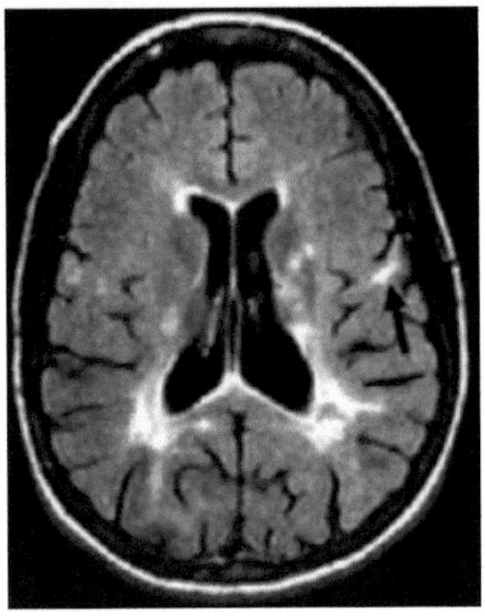

Fig. 3.11. Axial fluid attenuated inversion recovery (FLAIR) image of a patient with multiple sclerosis. A long inversion time (TI=2200 ms) almost completely suppresses the signal from the cerebrospinal fluid (CSF) such that the periventricular lesions are more conspicuous. In addition, several subcortical lesions (*arrow*) are seen that could not be demonstrated on standard T2-weighted images. (Image courtesy of Mark A. Horsfield)

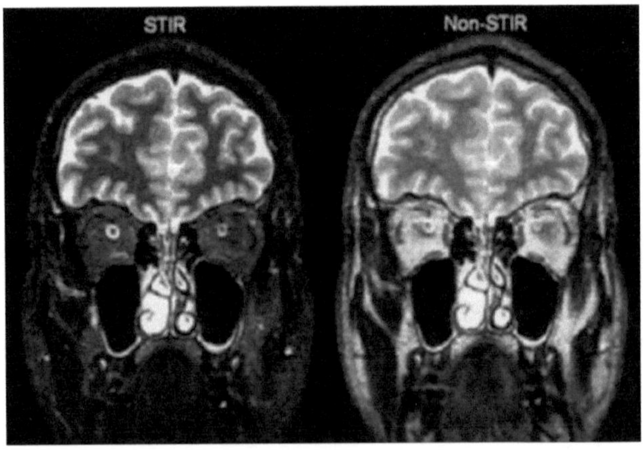

Fig. 3.10. Short tau inversion recovery (STIR) image (left) is used to suppress signal form the peri-orbital fat. In a non-STIR image (right), the details of the optic nerve cannot be seen due to the strong signal from peri-orbital fat. The inversion time of 170 ms in the STIR image causes the fat to pass through zero or be nulled. The echo time (TE=90 ms) is the same in both images. (Image courtesy of Mark A. Horsfield)

3.5 Artifacts

3.5.1 Metal Artifacts

Metal objects are well known to cause hypointense artifacts due to local distortions of the magnetic field (Laakman et al. 1985; Heindel et al. 1986; Shellock 2001). Dental implants, surgical clips, stents, and mascara can all be sources of ferromagnetic or paramagnetic materials (Sacco et al. 1987). The 180° refocusing pulse of spin-echo imaging tends to decrease the severity of artifacts relative to gradient-echo imaging (Fig. 3.12). If gradient-echo pulse sequences are used, shorter echo times will decrease the severity of artifacts from metal objects.

3.5.2 Chemical Shift Artifacts

The hydrogen signal that is measured by MRI is primarily composed of fat and water. At the clinical MR field strengths, fat and water precess at significantly different frequencies (e.g., 3.5 ppm at 1.5 T or 230 Hz). Since spatial mapping in one direction is done according to frequency (i.e., frequency encoding), the frequency difference with which water and fat precess causes fat and water signals in a single voxel to be mapped to different voxel locations (Fig. 3.13). This pixel shifting due to the chemical makeup is called a chemical shift artifact (Soila et al. 1984; Dwyer et al. 1985). The extent of misregistration of fat and water depends on the range of frequencies that can be assigned to spatial location (bandwidth). Low bandwidth imaging results in large degree of chemical shift artifacts. While higher bandwidth imaging will reduce chemical shift artifacts, low bandwidth imaging gives higher signal to noise and better image quality. Chemical shift artifacts increase with increasing field strength.

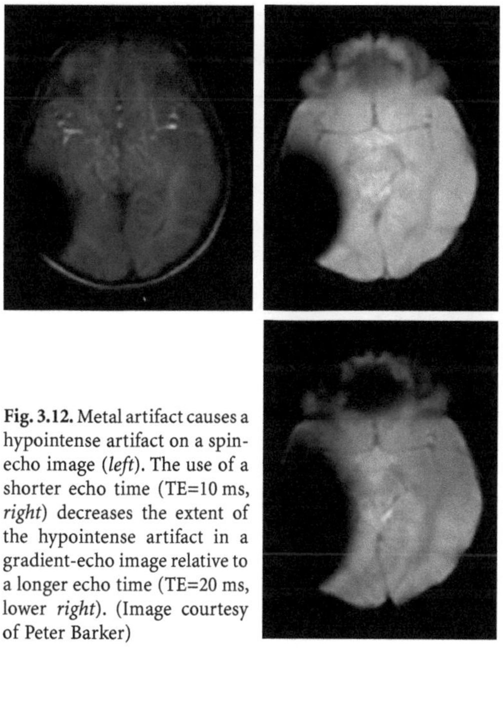

Fig. 3.12. Metal artifact causes a hypointense artifact on a spin-echo image (*left*). The use of a shorter echo time (TE=10 ms, *right*) decreases the extent of the hypointense artifact in a gradient-echo image relative to a longer echo time (TE=20 ms, lower *right*). (Image courtesy of Peter Barker)

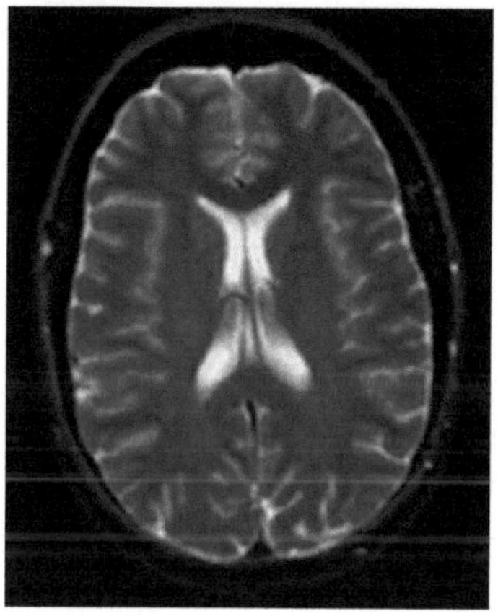

Fig. 3.13. A chemical shift artifact causes fat signal in the scalp to be mapped onto the posterior aspect of the brain in this low-bandwidth T2-weighted image. (Image courtesy of Peter Barker)

3.5.3 Motion Artifacts

Movement due to patient motion or pulsatile motion such as from blood and CSF can become mismapped which leads to artifacts in the image. Ghosting artifacts are seen in the phase encode direction due to periodic motion such as due to blood flow (Wood and Henkelman 1985). Image blurring occurs due to random motion from signal cancellation (Fig. 3.14).

Artifacts due to patient motion are minimized by immobilizing the patient. Gating to the cardiac cycle or respiratory cycle is used to minimize artifacts due to the heart beating or the patient breathing, respectively. Alternately, respiratory motion can be reduced by suspending respiration or performing a breath-hold (Paling and Brookeman 1986).

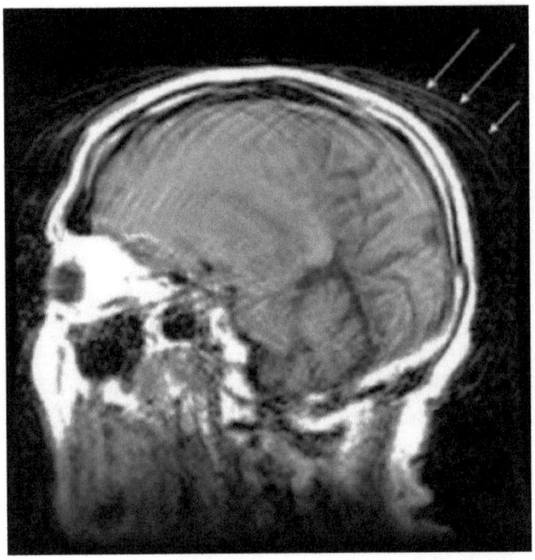

Fig. 3.14. The inability of a patient to remain still during a scan results in image blurring within the brain as well as ghosting artifacts (*arrows*) outside the head. (Image courtesy of Peter Barker)

One method for reducing the effect of motion artifacts due to blood flow into the imaging slice is to suppress the inflowing blood with spatial presaturation pulses. Spatially selective RF pulses in the regions adjacent to the imaging plane are used to saturate the unwanted inflowing blood.

Gradient moment nulling or flow compensation is used to compensate for phase shifts that occur due to motion during the application of the gradients (Dwyer et al. 1985; Haacke and Lenz 1987; Elster 1988; Ehman and Felmlee 1990). Typically additional pulses in the slice select and frequency encoding waveforms are incorporated. These pulses are equal but opposite in amplitude. Thus, motion of a constant velocity that would normally accumulate a net phase is rephased. The additional gradient pulses increase the TE, but can be a very effective method in gradient-echo pulse sequences of reducing CSF flow effects.

3.5.4 Wrap-Around Artifacts

Wrap-around artifact or aliasing (Fig. 3.15) occurs when a portion of the anatomy outside the field a view appears in the reconstructed image (Bellon et al. 1986; Pusey et al. 1988). Aliasing is purely a digitization phenomena that occurs when spatial locations outside the field of view are detected and than reconstructed as wrapped data in the image. Aliasing in the read direction may be prevented by increasing the field of view. The use of surface coils to prevent excitation of spins outside the field of view or spatial saturation (Edelman et al. 1988) to reduce signal from outside the field of view can also offer a method to minimize aliasing. Another method for minimizing or eliminating aliasing artifacts is to oversample the signal by increasing the number of phase encoding steps. However, more imaging time will be required if more phase encoding steps are obtained.

3.6 Gadolinium Contrast Studies

Gadolinium-based contrast agents, such as gadolinium diethylene triamine pentaacetic acid (Gd-DTPA) (Weinmann et al. 1984), belong to the class of paramagnetic contrast agents. Paramagnetic contrast agents contain unpaired electrons. When these exogenous paramagnetic agents are injected intravenously, the interaction of the unpaired electrons with the precessing nuclei increased the relaxation rate of the neighboring protons or tissue water. The effect of these paramagnetic agents is to shorten T1 and T2 relaxation. At low doses, gadolinium-based

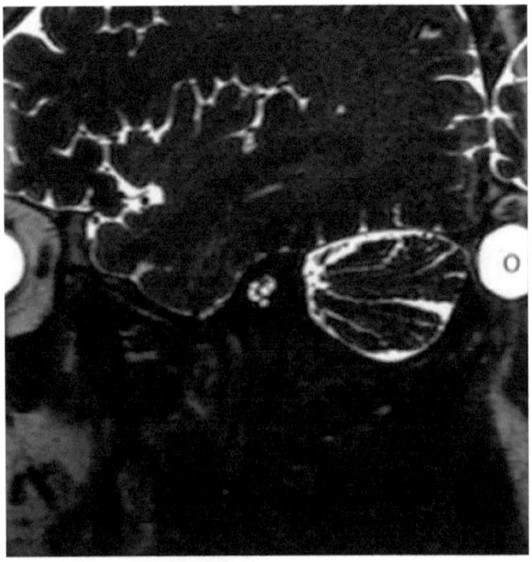

Fig. 3.15. Aliasing or wrap-around artifact occurred in this image when too small a field of view was chosen. Notice the fold-over artifact on the *right-hand side* of the image (letter *O* on eye). (Image courtesy of Peter Barker)

contrast agents exert their effects by primarily altering T1, which leads to an increase signal intensity in perfused tissues. At higher concentrations, the effect is primarily on T2 and leads to a signal loss or hypointense artifact when the contrast agent is present. Tissues that uptake gadolinium-based contrast agents appear darker on T2-weighted images.

First pass perfusion of bolus administration of gadolinium-based contrast agents leads to regional signal intensity changes that are related to tissue hemodynamics. Unlike conventional X-ray contrast agents where the concentration of the contrast agent directly affects the signal intensity, the gadolinium-based MR contrast agents exert their effects on the local protons or water. In the normal brain, due to the blood–brain barrier, the contrast agent is retained within the cerebral vascular. However, water from the blood pool that has experienced shortening of T1 and T2 due to the presence of the contrast agent may diffuse into to the surrounding extracellular space. If the blood–brain barrier is damaged, then the agents can leak out into the brain parenchyma. Thus, MR contrast kinetics can become quite complex.

Typically, the dosages of gadolinium-based contrast agents are chosen such that there is a linear relationship between contrast concentration and changes in T1 or T2 relaxation. In addition, tracer kinetic theory is applied during the first pass of the contrast agent through the brain to minimize any confounding effects of water diffusion. In perfusion imaging of the brain, T_2-weighted images are often obtained during the first transit or passage of the contrast agent bolus through the brain. As the contrast agent transits the brain vasculature, T_2^* effects predominate resulting in a negative signal intensity in perfused tissues (Fig. 3.16). By evaluating the concentration versus time curves of the first pass of the contrast bolus, regional cerebral blood volume can be estimated as the area under the curve (Rosen et al. 1991). Moreover, if the arterial input function is know, then other quantities such as mean transit time (MTT) and regional cerebral blood flow (rCBF) can be estimated. Other parameters such as contrast arrival time can also be evaluated from these curves.

Several gadolinium-based contrast agents that have a larger molecular structure either by the formation of dendrimers or binding to macromolecules such as albumin are under investigation for use in magnetic resonance angiography (MRA). Due to the large size of these agents, they cannot diffuse from the vascular space and thus remain intravascular.

Increases in vascularity and permeability as may occur in tumors as well as edema which may occur secondary to an ischemic event or with certain pathologies often results in an increased signal intensity of T1-weighted images.

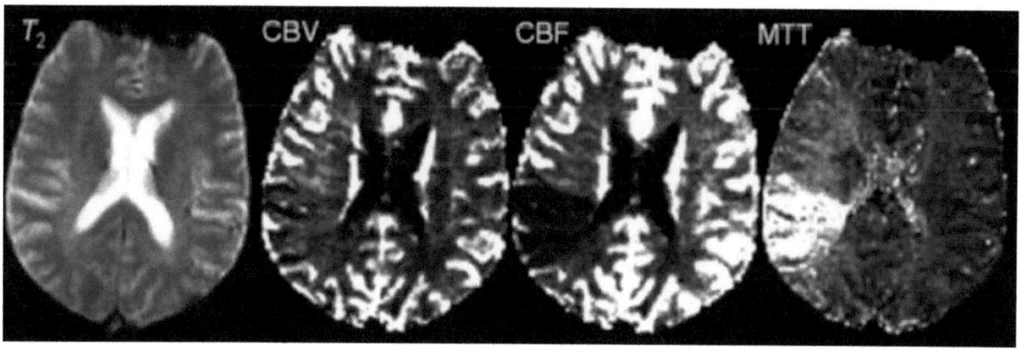

Fig. 3.16. Cerebral perfusion parameters can be estimated from analysis of the first passage of a contrast agent through the brain in a stroke patient. A single T2-weighted image (*left*) from a series of 100 images that were collected as the contrast bolus traverses the brain is shown. Parameters such as cerebral blood volume (*CBV*), cerebral blood flow (*CBF*), and mean transit time (*MTT*) can be calculated from the series of first pass images. In order to achieve a high temporal resolution of the scan, spatial resolution is decreased which results in poor image quality and image distortion. (Images courtesy of Mark A. Horsfield)

References

Atlas SW, Grossman RI, Hackney DB, Goldberg HI, Bilaniuk LT, Zimmerman RA (1988) STIR MR imaging of the orbit. AJR Am J Roentgenol 151:1025–1030

Bellon EM, Haacke EM, Coleman PE, Sacco DC, Steiger DA, Gangarosa RE (1986) MR artifacts: a review. Am J Roentgenol 147:1271–1281

Bulte JW, Zhang S, van Gelderen P, Herynek V, Jordan EK, Duncan ID, Frank JA (1999) Neurotransplantation of magnetically labeled oligodendrocyte progenitors: magnetic resonance tracking of cell migration and myelination. Proc Natl Acad Sci U S A 96:15256–15261

De Coene B, Hajnal JV, Gatehouse P, Longmore DB, White SJ, Oatridge A, Pennock JM, Young IR, Bydder GM (1992) MR of the brain using fluid-attenuated inversion recovery (FLAIR) pulse sequences. Am J Neuroradiol 13:1555–1564

Dwyer AJ, Knop RH, Hoult DI (1985) Frequency shift artifacts in MR imaging. J Comput Assist Tomogr 9:16–18

Edelman RR, Atkinson DJ, Silver MS, Loaiza FL, Warren WS (1988) FRODO pulse sequences: a new means of eliminating motion, flow, and wraparound artifacts. Radiology 166:231–236

Ehman RL, Felmlee JP (1990) Flow artifact reduction in MRI: a review of the roles of gradient moment nulling and spatial presaturation. Magn Reson Med 14:293–307

Elster AD (1988) Motion artifact suppression technique (MAST) for cranial MR imaging: superiority over cardiac gating for reducing phase-shift artifacts. AJNR Am J Neuroradiol 9:671–674

Frahm J, Haase A, Matthaei D (1986) Rapid NMR imaging of dynamic processes using the FLASH technique. Magn Reson Med 3:321–327

Haacke EM, Lenz GW (1987) Improving MR image quality in the presence of motion by using rephasing gradients. AJR Am J Roentgenol 148:1251–1258

Hajnal JV, Bryant DJ, Kasuboski L, Pattany PM, De Coene B, Lewis PD, Pennock JM, Oatridge A, Young IR, Bydder GM, Gatehouse P, Longmore DB, White SJ (1992) Use of fluid attenuated inversion recovery (FLAIR) pulse sequences in MRI of the brain. J Comput Assist Tomogr 16:841–844

Heindel W, Friedmann G, Bunke J, Thomas B, Firsching R, Ernestus RI (1986) Artifacts in MR imaging after surgical intervention. J Comput Assist Tomogr 10:596–599

Laakman RW, Kaufman B, Han JS, Nelson AD, Clampitt M, O'Block AM, Haaga JR, Alfidi RJ (1985) MR imaging in patients with metallic implants. Radiology 157:711–714

Paling MR, Brookeman JR (1986) Respiration artifacts in MR imaging: reduction by breath holding. J Comput Assist Tomogr 10:1080–1082

Pusey E, Yoon C, Anselmo ML, Lufkin RB, Stark DD, Brown R, Leikind B, Hanafee WN, Brown RK, Solomon MA, Tarr RW (1988) Aliasing artifacts in MR imaging. Comput Med Imaging Graph 12:219–224

Rosen BR, Belliveau JW, Buchbinder BR, McKinstry RC, Porkka LM, Kennedy DN, Neuder MS, Fisel CR, Aronen HJ, Kwong KK (1991) Contrast agents and cerebral hemodynamics. Magn Reson med 19:285–292

Sacco DC, Steiger DA, Bellon EM, Coleman PE, Haacke EM, Gangarosa RE (1987) Artifacts caused by cosmetics in MR imaging of the head. Am J Roentgenol 148:1001–1004

Shellock FG (2001) Metallic neurosurgical implants: evaluation of magnetic field interactions, heating, and artifacts at 1.5-Tesla. J Magn Reson Imaging 14:295–299

Soila KP, Viamonte M, Jr., Starewicz PM (1984) Chemical shift misregistration effect in magnetic resonance imaging. Radiology 153:819–820

Wehrli FW, MacFall JR, Glover GH, Grigsby N, Haughton V, Johanson J (1984) The dependence of nuclear magnetic resonance (NMR) image contrast on intrinsic and pulse sequence timing parameters. Magn Reson Imaging 2:3–16

Weinmann H, Brasch R, Press W, Wesbey G (1984) Characteristics of gadolinium-DTPA complex: a potential NMR contrast agent. AJR 142: 619–624

Wood ML, Henkelman RM (1985) MR image artifacts from periodic motion. Med Phys 12:143–151

Young IR, Bailes DR, Bydder GM (1985) Apparent changes of appearance of inversion-recovery images. Magn Reson Med 2:81–85

4 Fast Imaging with an Introduction to k-Space

Joseph C. McGowan

CONTENTS

4.1 Introduction

The quest for speed in diagnostic imaging is understandable from all perspectives. The physician desires a "snapshot" of the anatomy or process in question and is concerned about the effect of physiologic motion on the examination. Repetition of the examination is often indicated when the process to be investigated is dynamic. The patient may be limited in ability to remain still, or may be uncomfortable during the imaging procedure. All participants desire a quick answer to the questions being addressed by the study. Finally, economic imperatives often favor a rapid exam.

It has always been possible to trade quality for speed, or vice versa, in magnetic resonance imaging. For example, repeating an exam and averaging the results is a classic method of improving the quality of some images. This method may fail, however, in the presence of some types of physiologic motion. Fortunately, much attention has been focused on methods to improve imaging speed while maintaining quality. Some improvements have been realized via advances in technology. Specifically, improvements in signal preservation, noise rejection and gradient performance have allowed optimization of existing techniques with maximal yield of usable signal. The most impressive improvements, however, have been realized by finding means of circumventing the physical limitations imposed by relaxation, some of which will be explained below.

Gradient-echo imaging may be thought of as the "original" fast scan technique. It was known that the inherent spin dephasing via T2 decay was a relatively longer process compared to the signal decay due to the imperfections of the magnet. When magnet technology improved, it was found that sufficient signal to reconstruct an image could be obtained without refocusing the spins. Gradient-echo imaging could not, however, replace all conventional spin-echo imaging as it did not produce "pure" T2-weighting. Gradient and spin-echo techniques can be thought of as bases for all fast imaging techniques. In fact, it will be shown that all current fast imaging techniques are in some way hybrid forms of these two. To begin, we will trace the development of fast spin-echo imaging.

The success of magnetic resonance imaging (MRI) as a diagnostic modality can be attributed to a number of factors, but prominent among them is that in many disease states the observed transverse relaxation time (T2) is altered. Thus, the most clinically useful results in MRI are obtained with so-called T2 weighted contrast, where the intensity of an individual picture element (pixel) in the image reflects the observed T2 of the tissue. For many years these studies were performed with the spin-warp pulse sequence, discussed in an earlier chapter. Briefly, in that sequence one chooses principally the repetition rate (TR) and the echo time (TE). Using relatively long TR and TE values, the signal intensity in regions with long T2 is higher, causing those regions to appear hyperintense on the resulting images. The TR must be long enough so that progressive saturation, which would contribute T1 contrast, is minimized to the degree necessary. The compromise, of course, is that the

J. C. McGowan, PhD
Associate Professor of Electrical Engineering, Dept. of Electrical Engineering, United States Naval Academy, Annapolis, MD 21405-5025, USA

exam time increases linearly with TR. It is possible to perform more rapid imaging using short TR conventional spin-echo or gradient-echo sequences, but pure T2 contrast cannot be obtained. It should also be noted that the conventional spin-echo sequence is relatively inefficient in terms of data acquisition, because the majority of the time spent imaging is actually spent waiting for the decay of longitudinal magnetization.

The resolution to the quandary posed above was found in a pulse sequence that preserved the long time between excitations (TR) but made use of the "dead time" to acquire more data with which to construct an image. These data, taken together, constitute the "k-space" representation of the image. A basic understanding of this concept is easily gained and clearly illustrates the evolution from conventional to fast spin-echo imaging. Images obtained with fast spin-echo (FSE, also called RARE and turbo spin-echo) techniques are now the most clinically essential. The ability to interpret and manipulate the contrast obtained with FSE is requisite to effective exploitation of the diagnostic capability.

In earlier chapters the development of gradient-echo imaging was attributed in part to the advances in magnet and signal-processing technology that made it possible to obtain images without spin-echoes. In a similar manner, an ultra fast gradient-echo technique dubbed echo-planar imaging followed further technological developments. This again constituted a means of using most of the scan time to acquire data rather than wait for relaxation. It was also recognized that the spin- and gradient-echo techniques could be combined in a variety of methods that offer opportunities to optimize the trade-offs between speed and quality.

4.2 k-Space

During MRI or any imaging examination, data is collected for future display. The display can be visualized as a collection of numbers corresponding to brightness (or gray scale) arranged in a (typically) square array or matrix. A possible approach in imaging is to acquire an individual point of data representing some feature of anatomy or function and to use that data value to fill in the intensity on the image matrix. Clearly, conventional X-ray imaging works in this way, even as all of the points are acquired simultaneously. If, for example, a problem with the X-ray film caused only half of the image locations to be obtained, the part of the image that was obtained would be perfect and indistinguishable from the corresponding part of a control image. Mathematically, it is said that there is a one-to-one correspondence between individual data points and spatial locations. It might be surprising to know that in magnetic resonance imaging, although it still true that the number of data points is equal to the number of image locations (picture elements, pixels), there is not a one-to-one correspondence. Rather, each data point that is acquired influences the entire image in some way. The image cannot be fully reconstructed (formed) without all of the data. Further, a mathematical process called the Fourier transform must be employed to translate the data into an image. Figure 4.1 is a diagram of this process in a "black box" sense.

Consider any MR image. If one wanted to send a perfect description of that image to a colleague, it would be possible to write down each pixel intensity on a gray scale from 0-256, agree in which order the numbers would be sent, and proceed to transfer the

a

b

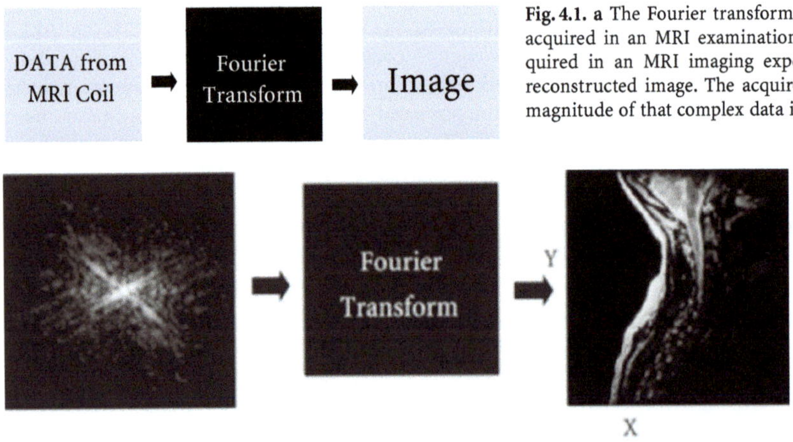

Fig. 4.1. **a** The Fourier transform is used to process the data acquired in an MRI examination into an image. **b** Data acquired in an MRI imaging experiment is shown with the reconstructed image. The acquired data is complex and the magnitude of that complex data is shown

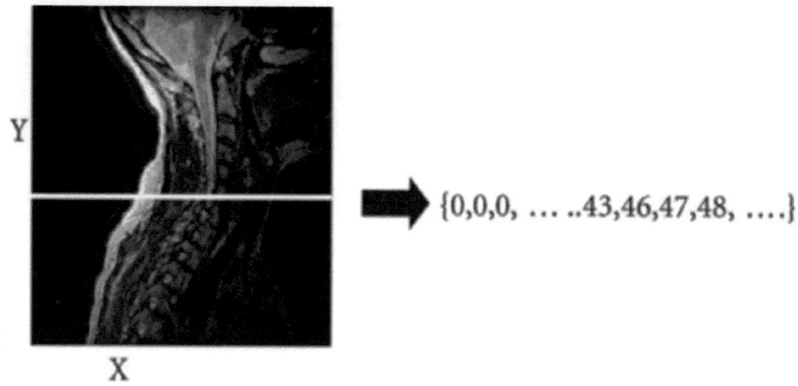

Fig. 4.2. An image is a matrix of gray scale values, or intensities

numbers one at a time. The colleague could receive the numbers, reassemble the image into a matrix form (Fig. 4.2), and then display them as the gray scale equivalent. Clearly, an image is nothing more or less than a matrix of gray scale values (Fig. 4.2). In “image space”, one can select a particular location and note the intensity. The coordinates in image space are simply the standard spatial coordinates in the image plane.

Similarly, the data collected in the MRI process is simply a list of numbers acquired over a length of time. During the examination, the voltages present in the RF coil are sampled and recorded by a computer. A voltage waveform of a particular frequency can be characterized by magnitude and phase and, typically, both parameters of the voltages are obtained using two radiofrequency channels. This is known as quadrature detection and results in data in so-called “complex” form. These data are assembled in what could be called the data matrix (Fig. 4.3). Each spin-echo can be recorded in this way as a collection of numbers including the approach to the echo as well as its decay. Successive spin-echoes with different strengths of phase encoding are recorded on their own line (Fig. 4.3c). Arranged in the data matrix (Fig. 4.3), the “locations” of individual data correspond to time, moving to the right with the progress of the spin-echo, and outward from the center with the integrated magnitude of the phase encoding gradient. Since the recording of the spin-echo is associated with the application of the “read” or frequency-encoding gradient, it is also correct to refer to the location with coordinates of integrated gradient magnitude. The center of the data matrix corresponds to zero gradient in both phase and frequency direction. It is the center, or peak, of the spin-echo acquired with zero phase encoding. Since stronger gradients contribute dephasing that in general lowers signal intensity, it is apparent that the center of the data matrix will have the largest intensity.

It may be seen at this point that the data matrix under discussion is no other than “k-space”, and that k-space is in some way an inverted form of image space. The coordinates of k-space can be thought of as times. The coordinates of image space are spatial in nature, but the gradients serve to establish a correspondence between frequency (or phase) and position. Thus, the coordinates of image space can be thought of as having units of frequency. It is useful to note that the k-space matrix is theoretically symmetric. Clearly, the ideal spin-echo is identical in build-up and decay, yielding, in conventional coordinates, the left-right symmetry of the matrix. Additionally, the magnitude of dephasing due to a phase encode gradient does not depend on the sign (direction) of the gradient. Thus, applying a “positive one unit” of phase encoding is theoretically identical to applying a “negative one unit”, and thus the matrix is symmetric top to bottom. This two-dimensional symmetry is exploited in some techniques that shorten acquisition time by acquiring only a part of the actual matrix and filling in missing data.

The Fourier transform, introduced above as a “black box” that changes the data matrix to the image, can be described in a number of ways. Fourier theory holds that any function in time (the signal, the spin-echo) can be exactly described as the sum of sinusoidal functions. The individual sinusoids (of particular frequency) constitute the frequency components of the signal (Fig. 4.4) and the Fourier transform is simply a mathematical tool used to convert one to the other. Thus, in terms of signal processing, the Fourier transform serves to relate the time domain representation of a signal to its frequency domain equivalent. The theory can be extended to more than one dimension. In two-dimensional (2D) MRI, the 2D Fourier

Fig. 4.3. **a** Intensity values represent signal strength at a point in time. A horizontal line in the data matrix represents a single spin-echo, with the center corresponding to the peak of the echo. **b** The spin-echo corresponding to the indicated line in the data matrix. **c** Different phase encode values correspond to different horizontal lines of the data matrix. The center in the vertical direction corresponds to the line obtained with zero phase encoding

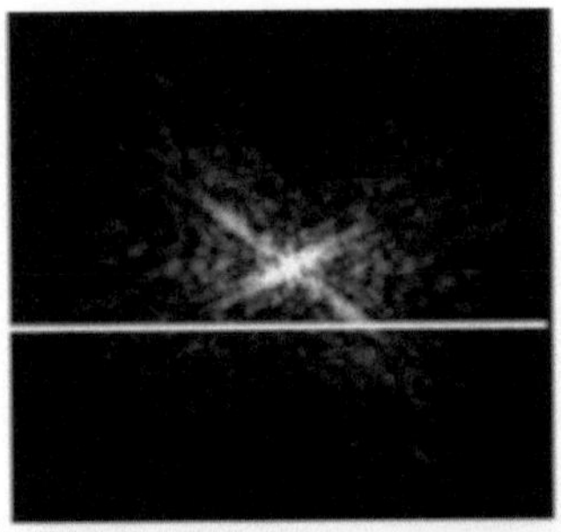

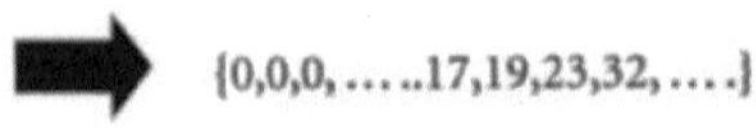

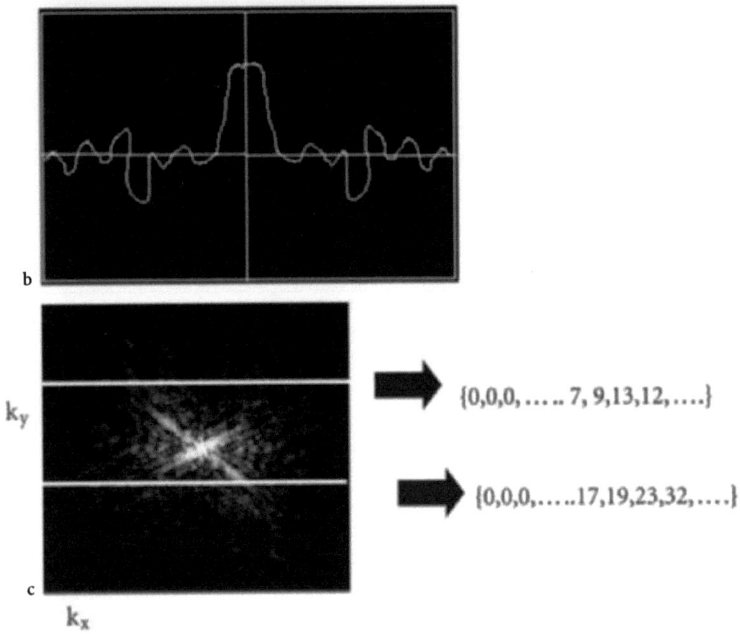

transform serves to translate k-space to image space. The mechanics of doing so are handled quite efficiently and rapidly by modern computers.

A pulse sequence for MRI can be thought of as a scheme for "covering" k-space, that is, for acquiring data such that all point of k-space are known. The spin-warp sequence is perhaps easiest to understand as each horizontal line of k-space is completely filled by the acquisition of one spin-echo. Successive spin-echoes with different phase encode values constitute the remaining lines and fill the matrix. When k-space is filled, the Fourier transform (albeit in two dimensions) of that matrix will directly yield the image (Fig. 4.5).

The k-coordinate, establishing the location in the k-space matrix, can be defined for constant gradients as:

$$k = \frac{\gamma G(t)}{2\pi} \tag{1}$$

where G is gradient strength as a function of time, γ is the gyromagnetic ratio, and t is the time of gradient application (Fig. 4.6). The read gradient controls k_x and is turned on in conjunction with the collection of data. With the passage of time, Eq. (1) can be continuously evaluated as the k coordinate increases linearly. Similar "motion" in k space is associated with all gradient manipulations in the pulse sequence.

The k-space matrix can be filled line-by-line, as has been described above, or via less conventional means, including as a spiral outward from the center, simply by varying the application of gradients. As noted, application of a constant read gradient in the absence of a phase encode gradient is equivalent to moving to the right with time in the k-space matrix. Application of a constant phase encode gradient along with the read gradient would provide a diagonal motion. To move back to the left one would apply a negative read gradient. Curved paths would be real-

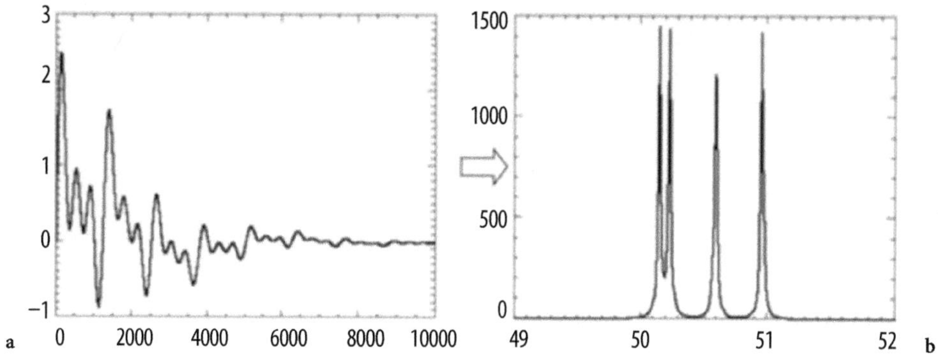

Fig. 4.4a,b. Time-domain and frequency domain plots are related by the Fourier transform. Fourier theory holds that any function may be represented by adding up a series of sin and cos functions. In MRI, the function is the echo, a complicated sum of components at different frequencies corresponding to the different spatial positions from which the signal is obtained. The echo is obtained in the time domain and depicted in (**a**), the time-domain plot. Recall that frequency encoding gradients establish a correspondence between frequency and spatial position. Extracting the signal that corresponds to a particular frequency is equivalent to isolating the signal from a particular position. In (**b**), the frequency-domain plot, the frequency components can be identified by frequency and magnitude. It is difficult to discern these individual behaviors from the time-domain depiction

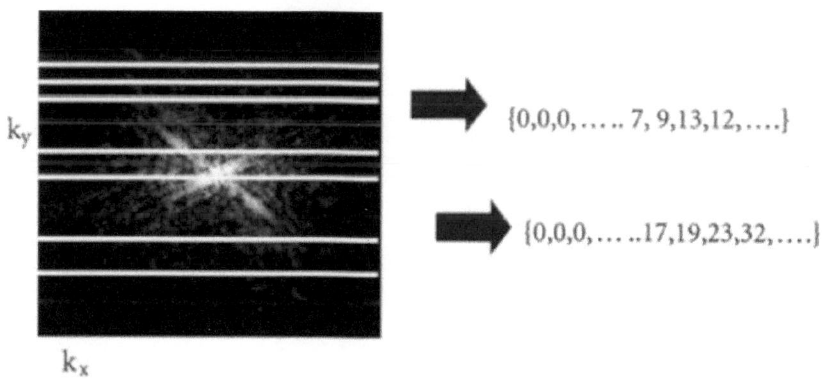

Fig. 4.5. When all echoes associated with all values of the phase encode gradient are acquired, k-space is covered and an image can be reconstructed. K-space can be covered by a variety of trajectories. A single echo in a spin-warp imaging sequence can be visualized as starting on the left edge of k-space and moving to the right edge

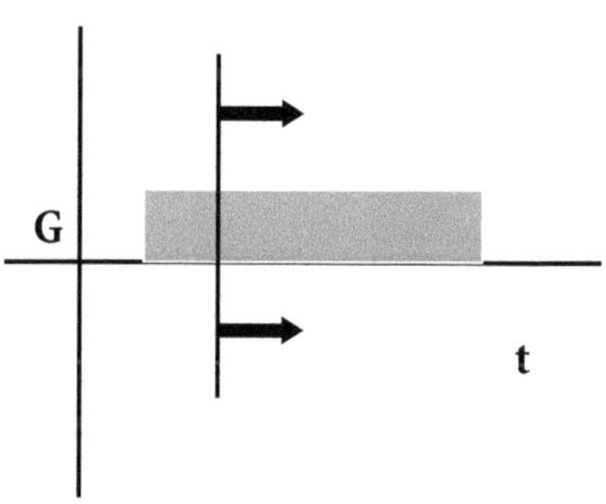

Fig. 4.6. The k-coordinate is proportional to the area under the gradient-time curve

ized by more complex time-varying gradients. Some of these are desirable from the standpoint of accurate and physically realizable fast gradient switching. That is, one may choose a k-space trajectory based upon the physical limitations of the gradient amplifiers. The original echo-planar implementation (discussed below) is based upon applying to the gradient amplifiers the most basic waveform possible, a sinusoid. Curved trajectories may be less intuitive than the visualization of individual spin-echoes, but from the standpoint of the cumulative gradient effect they are relatively straightforward to interpret. The complicated k-space trajectories that are employed by modern pulse sequences, and indeed any k-space trajectories, can be created by controlling the gradients in this manner.

The contribution to the final image of specific data points may not be intuitively obvious, because the form of the final image is not discernible from the appearance of the k-space matrix. However, the effect of a single data point on the entire image can be estimated and simulated. The nature of that effect is related to the position of the data point in the k-space matrix. The implications of this observation are profound and essential to the understanding of artifact as well as to the proper prescription of the imaging study. For example, an artifact featuring parallel stripes or a herringbone pattern may be seen on an image when a "pop" of static electricity is recorded during image data collection, and where only one or two points are abnormally high values. The orientation and number of the stripes are functions of the location of the bad point(s) in k-space (Fig. 4.7). This arises from the fact that each data point can be associated with a sinusoidal function that is part of the Fourier representation of the data, where the fre-

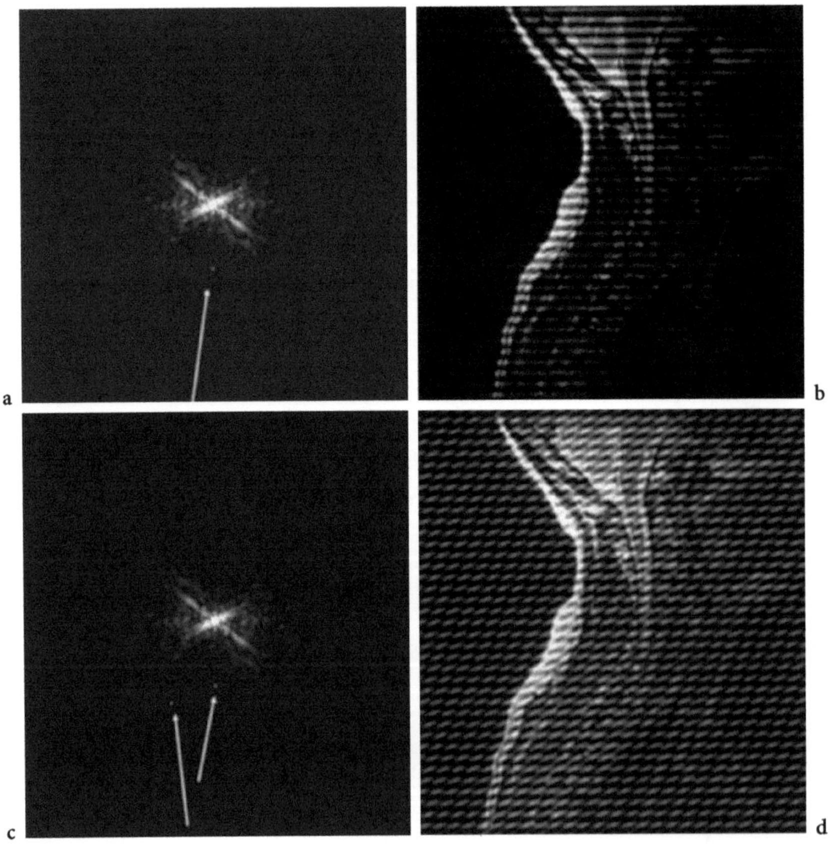

Fig. 4.7a–d. Striping (**a,b**) and Herringbone (**c,d**) artifacts result from a few "bad", that is, abnormally high values in the MRI acquisition. The number and orientation of stripes are determined by the position of the bad points (*arrows*) in k-space

quency of the sinusoid (striping function) is higher for larger values of the k-coordinate.

An accurate and simple generalization is that the central area of k-space contributes primarily to image contrast while the peripheral area of k-space contributes primarily to the definition of edges. This can be illustrated by the simulated reconstruction of an image using only a portion of the data, with the remaining data points set to zero. As can be seen in Fig. 4.8, a reconstruction using only 6% of the original data points results in a blurry yet interpretable image that would in some cases be diagnostic. Omitting the center data points yields an image that shows only edges (Fig. 4.8c). These observations give rise to some techniques for rapid image acquisition (for example, so-called keyhole imaging where outer points are "reused" in subsequent images).

To summarize, the signal is acquired over time by sampling the voltage present in the radiofrequency coil. The frequency content of that signal reflects the encoding of the gradients, which establish a correspondence between frequency and spatial position. The Fourier transform is employed to convert the time-domain signal into the frequency domain information that is decoded into spatial position.

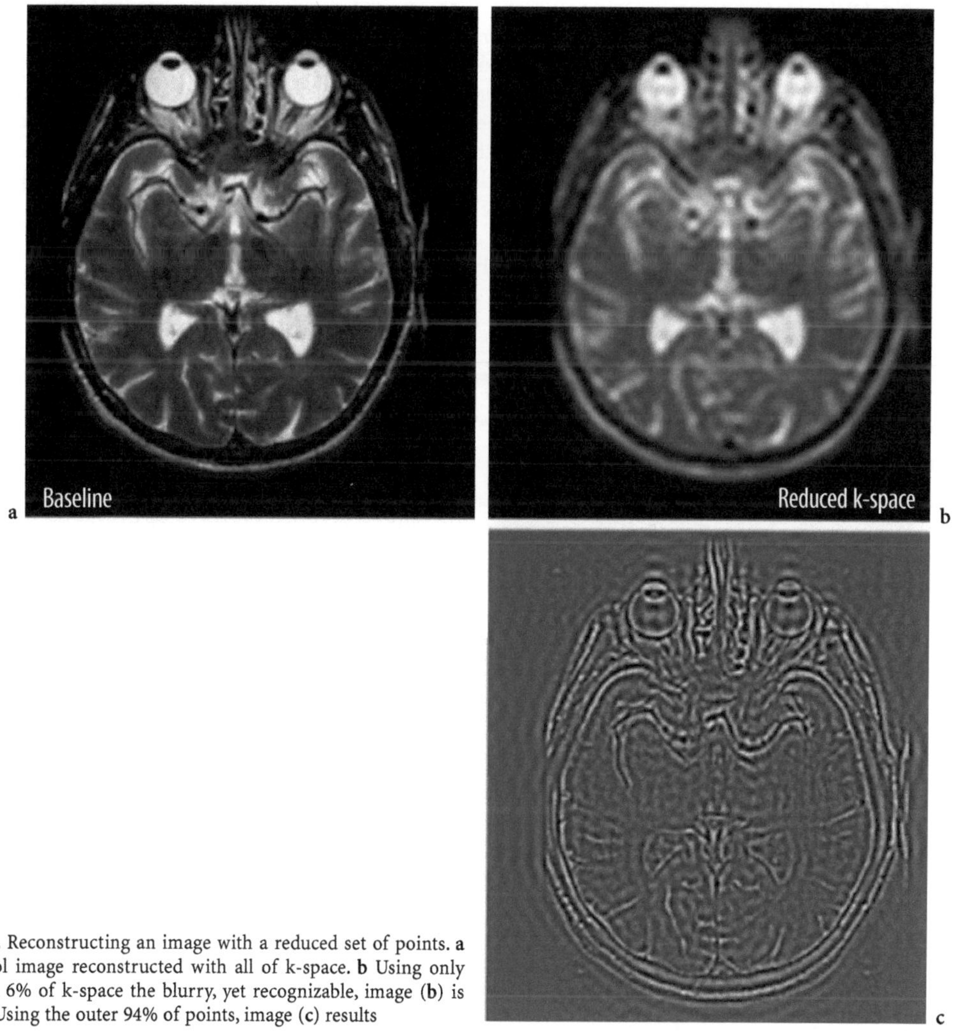

Fig. 4.8a–c. Reconstructing an image with a reduced set of points. **a** The control image reconstructed with all of k-space. **b** Using only the central 6% of k-space the blurry, yet recognizable, image (**b**) is formed. **c** Using the outer 94% of points, image (**c**) results

4.3 Spin-Echo Acquisition with Multiple Echoes

Recall that conventional spin-echo imaging can be used to obtain T2-weighted diagnostic images. A long repetition time (TR) must be used to allow for the recovery of longitudinal magnetization and to avoid T1 weighting. Proton density images are typically obtained in these studies because they come "free", that is, without any time penalty. Specifically, the time spent collecting the data to acquire proton density images is completely contained within the time spent waiting for T1 decay. A slight extension of this technique gives the general "multiple spin-echo" acquisition, as discussed in Chap. 3 and diagrammed in Fig. 4.9. In this technique, the spin magnetizations are repeatedly refocused by successive inversion pulses. In the example four echoes are produced but more or fewer are possible. During each TR period, multiple lines of k-space data are acquired, one for each spin-echo that is formed. Each of these echoes is associated with the same phase-encode gradient, but they differ in echo time (TE). Thus, in each of the k-space matrices that correspond to specific echo times, the same line is filled in during the TR. The k-space data are used to build up k-space matrices for each of the images as diagrammed in Fig. 4.9b. At the end of the acquisition there is enough information to reconstruct images for each of the TEs for which echoes were collected. A single completion of the acquisition sequence yields data for four images, and the time taken is the same as that required to collect data for the single longest image. This technique thus improves the efficiency of image data collection by yielding multiple images in the same time that would be required to obtain one. However, greater than two multiple spin-echo images, for example, series with TE values of 30, 60, 90, and 120 ms, have not typically been found to be clinically useful. The images that are most valuable are typically the long-TE (T2-weighted) images and perhaps the very short TE (or proton-density weighted) images. Standard imaging protocols for many years included proton-density images whenever T2-weighted images were obtained, even though they might have been considered of limited utility. These images were considered "free" in that no time was added to the study to obtain them.

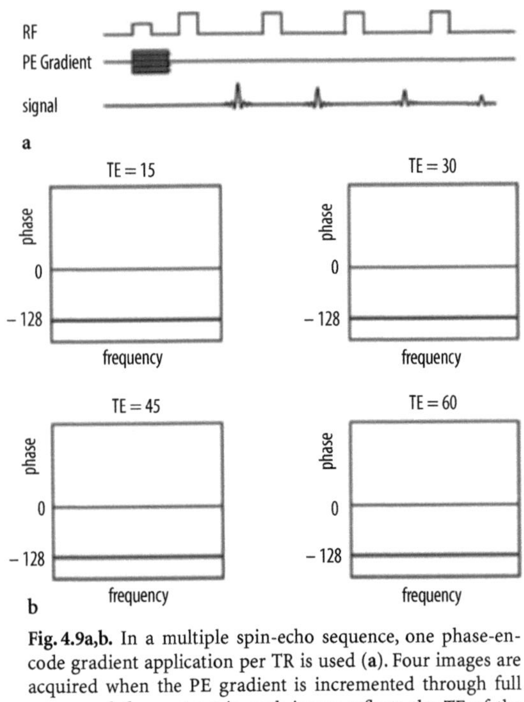

Fig. 4.9a,b. In a multiple spin-echo sequence, one phase-encode gradient application per TR is used (**a**). Four images are acquired when the PE gradient is incremented through full range, and the contrast in each image reflects the TE of the echo associated with that image. K-space maps are shown in (**b**) for the first TR period

4.4 Fast Spin-Echo

Fast spin-echo imaging (originally called RARE, rapid acquisition with relaxation enhancement and also "turbo spin-echo"; Hennig and Friedburg 1986) was introduced to exploit the "available" time in the TR period and to apply this time to the acquisition of a single image rather than acquisition of many images. In principle, the idea is to take a multiple echo sequence as illustrated above, and instead of writing the four lines of k-space in four separate k-space matrices, to use them all in a single k-space matrix, which thus is filled four times faster. In order to accomplish this the phase encoding must vary between each of the echoes – otherwise the four lines of k-space will occupy the same points.

Clearly, the difficulty with this idea is that the four echoes yielding data have different values of TE. In fact, in FSE imaging the k-space matrix is filled with lines representing echoes that differ widely in TE. To understand how this is possible one must recall that only a small portion of k-space determines the contrast in the image, and that the contrast is the parameter that is expected to change most dramatically between echoes with different TE values. On the other hand, if the subject is stationary, one does not expect the edge information to change. Thus, in FSE imaging there is not defined a single TE but rather an effective TE. The effective TE is the TE corresponding to the information obtained with low values of the phase encode (PE) gradient. Equivalently, the effective TE is the TE of the echoes where the dephasing due to the PE gradient is minimal, giving the higher intensity, central part of k-space. The decision regarding which echo to use for the contrast information is made automatically as part of the prescription of the pulse sequence when the effective TE is chosen.

Consider FSE acquisition with four echoes. The rf excitation part of the pulse sequence is essentially identical to the four-echo multiple spin-echo sequence discussed above. The essential difference between the sequences is in the phase encoding gradient, applied before every echo. In each TR period, four lines of k-space are filled in the same image. An example is depicted in Fig. 4.10. Note in the example that the overall signal intensity increases over the TR period, that is, that the strongest echo is the last one. That may be counter-intuitive given that T2 decay (dephasing) progresses during TR, an effect that contributes to loss of signal over time. Pure T2 decay is indeed present and is irreversible but it is relatively slow on the time scale of interest. In contrast a largely reversible dephasing is contributed by field gradients, and it is this type of dephasing, specifically that of the phase encode gradient, that dominates the overall strength of successive spin-echoes in FSE imaging. Smaller values of PE gradient contribute less dephasing and thus result in stronger signals. In the example of Fig. 4.10 the value of the PE gradient decreases with successive echoes and thus the signal strength increases. In viewing this example, recall that negative gradient application can be used to decrease the overall integrated magnitude of any gradient. For completeness we note that $T2^*$ decay, the observed signal decay during the echo, includes magnet inhomogeneities that make up most of the observed dephasing of the individual spin-echo. This dephasing is to a large degree reversible and is in fact reversed when each spin-echo is formed.

Fast spin-echo can be employed with as many echoes as desired, as long as the signal is sufficient at the end of the sequence to allow collection of data. The number of echoes collected in each TR period is known as the echo train length (ETL) and represents the factor by which the total image acquisition time is divided. Equivalently, it is the factor by which the exam is speeded up. Repetition time (TR) is defined as in any pulse sequence and effective TE is defined as noted above. Echo spacing is defined as the time between successive echoes and any of these factors are determined by the other three. A useful relationship is:

$$T_a = TR * \frac{\# PE}{ETL} \qquad (2)$$

where Ta is the acquisition time, #PE is the number of phase encode steps and ETL is echo train length.

FSE imaging is now routine clinical practice and produces diagnostic quality T2-weighted images in brain and spine (Fig. 4.11). The choice of ETL and other timing parameters is made with consideration of local equipment and constraints. Typically the

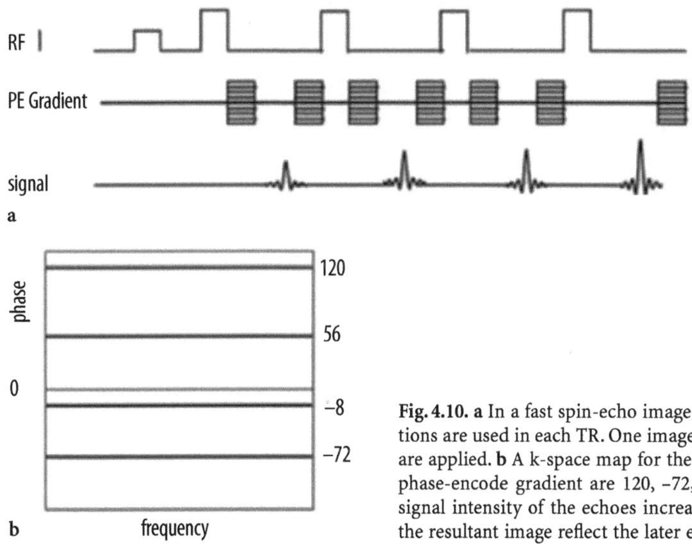

Fig. 4.10. a In a fast spin-echo image, multiple phase encode gradient applications are used in each TR. One image is acquired after all phase-encode values are applied. **b** A k-space map for the first TR is shown. Here, the values of the phase-encode gradient are 120, –72, 56, –8. Ordering in this way makes the signal intensity of the echoes increase during TR, and makes the contrast of the resultant image reflect the later echo

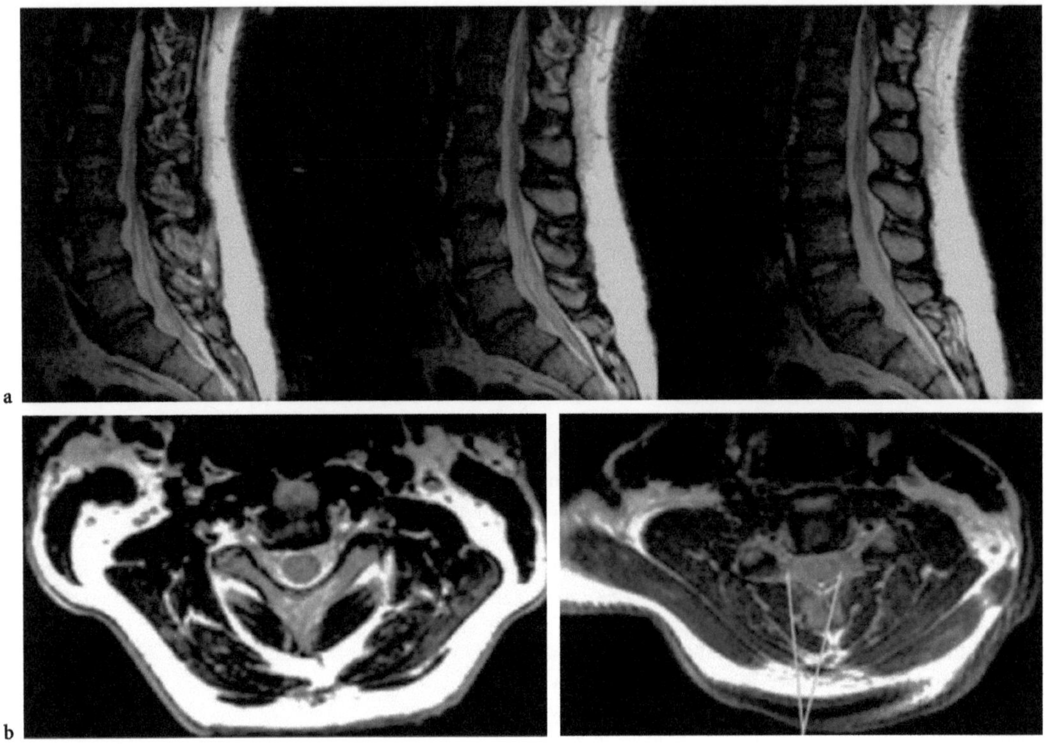

Fig. 4.11a,b. Spine FSE imaging with near-isotropic voxels (a) at 1.5 mm resolution and (b) demonstrating excellent resolution of nerve roots

quality of images obtained at any individual center will dictate the ETL, made, all else equal, as large as possible.

The ultimate extension of FSE is single-shot FSE (SSFSE), whereby the entirety of k-space is filled in following a single initial excitation ($\pi/2$) rf pulse. This pulse sequence actually has no TR value, since there is no repetition, but may require only tens of seconds. In current implementation the symmetry of k-space is exploited in SSFSE, with slightly more than half of the phase encode values sufficing to fill in the data matrix. The resulting images are of lower quality than generally expected for diagnostic images, but are highly useful for "go/no go" evaluation of certain lesions and particularly in patients whose ability to remain still is limited. As shown in Fig. 4.12, SSFSE was employed to produce a diagnostic image in an uncooperative patient where conventional SE and even FSE were simply too slow. Single-shot FSE in brain may not typically provide the quality needed by clinicians for routine evaluation, but continued improvements in scanner technology and signal processing should result in standard protocols featuring this technique.

4.5 Image Quality and Artifacts

A reasonable concern is the extent to which FSE images are equivalent to those acquired with conventional spin-echo techniques. Clearly, to make this comparison the images must be acquired with the FSE effective TE values equal to the conventional TE values. That being assumed, FSE images are in fact used like the conventional spin-echo images that they were designed to replace. However, some differences do arise from a number of physical factors. First, the signals that fill k-space do originate from spin-echoes with different values of TE, and the effects of pure T2 decay make those echoes different. In the case of FSE with the longest echoes assigned to the low phase encode values, the effect is minimized because the strongest echoes (low phase encoding) will be the least affected by T2 decay during the TR period. Thus, in FSE images with long effective TE, the image quality is highest because the high phase encode acquisitions, which are characterized by maximal dephasing and lowest signal strength, occur early in

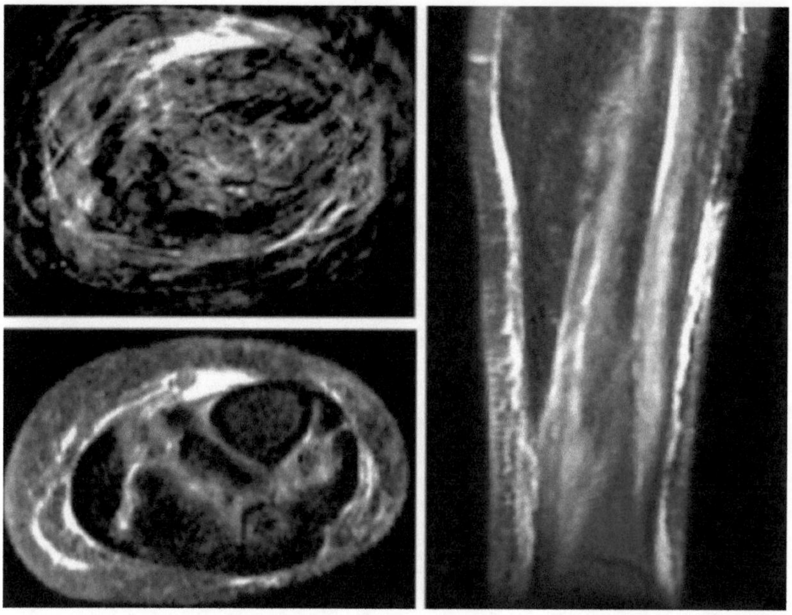

a

b

c

Fig. 4.12a–c. FSE (TR 4000 ms ETL 8) imaging was unsuccessful in an uncooperative patient (**a**). SSFSE with 19-s acquisition time (6-mm slices, TE 97) was diagnostic (**b,c**)

the T2 process. These acquisitions provide the high spatial frequency edge information. In the alternate scenario, PD-weighted FSE, the higher phase encode acquisitions must be assigned to the later echoes. If signal strength is insufficient at this point in the sequence, the information from those echoes will be contaminated or dominated by noise, disrupting the reconstruction of edge information. The resulting images will be relatively blurred.

Another source of blurring common to all imaging modalities is described by the point-spread function, which relates the theoretical distribution of signal originating within a single pixel to adjacent pixels. In FSE, the point-spread function takes the form:

$$FW_{1/2} = \frac{\Delta y * 2}{\pi} \frac{ETL * E_s}{T2} \tag{3}$$

with FW representing the full width and half height of the function, this being a standard measure of linewidth such that a wider line corresponds to more "spread" of the information, hence more blurring. In this equation, Δy is the pixel dimension, and the remaining parameters have been previously defined. A similar issue related to the point spread function is ringing artifact, manifest as repeating bands related to the discontinuous T2 weighting function. Again, this artifact results from the fact that significant T2 decay can occur on the time scale of the phase encoding. Methods have been proposed and implemented to reduce these effects. The importance of the point spread function to the physician prescribing the MR scan is that the amount of blurring and ringing due to T2 decay can be controlled through the ETL and the E_S.

Another concern in 2D FSE is magnetization transfer (MT). Consider that when multiple slices are prescribed, the data to reconstruct them is acquired in an interleaved fashion. Thus, the repetition time contains all of the echoes being acquired for one slice, and also the echoes for all slices in the study. For a given slice, the rf excitation for its adjacent slices can be considered "off-resonance" in the same sense as for the design of a magnetization transfer sequence. In conventional spin-echo, these effects are present but insignificant. In FSE, the rf pulses occur much more frequently. Here, the MT effects are measurable and tend to enhance the contrast achieved by T2 weighting. A related concern is the observation that many successive inversion pulses carry a heavy absorbed power load, and may be limited by United States Food and Drug Administration (FDA) or other government agency constraints. This limitation increases in severity with static magnetic field strength, and is of note as the number of higher field clinical scanners continues to rise. However, it is possible with current technology to acquire FSE data at high field with careful choice of scan parameters (Fig. 4.13).

Susceptibility artifact has been observed to be mitigated by FSE imaging as opposed to conventional spin-echo. This may be related to the information that is incorporated into the image from the short echo phase encodes, presumably less affected by susceptibility-induced dephasing. One application where this observation is important is in post-surgical spine imaging, where metallic fragments can cause difficulty in interpretation of conventional images. An example demonstrating the susceptibility advantage in the knee is provided in Fig. 4.14.

4.6 Echo-Planar Imaging

We have seen that acquiring more than one line of k-space from a single excitation pulse allows spin-echo to become "fast spin-echo". In a completely

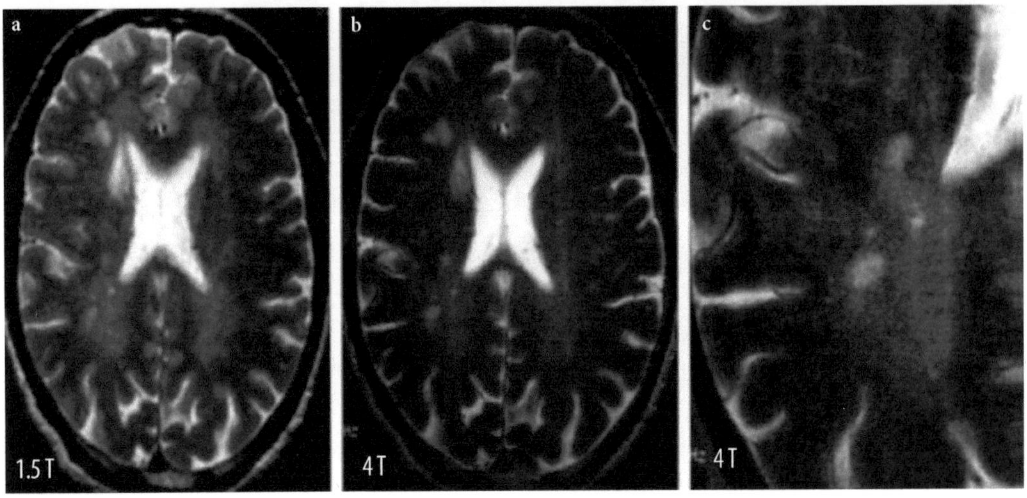

Fig. 4.13a–c. Imaging at high field in MS offers the potential for higher signal-to-noise ratio, better resolution and perhaps the detection of incipient MS lesions. A diagnostic scan at 1.5 T (**a**) is compared with a 4-T scan (**b**), also enlarged for clarity (**c**)

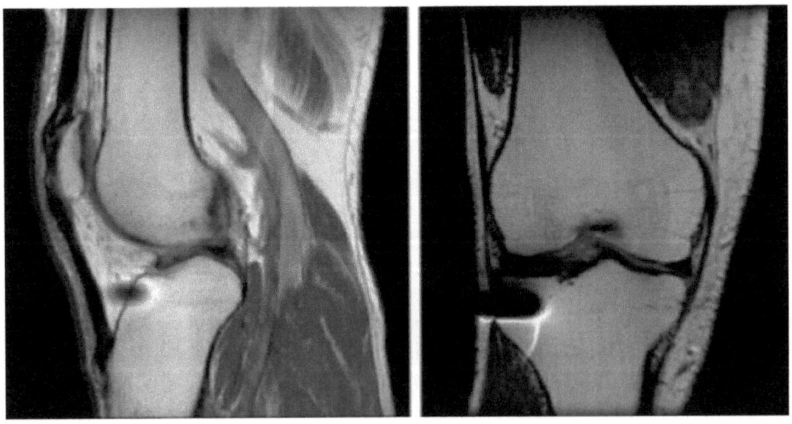

a b

Fig. 4.134,b. Susceptibility artifact is mitigated by FSE (**a**) compared with conventional spin-echo imaging of the same knee. A surgical pin demonstrates a much more severe artifact in the conventional spin-echo image (**b**) analogous manner, repeated gradient echoes can be refocused and obtained from a single excitation pulse resulting in so-called echo planar methods. As proposed in 1977 by MANSFIELD, the original echo-planar sequence was based upon a single excitation pulse (shot) and a zigzag trajectory through k-space brought about by the oscillation of one gradient (producing gradient-echoes) in the presence of a constant orthogonal gradient (Fig. 4.15). In current practice all similar techniques are referred to as EPI. A practical challenge with this technique is posed by the non-uniform coverage of k-space, but this is overcome by sophisticated reconstruction techniques. Other methods of covering k-space include the use of very rapid gradient switching (blipped gradients) to allow a k-space trajectory that is equivalent to spin-warp (at the cost of greater demands on system engineering). In yet another variation, spiral trajectories are achieved by oscillations of both x and y gradients at more reasonable speeds. This reduces the need for extremely rapid gradient switching at the cost of additional complexity in image reconstruction and sparser sampling of the higher k-space regions.

Echo-planar imaging (EPI) as originally implemented is the fastest of the fast techniques owing to its reliance on a single excitation and having no need for other rf pulses for refocusing. As a variation, the single excitation can be replaced by a spin-echo or by some other brief preparation of the magnetization. The EPI acquisition follows using all gradient-echoes and k-space is covered. Better quality can be obtained if necessary by performing two or more EPI acquisitions, with attendant linear increases in acquisition time. As with SSFSE, in single shot EPI the effective TR is infinitely long but the entire study is accomplished in just a few seconds. Contrast is characterized by T2* or by whatever magnetization preparation was employed. The most rapid echo-planar imaging is vulnerable to artifacts including significant blurring in the direction orthogonal to readout, as well as motion and susceptibility. These challenges may impose limitations on the brevity of the acquisition time.

4.7 Hybrid Techniques: GRASE

We have seen that all fast imaging techniques can be evaluated based upon the number of acquisitions and the number and type of refocusing rf pulses. In all cases it is possible to take more time to acquire the image in order to gain quality. In FSE one can incorporate more shots by acquiring less echoes per repetition period. The same is true in EPI. It is also possible to combine the techniques by, for example, incorporating a refocusing rf pulse into an EPI sequence in order to restore strength of signal. This is the basis of so-called GRASE (gradient-echo and spin-echo) and related techniques (FEINBERG and OSHIO 1991). All of the techniques can be viewed in light of their position on a 2D grid, with one axis assigned to the number of spin-echoes per shot (ranging from one to full k-space coverage) and the other axis assigned to the number of gradient-echoes per shot. Single shot techniques of FSE and EPI represent the maximum extent of the two axes, multi shot FSE and EPI occupy intermediate points on those axes, and hybrid techniques including GRASE can reside anywhere within the plane defined by the axes. It is reasonable to surmise that an optimal imaging protocol can be found on this grid for all possible constraints.

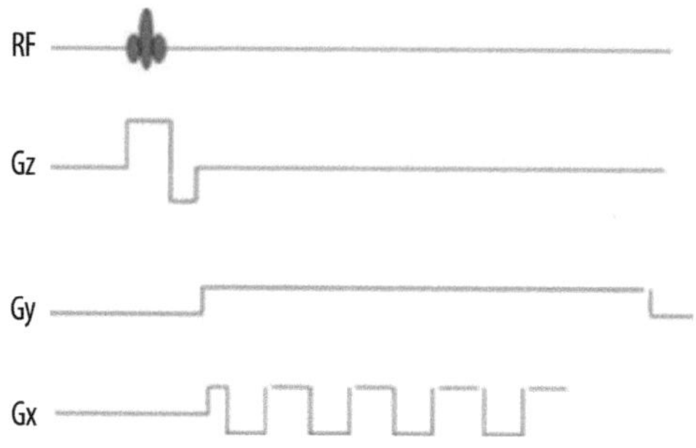

Fig. 4.15. Timing diagram example for echo planar imaging

4.8 Burst Imaging

Burst imaging is another class of ultra-fast imaging methodology, based upon the generation of a series of spin (and stimulated) echoes. A single shot technique; it differs from those discussed above by the employment of a burst pulse originated as DANTE (delays alternating with nutations for tailored excitation). In this composite pulse a large number of evenly spaced, low flip-angle individual pulses are used. The basic pulse sequence is known as DUFIS (DANTE ultrafast imaging sequence) and employs the burst pulse given in the presence of a constant gradient (HENNIG 1998). An inversion (180°) pulse follows to refocus (rephase) the transverse magnetization. Clearly, the train of excitation pulses creates a large number of echoes. However, as the spacing of the pulses is constant, many of the echoes are superimposed upon one another. Reconstruction algorithms account for the phase imposed by the constant gradient and assign the data to the proper location in k-space. Burst imaging is among the most quiet of MR sequences as it does not require rapid gradient switching.

4.9 Parallel Imaging

There has been a great deal of recent development and interest in parallel imaging, achieved by simultaneously acquiring additional signals from coils arranged in an array around the tissue of interest (Sodickson and Manning 1997; Pruessman et al. 1999). Although parallel imaging is not based upon rapidity of acquisition, it deserves mention in this chapter because any increase in quality may be "traded off" in an engineering sense to permit an increase in speed. Parallel imaging may be viewed as an evolution of the employment of phased array coils, such as those in common use to image long structures in the body (e.g. spinal cord). In pulse sequences that use these coils, each in turn acquires data from the area of the body in its vicinity. The reconstruction algorithm combines the data from coils to make a seamless image of the entire structure. Although there is overlap, it is generally true that each receive coil is "responsible" for a different part of the image. In contrast, parallel imaging uses multiple receive coils to provide simultaneous data on the same part of the anatomy, giving the benefit of a repeat study for averaging but taking effectively no more time. The reconstruction of this data into an image is challenging but has been accomplished using techniques known as SMASH and SENSE. An example of parallel imaging is given as Fig. 4.16 and was obtained using 12 signal processing channels and a purpose-built parallel imaging head coil with 12 coils.

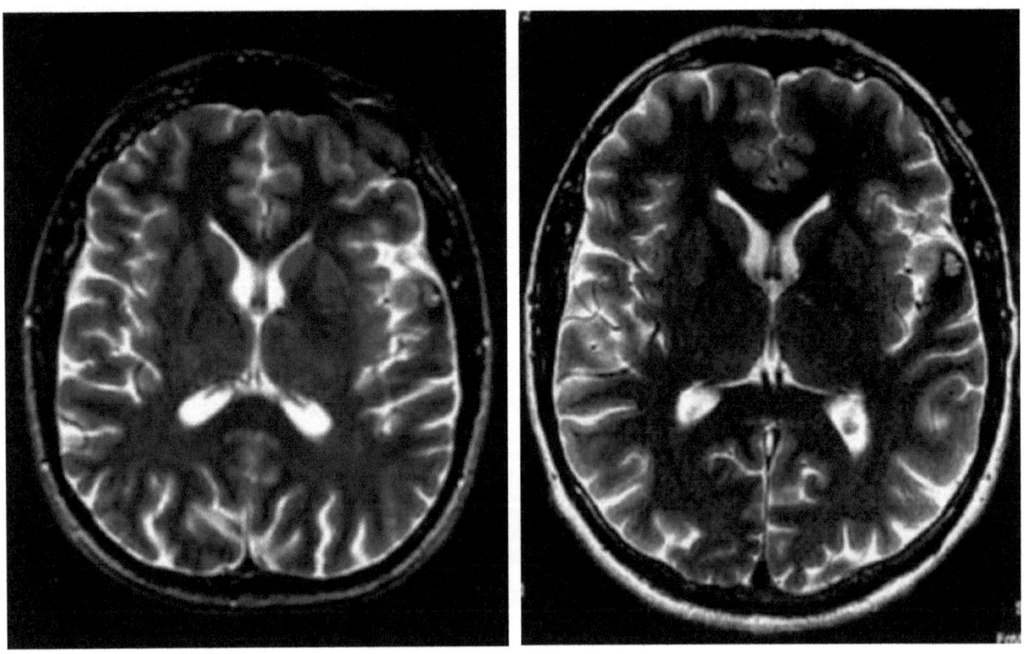

a b

Fig. 4.16a,b. Comparison of standard imaging (a) and parallel imaging (b)using a 12 channel head coil (courtesy E. Knopp, New York University)

4.10 Conclusion

Fast imaging is employed for much of the current clinical imaging in brain, offering the diagnostic power of long TE imaging, rapid acquisition times, and the ability to manipulate contrast as well as to tailor the study to the desired speed/quality compromise. An understanding of the essential parameters that define these techniques can enhance the ability of the physician to prescribe and interpret imaging studies. Novel scan sequences based upon FSE, EPI, and other techniques, coupled with continued advances in magnet and system technology, will continue to extend diagnostic capabilities.

Acknowledgments.
The author is grateful for magnetic resonance images provided by his clinical colleagues at the University of Pennsylvania, and in particular to Dr. Robert I. Grossman, friend and mentor.

References

Feinberg DA, Oshio K (1991) GRASE (gradient- and spin-echo) MR imaging: a new fast clinical imaging technique. Radiology 181:597–602
Hennig JHM (1998) Burst imaging. MAGMA 1:39-48
Hennig JNA, Friedburg H (1986) RARE imaging: a fast imaging method for clinical MR. Magn Reson Imag 3:823-833
Mansfield P (1977) Multi-planar image formation using NMR spin echoes. J Phys C Solid State Phys 10:L55-L58
Pruessman KP, Weiger M, Sheidegger MB, Boesiger P (1999) SENSE: sensitivity encoding for fast MRI. Magn Reson Med 42:952-962
Sodickson, DK, Manning WI (1997) Simultaneous acquisition of spatial harmonics (SMASH):fast imaging with radiofrequency coil arrays. Magn Reson Med 38:591-603

5 Magnetization Transfer

Joseph C. McGowan

CONTENTS

5.1 Introduction

One of several techniques that achieve contrast by preparing the magnetization in some way and then sampling the prepared magnetization via a conventional imaging sequence, magnetization transfer offers advantages that have proven valuable in the study of white matter disorders. In the most common implementation, the magnetization transfer preparation is integrated into a gradient echo pulse sequence, with a conventional gradient echo acquisition serving as a control study. The magnetization transfer (MT) effect can be expressed quantitatively and also evaluated using histogram measures. With the assumption of models for molecular behavior within tissue, fundamental relaxation parameters can theoretically be extracted by solving an inverse problem. Imaging sequences incorporating MT have proven to be relatively easy to implement and to interpret, and have become a common research tool for evaluation of brain disorders. This brief overview will lay out the fundamental assumptions regarding the MT model and will provide suggestions for implementation and analysis of MT studies.

5.2 Physical Basis

Conventional MRI techniques with relaxation-time weighting incorporate the implicit assumption that a quantity of a particular tissue may be fully characterized by use of T1, T2, and proton density. For example, if a particular tissue appears hypointense relative to another on a T1-weighted image, the difference may be attributed to the former tissue having a longer T1. Since conventional MRI is not typically used (or designed) to provide quantitative measurements on an absolute scale, a region may be described as hypo- or hyperintense without any conclusions being drawn about the magnitude of change in T1 that was responsible for the observation.

By comparison, the magnetization transfer (MT) model allows two (or more) components on the molecular level to each have their own relaxation parameters. This leads to the characterization of tissue with at least twice as many parameters as in the conventional MRI case. While in theory this represents an expansion in the ability to characterize tissue that is analogous to the advantage of MRI over X-ray, the full parameter space has yet to be exploited. What instead has arisen is a potentially novel contrast mechanism that can be used to make images reflecting in some way the exchange properties of magnetization between, in the limit, large and small molecules. Specifically, tissue is treated as a more complicated structure that includes not only protons in water molecules, but also bound-water protons associated with proteins and other large molecules. Since bound-water protons cannot be imaged directly via conventional means, the technique is constructed to sample them indirectly. In theory, advantage is taken of the wider frequency spectrum associated with short-T2 protons (bound water spins, macromolecular spins) that behave more solid-like when compared with protons of water. Thus, saturating radiofrequency energy is applied adjacent to, but not on, the resonance frequency of the free water protons. This tends to drive the short-T2 protons into saturation while leaving the free water protons untouched. A process of, most likely, cross relaxation, effectively "transfers" the magnetization of the saturated macromolecules to the free water protons. The effect of this transfer is seen as a reduction in available magnetization in the free water protons. Subsequent sampling of the free

---

J. C. McGowan, PhD
Associate Professor of Electrical Engineering, Department of Electrical Engineering, United States Naval Academy, Annapolis, MD 21405-5025, USA

water spin magnetization via any pulse sequence will elicit a relatively smaller signal. Translated into imaging terminology, regions where this mechanism are effective will be hypointense. A more rigorous treatment of this model and information on the foundation experiments of the technique may be found in the listed articles and reviews (McConnell 1958; Forsen and Hoffman 1963a,b, 1964; Edzes and Samulski 1977, 1978; McGowan 2001; Horská 1996).

The consequence of magnetization transfer in human MRI is that observed proton relaxation times may reflect not only the characteristics of free water protons, but also the characteristics of the macromolecular environment. MT analysis has been said to represent a window into the structure of tissue, and this idea has been borne out by studies relating MT observations to histopathology. The implementation of MT typically has included a control study, so that quantitative values can be obtained by comparing the two sets of images. MT analysis has been suggested to provide information complementary to T1, T2, and proton density.

5.3 Magnetization Transfer Imaging

Magnetic resonance imaging is based upon the supposition that rf excitation, applied off-resonance, exhibits a preferential saturation effect on the short-T2 macromolecules. The observed results of MT studies are consistent with this theory. The first reported study of MTI employed continuous rf excitation using a dedicated rf channel to saturate the macromolecular (bound) spins (Wolff and Balaban 1989), but subsequent experiments by Schnall and collaborators used the standard signal channel to excite the bound spins, as well as to perform the excitation required by the imaging pulse sequence (McGowan et al. 1994). Another approach was introduced and dubbed "on resonance" pulsed magnetization transfer (Hu et al. 1992). In this variant the effect of pulses applied at the proton resonance frequency is to leave the long T2 spins with magnetization intact while saturating the short T2 spins. This method can be shown to be equivalent via Fourier transform to the off-resonance approach, and can be shown to be equivalent to saturation at a certain off-resonance frequency (referred to as effective offset frequency). A theoretical treatment detailing off-resonance selective saturation has been provided (McGowan and Leigh 1994).

The above-listed experimental MT techniques all produce MT images where image intensity is reduced in regions where the MT effect is significant. As noted, control images are also obtained so that a comparison may be made between the two. The ratio of intensities of these two images is a natural measurement, but the most common measure of the MT effect is actually that ratio subtracted from unity, known as the magnetization transfer ratio (MTR). This measure was introduced as a value that increased in magnitude with increasing MT effect (Dousset et al. 1992). Assuming that the saturation provided to the short T2 spins is perfectly selective, meaning that the equilibrium magnetization of the macromolecular spins is reduced to zero while the water spin magnetization is not directly affected, the water-spin magnetization will be maintained at a reduced value in the steady-state, during the pulse sequence. The decrease in magnetization will be larger in regions where the exchange of magnetization is more "efficient", with efficiency potentially a function of one or more of the relaxation parameters that characterize either type of spin. In practice, selective saturation departs significantly from perfect selectivity in any pulsed experiments. However, rather than accept the additional complexity of adding a separate transmit channel to apply continuous wave rf energy, most researchers accept a smaller degree of saturation and rely upon an assumption that the behavior observed will be consistent with an equivalent continuous wave saturating power. Since the results of many experiments to date have been presented by comparison with controls, as relative differences between groups and individuals, this is a reasonable compromise.

It should be noted that contrast between areas exhibiting varying degrees of MT effect is developed and superimposed upon the intrinsic contrast of the baseline image. Thus the appearance of MT images is highly variable when the underlying images can be gradient echo, spin echo, or spin-echo with exogenous contrast. For quantitative study, many researchers have adopted gradient echo imaging as the control image, in order to superimpose the MT results on strictly proton density images. Magnetization transfer contrast is also used in a qualitative manner for applications including magnetic resonance angiography and as a means of enhancing contrast visibility when exogenous contrast agents are given. These techniques are successful because the MT effect is generally pronounced in relatively dense tissues and relatively ineffective in fluids. In MRA, tissue intensity is reduced while blood remains bright. In studies with exogenous contrast agents, incorporation of MT pulses into the imaging sequence can provide additional tissue suppression to allow the contrast-affected tissues to appear brighter. Appropriate control studies should be used in this case to ensure that the two independent effects are not confused. These applications of MT have been implemented on many commercial scanners and are used with both gradient-echo and spin-echo pulse sequences.

As has been described here, the MT experiment nearly always includes its own control study. A difficulty may arise when trying to compare MTR numbers between different scanners, over time, or between sites. This arises in part because scanners have never been designed to produce "reproducible" absolute values of image intensity. Rather, they must be able to reproduce contrast differences in reference phantoms. Coil loading with varying filling factors with different size patients is just one of several variables that are compensated for by the automatic "prescan" functions of clinical scanners. When obtaining quantitative MT studies, it may be necessary to override some of the automatic adjustments in order to minimize the differences between acquisition of the MT and control images.

Scanner manufacturers have employed a variety of ways to effect the prescription of MT images with clinical software. Some use the concept of "flip angle" (although this may not have meaning in the context of the off-resonance excitation of macromolecular spins) as power. This flip angle is understood as related to the power that the scanner provides to the rf coil to produce, for example, a 90° flip angle in proton spins of water. This is meaningful as a relative measure of saturating power, but may be difficult to convert to conventional power units without detailed knowledge of the scanner software and hardware. Offset frequency is self-explanatory when the pulse sequence incorporates pulsed off-resonance MT excitation, less so when "on-resonance" pulses are used. To compare studies, the experimental parameters should match exactly, as any MTR is a strong function of the experimental parameters. The choice of effective offset frequency may be controversial. The common wisdom is to avoid "direct saturation" of the water spins while still providing saturation to the macromolecular spins. In brief, this is unlikely to be achieved. There is no sharp line delineating the region of "direct saturation". Rather, it is reasonable to assume that there is always some direct effect on the water spins and always some indirect effect on the macromolecular spins. Perhaps the best compromise in the prescription of the scanning protocol is to choose experimental parameters to maximize the contrast, or MTR difference, between tissues of interest.

Magnetization transfer images may be acquired with control images to obtain MTR values for each image location. Additional images may also be acquired in order to obtain additional data points for later application to the inverse problem of determining fundamental tissue relaxation and exchange parameters. The additional images will often be prescribed using a programmed variation of the effective offset frequency or the effective saturation power, or both. A series of images at constant power with variable offset frequency yields data that is often referred to as a Z-spectrum (Grad and Bryant 1990).

5.4 Analysis of Magnetization Transfer Images

Images can be analyzed pixel-by-pixel or regions of interest (ROI) can be prescribed with the MTR calculated as an average of contained pixels. Most early MTR studies used ROI analysis as the calculation of individual pixel MTR values can be somewhat noisy. However, in some cases insight can be gained from MTR images constructed via pixel-by-pixel MTR calculation and if necessary ROI values can easily be obtained from those images. An example in MS demonstrating regions of interest is depicted in Fig. 5.1. Studies involving patients diagnosed with multiple

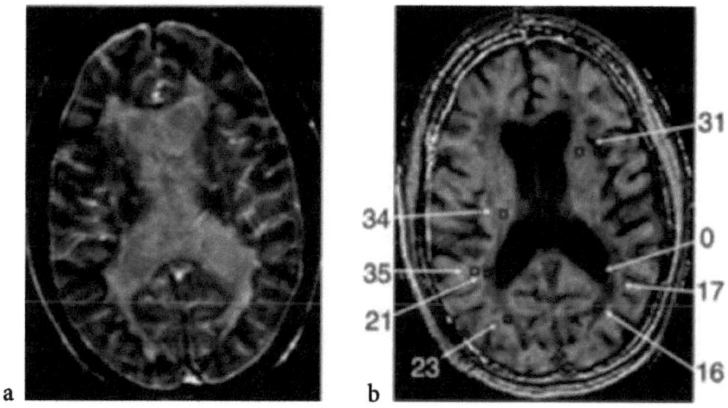

Fig. 5.1a,b. Magnetization transfer imaging in a patient with multiple sclerosis. **a** An image with MT contrast, where darker regions represent greater MT saturation effect. **b** The corresponding MT map, arrived at by normalizing the MT image using an image obtained without MT saturation, that is, by obtaining the MT ratio. Higher intensity corresponds to greater MTR on the MT map. Regions of interest are shown with regional average MT values depicted, demonstrating the range and variance of abnormal tissue in MS

sclerosis (MS) have led to increased understanding of the disease and in particular of the nature of lesion evolution (Petrella et al. 1996; Hiehle et al. 1994).

In response to the recognition of the diffuse nature of MS, and the concept of diseased "normal appearing white matter", McGowan and Grossman developed the MTR histogram which was applied by van Buchem et al in 1996 (van Buchem et al. 1996). This method of analysis was designed to be applicable to MS because it was responsive to the large scale variation of MTR in lesions as well as to the small scale variation in what was to be dubbed "normal appearing white matter." A histogram is simply a graph depicting the number of pixels with a certain value of, in this case, MTR. The height of the histogram at any MTR value represents the frequency with which that value occurs in the underlying data. The range of MTR values is divided into "bins" and the choice of bin size is important to the character of the histogram. Specifically, too-large bins tend to overly smooth the data and too-small bins provide a noisy appearance that masks the features within that are being sought. The optimum size is a function of the quality (signal-to-noise ratio) of the raw data. Figure 5.2 is the first comparison of MTR histograms, obtained from human subjects. Figure 5.3 shows a series of MTR histograms obtained in a rat spinal cord injury model and serves to identify some of the histogram parameters that may be studied and compared. MTR values have also been presented using a contour map technique (Fig. 5.4) and this showed promise for identification of patterns of abnormality that were consistent with pathology studies yet inapparent on conventional MRI (McGowan et al. 1999).

a
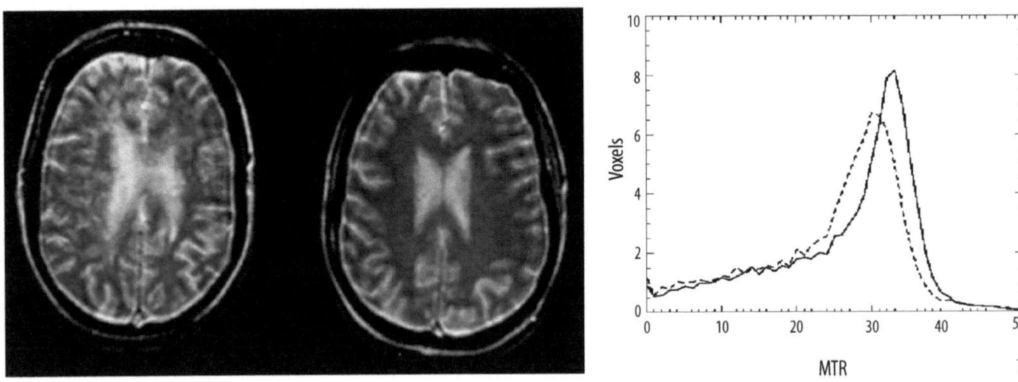

b

Fig. 5.2. a MT images obtained in a patient with MS (*left*) and a normal volunteer. **b** MT histogram corresponding to the images. A decrease and shift of the characteristic peak associated with white matter is seen

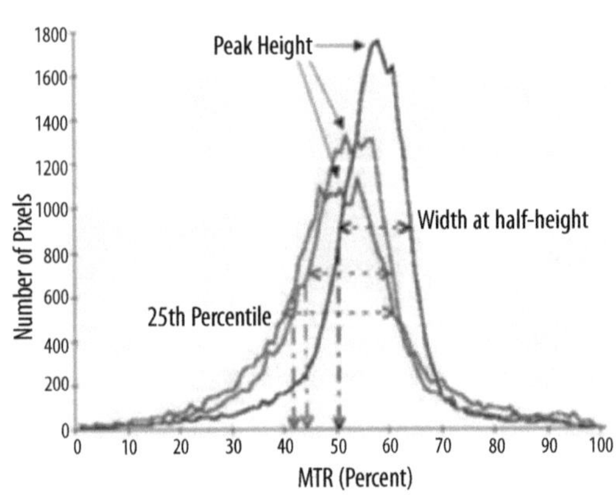

Fig. 5.3. MTR histograms in a rat spinal cord injury model, including an average control histogram and average histograms corresponding to weight-drop injuries with 2.5 and 15 cm drop-heights

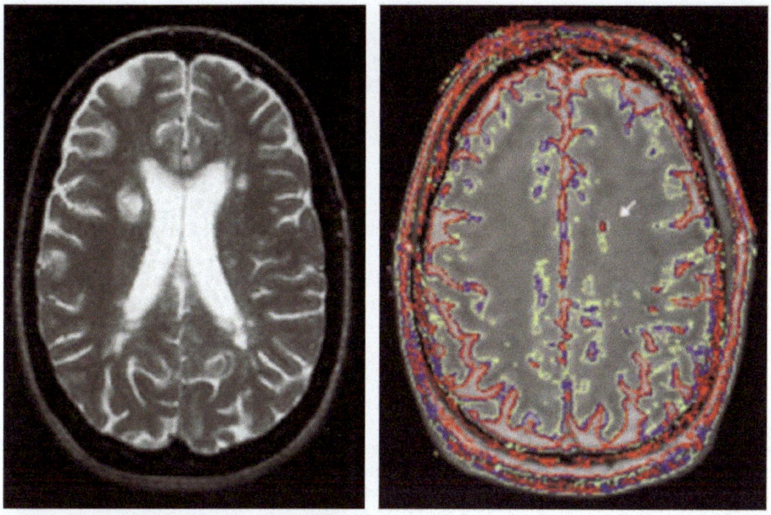

a c

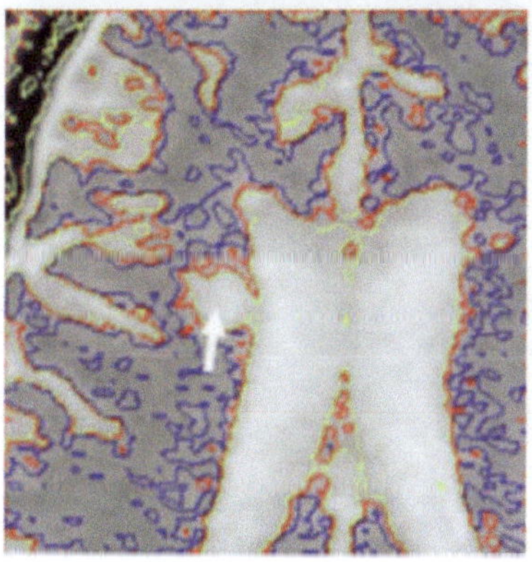

b

Fig. 5.4. a An example MTI image in multiple sclerosis with focal lesions in the periventricular white matter. **b** An MT contour plot demonstrates the gradation of MTR values from the low-MTR center of the large focal lesion (*thick arrow*) to the normal-appearing white matter. The contours are drawn at 2, 4, and 6 standard deviations (SD) below normal values as obtained from age-matched control subjects. A smaller lesion on the contralateral side is shown to be asymmetric with regard to MTR. **c** In another patient, a small focal MS lesion (*red contours,* 6 SD below normal MTR, *arrow*) is shown to be extended into normal-appearing tissue by MT contours at 2 SD below normal

5.5 The Inverse Problem

Some researchers have investigated models of increased complexity compared to the simple binary spin bath model discussed above. Impressive results have been obtained by treating the macromolecular fraction as characterized by other than Bloch equation (i.e., T1 and T2) behavior (Morrison et al. 1997; Li et al. 1997; Henkelman et al. 1993). Implementation of this assumption was achieved by substituting a Gaussian or superlorentzian line shape to describe the behavior of the macromolecular magnetization, where the Bloch equations would predict a lorentzian line shape. To pursue these models, additional data points must be gathered and the resulting Z-spectra fitted to appropriate line shapes. The results of fitting are model parameters including relaxation times associated with the macromolecular component and characteristic exchange (transfer) rates. The time cost of these experiments is high, even though a single control study can be used for many values of effective offset frequency. When the studies are completed, however, results include images based upon one parameter of the MT model. Such images are being investigated in light of the potential clinical value of an additional MRI contrast parameter. Current studies also attempt to optimize the number of data points gathered with the aim of a reasonable study time for application to human subjects.

References

Dousset V, Grossman RI, Ramer KN et al (1992) Experimental allergic encephalomyelitis and multiple sclerosis: lesion characterization with magnetization transfer imaging (published erratum appears in Radiology 1992, 183:878). Radiology 182:483-491

Edzes HT, Samulski ET (1977) Cross relaxation and spin dif-

fusion in the proton NMR of hydrated collagen. Nature 265:521-523
Edzes HT, Samulski ET (1978) The measurement of cross-relaxation effects in the proton NMR spin-lattice relaxation of water in biological systems: hydrated collagen and muscle. J Magn Res 31:207-229
Forsen S, Hoffman R (1963a) A new method for the study of moderately rapid chemical exchange rates employing nuclear magnetic double resonance. Acta Chem Scand 17:1787-1788
Forsen S, Hoffman R (1963b) Study of moderately rapid chemical exchange reactions by means of nuclear magnetic double resonance. J Chem Phys 39:2892-2901
Forsen S, Hoffman R (1964) Exchange rates by nuclear magnetic multiple resonance. III. Exchange reactions in systems with several nonequivalent sites. J Chem Phys 40:1189-1196
Grad J, Bryant RG (1990) Nuclear magnetic cross-relaxation spectroscopy. J Magn Res 90:1-8
Henkelman RM, Huang X, Xiang Q, Stanisz GJ, Swanson S, Bronskill MJ (1993) Quantitative interpretation of magnetization transfer. Magn Reson Med 29:759-766
Hiehle JFJ, Lenkinski RE, Grossman RI et al (1994) Correlation of spectroscopy and magnetization transfer imaging in the evaluation of demyelinating lesions and normal appearing white matter in multiple sclerosis. Magn Reson Med 32:285-293
Horská A (1996) SRGS. Measurement of spin-lattice relaxation times and kinetic rate constants in rat muscle using progressive partial saturation and steady-state saturation transfer. Magn Reson Med 36:232-240
Hu BS, Conolly SM, Wright GA, Nishimura DG, Macovski A (1992) Pulsed saturation transfer contrast. Magn Reson Med 26:231-240
Li JG, Graham SJ, Henkelman RM (1997) A flexible magnetization transfer line shape derived from tissue experimental data. Magn Reson Med 37:866-871
McConnell HM (1958) Reaction rates by nuclear magnetic resonance. J Chem Phys 28:430-431
McGowan JC, Leigh JS Jr (1994) Selective saturation in magnetization transfer experiments. Magn Reson Med 32:517-522
McGowan JC, Schnall MD, Leigh JS (1994) Magnetization transfer imaging with pulsed off-resonance saturation: contrast variation with saturation duty cycle. J Magn Res 4:79-82
McGowan JC, McCormack TM, Grossman R et al (1999) Diffuse axonal pathology detected with magnetization transfer imaging following brain injury in the pig. Magn Reson Med 41:727-733
McGowan JC (2001) Magnetic resonance imaging and magnetization transfer. Academic, New York (Advances in imaging and electron physics, vol 118)
Morrison C, Stanisz G, Henkelman RM (1995) Modeling magnetization transfer for biological-like systems using a semi-solid pool with a super-Lorentzian lineshape and dipolar reservoir. J Magn Reson Ser B 108:103-113
Petrella JR, Grossman RI, McGowan JC, Campbell G, Cohen JA (1996) Multiple sclerosis lesions: relationship between MR enhancement pattern and magnetization transfer effect. AJNR Am J Neuroradiol 17:1041-1049
Van Buchem MA, McGowan JC, Kolson DL, Polansky M, Grossman RI (1996) Quantitative volumetric magnetization transfer analysis in multiple sclerosis: estimation of macroscopic and microscopic disease burden. Magn Reson Med 36:632-636
Wolff SD, Balaban RS (1989) Magnetization transfer contrast (MTC) and tissue water proton relaxation in vivo. Magn Reson Med 10:135-144

6 Quantitative Diffusion Imaging

Peter C.M. van Zijl, Lidia Nagae-Poetscher and Susumu Mori

CONTENTS

6.1 Introduction

The basic principles of diffusion magnetic resonance imaging (MRI) were established in the mid 1980s (for recent reviews see Le Bihan 2003; Le Bihan and van Zijl 2002), combining principles of MRI with principles of diffusion sensitization through the use of pairs of magnetic field gradient pulses. The potential of diffusion MRI is based on the notion that, while diffusing, water molecules probe tissue structure at a microscopic scale well beyond the usual image resolution. During typical diffusion periods of about 50–100 ms, water molecules (water is the most convenient molecular species to study with diffusion MRI, but some metabolites may also be studied with spectroscopy; Moonen et al. 1990; van Zijl et al. 1994) move in the brain on average over distances of around 10–20 ìm, bouncing, crossing, or interacting with many tissue components, such as cell membranes, fibers, or macromolecules. The overall effect observed in a diffusion MRI image volume element (voxel) therefore reflects, on a statistical basis, the displacement distribution of the water molecules present within this voxel. The non-invasive observation of this displacement distribution in vivo thus provides unique clues on the structure and geometric organization of tissues. Since the initial work by Le Bihan, the developments in the application of diffusion imaging and spectroscopy in vivo have been rapid (Table 6.1). The most successful application of diffusion MRI since the early 1990s has been acute brain ischemia (Moseley et al. 1990a; van Gelderen et al. 1994; Baird and Warach 1998; Sotak 2002). Brain data show that diffusion is anisotropic in white matter (Moseley et al. 1990b), leading to the opportunity to probe the cumulative effect via so-called trace imaging (van Gelderen et al. 1994; Mori and van Zijl 1995) (or isotropic diffusion imaging) or to develop a formalism to quantify this anisotropy in an orientationally independent manner (Basser et al. 1994a; Basser and Pierpaoli 1996; Basser and Jones 2002; Pierpaoli and Basser 1996). This latter formalism has provided not only a means to study the magnitude of diffusion anisotropy (Pierpaoli and Basser 1996; Pierpaoli et al. 1996; Ulug and van Zijl 1999), but also the possibility to acquire orientational information from two-dimensional color maps (Pajevic and Pierpaoli 1999) or from three-dimensional tracking of major white matter fibers (Mori et al. 1999; Conturo 1999; Jones et al. 1999a; Basser et al. 2000; Poupon et al. 2000; Mori and van Zijl 2002). This development has started a new era of connectivity imaging that is presently making rapid progress.

In this chapter, we will first describe the principles of isotropic and anisotropic diffusion, together with approaches to create image contrast based on these properties. The basics of why it is needed to use a ten-

P. C. M. van Zijl
Johns Hopkins University Medical School, Department of Radiology, 217 Traylor Bldg., 720 Rutland Ave., Baltimore, MD 21205, USA
L. Nagae-Poetscher; S. Mori
F. M. Kirby Research Center for Functional Brain Imaging, Kennedy Krieger Institute, 707 N. Broadway, Baltimore, MD 21205, USA

Table 6.1. History of some important in vivo diffusion MRI and MRS developments[a]

Year	Advance	Reference(s)
1986	Le Bihan et al. report first in vivo diffusion images	Le Bihan et al. (1986)
1990	Moonen et al. report first in vivo diffusion spectroscopy	Moonen et al. (1990)
1990	Moseley et al. show early ADC changes in acute stroke	Moseley et al. (1990a)
1990	Moseley et al. show diffusional anisotropy in cat brain	Moseley et al. (1990b)
1992	Warach et al. first measure stroke patients using DWI	Warach et al. (1992)
1994	Van Gelderen et al. suggest use of tensor trace to better observe ischemic lesions through removal of the diffusion anisotropy	Van Gelderen et al. (1994)
1994	Davis et al. show ADC changes within 2–3 min of ischemic onset	Davis et al. (1994)
1994	Basser et al. introduce theory for diffusion tensor imaging	Basser et al. (1994a,b)
1996	Basser and Pierpaoli design orientation-independent anisotropy indices	Pierpaoli et al. (1996); Pierpaoli and Basser (1996)
1997	Makris uses DTI to design fiber color scheme	Makris et al. (1997)
1999	Mori et al. report successful tracking of white matter fibers; Conturo et al. and Jones et al. report first human data	Mori et al. (1999); Conturo et al. (1999); Jones et al. (1999)
1999	Jones et al. discuss importance of multi-directional diffusion acquisition	Jones et al. (1999)
2000	Wiegell et al. report imaging of fiber crossings	Wiegell et al. (2000)

[a]The above table focuses on medical technology rather than NMR literature and clinical discoveries. Notice that in the 1960s, 1970s and 1980s, much NMR literature appeared on excised tissue diffusion properties and anisotropy determination. This literature is not included here because we focus on in vivo work, but a comprehensive review of this early work is available from Karger et al. (1988).

sor to describe diffusion in tissue will be explained, and schemes to generate orientation-independent diffusion tensor descriptions will be discussed. Subsequently, it will be discussed how to optimally acquire the experimental data needed for the tensor description and how the results will depend on the range of b-values and the number of directions used. This will be followed by a brief overview of recent applications.

6.2 Diffusion Basics

Diffusion is defined as a process by which random molecular motion transports matter from one part of a system to another. In an isotropic medium such as neat water, this process can be described by a single coefficient, i.e., the diffusion constant *D*, and a characteristic equation of motion. This diffusion equation, also known as Fick's second law, states that the change in the concentration *C* (or the amount of matter transported) in time is proportional to the change in the concentration gradient with respect to the positional coordinates:

$$\frac{\partial C}{\partial t} = D\nabla^2 C \qquad [6.1]$$

in which $\nabla^2 = \frac{\delta^2}{\delta r^2}$. The magnitude of diffusion is thus defined as the flux of molecules per time unit (m^2/s). MRI can measure diffusion through application of self-refocusing pairs of magnetic field gradients (Fig. 6.1) (Stejskal and Tanner 1965). The random phase loss due to diffusion between different spatial locations can not be refocused and a signal loss is found that will depend on the gradient strength G, gradient length δ, and the time over which diffusion is measured, the diffusion time t_{dif}, which depends both on the time period between the starts of the two diffusion gradients (Δ) as well as on their length and shape. For rectangular gradients and free (isotropic) Gaussian diffusion, this is described by the basic Stejskal-Tanner equation:

$$S/S_0 = e^{-\gamma^2 G^2 \delta^2 t_{dif} D} = e^{-\gamma^2 G^2 \delta^2 (\Delta - \delta/3) D} = e^{-bD} \qquad [6.2]$$

The b-value, describing the product of the gradient and timing constants, was introduced by Le Bihan et al. (1986). When combining diffusion weighting with imaging, the results are known as *diffusion-weighted imaging* (DWI), a term now common in clinical imaging. The DW contrast adds to other contrast in the image, including spin density, T1, and T2 contrast. To obtain pure diffusion information, it is necessary to acquire the diffusion-based signal decay as a function of b-value (at least two in an isotropic system), leading to *absolute*

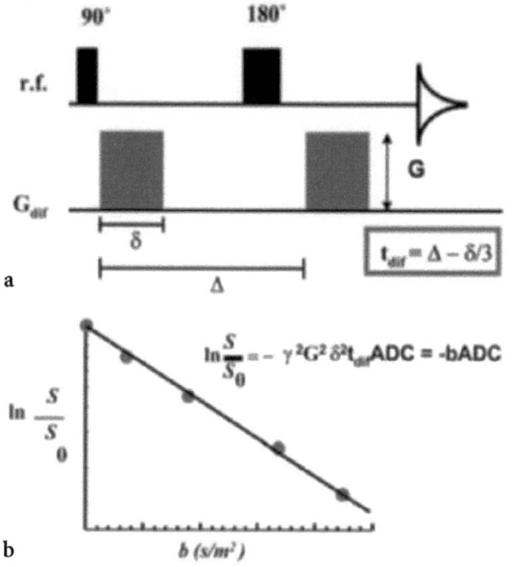

Fig. 6.1a,b. **a** Typical spin-echo Stejskal Tanner pulse sequence for diffusion weighting with a pair of pulsed field gradients of strength G and length d. Data acquisition is denoted by a free induction decay. **b** Calculation of the apparent diffusion constant (*ADC*) from a linear fit of the normalized logarithmic signal decay as a function of b-factor. The diffusion time and signal decay are defined for a pair of square field gradients

diffusion images, in which the D-value is displayed as a function of space.

When studying biological systems, the environment is in general anisotropic and the imaging volume will reflect a weighted average of multiple compartments with different diffusion constants. This weighting will depend on the size of the compartments, their properties (viscosity, binding with macromolecular structures, etc.), as well as on the barriers between them (exchange). Due to this environmental dependence, it is common to speak of the *apparent diffusion coefficient* (ADC). This situation provides the opportunity to study tissue microstructure by varying the length of the diffusion time. For instance, under the condition of permeable compartment separations, two extreme situations can be distinguished. For very long diffusion times, water molecules can probe most compartments "i" with populations p_i, which can be seen as fast exchange on the measurement time scale:

$$S/S_0 = e^{-b\sum_i p_i D_i} = e^{-b(ADC)} \quad [6.3a]$$

For very short diffusion times (or very impermeable barriers) water molecules most probably stay within their compartments and the condition of slow exchange is approached, under which the measured "approximately-exponential" signal decay at low b-values is built up of contributions of the signal decays in individual compartments. Neglecting relaxation contributions, one has:

$$S/S_0 = \sum_i p_i e^{-bD_i} \cong e^{-b(ADC)} \quad [6.3b]$$

As a consequence, classical (Gaussian) treatment of the diffusion process may not properly reflect the tissue properties. Interestingly, the practical situation is that, at sufficiently low b-values (< ~1000 s/mm²) and within experimental accuracy, the in vivo situation can generally be described by a single exponential, as used in Eq. 6.3a,b. This simple "single-exponential" situation is no longer valid when going to higher b-values as has been demonstrated in cell systems (van Zijl et al. 1991, 1994; Andrasko 1976b), as well as in vivo (for a recent review see Cohen and Assaf 2002). In cell suspensions or perfused cell systems, this situation can generally be approximated by a biexponential description for intra- and extracellular diffusion, including the membrane transport if necessary. In tissue, despite the appearance of a bi-exponential, the situation is probably more complex. Attempts to understand this in vivo behavior are now a hot topic of discussion.

To get an impression of the distance scale measured by diffusion imaging, it is convenient to start with free diffusion, in which the radius of the diffusion sphere is given by the standard deviation of the Gaussian displacement profile. This is reflected by the well-known Einstein equation for the mean square displacement:

$$\sigma = r_{rms} = \sqrt{x^2 + y^2 + z^2} = \sqrt{2Dt_{dif}} \quad [6.4]$$

Free water diffusion at 37°C corresponds to D=3 × 10^{-9} m²/s, which can be taken as an upper limit in vivo and is closely approximated in cerebral spinal fluid (CSF). In tissue, a D-value of about 1.5 × 10^{-9} m²/s is a frequent estimate for free cellular diffusion. In a clinical scanner, available gradient strengths limit diffusion times to the order of about 40–50 ms, corresponding to a free diffusion distance of about 12 µm. Cellular restrictions in the brain (membranes, organelles, macromolecules) are found over much smaller distances, and reduced diffusion constants are measured for both gray and white matter. One way to probe the spatial boundaries is by assessing displacement probabilities using so-called q-space imaging (Callaghan et al. 1991, 1999; Cory and

GARROWAY 1990), in which $\overline{q}$ is the reciprocal spatial vector (units of m^{-1}), defined as $(\gamma\overline{G}\delta/2\pi)$. Under the conditions of $\delta<\Delta$, the magnitude of $\overline{q}$ controls the signal decay via:

$$S(\overline{q})/S_0 = \int P(\overline{R},\Delta)e^{(i2\pi\overline{q}\cdot\overline{R})}d\overline{R} \quad [6.5]$$

in which $\overline{R}$ is the average displacement vector and $P(\overline{R},\Delta)$ the displacement probability distribution function. Recent work by ASSAF and COHEN (2000) indicates that the slower component (i.e., the one remaining at high b-value) measured from biexponential analysis of the diffusion decay in the brain has a displacement probability of about 2 μm, and concluded that this is probably due to the brain fibers, where restrictions are formed by axonal (~3 μm) and myelin diameters (1–2 μm), leading to orientationally restricted diffusion. However, such orientational restrictions can also be detected using lower b-values (BEAULIEU 2002), as has been demonstrated in recent years using diffusion tensor imaging.

6.3 Diffusion Tensor Imaging (DTI)

6.3.1 Tensor Properties and Calculations

The presence of spatial restrictions in tissue causes water diffusion to be orientationally dependent. This is illustrated in Fig. 6.2. Diffusion is measured in the so-called laboratory frame, defined by the axes of the MRI scanner (z-axis along the field, x and y perpendicular and given by the gradient directions). When diffusion is isotropic (Fig. 6.2a), measurement of diffusion constants using the x, y, or z-gradients will all give the same value. If diffusion is anisotropic, this is no longer the case. For instance, in Fig. 6.2b diffusion is restricted by a cylinder along the z-axis, leading to the measurement of two different diffusion constants ($ADC_{||}$ and $ADC_{\perp}$). Obviously, in practice, such a situation will not occur and the restrictions will be randomly oriented in the laboratory frame. As a consequence, diffusion is generally described by a tensor (Fig. 6.2c) (VAN ZIJL et al. 1994; VAN GELDEREN et al. 1994; KARGER et al. 1988; BASSER et al. 1994b). As diffusion constants are real values, this is a symmetric tensor ($ADC_{\alpha\beta} = ADC_{\beta\alpha}$; $\alpha \neq \beta$; $\alpha, \beta, \in \{x,y,z\}$) characterized by six unique diffusion constants. Consequently, the signal decay is not described by the simple equation [2] above, but rather by:

$$S/S_0 = e^{-\gamma^2\delta^2 t_{dif}\overline{\mathbf{G}}\cdot\overline{\overline{\mathbf{D}}}\cdot\overline{\mathbf{G}}} = e^{-\gamma^2\delta^2 t_{dif}\sum_{\alpha,\beta} G_\alpha G_\beta ADC_{\alpha\beta}} = e^{-\sum_{\alpha,\beta} b_{\alpha\beta} ADC_{\alpha\beta}} \quad \alpha, \beta \in \{x,y,z\} \quad [6.6]$$

Thus, at least seven measurements are needed to determine these tensor elements (one at low b-value and six directions at high b-value). This complicates and slows down image analysis. For instance, when trying to identify stroke lesions, anisotropy effects may be very cumbersome and confusing in ischemic regions. As a consequence, the first practical application of diffusion tensor imaging involved the acquisition of a reduced data set, removing the anisotropy information inherent in the tensor and creating an image representing the trace of the tensor at any given point (VAN GELDEREN et al. 1994; MORI and VAN ZIJL 1995), which is a rotationally invariant quantity. This has become especially important in the clinic for detection of ischemic lesions (BAIRD and WARACH 1998; SOTAK 2002; ULUG et al. 1997). On the other hand, the analysis of diffusion anisotropy in vivo may provide important new information regarding tissue microstructure. This field was pioneered by PIERPAOLI and BASSER (1996) and PIERPAOLI et al. (1996), who defined orientationally independent anisotropy indices based on intrinsic structural properties of ellipsoids (magnitude, volume, etc.) that can be used to quantify the tissue anisotropy properties in an unbiased manner between subjects.

In order to assess such diffusion anisotropy in an orientation-independent manner, the diffusion tensor (measured in the laboratory frame, as detailed in the next section on data acquisition) needs to be diagonalized to determine the magnitude of the apparent diffusion constants in each voxel. The magnitude of the three resulting ADCs, the eigenvalues $\gamma_1, \gamma_2, \gamma_3$, determine the shape of the so-called diffusion ellipsoid. The orientation of the ellipsoid in the laboratory frame is determined by the rotation matrix, R, containing the three eigenvectors

$$\begin{bmatrix} ADC_{xx} & ADC_{xy} & ADC_{xz} \\ ADC_{xy} & ADC_{yy} & ADC_{yz} \\ ADC_{xz} & ADC_{yz} & ADC_{zz} \end{bmatrix} \xrightarrow{\text{diagonalize}} R^{-1} \begin{bmatrix} \lambda_1 & 0 & 0 \\ 0 & \lambda_2 & 0 \\ 0 & 0 & \lambda_3 \end{bmatrix} R \quad [6.7]$$

Laboratory frame diagonal frame

After diagonalizing the tensor, the eigenvalues can be used to calculate a multitude of diffusion anisotropy indices. However, there are some potential problems. For most of these indices, the eigenvalues

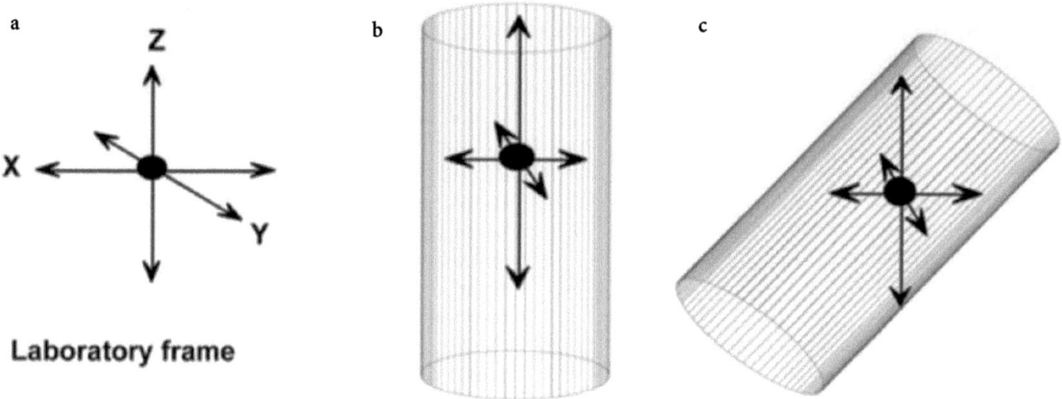

$$\begin{bmatrix} ADC & 0 & 0 \\ 0 & ADC & 0 \\ 0 & 0 & ADC \end{bmatrix} \qquad \begin{bmatrix} ADC_{xx} & 0 & 0 \\ 0 & ADC_{yy} & 0 \\ 0 & 0 & ADC_{zz} \end{bmatrix} \qquad \begin{bmatrix} ADC_{xx} & ADC_{xy} & ADC_{xz} \\ ADC_{xy} & ADC_{yy} & ADC_{yz} \\ ADC_{xz} & ADC_{yz} & ADC_{zz} \end{bmatrix}$$

$$ADC_{xx} = ADC_{yy} = ADC_{zz} = ADC \qquad ADC_{zz} = ADC_{//}; \; ADC_{xx} = ADC_{yy} = ADC_{\perp} \qquad ADC_{\alpha\beta} = ADC_{\beta\alpha}$$

Fig. 6.2a–c. **a** Laboratory frame in a diffusion experiment. The z-axis is along the magnetic field; x,y,z are the gradient directions. For isotropic diffusion (**a**), all tensor elements are equal. **b** For diffusion in a tube with cylindrical symmetry oriented along the field, there are two different diffusion constants, namely parallel to the tube and perpendicular. **c** In vivo, the orientation of fibers or other structures may not be along the field, and the diffusion has to be described by a symmetric tensor with six different elements. Average local geometry can be deduced using a diagonalization procedure

need to be ranked by magnitude, which may introduce a bias in the presence of noise (Pierpaoli and Basser 1996; Pierpaoli et al. 1996). To avoid this, Pierpaoli et al. (1996) and Pierpaoli and Basser 1996 designed indices that combine tensor elements to represent ellipsoid properties that are invariant with respect to such ordering. These properties are based on three basic invariants of a tensor, which are (Ulug and van Zijl 1999):

1st invariant (trace):

$$I_1 = ADC_{xx} + ADC_{yy} + ADC_{zz} = \lambda_1 + \lambda_2 + \lambda_3 \qquad [6.8a]$$

2nd invariant:

$$\begin{aligned} I_2 &= ADC_{xx}ADC_{yy} + ADC_{xx}ADC_{zz} + ADC_{yy}ADC_{zz} \\ &\quad - ADC_{xy}^2 - ADC_{xz}^2 - ADC_{yz}^2 = \lambda_1\lambda_2 + \lambda_1\lambda_3 + \lambda_2\lambda_3 \end{aligned} \qquad [6.8b]$$

3rd invariant (determinant):

$$\begin{aligned} I_3 &= ADC_{xx}(ADC_{yy}ADC_{zz} - ADC_{yz}^2) - ADC_{xy}(ADC_{xy}ADC_{zz} - ADC_{xz}ADC_{yz} \\ &\quad + ADC_{xz}(ADC_{xy}ADC_{yz} - ADC_{xz}ADC_{yy}) = \lambda_1\lambda_2\lambda_3 \end{aligned} \qquad [6.8c]$$

These three invariants are sufficient to completely describe the tensor. Further invariants can be constructed from the basic three above. A common one is:

Square of tensor magnitude:

$$\begin{aligned} I_4 &= ADC_{xx}^2 + ADC_{yy}^2 + ADC_{zz}^2 + ADC_{xy}^2 + ADC_{xz}^2 + ADC_{yz}^2 \\ &= \lambda_1^2 + \lambda_2^2 + \lambda_3^2 \end{aligned} \qquad [6.8d]$$

6.3.2 Diffusion Anisotropy Definitions

As can be seen from the equations, the invariant properties have units of *ADC*, *ADC*^{2}, and *ADC*^{3}, which relate to the average *ADC*, the surface, and the volume of the ellipsoid (Ulug and van Zijl 1999). Thus, a set of diffusion constants can be defined describing such inherent properties of the ellipsoid. Alternatively, one can define diffusion anisotropies reflecting such ellipsoid properties, as done by Basser and Pierpaoli. Such anisotropies are now being used as clinical indicators of tissue status in different pathologies. The most important ones of these are the fractional anisotropy (FA), relative anisotropy (RA), and volume ratio (VR), which relate to the invariants via:

$$FA = \sqrt{\tfrac{3}{2}\left(1 - \frac{I_1^2}{3I_4}\right)} = \sqrt{1 - \frac{I_2}{I_4}} = \sqrt{1 - \frac{\lambda_1\lambda_2 + \lambda_1\lambda_3 + \lambda_2\lambda_3}{\lambda_1^2 + \lambda_2^2 + \lambda_3^2}}$$

range: 0 (isotropic) - 1(anisotropic) [6.9a]

$$RA = \sqrt{\frac{3I_4}{I_1^2} - 1} = \sqrt{2}\sqrt{\left(1 - \frac{3I_2}{I_1^2}\right)} = \sqrt{2}\sqrt{\left(1 - \frac{3(\lambda_1\lambda_2 + \lambda_1\lambda_3 + \lambda_2\lambda_3)}{(\lambda_1 + \lambda_2 + \lambda_3)^2}\right)}$$

range: 0 (isotropic) $-\sqrt{2}$ (anisotropic) [6.9b]

$$VR = 27I_3 / I_1^3 = 27(\lambda_1\lambda_2\lambda_3)/(\lambda_1 + \lambda_2 + \lambda_3)^3$$

range: 1 (isotropic) – 0 (anisotropic) [6.9c].

Of these, the most commonly used one is the FA, but in principle any of them can be used as they are inherently related (Ulug and van Zijl 1999). Another measure that has been suggested is the so-called lattice anisotropy index (LI) (Pierpaoli and Basser 1996; Pierpaoli et al. 1996), which is an inter-voxel (lattice) measure in which voxel anisotropies are compared to those of neighboring voxels. Obviously, such a comparison depends on spatial resolution and the distance from the voxel and is more complex than the intra-voxel quantities in Eq. 6.9. Another very useful index, which is directly related to the cylindrical symmetry of diffusion is the fiber anisotropy (Ulug and van Zijl 1999), also called the total anisotropy (A_σ) (Conturo et al. 1996) or the standard deviation anisotropy (A_{sd}):

$$A_{fiber} = A_\sigma = A_{sd} = \frac{ADC_{//} - ADC_{\perp}}{ADC_{//} + 2ADC_{\perp}} = \frac{\lambda_1 - \frac{1}{2}(\lambda_2 + \lambda_3)}{\lambda_1 + \lambda_2 + \lambda_3} \qquad [6.10]$$

Prolate diffusion range:
1 (anisotropic) – 0 (isotropic): A_{fiber} = RA / $\sqrt{2}$

Oblate diffusion range:
0 (isotropic) – –0.5 (anisotropic)

An anisotropy index should preferably have the following properties: (a) to have a physical meaning, it should represent inherent diffusion ellipsoid properties; (b) to be measured reproducibly in vivo, it should be orientation independent; (c) to reduce bias and sensitivity to noise, it should not require eigenvalue sorting i.e., the ordering by magnitude; (d) to avoid introduction of additional noise, it should be obtainable without tensor diagonalization; (e) for improved understanding and convenience, it should be normalized between 0 (isotropic) and 1 (fully anisotropic). These conditions are met by FA, RA / $\sqrt{2} = A_{fiber}$, and $1-VR$. One important question relates to the sensitivity of these related indices to tissue differences in cylindrical anisotropy. Based on their definitions, FA is most sensitive for cylindrical anisotropy below 0.5, RA / $\sqrt{2} = A_{fiber}$ is linear over the full range, and $1-VR$ is the most sensitive above 0.85. A better index in the above-0.5 range would therefore be the so-called ultimate volume anisotropy: $UA_{vol} = \sqrt{(3\sqrt[3]{I_3}/I_1 - 1)^2}$ (Ulug and van Zijl 1999), which is more sensitive above about 0.6.

Anisotropy measurements are now starting to be used in clinical application. It may not be well realized that these anisotropy numbers can be obtained without tensor diagonalization, but this may lead to simpler techniques in the future. When fiber tracking is the goal of the experiments (see Sect. 6.5), diagonalization of the tensor is still necessary to obtain the eigenvectors.

6.4 DTI Data Acquisition

In a diffusion experiment, magnetic field gradients are used to sensitize the experiment to microscopic tissue water motion. As such, the experiments are extremely sensitive to motion as well as to the performance of the gradients (stability, eddy currents). Most modern imagers have high-quality shielded gradients and can perform excellent single-shot echo planar imaging (EPI). Thus, previous approaches to avoid motion influences, such as the use of navigator echoes and cardiac gating are less common. Recently, the quality of EPI data was further improved by the use of parallel imaging (SENSE, Pruessmann et al. 1999; SMASH, Sodickson and Manning 1997) which can remove much of the image distortions due to local field inhomogeneities (Bammer et al. 2002). This has become especially important with the recent more common availability of clinical 3T scanners, because magnetic field inhomogeneity effects scale with the field. Another effect of magnetic field inhomogeneities is the presence of background gradients that interfere with the imaging gradients as well as the diffusion quantification. The imaging gradients themselves can also interfere with the diffusion quantification. This latter problem can simply be solved by placing the dephasing gradients directly next to the encoding and slice-selection gradients, avoiding interference. In the following, we will assume all of these parameters to be acceptable and focus only on the diffusion weighting to be attained for the purpose of trace imaging and the more involved anisotropy imaging and fiber tracking.

For a recent review of DTI data acquisition, see Basser and Jones (2002)

6.4.1 Trace Imaging

Trace imaging (van Gelderen et al. 1994) is currently the most common application of DTI. In most clinics, this consists of three measurements (x,y,z weighting) and addition of the scans. This will work well, as long as interference with imaging gradients is avoided (see above) and background gradients are limited. Actually, it is possible to perform trace imaging in a single scan in which most interference with background gradients is removed (Mori and van Zijl 1995; Wong et al. 1995; Chung et al. 1998). For correct quantification, it is prerequisite that no interfering imaging gradients are present during diffusion encoding, but this can be easily accomplished as outlined above. The recent availability of imaging gradients as strong as 8 G/cm on whole-body systems may make this sequence more popular, especially in view of the high quality images that can be attained

6.4.2 Anisotropy Imaging

In DTI, acquisition schemes need to be used that acquire all elements of this diffusion tensor in an optimal manner, i.e., as fast as possible and with the highest signal to noise ratio (SNR). Because the tensor is symmetric, DTI requires diffusion weighting along at least six independent axes plus a reference image. The latter should employ some minimal diffusion weighting to remove some unwanted coherence pathways as well as some flowing components (b-value of 50-100 s/mm^2). At the high value, weighting in all directions should be sufficient to obtain a well-measurable difference. This is not trivial, as signal loss due to weighting may be easily achieved along the fiber direction, but not as easily perpendicular to it. At present, b-values from 600-1000 s/mm^2 are most routinely used. Another factor that has to be optimized is the orientation of the gradients. As one can easily understand, the best combination of gradient orientations, without a priori knowledge of tensor orientation and any bias, is to distribute them uniformly in the 3D space. For example, for six orientations, it becomes an octahedral configuration. Recent important work by Jones et al. (1999b) has shown that optimum acquisition scheme for tensor component determination uses more than six directions, namely about 20-30 (Skare et al. 2000). Importantly, the number of reference scans should also be increased in proportion in order to maintain optimum SNR properties, namely about 1:6 (Skare et al. 2000). At our scanner we presently use 32 directions and 5 references. To avoid motion artifacts, it helps to acquire all directions separately and to align the individual diffusion-weighted images before performing the tensor analysis using multi-variate fitting.

Finally, two important issues have to always be kept in mind. First of all, when working at limited SNR, anisotropy values may increase and thus lead to erroneous interpretation of the data. Secondly, partial volume effects (with CSF or gray matter structures; Alexander et al. 2001; Pfefferbaum et al. 2003) may change the measured anisotropies, which consequently may show a resolution dependent effect. This may cause problems when comparing anisotropies between different research groups or even between normal controls and patients, where some atrophy or different choice of reference slice may be misinterpreted for a lesion. Such problems will obviously worsen for smaller brain structures.

Figure 6.3 demonstrates the types of images that are usually acquired and how the appearance of the image typically changes during data analysis.

The reader is also referred to the works by Pierpaoli and Basser (1996) and Pierpaoli et al. (1996) for further discussion of anisotropy imaging.

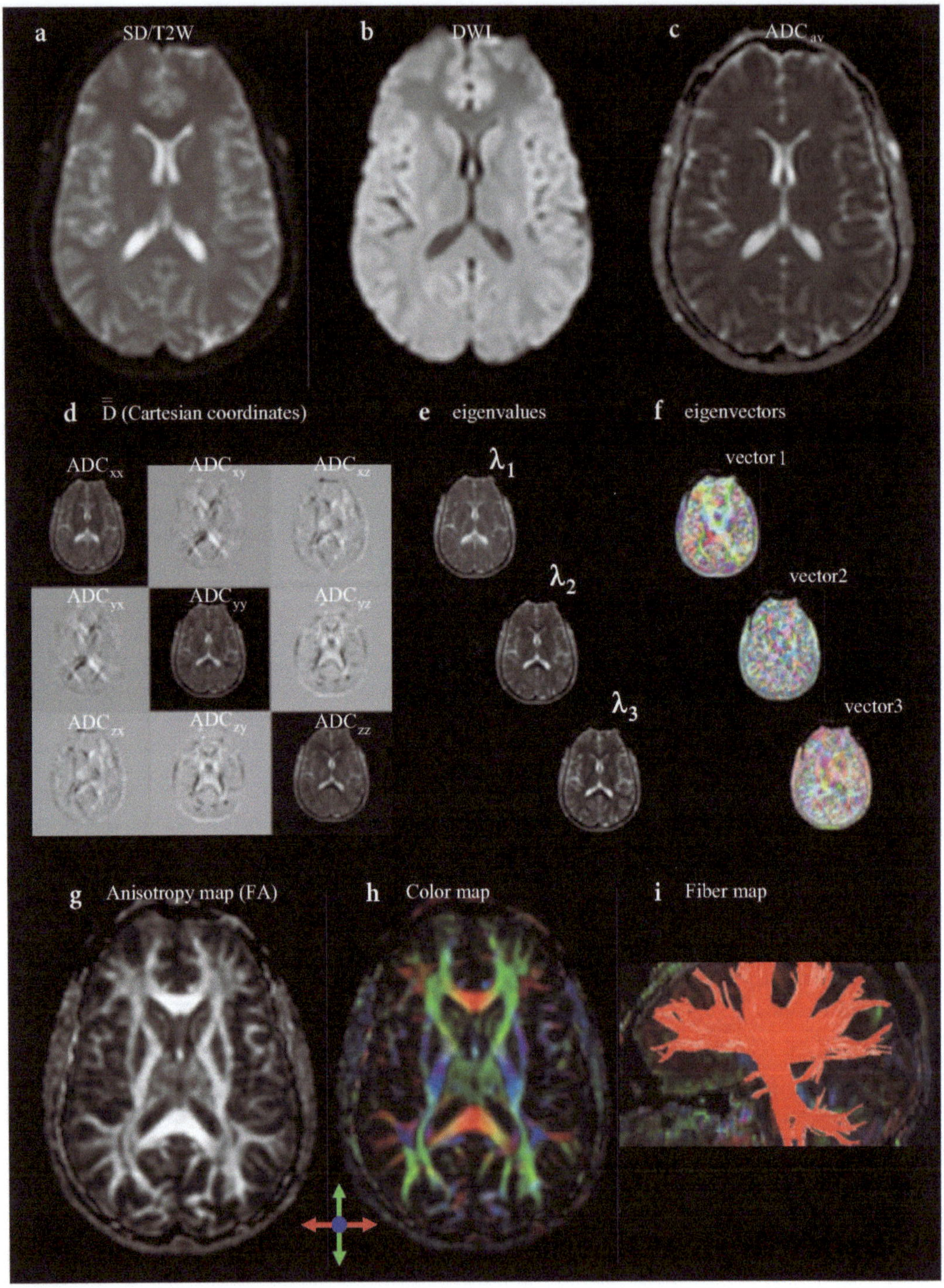

Fig. 6.3a–i. Different image types used in DTI. **a** b0 map (actually b ~ 50 s/mm^2); **b** DWI (b ~ 700 s/mm^2); **c** ADC$_{av}$ map; **d** tensor images in the cartesian (laboratory) reference frame; **e** tensor elements remaining after diagonalization, namely the eigenvalues: l_1, l_2, l_3; **f** eigenvectors; **g** FA map; **h** color-coded map showing fibers oriented right–left as *red*, anterior-posteriorly as *green*, and perpendicular to the plane as *blue*; intensity is proportional to FA; **i** fiber-tracking of the fibers passing through the left middle cerebral peduncle

6.5 Axonal Mapping/Fiber Tracking

Another parameter that can be obtained from DTI is the orientation of diffusion ellipsoids (eigenvectors). The most intuitive way to show the orientation is the vectors presentation, in which small lines (vector) indicate the orientations of the longest axis of diffusion ellipsoids. However, unless a small region is magnified, the vector orientation is often difficult to see. To overcome this problem, a color-coded scheme is used (Pajevic and Pierpaoli 1999; Makris et al. 1997). Examples are shown in Fig. 6.4 (left). In the color map, three orthogonal axes (e.g., right–left, superior–inferior, and anterior–posterior) are assigned to three principal colors (red, green, and blue). If a fiber is running at 45° from red and blue axes, it is assigned magenta, which is mixture of red and blue.

Assuming that the orientation of the largest component of the diagonalized diffusion tensor represents the orientation of dominant axonal tracts, DTI can provide a 3D vector field, in which each vector presents the fiber orientation (Fig. 6.4). Currently, there are several different approaches to reconstruct white matter tracts, which can be roughly divided into two types. Techniques classified in the first category are

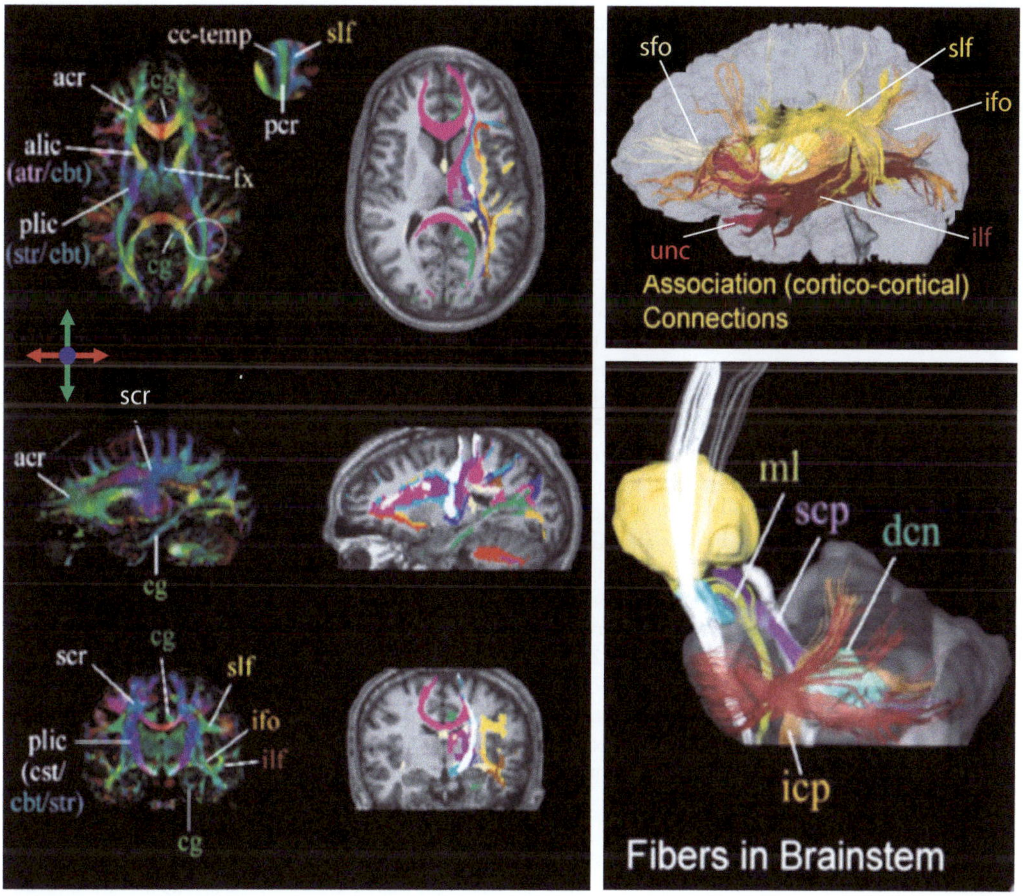

Fig. 6.4. Examples of brain fiber color maps (*left column*) and 3D-based fiber tracts projected in a plane (*middle column*) or shown in 3D space (*right column*). In the color maps, *blue*, *red*, and *green* indicate inferior (*i*)–superior (*s*), left–right, and anterior (*a*)–posterior, respectively. The 3D fiber tracts in the middle column are superimposed on MPRAGE images, showing that axonal mapping can be used to parcelate the white matter. *acr*, Anterior corona radiata; *alic*, anterior limb internal capsule; *atr*, anterior thalamic radiation; *cbt*, corticobulbar tract; *cg*, cingulum; *cp*, cerebellar peduncle; *cst*, corticospinal tract; *dcn*, deep cerebellar nuclei; *fx*, fornix; *icp*, inferior cerebellar peduncle; *ifo*, inferior fronto-occipital fasciculus; *ilf*, inferior longitudinal fasciculus; *ml*, medial lemniscus; *pcr*, posterior corona radiate; *plic*, posterior limb internal capsule; *scp*, superior cerebellar peduncle; *scr*, superior corona radiata; *sfo*, superior fronto-occipital fasciculus; *slf*, superior longitudinal fasciculus; *str*, superior thalamic radiation; *unc*, uncinate fasciculus. [Data reproduced with permission from Wakana et al. (2004)]

based on line propagation algorithms that use local tensor information for each step of the propagation. The main differences among techniques in this class stem from the way information from neighboring pixels is incorporated to define smooth trajectories or to minimize noise contributions. The second type of approach is based on global energy minimization to find the energetically most favorable path between two predetermined pixels. These methods have been recently reviewed (Mori and van Zijl 2002), but many more innovations and improvements are expected in the coming years. When designing or using such technologies, it is important to understand the basis of the anisotropy contrast in DTI and the limitations imposed by using a macroscopic technique to visualize microscopic restrictions. For instance, when using such vector fields to track axonal pathways, one must always be aware of the influence of noise, partial volume effects and the effect of termination criteria (Mori and van Zijl 2002; Lori et al. 1999, 2002; Mangin et al. 2002; Lazar and Alexander 2001). The following main points should be kept in mind. First, conventional DTI data acquisition and processing methods are challenged by a voxel containing more than one population of axonal tracts with different orientations. Second, DTI cannot provide information on cellular-level axonal connectivity. Multiple axons from individual cells may merge into or branch out from one voxel. Within a voxel, cellular-level axonal information of multiple compartments is averaged. The third important limitation is that afferent and efferent pathways of axonal tracts cannot be judged from the direction of water diffusion in a voxel. The question that often arises is therefore what tractography will be able to provide. Based on the relative size of the voxel and the human brain and recent experimental results (Wakana et al. 2004), it should be safe to say that it can rev matter tracts (e.g., see the atlas data in Fig. 6.3). The possibility to study crossing fibers has also been suggested (Frank 2001; Tuch et al. 2001; Wiegell et al. 2000), but more research is needed in this area.

6.6 Applications of Quantitative DWI/DTI to the Brain

Most applications were recently reviewed in an article by Dong et al. (2004), and in special issues of *NMR in Biomedicine* (Vol. 15, issues 7,8, 2002) and the *European Journal of Radiology* (Vol. 45, issue 3, 2003). As mentioned in the introduction, the structural organization of the brain comprises multiple microscopic components, including microtubules, cell membranes, axons, myelin, and macromolecules arranged into macroscopically identifiable structures such as the fiber bundles. This architecture restricts the Brownian motion of water, superimposing varying degrees of anisotropy depending on the location in the brain. Diffusion, probing this water motion, therefore yields an in vivo measurement of a physical property rather than an MRI property such as T1, T2 and magnetization transfer (Horsfield and Jones 2002). An alteration of such a physical property in case of disease can represent a distinct and advantageous window for clinical analysis. Thus, because microscopic information is provided by this technique, a higher sensitivity for lesion detection is expected, either in diseases bearing focal lesions or diffuse abnormalities. Such a higher sensitivity compared to conventional MRI would allow early intervention, which is considered to be crucial in diseases such as stroke. Refinement of diagnosis with more precise anatomical information, for instance, involvement of surrounding anatomical structures in tumors and more precise localization of lesions will lead to better correlations with clinical scales. This may offer substantial benefits to patients including potentially better treatment choices and improved follow-up information.

6.6.1 Normal Control Values of Diffusion Parameters During Early Development and Aging

Although studies that evaluate focal lesions usually use the correspondent contralateral areas for comparison, studies that include more diffuse lesions commonly need their own group of normal controls. Tables 6.2 and 6.3 summarize normative anisotropy (FA and $A_{fiber} = RA / \sqrt{2}$) and average apparent diffusion coefficient (ADC_{av}) values reported in the literature for several structures in white matter (WM) and gray matter (GM), respectively. The average diffusion constant was first used in the stroke literature (Mori and van Zijl 1995; Decanniere et al. 1995) and is defined by:

$$ADC_{av} = Tr(\overline{\overline{D}})/3 \qquad [6.11]$$

Even though (ADC_{av}, FA, and A_{fiber} are orientation-independent quantities, care has to be taken in their interpretation. The reason is the influence of partial

Table 6.2. Diffusion parameters in some normal brain white matter regions

	Age	ADC_{av}	FA	Afiber=A = RA / √2	Nominal voxel volume (μl)	Reference
	27–36 years	0.69[e]	0.87[e]		8.7	PIERPAOLI et al. (1996)
	~25–40	0.75–0.88	0.78–0.81	0.55–0.63	18.1	ULUG and VAN ZIJL (1999)
	23–47 years	0.72[e]	0.71[e]	0.50	11–18	SHIMONY et al. (1999)
cc	23–76 years		0.57–0.70[f]		6.9	PFEFFERBAUM et al. (2000)
	Mean age 28±11 years	0.74–0.80[$]	0.65–0.71		17	ARFANAKIS et al. (2002)
	Mean age 26±8 years		0.70–0.72		4.4	SUN et al. (2003)
	19–34 years	0.79–0.81		0.64–0.66	9.3	WESTERHAUSEN et al. (2003)
	Preterm[a]; full term[a]	1.0–1.3 (plic) 1.1 (plic)		0.07–0.16 0.23	28	HUPPI et al. (1998, 2001)
	Full term[b]	1.0–1.2		0.13–0.21	11–28	NEIL et al. (1998, 2002)
	0 years[c] 2–10 years[c]	0.9–1.4 0.6–0.8		0.14–0.30 0.47–0.55	N/A	NEIL et al. (2002); MUKHERJEE et al. (2002)
	27–36 years	0.64e	0.76[e]		8.7	PIERPAOLI et al. (1996)
ic	~25–40	0.69–0.70	0.71–0.74	0.50–0.52	18	ULUG and VAN ZIJL (1999)
	23–47 years	0.70–0.72[e]	0.59–0.65[e]	0.39–0.45	10-18	SHIMONY et al. (1999)
	Mean age 28±11 years	0.65–0.67[$]	0.54–0.64		17	ARFANAKIS et al. (2002)
	Mean age 26±8 years		0.46–0.57		4.4	SUN et al. (2003)
	Preterm[a]; full term[a]	1.5–2.0 1.2		0.04–0.13 0.17	28	HUPPI et al. (1998, 2001)
	Preterm[d]; full term[b]	1.4–1.9 1.0–1.5		0.07–0.12	11–28	NEIL et al. (1998)
	7–30 years	0.84	0.46		18	EICHLER et al. (2002)
	27–36 years	0.65–0.72[e]	0.46–0.87[e]		8.7	PIERPAOLI et al. (1996)
wm	~25–40	0.75	0.70	0.48	18	ULUG and VAN ZIJL (1999)
	23–47 years	0.78–0.80[e]	0.33–0.42[e]	0.21–0.26	10–18	SHIMONY et al. (1999)
	23–37 years 56–85 years	0.81 0.91	0.24 0.22		31	O'SULLIVAN et al. (2001)
	23–76 years		0.35–0.44[e]		6.9	PFEFFERBAUM et al. (2000)
	35±7 years		0.42–0.45		63	STEEL et al. (2001)
	Mean age 26±8 years		0.42–0.64		4.4	SUN et al. (2003)

cc, Corpus callosum; ic, internal capsule; plic, posterior limb; wm, white matter.

[a] Preterm <38 weeks; full term ≥38 weeks; taken from Figs. 3 and 4 and Table 6.2 in HUPPI et al. (1998); HUPPI et al. (1998, 2001) gave RA as a percentage. We have recalculated this to A_{fiber} by dividing by 100* $\sqrt{2}$

[b] Table 6.2, NEIL et al. (1998).

[c] From Fig. 6.1 in NEIL et al. (2002).

[d] Figs. 4 and 5, NEIL et al. (1998).

[e] Calculated from the eigenvalues given in the chapter.

[f] Deduced from graph; these values are after spatial warping, a procedure that increases the measured FA by about 10%.

Table 6.3. Diffusion parameters in some normal brain gray matter regions

	Age	ADCav	FA	Afiber=A = RA / $\sqrt{2}$	Nominal voxel volume (μl)	Reference
	Full term[a]	1.16-1.18		0.06	11–28	NEIL et al. (1998)
GM (cortex)	27–36 years	0.83[b]	0.20[b]		8.7	PIERPAOLI et al. (1996)
	~25-40	0.93	0.39	0.22	18	ULUG and VAN ZIJL (1999)
	23–47 years	0.93[b]	0.09-0.15[b]	0.05-0.09	10–18	SHIMONY et al. (1999)
	Full term[a]	1.08		0.08	11–28	NEIL et al. (1998)
tha	~25–40	0.73	0.43	0.25	18	ULUG and VAN ZIJL (1999)
	23–47 years	0.72[b]	0.30[b]	0.19	10–18	SHIMONY et al. (1999)
	Full term[a]	1.24		0.07	11–28	NEIL et al. (1998)
hcn	27–36 years	0.67[b]	0.17[b]		8.7	PIERPAOLI et al. (1996)
	~25–40	0.68	0.41	0.22	1.9×1.9×5	Ulug and VAN ZIJL (1999)
	23–47 years	0.80[b]	0.17[b]	0.10	10–18	SHIMONY et al. (1999)
	Full term[a]	1.18		0.07	11–28	NEIL et al. (1998)
put	~25–40	0.72	0.42	0.23	18	Ulug and VAN ZIJL (1999)
	23-47 years	0.73[b]	0.14[b]	0.08	10-18	SHIMONY et al. (1999)
hf	24-49 years	0.28[b]	0.01		8.7	ASSAF et al. (2003)

gm, Gray matter; tha, thalamus; hcn, head of caudate nucleus; put, putamen; hf, hippocampal formation.
[a] Tables 6.1 and 6.2, NEIL et al. (1998).
[b] Calculated from the eigenvalues given in the chapter.

volume effects, which may appear in more or less fashion depending on the voxel size, b-value, size of region of interest, and encoding and slice directions. An excellent overview of the effect of these factors on DTI calculations has been given by ALEXANDER et al. (2001). At commonly used b-values, anisotropy values for large WM structures will be less affected by partial volume errors and thus more reliable and probably higher than those in smaller structures, where resolution limitations prohibit good definition of the structure in a DTI map. This could for instance explain why the FA values by PIERPAOLI et al. (1996) and ULUG et al. (1999) are consistently higher than by other groups. On the other hand, the data by these two groups are older (acquired around 1995–1997) and may have had lower SNR, thereby increasing the anisotropy. For smaller structures than the corpus callosum, partial volume effects with crossing fibers, some gray matter, and/or CSF will reduce anisotropy. To get an impression of the accuracy of the anisotropy values for a certain ROI, some authors evaluate the agreement in value between the anisotropies in the comprising voxels. A large variation would indicate involvement of many different structures, while a high coherence would support the anisotropy value for a single structure (PFEFFERBAUM et al. 2000). Thus, the present tables should only be used as a general guideline for trends, while better numbers at smaller voxel size (more homogeneous voxel composition per voxel) are to be expected in the near future due to the availability of much higher signal-to-noise ratio (SNR) through the advent of stronger gradients (already up to 8 G/cm for whole-body gradients) and higher magnetic field strengths (3 Tesla) in the clinic. Further improvement in accuracy will occur when individual structures in white matter are selected though fiber tracking, such as performed by STIELTJES et al. (2001) for the brainstem. However,

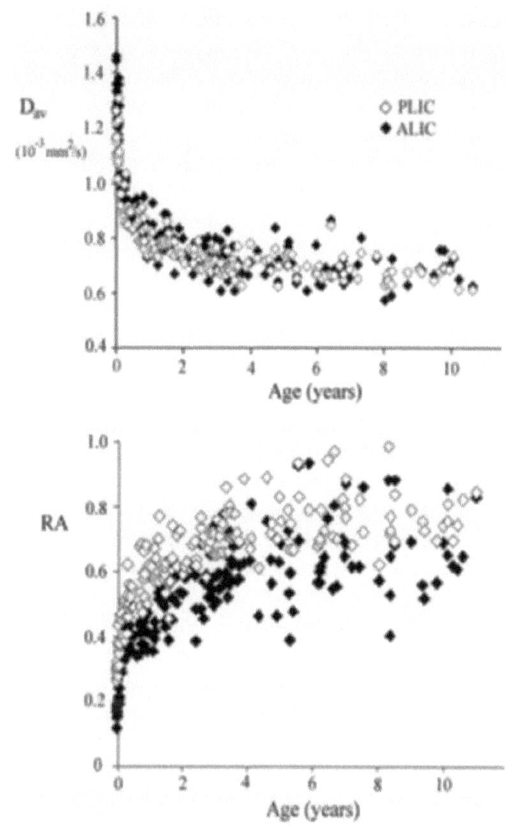

Fig. 6.5. Plots of ADC_{av} and RA of the posterior (*PLIC*) and anterior lobes (*ALIC*) of internal capsule as a function of age for the first 10 years of life. The data start at 26 weeks of gestational age (very high ADC_{av} and very low RA) (see also Table 6.2) and the values quickly normalize a few months after birth and are almost completely settled after two years. [Data reproduced with permission from Neil et al. (2002)]

even in that situation, the final anisotropy will depend on the thresholds chosen for tracking.

In pre-term and full-term newborn brain, ADC_{av} values are considerably higher and anisotropy values considerably lower than in adults (Huppi et al. 1998, 2001; Neil et al. 1998, 2002). During development (preterm-full-term-adult), the ADC_{av} of white matter (Table 6.2) decreases with age whereas anisotropy increases reflecting regional differences (Huppi et al. 1998; Neil et al. 1998, 2002). An example is shown for the internal capsule in Fig. 6.5 (Neil et al. 2002). The anisotropy increase in white matter has been described to happen in two distinct phases. The first, called "pre-myelinating state", has thus far only been detected by DTI, as T1 and T2-weighted sequences are not sensitive to these changes. The second phase of increase in RA corresponds with myelin production and maturation. The pre-myelination phase was attributed to changes in the cytoarchitecture of the axons. In this respect it is important to consider recent work by Beaulieu (2002) and Beaulieu and Allen (1994) showing that the magnitude of the diffusion anisotropy correspond to restrictions imposed by the axonal membrane and not by the smaller structures within the axon. The rate of anisotropy change differs between different white matter structures (Neil et al. 2002). This was for instance found for the internal capsule, where the posterior lobe (PLIC) myelinates before the anterior lobe (ALIC), leading to differences in anisotropy and average diffusion constants between these structures during early development. Another interesting insight into the physiology of the developing brain provided by DTI is the observation of transient high anisotropy in the cortical gray matter during the period from 26–32 weeks of gestation, similar to what is observed in the developing mouse brain (Mori et al. 2001). A good correlation with the period of intense neuronal migration, in which the cytoarchitecture of the cortex includes radial glial fibers and radially oriented dendrites of the pyramidal cells was noticed.

A decrease in FA and increase in ADC_{av} are seen with normal aging (Pfefferbaum et al. 2000; Moseley 2002; Nusbaum et al. 2001; O'Sullivan et al. 1999). Especially important in such aging studies is the analysis of preservation of the white matter volume. Atrophy may lead to an artificial reduction in anisotropy and increase in the average diffusion constant. To assess this, Pfefferbaum et al. (2000) measured so-called intervoxel coherence, which reflects the agreement between anisotropy values of the voxels included in the ROIs chosen for the different structures. Such coherence could be shown to be preserved along normal aging, indicating that the DTI changes are related to microstructural deterioration.

6.6.2 Diffusion Imaging of Acute Ischemia

The possibility of early (Moseley et al. 1990a; Baird and Warach 1998; Warach et al. 1995; Lutsep et al. 1997; Sorenson et al. 1996; Ricci et al. 1999) and accurate (Gonzalez et al. 1999) detection of stroke, along with the distinction of potentially salvageable ischemic tissue (penumbra) (Baird and Warach 1998; Donnan and Davis 2002) has aroused intense research and patient management change in the area, leading to the concept that "time is brain".

DWI shows conspicuous hypersignal intensity within minutes after the onset of ischemia (MOSELEY et al. 1990a; MINEMATSU et al. 1992; DAVIS et al. 1994; PROVENZALE and SORENSEN 1999), believed to be caused by cytotoxic edema due to failure of Na^{+}/K^{+} membrane pump, which occurs after disruption of oxidative energy metabolism. As explained earlier, the ADC maps have to be analyzed in conjunction with DWI, as the hypersignal on the latter can be due to residual T2 contrast, described as "T2 shine-through" phenomena (ULUG et al. 1997; PROVENZALE and SORENSEN 1999; HUISMAN 2003). A true restricted-diffusion image displays hypersignal on DWI and hyposignal on ADC maps. Employing these images, early detection of stroke is usually straightforward, despite the description of some pitfalls such as reversibility of DWI changes as well as variation on the signal behavior of DWI and ADC along the time course of stroke (PROVENZALE and SORENSEN 1999; SCHLAUG et al. 1997). The mismatch between perfusion weighted image (PWI) and DWI indicates the presence of a penumbra of reduced flow around the ischemic core identified by the diffusion deficit (SORENSON et al. 1996; SCHLAUG et al. 1999). Such a region contains potentially salvageable tissue, allowing prompt intervention with thrombolytic therapy if diagnosed within the first few hours of onset. The role of DTI in the acute stroke scenario has gained importance through the realization that the acquisition of a diffusion constant in a single direction may lead to erroneous and confusing interpretation of stroke pathology and lesion evolution. This issue came about in the human literature when confusion arose about the length of the diffusion-constant normalization period after ischemia (SORENSON et al. 1996; WELCH et al. 1995; WARACH et al. 1996a,b), a problem that was due to choice of different directions of the diffusion-weighting gradients by different groups. This confusion could be addressed by using the trace of the tensor (WARACH et al. 1997), as first suggested in animal studies (VAN GELDEREN et al. 1994; MORI and VAN ZIJL 1995; ULUG et al. 1997).

One point that is a topic of much discussion is whether the magnitude of the diffusion drop is an indicator of the salvageability of the tissue in the penumbra. Based on animal studies, we do not believe that this is the case. For instance, cat studies at high time resolution (DECANNIERE et al. 1995; DAVIS et al. 1994) show that the average diffusion constant drops about 30% during cardiac arrest. A small initial drop of a few percent was noticed in the diffusion constant upon occlusion in an ischemia model (DAVIS et al. 1994), but this was followed by an almost instantaneous steep large drop after 2 min, presumably upon depolarization. No correlation between the severity of penumbral involvement and the absolute value of the diffusion constant has been found in humans, and it is probably the case that variation in ADC_{av} values reflects partial voluming between fully depolarized and polarized cells with normal ADCs.

The role of anisotropy measurements is not defined yet, although some evidence points to DTI as a more refined prognostic tool potentially yielding better clinical correlation (SOTAK 2002; SORENSEN et al. 1999; YANG et al. 1999; GILLARD et al. 2001; KUNIMATSU et al. 2003). Similar to ADC_{av} values, anisotropy values also appear to vary depending on the time course of stroke (YANG et al. 1999) with some patients presenting with increased values in the acute and subacute phase (relative to contralateral), others with increased values acutely and reduced values subacutely, and a third group with reduced values both acutely and subacutely. All patients had reduced anisotropy in the chronic phase. Increased values in the acute phase have been explained on the basis of reduction of the extracellular space after intracellular accumulation of water with increased tortuosity of membranes leading to greater restriction of water, whereas, decreased values may reflect extracellular edema and cell lysis. Anisotropy values within 12 h of stroke correlated well with clinical and outcome scales. Evaluation with the full-tensor approach theoretically improves lesion detection and gives better discrimination on white and gray matter lesions (SORENSEN et al. 1999; MUKHERJEE et al. 2000). Assessment of chronic infarcts and correlation with prognosis and follow-up is another potential field for DTI (KUNIMATSU et al. 2003; PIERPAOLI et al. 2001). DWI (LIU et al. 1999) and DTI (ARFANAKIS et al. 2002) have also been employed as a very sensible method for early detection and evaluation of diffuse axonal injury, such as experienced after trauma. The use of DTI for identification of salvageable tissue and subsequent intervention in cases of trauma has also approached (JONES et al. 2000). Recently, a fast clinician-friendly approach (C-FAST) to score six bilateral white matter regions (in the centrum semiovale, genu and splenium of the corpus callosum, anterior and posterior limbs of the internal capsules) on anisotropy maps was proposed as a prognostic tool (PTAK et al. 2003).

DWI and DTI have also been shown to detect hypoxic-ischemic lesions early in the neonatal period (HUPPI et al. 2001; INDER et al. 1999), although a pseudonormalization of diffusion parameters at about 1 week after injury has to be taken into account (McKinstry et al. 2002). DTI acquired on the first day may therefore lead to misleading results. In the chronic phase, DTI with color-coded maps and fiber-tracking has shown that there may be variability in the involvement of pathways in patients with the same diagnosis, as in periventricular leukomalacia (PVL) (Hoon et al. 2002). This information could be helpful to provide a more specific localization of lesions in the white matter, better understanding of the pathophysiology of the disease what would lead to better clinical correlation and better oriented therapeutic intervention. DTI parameters and fiber-tracking were also tested in patients with congenital hemiplegia (Glenn et al. 2003) and stands as a promising technique for the assessment of motor dysfunction in the pediatric population.

6.6.3
Initial Applications in Other Diseases

As DTI reflects both axonal and myelin restrictions, DTI and DWI are expected to be very useful in the assessment of disorders in which these microstructures are changed. This is especially so for white matter diseases (Horsfield and Jones 2002), which are expected to show an increase in average apparent diffusion constant and/or a decrease in diffusion anisotropy. The availability of fiber tracking technologies (Mori and van Zijl 2002) may make it possible to relate such diseases to specific fiber bundles. For instance, the cingulum (Sun et al. 2003) and frontotemporal and frontoparietal tracts (Burns et al. 2003) have been sought for in schizophrenic patients, the cortical-spinal tracts in multiple sclerosis (MS) (Wilson et al. 2003) and amyotrophic lateral sclerosis (ALS) (Sach et al. 2004), and the temporal-parietal white matter in dyslexia (Klingberg et al. 2000).

Leukodystrophies, as primary white matter diseases, comprise a very appealing group to be evaluated by DTI. Although one study suggested that DWI could differentiate dysmyelinating (primary problem with myelin production) from demyelinating (secondary destruction of myelin) diseases (Ono et al. 1997), which would potentially contribute to the diagnosis of this challenging group of diseases, this still has to be confirmed by other studies. Decreases in FA and increases in ADC_{av} were able to reproduce the histopathological classification that is currently used in adrenoleukodystrophy (ALD), suggesting that DTI can be helpful to follow progression of the disease (Ito et al. 2001; Eichler et al. 2002). Abnormal fiber-tracking of the genu of the corpus callosum has been demonstrated in a patient with X-ALD, in agreement with lesions shown by conventional MRI and neuropsychological evaluation (Mori et al. 2002).

The use of DWI to differentiate tumor from abscesses and arachnoid cysts from epidermoid cysts are well recognized in clinical practice, despite some pitfalls (Bergui et al. 2001). Abscesses, with their high content of macromolecules, cause restriction of diffusion, while tumors usually do not. Exceptions to this rule would be tumors with high cellularity that would also lead to decrease in diffusivity. Epidermoid cysts present with restricted diffusion signs, whereas arachnoid cysts display signal that follows CSF. For tumors, besides the attempts on quantification for differentiation of tumor infiltration versus edema and even for tumor grading and histologic typing (Dong et al. 2004; Sinha et al. 2002; Bastin et al. 2002), DTI and fiber-tracking can be used to better localize eloquent tracts and help the planning of maximum function-preserving surgeries (Tummala et al. 2003). Along with tumors, epilepsy presents with the option of surgical management and DTI has contributed to evaluate the lesion itself as well as the extension of abnormal tissue (Arfanakis et al. 2002; Eriksson et al. 2001).

A final application of DTI that looks promising is the assessment of the spine. This work is just starting and still has to resolve many issues, especially related to motion artifacts and the low SNR in the small spinal structures that need to be acquired at high spatial resolution (Ries et al. 2000; Demir et al. 2003; Clark and Werring 2002).

6.7
Conclusions

In the mid 1990s, DWI developed from a technically difficult and novel approach to a routine acquisition technique on clinical scanners. It now takes under 1 min to be acquired and can bring valuable information and pathophysiologic insight in many diseases. The same transition is currently happening in DTI, which is expected to contribute much novel clinical and neuroscientific information presently not accessible by other technologies. For instance, DTI is the only approach for tracking brain white matter fibers non-invasively in the human brain. In combination with functional MRI, which can outline activated cortical networks, DTI may thus provide clues on functional connectivity. DTI is also increasingly been used to demonstrate subtle connectivity anomalies in a variety of dysfunctions, such as cerebral palsy, cancer, stroke, dyslexia, or diseases including multiple sclerosis and schizophrenia. Before DTI can become true clinical routine, some progress is still needed. This relates to factors such as scan time and therefore, patient tolerance, and the complexity of post-processing (now mostly off-line) required for the method. These issues are already being addressed. For instance, clinical equipment with whole-body gradients of up to 8 G/cm is becoming available, which, together with the clinical availability of 3-Tesla magnets will allow the use of multi-directional DTI at high spatial resolution (around 2×2×2 mm^3) in a few minutes. Another issue that is often discussed is which quantitative parameter to choose, FA, RA, etc. Actually, these anisotropies are all related and the only advantage of using one versus the other will be based on contrast to noise, which depends on anisotropy of the particular structure being studied. It would be most helpful if all researchers would report the eigenvalues so that others can calculate any parameter they want. A further essential consideration for data analysis and reporting is the influence of partial volume effects between different structures. This is especially problematic for group studies or development studies.

However, it is safe to say that DTI and tractography provide us with a new opportunity for quantitative diagnosis of white matter structures in living humans and to assess changes due to brain disease.

References

Alexander AL, Hasan KM, Lazar M, Tsuruda JS, Parker DL (2001) Analysis of partial volume effects in diffusion-tensor MRI. Magn Reson Med 45:770-780

Andrasko J (1976b) Water diffusion permeability of human erythrocytes studied by a pulsed gradient NMR technique. Biochim Biophys Acta 428:304-311

Arfanakis K et al (2002) Diffusion tensor MR imaging in diffuse axonal injury. AJNR Am J Neuroradiol 23:794-802

Arfanakis K et al (2002) Diffusion tensor MRI in temporal lobe epilepsy. Magn Reson Imaging 20:511-519

Assaf BA et al (2003) Diffusion tensor imaging of the hippocampal formation in temporal lobe epilepsy. AJNR Am J Neuroradiol 24:1857-1862

Assaf Y, Cohen Y (2000) Assignment of the water slow-diffusing component in the central nervous system using q-space diffusion MRS: implications for fiber tract imaging. Magn Reson Med 43:191-199

Baird AE, Warach S (1998) Magnetic resonance imaging of acute stroke. J Cereb Blood Flow Metab 18:583-609

Bammer R et al (2002)Diffusion tensor imaging using single-shot SENSE-EPI. Magn Reson Med 48:128-136

Basser PJ, Jones DK (2002) Diffusion-tensor MRI: theory, experimental design and data analysis - a technical review. NMR Biomed 15:456-467

Basser PJ, Pierpaoli C (1996) Microstructural and physiological features of tissues elucidated by quantitative-diffusion-tensor MRI. J Magn Reson B 111:209-219

Basser PJ, Mattiello J, LeBihan D (1994a) MR diffusion tensor spectroscopy and imaging. Biophys J 66:259-267

Basser PJ, Mattiello J, LeBihan D (1994b) Estimation of the effective self-diffusion tensor from the NMR spin echo. J Magn Reson B 103:247-254

Basser PJ, Pajevic S, Pierpaoli C, Duda J, Aldroubi A (2000) In vitro fiber tractography using DT-MRI data. Magn Reson Med 44:625-632

Bastin ME, Sinha S, Whittle IR, Wardlaw JM (2002) Measurements of water diffusion and T1 values in peritumoural oedematous brain. Neuroreport 13:1335-1340

Beaulieu C (2002) The basis of anisotropic water diffusion in the nervous system – a technical review. NMR Biomed 15:435-455

Beaulieu C, Allen PS (1994) Determinants of anisotropic water diffusion in nerves. Magn Reson Med 31:394-400

Bergui M, Zhong J, Bradac GB, Sales S (2001) Diffusion-weighted images of intracranial cyst-like lesions. Neuroradiology 43:824-829

Burns J et al (2003) Structural disconnectivity in schizophrenia: a diffusion tensor magnetic resonance imaging study. Br J Psychiatry 182:439-443

Callaghan PT, Coy A, MacGowan D, Packer KJ, Zelaya FO (1991) Diffraction-like effects in NMR diffusion studies of fluids in porous solids. Nature 351:467-469

Callaghan PT, Codd SL, Seymour JD (1999) Spatial coherence phenomena arising from translational spin motion in gradient spin echo experiments. Concepts Magn Reson 11:181-202

Chun T, Ulug AM, van Zijl PC (1998) Single-shot diffusion-weighted trace imaging on a clinical scanner. Magn Reson Med 40:622-628

Clark CA, Werring DJ (2002) Diffusion tensor imaging in spinal cord: methods and applications - a review. NMR Biomed 15:578-586

Cohen Y, Assaf Y (2002) High b-value q-space analyzed diffusion-weighted MRS and MRI in neuronal tissues - a technical review. NMR Biomed 15:516-542

Conturo TE, McKinstry RC, Akbudak E, Robinson BH (1996) Encoding of anisotropic diffusion with tetrahedral gradients: a general mathematical diffusion formalism and experimental results. Magn Reson Med 35:399-412

Conturo TE et al (1999) Tracking neuronal fiber pathways in the living human brain. Proc Natl Acad Sci USA 96:10422-10427

Cory DG, Garroway AN (1990) Measurement of translational displacement probabilities by NMR – an indicator of compartmentation. Magn Reson Med 14:435-444

Davis D et al (1994) Rapid monitoring of changes in water diffusion coefficients during reversible ischemia in cat and rat brain. Magn Reson Med 31:454-460

Decanniere C, Eleff S, Davis D, van Zijl PCM (1995) Correlation of rapid changes in the average water diffusion constant and the concentrations of lactate and ATP breakdown products during global ischemia in cat brain. Magn Reson Med 34:343-352

Demir A et al (2003) Diffusion-weighted MR imaging with apparent diffusion coefficient and apparent diffusion tensor maps in cervical spondylotic myelopathy. Radiology 229:37-43

Dong Q et al (2004) Clinical applications of diffusion tensor imaging. J Magn Reson Imaging 19:6-18

Donnan GA, Davis SM (2002) Neuroimaging, the ischaemic penumbra, and selection of patients for acute stroke therapy. Lancet Neurol 1:417-425

Eichler FS et al (2002) Proton MR spectroscopic and diffusion tensor brain MR imaging in X-linked adrenoleukodystrophy: initial experience. Radiology 225:245-252

Eriksson SH, Rugg-Gunn FJ, Symms MR, Barker GJ, Duncan JS (2001) Diffusion tensor imaging in patients with epilepsy and malformations of cortical development. Brain 124:617-626

Frank LR (2001) Anisotropy in high angular resolution diffusion-weighted MRI. Magn Reson Med 45:935-939

Gillard JH et al (2001) MR diffusion tensor imaging of white matter tract disruption in stroke at 3 T. Br J Radiol 74:642-647

Glenn OA et al (2003) DTI-based three-dimensional tractography detects differences in the pyramidal tracts of infants and children with congenital hemiparesis. J Magn Reson Imaging 18:641-648

Gonzalez RG et al (1999) Diffusion-weighted MR imaging: diagnostic accuracy in patients imaged within 6 hours of stroke symptom onset. Radiology 210:155-162

Hoon AH Jr et al (2002) Diffusion tensor imaging of periventricular leukomalacia shows affected sensory cortex white matter pathways. Neurology 59:752-756

Horsfield MA, Jones DK (2002) Applications of diffusion-weighed and diffusion tensor MRI to white matter diseases. NMR Biomed 15:570-577

Huisman TA (2003)Diffusion-weighted imaging: basic concepts and application in cerebral stroke and head trauma. Eur Radiol 13:2283-2297

Huppi PS et al (1998) Microstructural development of human newborn cerebral white matter assessed in vivo by diffusion tensor magnetic resonance imaging. Pediatr Res 44:584-590

Huppi PS et al (2001) Microstructural brain development after perinatal cerebral white matter injury assessed by diffusion tensor magnetic resonance imaging. Pediatrics 107:455-460

Inder T et al (1999) Early detection of periventricular leukomalacia by diffusion-weighted magnetic resonance imaging techniques. J Pediatr 134:631-634

Ito R et al (2001) Diffusion tensor brain MR imaging in X-linked cerebral adrenoleukodystrophy. Neurology 56:544-547

Jones DK, Simmons A, Williams SC, Horsfield MA (1999a) Non-invasive assessment of axonal fiber connectivity in the human brain via diffusion tensor MRI. Magn Reson Med 42:37-41

Jones DK, Horsfield MA, Simmons A (1999b) Optimal strategies for measuring diffusion in anisotropic systems by magnetic resonance imaging. Magn Reson Med 42:515-525

Jones DK et al (2000) Cluster analysis of diffusion tensor magnetic resonance images in human head injury. Neurosurgery 47:306-313; discussion 313-314

Karger J, Pfeifer H, Heink W (1988) Principles and application of self-diffusion measurements by nuclear magnetic resonance. Adv Magn Reson 12:1-89

Klingberg T et al (2000) Microstructure of temporo-parietal white matter as a basis for reading ability: evidence from diffusion tensor magnetic resonance imaging. Neuron 25:493-500

Kunimatsu A et al (2003) Three-dimensional white matter tractography by diffusion tensor imaging in ischaemic stroke involving the corticospinal tract. Neuroradiology 45:532-535

Lazar M, Alexander AL (2001) Proceeding of International Society of Magnetic Resonance in Medicine 506, Glasgow, UK

Le Bihan D (2003)Looking into the functional architecture of the brain with diffusion MRI. Nat Rev Neurosci 4:469-480

Le Bihan D, van Zijl P (2002) From the diffusion coefficient to the diffusion tensor. NMR Biomed 15:431-434

Le Bihan D et al (1986) MR imaging of intravoxel incoherent motions: application to diffusion and perfusion in neurologic disorders. Radiology 161:401-407

Lim KO, Helpern JA (2002) Neuropsychiatric applications of DTI - a review. NMR Biomed 15:587-593

Liu AY, Maldjian JA, Bagley LJ, Sinson GP, Grossman RI (1999) Traumatic brain injury: diffusion-weighted MR imaging findings. AJNR Am J Neuroradiol 20:1636-1641

Lori NF, Akbuda E, Snyder AZ, Shimony JS, Conturo TE (1999) International Society of Magnetic Resonance in Medicine 775, Denver, CO

Lori NF, Akbudak JS, Shimony TS, Snyder RK, Conturo TE (2002) Diffusion tensor fiber tracking of brani connectivity: reliability analysis and biological results. NMR Biomed 15:494-515

Lutsep HL et al (1997) Clinical utility of diffusion-weighted magnetic resonance imaging in the assessment of ischemic stroke. Ann Neurol 41:574-580

Makris N et al (1997) Morphometry of in vivo human white matter association pathways with diffusion weighted magnetic resonance imaging. Ann Neurol 42:951-962

Mangin JF, Poupon C, Clark C, Le Bihan D, Bloch I (2002) Distortion correction and robust tensor estimation for MR diffusion imaging. Med Image Anal 6:191-198

McKinstry RC et al (2002) A prospective, longitudinal diffusion tensor imaging study of brain injury in newborns. Neurology 59:824-833

Minematsu K et al (1992) Diffusion-weighted magnetic resonance imaging: rapid and quantitative detection of focal brain ischemia. Neurology 42:235-240

Moonen CT, van Zijl PC, Le Bihan D, DesPres D (1990) In vivo NMR diffusion spectroscopy: 31P application to phosphorus metabolites in muscle. Magn Reson Med 13:467-477

Mori S, van Zijl PC (2002) Fiber tracking: principles and strategies - a technical review. NMR Biomed 15:468-480

Mori S, van Zijl PCM (1995) Diffusion weighting by the trace of the diffusion tensor within a single scan. Magn Reson Med 33:41-52

Mori S, Crain BJ, Chacko VP, van Zijl PCM (1999) Three dimensional tracking of axonal projections in the brain by magnetic resonance imaging. Ann Neurol 45:265-269

Mori S et al (2001) Diffusion tensor imaging of the developing mouse brain. Magn Reson Med 46:18-23

Mori S et al (2002) Imaging cortical association tracts in human brain. Magn Reson Med 47:215-223

Moseley M (2002) Diffusion tensor imaging and aging - a review. NMR Biomed 15:553-560

Moseley ME et al (1990a) Early detection of regional cerebral ischemia in cats: comparison of diffusion- and T2-weighted MRI and spectroscopy. Magn Reson Med 14:330-346
Moseley ME et al (1990b) Diffusion-weighted MR imaging of anisotropic water diffusion in the cat central nervous system. Radiology 176:439-445
Mukherjee P et al (2000) Differences between gray matter and white matter water diffusion in stroke: diffusion-tensor MR imaging in 12 patients. Radiology 215:211-220
Mukherjee P et al (2002) Diffusion-tensor MR imaging of gray and white matter development during normal human brain maturation. AJNR Am J Neuroradiol 23:1445-1456
Neil J et al (1998) Normal brain in human newborns: apparent diffusion coefficient and diffusion anisotropy measured by using diffusion tensor MR imaging. Radiology 209:57-66
Neil J, Miller J, Mukherjee P, Huppi PS (2002) Diffusion tensor imaging of normal and injured developing human brain - a technical review. NMR Biomed 15:543-552
Nusbaum AO, Tang CY, Buchsbaum MS, Wei TC, Atlas SW (2001) Regional and global changes in cerebral diffusion with normal aging. AJNR Am J Neuroradiol 22:136-142
Ono J, Harada K, Mano T, Sakurai K, Okada S (1997) Differentiation of dys- and demyelination using diffusional anisotropy. Pediatr Neurol 16:63-66
O'Sullivan M et al (2001) Evidence for cortical "disconnection" as a mechanism of age-related cognitive decline. Neurology 57:632-638
Pajevic S, Pierpaoli C (1999) Color schemes to represent the orientation of anisotropic tissues from diffusion tensor data: application to white matter fiber tract mapping in the human brain. Magn Reson Med 42:526-540
Pfefferbaum A et al (2000) Age-related decline in brain white matter anisotropy measured with spatially corrected echo-planar diffusion tensor imaging. Magn Reson Med 44:259-268
Pfefferbaum A, Adalsteinsson E, Sullivan EV (2003) Replicability of diffusion tensor imaging measurements of fractional anisotropy and trace in brain. J Magn Reson Imaging 18:427-433
Pierpaoli C, Basser PJ (1996) Toward a quantitative assesment of diffusion anisotropy. Magn Reson Med 36:893-906
Pierpaoli C, Jezzard P, Basser PJ, Barnett A, DiChiro G (1996) Diffusion tensor MR imaging of the human brain. Radiology 201:637-648
Pierpaoli C et al (2001) Water diffusion changes in Wallerian degeneration and their dependence on white matter architecture. Neuroimage 13:1174-1185
Poupon C et al (2000) Regularization of diffusion-based direction maps for the tracking of brain white matter fascicules. NeuroImage 12:184-195
Provenzale JM, Sorensen AG (1999) Diffusion-weighted MR imaging in acute stroke: theoretic considerations and clinical applications. AJR Am J Roentgenol 173:1459-1467
Pruessmann KP, Weiger M, Scheidegger MB, Boesiger P (1999) SENSE: sensitivity encoding for fast MRI. Magn Reson Med 42:952-962
Ptak T et al (2003) Cerebral fractional anisotropy score in trauma patients: a new indicator of white matter injury after trauma. AJR Am J Roentgenol 181:1401-1407
Ricci PE, Burdette JH, Elster AD, Reboussin DM (1999) A comparison of fast spin-echo, fluid-attenuated inversion-recovery, and diffusion-weighted MR imaging in the first 10 days after cerebral infarction. AJNR Am J Neuroradiol 20:1535-1542
Ries M, Jones RA, Dousset V, Moonen CT (2000) Diffusion tensor MRI of the spinal cord. Magn Reson Med 44:884-892
Sach M et al (2004) Diffusion tensor MRI of early upper motor neuron involvement in amyotrophic lateral sclerosis. Brain 127:340-350
Schlaug G et al (1999) The ischemic penumbra: operationally defined by diffusion and perfusion MRI. Neurology 53:1528-1537
Schlaug G, Siewert B, Benfield A, Edelman RR, Warach S (1997) Time course of the apparent diffusion coefficient (ADC) abnormality in human stroke. Neurology 49:113-119
Shimony JS et al (1999) Quantitative diffusion-tensor anisotropy brain MR imaging: normative human data and anatomic analysis. Radiology 212:770-784
Sinha S, Bastin ME, Whittle IR, Wardlaw JM (2002) Diffusion tensor MR imaging of high-grade cerebral gliomas. AJNR Am J Neuroradiol 23:520-527
Skare S, Hedehus M, Moseley ME, Li TQ (2000) Condition number as a measure of noise performance of diffusion tensor data acquisition schemes with MRI. J Magn Reson 147:340-352
Sodickson DK, Manning WJ (1997) Simultaneous acquisition of spatial harmonics (SMASH): fast imaging with radiofrequency coil arrays. Magn Reson Med 38:591-603
Sorenson AG et al (1996) Hyperacute stroke: evaluation with combined multisection diffusion-weighted and hemodynamically weighted echo-planer MR imaging. Radiology 199:391-401
Sorensen AG et al (1999) Human acute cerebral ischemia: detection of changes in water diffusion anisotropy by using MR imaging. Radiology 212:785-792
Sotak CH (2002) The role of diffusion tensor imaging in the evaluation of ischemic brain injury. NMR Biomed 15:561-569
Steel RM et al (2001) Diffusion tensor imaging (DTI) and proton magnetic resonance spectroscopy (1H MRS) in schizophrenic subjects and normal controls. Psychiatry Res 106:161-170
Stejskal EO, Tanner JE (1965) Spin diffusion measurements: spin echoes in the presence of a time-dependent field gradient. J Chem Phys 42:288-292
Stieltjes B et al (2001) Diffusion tensor imaging and axonal tracking in the human brainstem. Neuroimage 14:723-735
Sun Z et al (2003) Abnormal anterior cingulum in patients with schizophrenia: a diffusion tensor imaging study. Neuroreport 14:1833-1836
Tuch DS, Wiegell MR, Reese TG, Belliveau JW, Wedeen V (2001) Proceeding of International Society of Magnetic Resonance in Medicine 502, Glasgow, UK
Tummala RP, Chu RM, Liu HTT, Hall WA (2003) Application of diffusion tensor imaging to magnetic-resonance-guided brain tumor resection. Pediatr Neurosurg 39:39-43
Ulug A, van Zijl PCM (1999) Orientation-independent diffusion imaging without tensor diagonalization: anisotropy definitions based on physical attributes of the diffusion ellipsoid. J Magn Reson Imaging 9:804-813
Ulug AM, Beauchamp N, Bryan RN, van Zijl PCM (1997) Absolute quantitation of diffusion constants in human stroke. Stroke 28:483-490

Van Gelderen P et al (1994) Water diffusion and acute stroke. Magn Reson Med 31:154-163
Van Zijl PC et al (1991)Complete separation of intracellular and extracellular information in NMR spectra of perfused cells by diffusion-weighted spectroscopy. Proc Natl Acad Sci USA 88:3228-3232
Van Zijl PCM, Davis D, Moonen CTW (1994) Diffusion spectroscopy in living systems. In: Gillies RJ (ed) NMR in physiology and biomedicine. Academic Press, San Diego, pp 185-198
Wakana S, Jiang H, Nagae-Poetscher LM, van Zijl PC, Mori S (2004) Fiber tract-based atlas of human white matter anatomy. Radiology 230:77-87
Warach S, Chien D, Li W, Ronthal MM, Edelman RR (1992) Fast magnetic resonance diffusion-weighted imaging of acute human stroke. Neurology 42:1717-1723
Warach S, Gaa D, Siewert B, Wielopolski P, Edelman RR (1995) Acute human stroke studied by whole brain echo planar diffusion-weighted magnetic resonance imaging. Ann Neurol 37:231-241
Warach S, Mosley M, Sorensen AG, Koroshetz W (1996a) Time course of diffusion imaging abnormalities in human stroke. Stroke 27:1254-1256
Warach S, Dashe JF, Edelman RR (1996b) Clinical outcome in ischemic stroke predicted by early diffusion-weighted and perfusion magnetic resonance imaging: a preliminary analysis. J Cereb Blood Flow Metab 16:53-59
Warach S, Boska M, Welch KM (1997) Pitfalls and potential of clinical diffusion-weighted MR imaging in acute stroke. Stroke 28:481-482
Welch KM et al (1995) A model to predict the histopathology of human stroke using diffusion and T2-weighted magnetic resonance imaging. Stroke 26:1983-1989
Westerhausen R et al (2003) The influence of handedness and gender on the microstructure of the human corpus callosum: a diffusion-tensor magnetic resonance imaging study. Neurosci Lett 351:99-102
Wiegell M, Larsson H, Wedeen V (2000) Fiber crossing in human brain depicted with diffusion tensor MR imaging. Radiology 217:897-903
Wilson M, Tench CR, Morgan PS, Blumhardt LD (2003) Pyramidal tract mapping by diffusion tensor magnetic resonance imaging in multiple sclerosis: improving correlations with disability. J Neurol Neurosurg Psychiatry 74:203-207
Wong EC, Cox RW, Song AW (1995) Optimized isotropic diffusion weighting. Magn Reson Med 34:139-143
Yang Q et al (1999) Serial study of apparent diffusion coefficient and anisotropy in patients with acute stroke. Stroke 30:2382-2390

7 MR Methods to Measure Cerebral Perfusion

Scott D. Swanson

CONTENTS

7.1 Introduction

More than 100 years ago, Roy and Sherrington (1890) showed that stimulation of peripheral nerves creates a change in local cerebral perfusion. Their setup was simple; the exposed cerebral surface of a dog brain and the means to provide sensory stimulation. Though not complicated, this experiment allowed them to directly visualize changes in blood flow with stimulation. Kety and Schmidt (1945) and Meier and Zierler (1954) developed methods and analysis for perfusion imaging of diffusible and non-diffusible tracers, respectively. These ideas revolutionized perfusion imaging and form the scientific foundation for MR imaging of perfusion. Today, MR has the ability to monitor blood flow with sophisticated methods that are either effectively or entirely noninvasive. Lost, however, is the direct and emphatic visualization of perfusion experienced by Roy and Sherrington (1890). The recording of quantitative blood flow by MRI is hidden behind complicated mathematical formulas and arcane pulse sequences.

The purpose of this chapter is to present a general description of the two methods that have come to dominate the measurement of cerebral perfusion with MRI: dynamic susceptibility contrast (DSC) and arterial spin labeling (ASL). In doing so, I hope to unravel some of the complicated mathematics so that the reader has a more general understanding of the procedures needed to obtain either a qualitative or a quantitative map of cerebral blood flow (CBF). In addition, I will present the possibility of measuring CBF with laser polarized xenon.

S. D. Swanson
Research Assistant Professor, Department of Radiology, University of Michigan, 200 Zina Pitcher Place, Ann Arbor, MI 48109-0553, USA

7.2 Background

Cerebral perfusion is a measure of the rate of blood flow through the capillary bed in a given mass of tissue and is a primary indicator of tissue health. The means to non-invasively image tissue perfusion has long been a goal in neuroscience. Perfusion imaging maps parameters related to the delivery of blood to the brain. These parameters include the mean transit time (MTT): the average time it takes a tracer to travel through the tissue, cerebral blood volume (CBV): the volume percent of blood in a voxel, and cerebral blood flow (CBF): the rate of blood flow per unit tissue. The cerebral blood volume in gray matter is 4%–7% and 2%–3% in white matter (Thomas et al. 2000). The units of CBF are commonly expressed in ml/min/100 g of tissue. Typical values of cerebral perfusion are 20–25 ml/min/100 g in white matter and 45–70 ml/min/100 g in gray matter (Calamante et al. 1999).

A variety of imaging modalities are able to measure cerebral perfusion. PET studies of ^{15}O labeled water (PHELPS 1991), nuclear medicine SPECT studies of ^{133}Xe (JAGGI et al. 1993), and X-ray CT studies of stable xenon (WINTERMARK et al. 2001) all provide maps of rCBF. The American Heart Association has recently compiled guidelines and recommendations for perfusion imaging in ischemic brain disease (LATCHAW et al. 2003).

In the last 15 years, advances in MRI have led to more and more routine and common measures to assess of CBF by MRI. Within MRI, DSC and ASL account for the vast majority of studies in the literature. DSC imaging uses a bolus injection of contrast agent and measures rCBF by following the time course of signal change in the brain caused by the passing of the bolus through an imaging voxel (VILLRINGER et al. 1988; ROSEN et al. 1989; BELLIVEAU et al. 1990, 1991). DSC MRI is used in most clinical MRI studies because of the high signal-to-noise ratio of the method and the ease of obtaining a relative (as opposed to absolute) measure of CBF. ASL methods magnetically label the blood flowing into the brain and create a new steady-state level of magnetization (DETRE et al. 1992; WILLIAMS et al. 1992; KIM 1995). ASL has the advantage that it uses no contrast agent but labels or tags water molecules by RF saturation. Because ASL does not use contrast agents, it is entirely non-invasive and may be repeated often. ASL is used in animal studies and in volunteer, or task activation functional imaging studies. There is a price to pay, however, as the signal-to-noise ratio (SNR) of the ASL perfusion image is approximately ten times less than the SNR of the DSC perfusion image. Other MRI methods are also being developed to measure rCBF. One promising technique is laser polarized xenon MRI (SWANSON et al. 1997). Xenon has long been used to measure CBF with SPECT or X-ray CT. Laser polarized xenon MRI has recently been used to measure CBF by DUHAMEL et al. (2002).

7.3 Dynamic Susceptibility Contrast

DSC MRI measures the passage of a bolus of non-diffusible contrast through the brain. A bolus of contrast is injected into a vein and travels through the vasculature into the brain where the change in MRI signal is recorded. The signal decreases as the bolus passes through the imaging slice. The decreased signal change is mathematically converted to a change in the concentration of contrast agent. The time course of the rate of change of contrast agent is integrated to yield the relative cerebral blood volume (relCBV). The arterial signal is also recorded and used to compute the mean transit time (MTT) and rCBF (regional cerebral blood flow).

7.3.1 What Causes the Signal to Change?

Signal intensity decreases because the paramagnetic contrast disrupts the magnetic fields in a small region surrounding the capillaries as it passes through the tissue. Disruption of the magnetic field decreases T_2^* (or increases $R_2^* = 1/T_2^*$) of water protons in tissue near the contrast agent. Since the echo of the spins is recorded at a time TE following the pulse, the change in T_2^* will result in a decrease in the signal intensity of the water proton spins.

The intensity of the water proton signal at time TE will be given by:

$$S_{TE} = S_0 e^{-R_2 TE} \tag{7.1}$$

where R_2 is the transverse relaxation rate ($1/T2$) of tissue. R_2^* is the effective transverse relaxation rate ($1/T_2^*$) in the presence of contrast agent.

If contrast agent is added to the tissue, an additional relaxation occurs due to the susceptibility induced dispersion created by addition of paramagnetic ions. The new relaxation rate can be defined as:

$$R_2^* = R_2 + r_2^* C_{Gd}(t) \tag{7.2}$$

where r_2^* is the relaxivity (relaxation rate per unit concentration of gadolinium) and $C_{Gd}(t)$ is the time dependent concentration of the gadolinium contrast agent. Rate constants (rather that the time constants such as $T2$ are used because the rates are additive and simplify the math. The signal intensity at time TE is now defined as:

$$S_{TE}^{Gd}(t) = S_0 e^{-R_2^*(t)TE} = S_0 e^{-R_2 TE} e^{-r_2^* C_{Gd}(t)TE} \tag{7.3}$$

7.3.2 How Does the Signal Change Correspond to Tracer Concentration?

The goal of this procedure is to calculate the concentrate of the concentration of the tracer. This can be done by taking the logarithm of the ratio of the signal with and without contrast agent.

$$\frac{S_{TE}^{Gd}(t)}{S_{TE}} = \frac{S_0 e^{-R_2 TE} e^{-r_2^* C_{Gd}(t) TE}}{S_0 e^{-R_2 TE}} = e^{-r_2^* C_{Gd}(t) TE} \quad (7.4)$$

$$C_{Gd}(t) \propto r_2^* C_{Gd}(t) = -\frac{\ln\left(\frac{S_{TE}^{Gd}(t)}{S_{TE}}\right)}{TE} \quad (7.5)$$

Figure 7.1a shows a representative curve of the signal intensity in a voxel as the contrast agent passes through the volume. These data are processed with Eq. (7.5) to generate the time–concentration curve shown in Fig. 7.1b. The arterial input function (AIF) (Fig. 7.1c) is measured from voxels near a major artery such as the MCA.

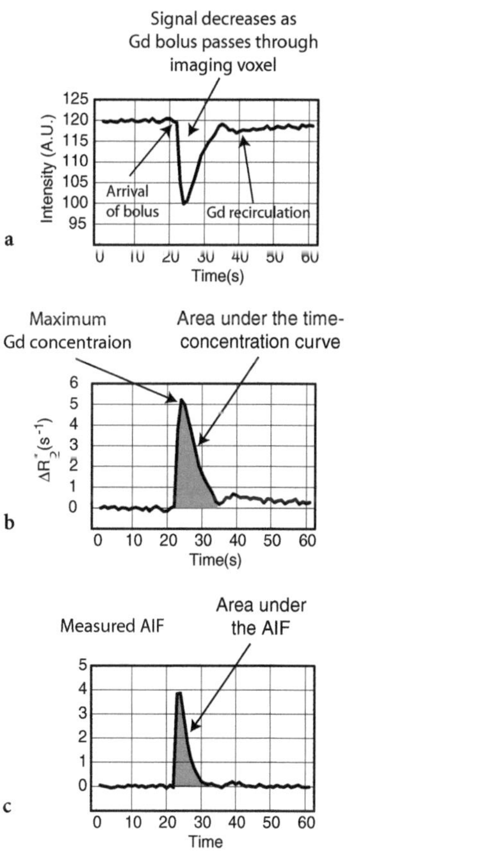

Fig. 7.1a–c. Generation of the concentration–time curve. The passage of contrast agent through the voxel causes the signal to decrease due to a decrease in T2* (an increase in R2*) resulting in a decrease in the MR signal (**a**). The signal–time curve is turned into a concentration–time curve by using equations 7.4 and 7.5. The arterial input function (**c**) is created in a similar manner, using these same equations to transform the signal–time curve measured near a major artery into a concentration–time curve.

Because the bolus passes through the tissue in a very short time, echo planer imaging (EPI) methods are needed to image the profile seen in Fig. 7.1a (Kwong et al. 1995).

This procedure assumes that the contrast agent does not leak out of the vessels into the tissue and that the contrast agent causes insignificant *T*1 enhancement.

7.3.3 How Is the Time–Concentration Tracer Curve Turned into a Measure of Perfusion?

After recording the images and creating the time–concentration curves for each voxel or region of interest, the data needs to be further analyzed to create maps of perfusion (rCBF), MTT, and CBV. At this stage the investigator needs to decide whether he or she desires a relative or a quantitative map of perfusion. There are basically three paths: (1) numerical integration (or summing up) of the data to create relative maps of CBV; (2) fitting the data to a gamma-variant function; or (3) deconvolution of the data using the AIF (Perkio et al. 2002). Of these three methods we will consider numerical integration and deconvolution.

7.3.3.1 Numerical Integration

The easiest method to create a measure of perfusion is to measure the area of the time–concentration curve (Fig. 7.1b).

$$relCBV = \int C_{tissue}(t)dt \quad (7.6)$$

This will provide an index that is proportional to the relative cerebral blood volume (relCBV) of a given pixel. Because of the ease of performing the numerical integration, this method is perhaps the most used in clinical application of MR perfusion imaging. It should be noted that this does not provide an absolute, quantitative measure of cerebral blood volume, but yields an image that may be useful for comparing normal to ischemic or diseased tissue.

7.3.3.2 Deconvolution

Indicator-dilution theory of perfusion imaging for non-diffusible tracers states that the time–concentration profile is equal to the cerebral blood flow times the convolution of the AIF and the tissue residue function (MEIER and ZIERLER 1954; ZIERLER 1965).

$$C_{Gd}(t) = CBF \int_{u=0}^{t} AIF(u)R(t-u)du \tag{7.7}$$

If the reader understands this equation and all of its implications, then read no further. If, however, one is trying to gain an understanding of how this convolution integral can be used to measure perfusion, then this section should be very helpful.

This statement leads to three obvious questions: What is the arterial input function? What is a convolution integral? What is a residue function?

The arterial input function was introduced previously and is simply the concentration of contrast agent in the arteries as a function of time. In a perfect world, one could shape the arterial input function so that it would be a delta function, or instantaneous spike of contrast agent. This would greatly simplify the mathematics and make quantitative perfusion imaging trivial. Because of the realities of injection and diffusion of contrast agent within the blood, this ideal function can never be achieved in practice. In general the AIF is a broad, Gaussian-like function determined by the rate at which contrast agent is injected and by the spread of the contrast agent that occurs as the blood flows from the injection site to the brain.

The second term, the residue function, is the manner in which contrast agent is retained by the tissue. Because there are many pathways that molecules of Gd chelates can follow through the capillary bed to leave the tissue, the residue function is a statistical probability of how it is retained in the tissue. The residue function is determined by deconvolving the time–concentration function with the arterial input function.

Figure 7.2 demonstrates convolution. The left column contains different arterial input functions ranging from a delta function in Fig. 7.2a to a Gaussian function in Fig. 7.2e. The center column contains an exponentially decaying residue function and is the same for each row. The right column shows what the detected tissue MRI signal would be measured for these combinations of AIF and residue functions. The delta function AIF in Fig. 7.2a is shifted by 10 s. Convolution of this function with the exponentially decaying residue function simply shifts the residue function by 10 s. In Fig. 7.2b, the AIF contains three well separated delta functions. Convolution with the residue function creates three well-separated exponentially decaying functions. As the delta functions become closer in time (Fig. 7.2c), the measured response does not decay to zero before another bolus of signal arrives. Therefore, the signal builds up with each additional arrival of bolus. In Fig. 7.2d, the AIF is a square wave (a series of back-to-back delta functions). The measured tissue response builds up while the AIF has a value of 1, and decays when the AIF = 0. Note change in scale in the value of the measured response in Fig. 7.2d. Finally, a more realistic Gaussian function is used in Fig. 7.2e for the AIF.

The demonstration of convolution in Fig. 7.2 does not show one how to deconvolve. Deconvolution is a much more complicated process and beyond the scope of this chapter. In summary, deconvolution uses an iterative process to create an estimate of the residue function if one is given the AIF and the time-concentration curve in the tissue of interest (OSTERGAARD et al. 1999). From Eq. (7.7), one can see that once the AIF and the residue function are known, then one can calculate a quantitative estimate of CBF.

$$CBF = \frac{C_{Gd}(t)}{\int_{u=0}^{t} AIF(u)R(t-u)du} \tag{7.8}$$

Since we have measured the time-concentration curve and the AIF, a quantitative estimate of CBF can be made.

$$CBV = \kappa \frac{\int C_{Gd}(t)dt}{\int AIF(t)dt} \tag{7.9}$$

Where κ is a scaling factor depending on the hematocrit and vessel geometry. Moreover, from the central volume theorem (MEIER and ZIERLER 1954), one can calculate the mean transit time (MTT).

$$MTT = \frac{CBV}{CBF} \tag{7.10}$$

Deconvolution of the time–concentration curve with the AIF provides quantitative estimates of CBF, CBV, and MTT.

7.4 Arterial Spin Labeling

Arterial spin labeling (ASL) magnetically labels the water proton spins in blood that is flowing into the brain (DETRE et al. 1992). Either continuous wave (CW) or pulsed (KIM 1995) RF energy is used to selec-

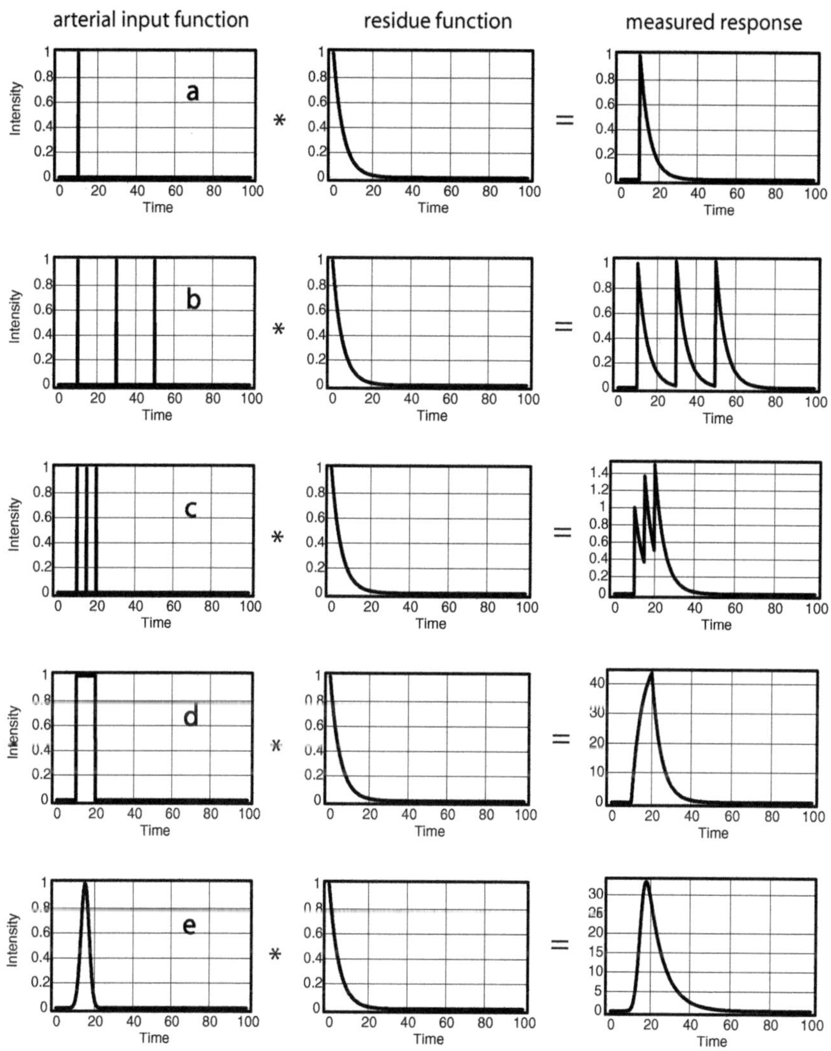

Fig. 7.2a–e. Convolution of the arterial input function with the tissue residue function yields the tissue concentration curve. An ideal delta function at time 10 s is used as the AIF and convoluted with the exponentially decaying residue function. This procedure shifts the residue function in time (**a**). Three delta functions separated by 20 s convoluted with the residue function yields three exponential decays at the appropriate time points (**b**). As the time between the three delta functions decreases, the tissue concentration does not decay to zero and the tissue concentration curve will begin to increase (**c**). A square AIF seen in (**d**) is 200 back-to-back delta functions. The convolution of a square AIF with the exponentially decaying residue function will result in a tissue concentration curve that first increases with a positive exponential and then decreases with a negative exponential (**d**). [Note the change in vertical scale in (**d**)]. A more realistic shape for an AIF is a Gaussian function as seen in (**e**)

tively invert magnetization in the arteries. Numerous methods have been developed over the last 10 years and are well reviewed in Calamante et al. (1999) and Barbier et al. (2001). This work focuses on the fundamental equations of sources and sinks of magnetization in the brain and illustrates the complicated coupled differential equations describing ASL imaging with simple pictures of coupled reservoirs.

7.4.1 What Causes the Signal to Change?

In order to be effective, ASL methods label the water proton magnetization in the blood stream to create a signal difference in the region of interest. The labeling is done with either CW RF excitation or with a pulsed RF excitation.

7.4.1.1 Spin-Lattice Relaxation

To gain an understanding of how ASL methods work, one must first examine the basic equations of magnetization. The Bloch equations state that the rate of change of magnetization is proportional to the difference between the equilibrium magnetization and the current level of magnetization. In a static sample, with no inflowing water molecules, magnetization is restored to equilibrium values by random motions of the nuclear spins. The time constant for this process is, of course, $T1$. Mathematically, this is written as a first order differential equation.

$$\frac{dM_z(t)}{dt} = \frac{\{M_0 - M_z(t)\}}{T_1} = R_1\{M_0 - M_z(t)\} \qquad (7.11)$$

where $M_z(t)$ is the time-dependent value of longitudinal magnetization, M_0 is the equilibrium value, and $T1$ is the spin-lattice relaxation time constant. Figure 7.3 shows a schematic of Eq. (7.11), where the reservoir of tissue magnetization is coupled to an infinite "lattice" by the rate constant R_1.

Figure 7.4a demonstrates what happens when the tissue magnetization is saturated by an RF pulse. Magnetization will flow from the lattice, with rate constant R_1, until the tissue reservoir is filled to M_0. Figure 7.4b shows that if $M_z(t)$ is sampled at times TR with a pulse of flip angle δ, the steady-state, longitudinal magnetization will be

$$M_{s.s.} = M_0 \frac{1 - e^{-TR/T_1}}{1 - e^{-TR/T_1} \cos\vartheta} \qquad (7.12)$$

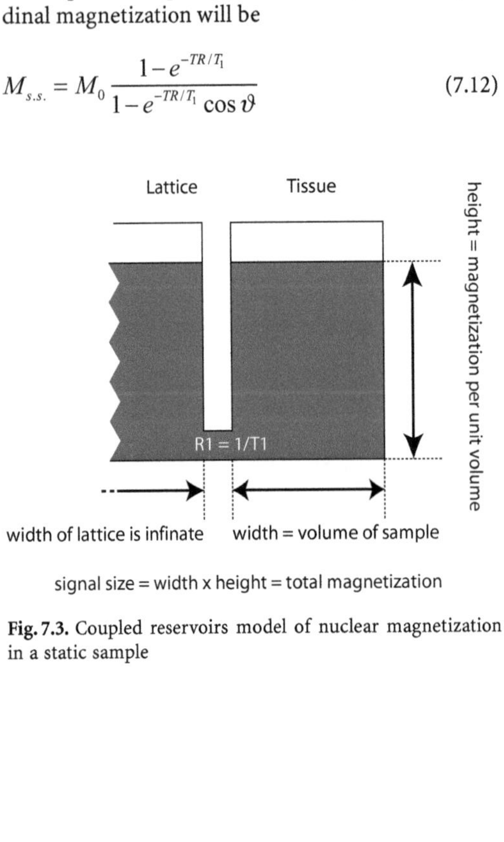

Fig. 7.3. Coupled reservoirs model of nuclear magnetization in a static sample

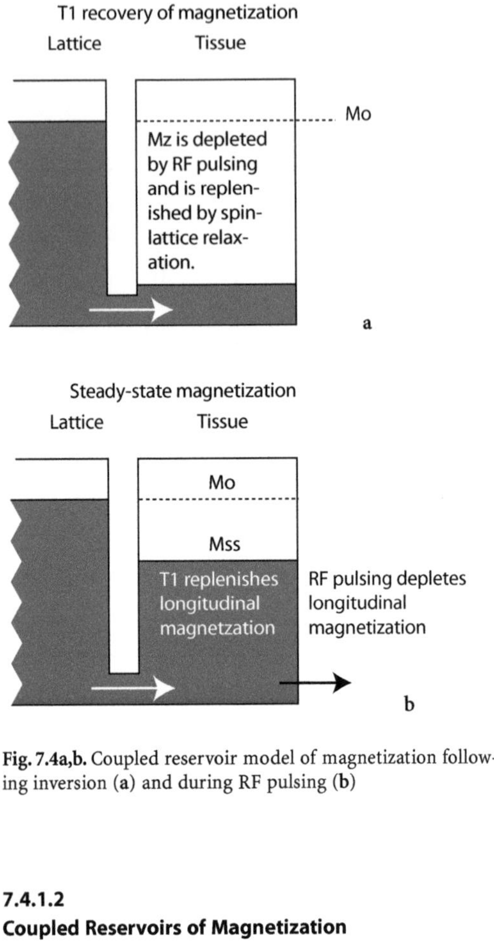

Fig. 7.4a,b. Coupled reservoir model of magnetization following inversion (**a**) and during RF pulsing (**b**)

7.4.1.2 Coupled Reservoirs of Magnetization

In vivo, there are other sources and sinks of water proton magnetization. One source would be the arterial blood flowing into a region of tissue and one sink would be the flow of venous blood exiting the tissue. The differential equation could then be written as,

$$\frac{dM_{brain}(t)}{dt} = \frac{\{M_0 - M_{brain}(t)\}}{T_1} + FM_{art.}(t) - FM_{ven.}(t) \qquad (7.13)$$

Because water is a freely diffusible tracer, the value of the magnetization in the venous blood can is given by the magnetization in the brain divided by the partition coefficient.

$$\frac{dM_{brain}(t)}{dt} = R_1\{M_0 - M_{brain}(t)\} + F\left\{M_{art.}(t) - \frac{M_{brain}(t)}{\lambda}\right\}, \qquad (7.14)$$

where F is the blood flow in ml/100g/min, λ is the blood/brain partition coefficient for water.

An additional magnetic coupling in brain tissue is the magnetization transfer that occurs between the mobile water protons and the immobile lipid bilayer protons of white and gray matter. MT is generated by applying RF energy off-resonance from the narrow water proton line but within the linewidth of the broad lipid proton resonance. The RF energy partially saturates the magnetization of the solid-like protons. This saturation is transferred to the water protons by magnetic cross-relaxation and exchange. MT occurs in ASL because the CW RF needed to invert magnetization in the carotid arteries causes significant MT in the brain. Therefore a control RF pulse is needed that generates MT but does not label arterial blood (McLaughlin et al. 1997). Pulsed methods minimize, but do not eliminate, MT effects in ASL. MT can be included by adding a term for cross-relaxation between the mobile and immobile protons

$$\frac{dM_{brain}(t)}{dt} = R_1\{M_0 - M_{brain}(t)\} + F\left\{M_{art.}(t) - \frac{M_{brain}(t)}{\lambda}\right\} + R_1\{M_{solid} - M_{brain}, \qquad (7.15)$$

where R_1 is the cross relaxation rate.

Figure 7.5 provides a picture of all of the magnetic couplings and magnetization flow patterns that are described mathematically in Eq. (7.15).

7.4.2 Measurement of Flow with ASL

Figure 7.6 demonstrates the conditions for CW ASL. In Fig. 7.6a, a control RF pulse is applied along with a magnetic field gradient. The pulse is off-resonance for spins in the brain and creates significant MT effect, resulting in a decrease in brain tissue signal. In Fig. 7.6b, the same RF energy is applied to the brain causing the same MT effect. This pulse, however, is on-resonance for spins in the carotid arteries and inverts the magnetization of the spins flowing into the brain. Because the level of magnetization in the arteries is less than the level of magnetization in the brain, the net flow of magnetization is out of the brain causing an additional decrease in the brain signal. The difference between the saturation in Fig. 7.6a and Fig. 7.6b is given by Williams et al. (1992):

$$F = \lambda R_{1app} \frac{M_{brain}^{cont} - M_{brain}^{ASL}}{2M_{brain}^{cont}} \qquad (7.16)$$

where $R_{1app} = R_1 + \frac{F}{\lambda}$.

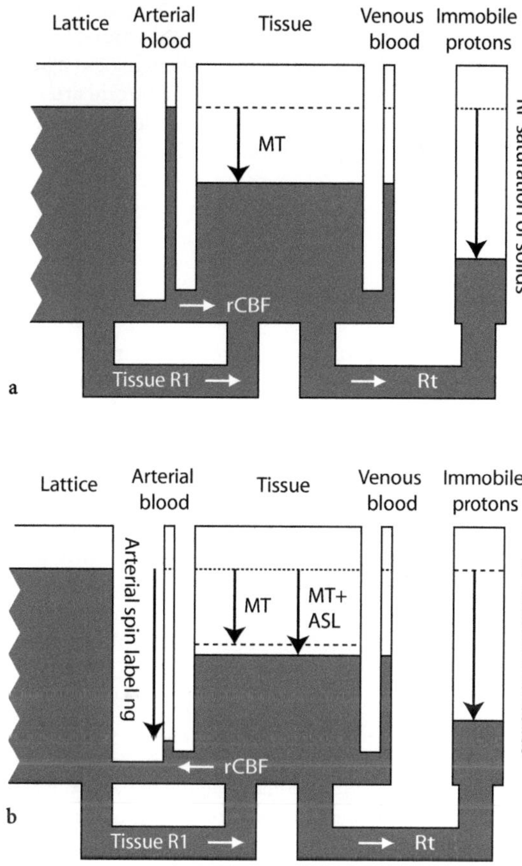

Fig. 7.6a,b. Behavior of magnetization during the control CW RF irradiation (a) and ASL of the carotid arteries (b)

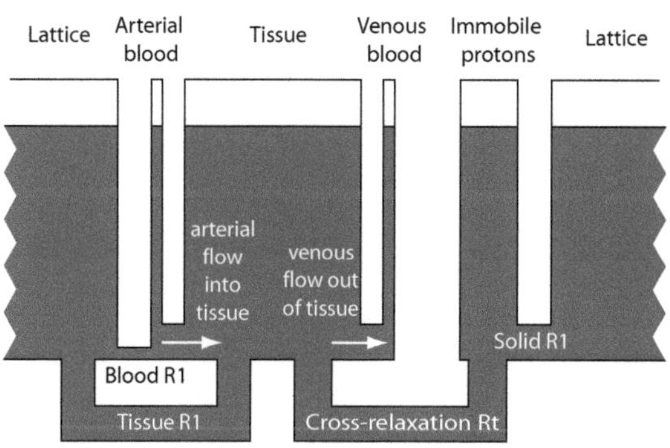

Fig. 7.5. A complete model of the coupled reservoirs of magnetization in the brain

To obviate the problems of MT, one needs to use a separate RF surface coil on the carotid arteries (Silva et al. 1995). This is technically challenging but allows one to label the water protons in the carotid arteries without causing MT in the brain. A schematic example of this technique is shown in Fig. 7.7.

7.5 Laser Polarized Xenon

Alternative means to measure CBF using MRI are also being explored. One promising technique that has been used in small animal models is laser polarized or hyperpolarized ^{129}Xe (Fig. 7.8) (Swanson et al. 1997; Duhamel et al. 2002). Xenon is a freely diffusible tracer and has been used by both CT (by attenuation of X-rays) and SPECT (as radioactive ^{133}Xe) to measure rCBF. Laser polarization increases the nuclear polarization (the percent of xenon in the spin up state) from normal levels of about 0.0001% to approximately 50% in ideal cases. With increased MR signal and near ideal tracer kinetics, it should be possible to use MRI of laser polarized xenon to measure perfusion.

For a freely diffusible tracer, such as xenon, the time-concentration profile of xenon in the tissue will be given by the same convolution integral [Eq. (7.7)] examined earlier.

$$M_T(t) = F\int_0^t M_A(u)\exp\left[-\left(\frac{F}{\lambda_{bt}}+\frac{1}{T_1}\right)(t-u)\right]du. \quad (7.17)$$

Though it is informative to evaluate the longitudinal magnetization, as done in Eq. (7.17), the imaging experiment will measure the transverse magnetization and it is necessary to determine the transverse magnetization. This is especially critical for polarized gas MRI, as the MR signal will be destroyed with each additional pulse. This fact is both a disadvantage and an advantage when attempting to measure flow with polarized gas MRI. It is a disadvantage in that once the magnetization is destroyed, it is gone and will not be replaced by T1 processes. It is an advantage because the ability to destroy the signal of the tracer that we are using to measure flow means that there will be no problem with recirculation of tracer. Once the signal is used, it is gone.

With a constant arterial input function, one can show that the transverse xenon magnetization will be:

$$M_T^{xy} = \sin\alpha \frac{M_A F\left\{1-\exp\left[-\left(\frac{F}{\lambda_{bt}}+\frac{1}{T_1}\right)\tau\right]\right\}}{\left(\frac{F}{\lambda_{bt}}+\frac{1}{T_1}\right)\left\{1-\cos\alpha\exp\left[-\left(\frac{F}{\lambda_{bt}}+\frac{1}{T_1}\right)\tau\right]\right\}} \quad (7.18)$$

With appropriate RF pulsing, the detected xenon signal in Eq. (7.18) linearly proportional to flow. Though rCBF measurements with laser polarized xenon are currently challenging, further advances in polarization technology and delivery may show that this historically important atom may yet have a role to play in MR methods to measure cerebral perfusion.

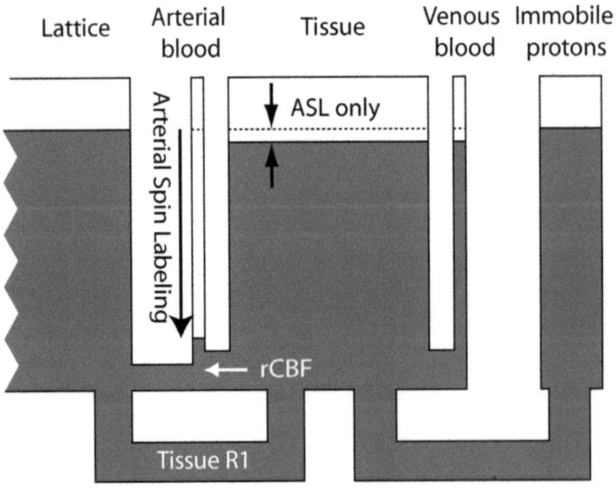

Fig. 7.7. Behavior of magnetization during CW RF irradiation using a dedicated surface coil in the neck. MT effects are eliminated.

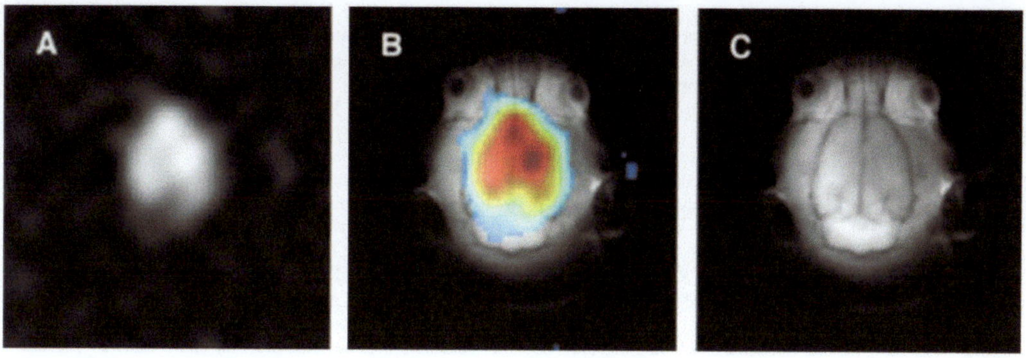

Fig. 7.8a–c. Image of laser polarized xenon dissolved in the brain of a rat (**a**), proton spin-echo image (**c**), and overlay (**b**). Each image has a FOV of 50×50 mm and a slice thickness of 10 mm. The xenon image was acquired with a 16×16 2D CSI pulse sequence and was zero-filled to 64×64 pixels

References

Barbier E, Lamalle L, Decorps M (2001) Methodology of brain perfusion imaging. J Magn Reson Imaging 13:496-520

Belliveau J, Rosen B, Kantor H, Rzedzian R, Kennedy D, Mckinstry R, Vevea J, Cohen M, Pykett I, Brady T (1990) Functional cerebral imaging by susceptibility-contrast NMR. Magn Reson Med 14:538-546

Belliveau J, Kennedy DJ, Mckinstry R, Buchbinder B, Weisskoff R, Cohen M, Vevea J, Brady T, Rosen B (1991) Functional mapping of the human visual cortex by magnetic resonance imaging. Science 254:716-719

Calamante F, Thomas D, Pell G, Wiersma J, Turner R (1999) Measuring cerebral blood flow using magnetic resonance imaging techniques. J Cereb Blood Flow Metab 19:701-735

Detre J, Wang J (2002) Technical aspects and utility of fMRI using bold and ASL. Clin Neurophysiol 113:621-634

Detre J, Leigh J, Williams D, Koretsky A (1992) Perfusion imaging. Magn Reson Med 23:37-45

Duhamel G, Choquet P, Grillon E, Leviel J, Decorps M, Ziegler A, Constantinesco A (2002) Global and regional cerebral blood flow measurements using NMR of injected hyperpolarized xenon-129. Acad Radiol 9 [Suppl 2]:S498-500

Hunsche S, Sauner D, Schreiber W, Oelkers P, Stoeter P (2002) Fair and dynamic susceptibility contrast-enhanced perfusion imaging in healthy subjects and stroke patients. J Magn Reson Imaging 16:137-146

Jaggi JL, Obrist WD, Noordergraaf A (1993) Signal analysis of noninvasive xenon-133 cerebral blood flow measurements. Ann Biomed Eng 21:85-95

Kety SS, Schmidt CF (1945) The determination of cerebral blood flow in man by the use of nitrous oxide in low concentrations. Am J Physiol 143:53-66

Kim S (1995) Quantification of relative cerebral blood flow change by flow-sensitive alternating inversion recovery (FAIR) technique: application to functional mapping. Magn Reson Med 34:293-301

Kwong K, Chesler D, Weisskoff R, Donahue K, Davis T, Ostergaard L, Campbell T, Rosen B (1995) MR perfusion studies with T1-weighted echo planar imaging. Magn Reson Med 34:878-887

Latchaw R, Yonas H, Hunter G, Yuh W, Ueda T, Sorensen A, Sunshine J, Biller J, Wechsler L, Higashida R, Hademenos G (2003) Guidelines and recommendations for perfusion imaging in cerebral ischemia: a scientific statement for healthcare professionals by the writing group on perfusion imaging, from the council on cardiovascular radiology of the american heart association. Stroke 34:1084-1104

Mclaughlin A, Ye F, Pekar J, Santha A, Frank J (1997) Effect of magnetization transfer on the measurement of cerebral blood flow using steady-state arterial spin tagging approaches: a theoretical investigation. Magn Reson Med 37:501-510

Meier P, Zierler K (1954) On the theory of the indicator-dilution method for measurement of blood flow and volume. J Appl Physiol 6:731-744

Ostergaard L, Weisskoff R, Chesler D, Gyldensted C, Rosen B (1996) High resolution measurement of cerebral blood flow using intravascular tracer bolus passages, part I: mathematical approach and statistical analysis. Magn Reson Med 36:715-725

Ostergaard L, Sorensen A, Kwong K, Weisskoff R, Gyldensted C, Rosen B (1996) High resolution measurement of cerebral blood flow using intravascular tracer bolus passages, part II: experimental comparison and preliminary results. Magn Reson Med 36:726-736

Ostergaard L, Chesler D, Weisskoff R, Sorensen A, Rosen B (1999) Modeling cerebral blood flow and flow heterogeneity from magnetic resonance residue data. J Cereb Blood Flow Metab 19:690-699

Perkio J, Aronen H, Kangasmaki A, Liu Y, Karonen J, Savolainen S, Ostergaard L (2002) Evaluation of four postprocessing methods for determination of cerebral blood volume and mean transit time by dynamic susceptibility contrast imaging. Magn Reson Med 47:973-981

Phelps ME (1991) PET - a biological imaging technique. Neurochem Res 16:929-940

Rosen B, Belliveau J, Chien D (1989) Perfusion imaging by nuclear magnetic resonance. Magn Reson Q 5:263-281

Rosen B, Belliveau J, Vevea J, Brady T (1990) Perfusion imaging with NMR contrast agents. Magn Reson Med 14:249-265

Roy C, Sherrington CS (1890) On the Regulation of the blood supply of the brain. J Physiol 11:85-108
Silva A, Zhang W, Williams D, Koretsky A (1995) Multi-slice MRI of rat brain perfusion during amphetamine stimulation using arterial spin labeling. Magn Reson Med 33:209-214
Sorensen A, Copen W, Ostergaard L, Buonanno F, Gonzalez R, Rordorf G, Rosen B, Schwamm L, Weisskoff R, Koroshetz W (1999) Hyperacute stroke: simultaneous measurement of relative cerebral blood volume, relative cerebral blood flow, and mean tissue transit time. Radiology 210:519-527
Swanson S, Rosen M, Agranoff B, Coulter K, Welsh R, Chupp T (1997) Brain MRI with laser-polarized ^{129}Xe. Magn Reson Med 38:695-698
Thomas D, Lythgoe M, Pell G, Calamante F, Ordidge R (2000) The measurement of diffusion and perfusion in biological systems using magnetic resonance imaging. Phys Med Biol 45:R97-R138
Villringer A, Rosen B, Belliveau J, Ackerman J, Lauffer R, Buxton R, Chao Y, Wedeen V, Brady T (1988) Dynamic imaging with lanthanide chelates in normal brain: contrast due to magnetic susceptibility effects. Magn Reson Med 6:164-174
Weber M, Gunther M, Lichy M, Delorme S, Bongers A, Thilmann C, Essig M, Zuna I, Schad L, Debus J, Schlemmer H (2003) Comparison of arterial spin-labeling techniques and dynamic susceptibility-weighted contrast-enhanced MRI in perfusion imaging of normal brain tissue. Invest Radiol 38:712-718
Williams D, Detre J, Leigh J, Koretsky A (1992) Magnetic resonance imaging of perfusion using spin inversion of arterial water. Proc Natl Acad Sci USA 89:212-216
Wintermark M, Maeder P, Thiran JP et al (2001) Quantitative assessment of regional cerebral blood flows by perfusion CT studies at low injection rates: a critical review of the underlying theoretical models. Eur Radiol 11:1220-1230
Zierler KL (1965) Equations for measuring blood flow by external monitoring of radioisotopes. Circ Res 16:309-321

8 Functional MRI

Peter Jezzard and Ahmed Toosy

CONTENTS

8.1 Introduction

Developments in magnetic resonance imaging (MRI) over the past decade have demonstrated that MRI, a non-invasive and widespread technology, can also report on human brain function via the correlate of the brain's associated local haemodynamic response (Belliveau et al. 1991; Ogawa et al. 1992; Kwong et al. 1992; Bandettini et al. 1992). The most common haemodynamic variable to be accessed by functional MRI (fMRI) is the level of blood oxygenation (in fact the MRI signal is sensitive to the level of blood *deoxygenation*), although MRI is able to access other markers of brain activity.

The majority of fMRI studies to date have addressed questions in basic neuroscience, and have studied the operation of the healthy brain in normal volunteers. A small, but increasing, number of studies have addressed questions in clinical neuroscience, and some of this work has gone on to find application in the clinic (Thulborn and Gisbert 2001). Of this work, little has been directed towards white matter diseases. This is presumably because fMRI methods are generally only sensitive to metabolic, and hence signalling, activity that occurs within the grey matter, and is unable to detect directly the transmission of signal within white matter fibres. Nevertheless, an important new insight into white matter disorders can be achieved by studying the effects on grey matter networks arising from disorders of the white matter.

8.2 Physiological and Biophysical Origins of fMRI

8.2.1 Metabolic and Haemodynamic Correlates of Brain Activity

Neurons communicate via small electrical impulses, receiving signals from other neurons via their dendrites, and sending impulses to other neurons via their axon. The signals received via the dendrites may either be excitatory (in which case there is an increased tendency for the neuron to relay the electrical signal further via its axon), or may be inhibitory (in which case there is a decreased tendency for the neuron to relay the electrical signal). Figure 8.1 shows a schematic diagram of a neuron, showing its

P. Jezzard, PhD
FMRIB Centre, Department of Clinical Neurology, John Radcliffe Hospital, Oxford, OX3 9DU, UK
A. Toosy, MD
Department of Headache, Brain Injury and Rehabilitation, Institute of Neurology, Queen Square, London, WC1N 3BG, UK

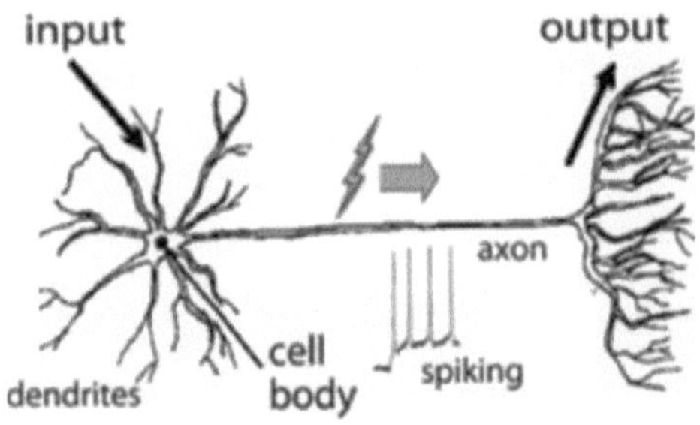

Fig. 8.1. Schematic diagram of a neuron, showing its dendrites, which receive electrical signals from other neurons, and its axon, which relays signals on to other neurons. Connection between neurons occurs across synapses.

principal elements. Surrounding the neurons are glia, which are cells involved in energy metabolism, storage, and maintenance of ionic balance.

The metabolic turnover of glia, activation of neurons, and establishment of the ion potentials in the cells of the brain all require a supply of energy. Current evidence suggests that most of the metabolic demands of brain signalling involve presynaptic activity (input and intracortical processing) rather than soma spiking activity (Logothetis et al. 2001). This energy is supplied in the form of adenosine triphosphate (ATP) generated in the mitochondria within cells. Under normal conditions ATP is formed via glucose consumption in the presence of oxygen (via aerobic glycolysis), and this glucose and oxygen is supplied by blood perfusing the tissue. Previous experiments involving a number of modalities have shown that local glucose consumption rises sharply when neuronal activation takes place. This is accompanied by an increase in local blood flow, and in local blood volume. From the perspective of fMRI, however, it is the balance of oxygen delivery and utilization that results in the observed signal changes. This is because blood oxygen is predominantly transported within red blood cells, bound to the large iron-containing molecule, haemoglobin. As is discussed below, it is the changing magnetic properties of haemoglobin as it gives up its oxygen that provides the most utilized contrast mechanism in functional MRI. Other related physiological parameters that can be accessed by MRI include cerebral blood flow, cerebral blood volume and, in animal models, glucose turnover via carbon-13 spectroscopy.

When considering the oxygen requirements of the brain it is informative to consider a formulation of the Fick principle that relates consumption of a nutrient by a tissue to the arteriovenous difference in the concentration of the nutrient in the blood. In this case oxygen is assumed to be consumed metabolically, and the Fick principle can be expressed as:

$$CMRO_2 = CBF \times 4\,[Hb^{TOT}]\,(Y_a\text{-}Y_v) \qquad [1]$$

where $CMRO_2$ is the metabolic rate of oxygen consumption, CBF is the cerebral blood flow, $[Hb^{TOT}]$ is the total (oxygenated or deoxygenated) concentration of haemoglobin, and the factor 4 accounts for the fact that four oxygen molecules can bind to each haemoglobin molecule. Y_a and Y_v are the oxygen saturation values (range 0 to 1) for arterial and venous blood (oxygen saturation is the fraction of haemoglobin molecules that are in the oxygenated state), and hence $(Y_a - Y_v)$ is a measure of the oxygen extraction fraction (OEF).

The hypothesized relationship between local $CMRO_2$ and CBF during neuronal stimulation is shown in Fig. 8.2. The increase in local $CMRO_2$ is thought to be rather modest (5–20%) and is coincident with the period of neuronal activity. The increased metabolic demand causes the CBF to increase quite markedly (albeit sluggishly), yielding a peak CBF demand some 5–10 seconds after the onset of stimulation. The increase in local CBF is much more significant (typically 30–100%), a necessary overcompensation that is likely to be due to the limited oxygen diffusion capacity from the blood to the mitochondria (Buxton and Frank 1997). Through Eq. 1 it can be seen that since CBF rises more than $CMRO_2$ during stimulation there is predicted to be a decrease in OEF (i.e. Y_v is increased). This is the effect that is used in blood oxygenation level dependent (BOLD) fMRI experiments.

Also shown in Fig. 8.2 is a representation of the associated change in local cerebral blood volume (CBV), along with the observed BOLD fMRI response, for both a short duration and a long duration stimulus. It can be seen that the CBV haemodynamic response is even more sluggish than the CBF haemodynamic response, and indeed contributes to the non-linear overshoot and post-stimulus undershoot that is frequently observed in practical fMRI data sets. The initial dip that is occasionally observed immediately following stimulus onset (Ernst and Hennig 1994; Menon et al. 1995) is postulated to be evidence of the brief temporal uncoupling of oxygen consumption (associated with the $CMRO_2$ increase) and oxygen delivery (associated with the more sluggish CBF increase) leading to a transient blood deoxygenation. The initial dip has proved to be very elusive, however, and is rarely observed at clinical field strengths.

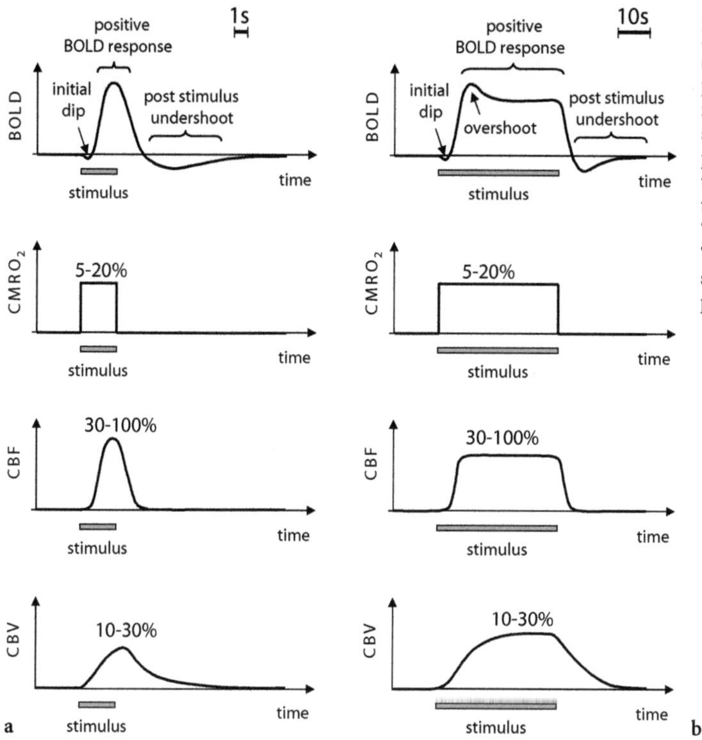

Fig. 8.2a, b. Diagram showing the BOLD signal, $CMRO_2$ (oxygen consumption), CBF (i.e. blood flow or perfusion) and CBV (blood volume) responses to a brief period of neuronal stimulation (**a**) and a more sustained period of neuronal stimulation (**b**). The typical features of the BOLD signal time course are shown, including the 'initial dip' (rarely seen below 4 T), the 'positive BOLD response', and the 'post-stimulus undershoot'. An 'overshoot' period is also sometimes seen.

8.2.2 BOLD Mechanisms

As alluded to above, the origin of the BOLD fMRI effect lies in the different magnetic properties of haemoglobin that has oxygen attached to it (oxyHb) versus haemoglobin that does not have oxygen attached (deoxyHb). Pauling and Coryell (1936) found that deoxyHb was slightly paramagnetic relative to tissue, whereas oxyHb was isomagnetic relative to tissue. The difference in magnetic susceptibility between whole blood that is fully deoxygenated and whole blood that is fully oxygenated has been measured to be approximately $\Delta\chi=0.2$ ppm×Hct (Thulborn et al. 1982), where Hct is the blood haematocrit (range 0.0–1.0). Since fully oxygenated blood is isomagnetic relative to tissue, vessels containing arterial blood cause little or no distortion to the magnetic field in the surrounding tissue. Conversely, capillary and venous vessels containing blood which is partially or significantly deoxygenated will distort the magnetic field in their vicinity (Ogawa et al. 1990; Turner et al. 1991). It is this local distortion of the magnetic field homogeneity, occurring on a microscopic scale, that provides the contrast mechanism in the BOLD fMRI experiment and enables changes in blood oxygenation level to be detected. This is shown schematically in Fig. 8.3 where the simulated magnetic field is shown for a blood vessel that contains partially deoxygenated blood. Figure 8.3a shows the case of the vessel being aligned with the main static B_0 field. In this case there is a shift in the magnetic field within the vessel, but little distortion of the field surrounding the vessel. As the angle between the blood vessel and the main B_0 field is altered to 45° (Fig. 8.3b) and 90° (Fig. 8.3c) it can be seen that the intravascular magnetic field is altered, and there is a progressively larger effect outside the blood vessel. In a representative tissue voxel there will be a random distribution of microvascular orientations resulting in a complex field distribution both for the intravascular water spins, and the extravascular (tissue) water spins. These field distributions lead to the T2* shortening that is the origin of the BOLD effect.

In practice both the water molecules in the blood itself (the intravascular compartment) and the water molecules in the tissue space that surrounds the vessels (the extravascular compartment) contribute to the MRI signal that is measured. Since the arte-

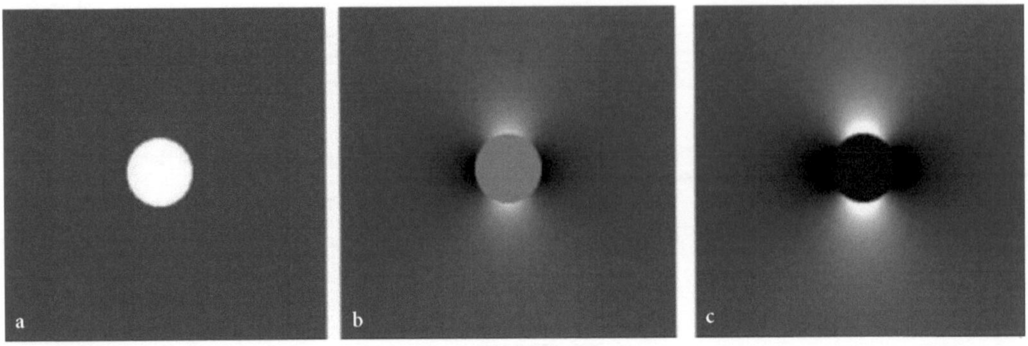

Fig. 8.3a–c. Simulated magnetic field variations within and surrounding a blood vessel orientated at various angles with respect to the static magnetic field. **a** Field variations for a vessel that is parallel to the static (B_0) field. **b** Field variations for a vessel at 45° to B_0. **c** Field variations for a vessel orientated perpendicular to B_0.

rial blood is fully oxygenated under normal circumstances, and since this does not change during periods of neuronal activity, it is only necessary to consider the signal changes that originate within and around the capillary and venous vessels. Various authors have conducted theoretical and numerical calculations which show that the extravascular signal contribution is given by the following formula (Ogawa et al. 1993):

$$R2^*_{BOLD} = k v_B^{max} (1-Y)\, CBV_v \qquad [2]$$

where $R2^*_{BOLD}$ is the BOLD relaxation contribution to $R2^*$ (=1/T2*), $v_B^{max} = 2\pi\gamma\Delta\chi B_0$, and CBV_v is the fractional blood volume of capillaries and venules in grey matter. Hence there will be a change in the signal intensity in a T2*-weighted image if either the blood oxygenation term (Y) changes, and/or if the CBV changes. It is instructive to compare the form of Eq. 2 with the CBV and BOLD plots shown in Fig. 8.2. Note that the increase in CBV during neuronal activation leads to an increase in $R2^*_{BOLD}$ (via Eq. 2) and hence to a signal decrease (T2* shortening). However, the increased oxygenation level of the blood (Y) that indirectly results from the increase in CBF leads to a decrease in $R2^*_{BOLD}$ (and hence to a signal increase). As can be seen in Fig. 8.2, these two effects compete with one another to yield a complex BOLD time-course that may have both positive and negative epochs.

A summary of these effects is shown in Fig. 8.4, demonstrating how shifts in the haemodynamic variables during neuronal stimulation lead to changes in the concentration of deoxyhaemoglobin in the tissue voxel, and hence to a signal change in a T2*-weighted image.

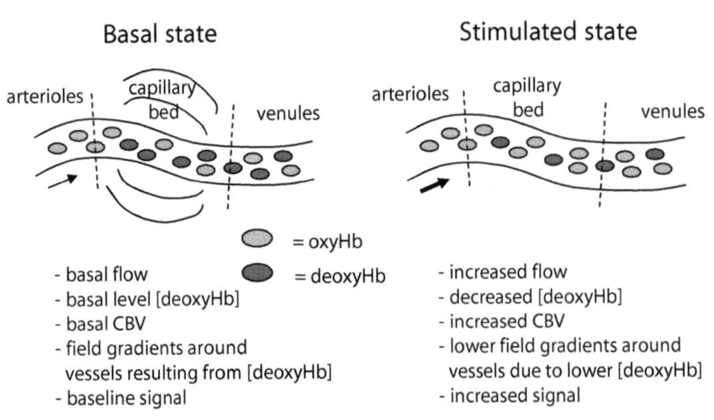

Fig. 8.4. Diagram showing the haemodynamic variables that change during neuronal activity. In the basal state deoxyhaemoglobin in the capillaries and venules causes microscopic field gradients to be established around the blood vessels. This in turn leads to a decreased signal in a gradient-echo MRI sequence. In the activated state the significant increase in flow and modest increase in oxygen demand result in a lower concentration of deoxyhaemoglobin in the capillaries and venules. As a result the field gradients around the vessels are diminished and the gradient echo signal is restored.

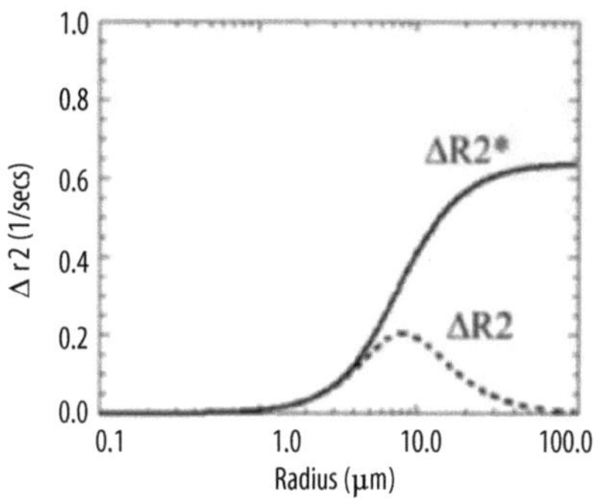

Fig. 8.5. Extravascular ΔR2* and ΔR2 changes versus vessel radius for a gradient-echo sequence (*solid line*) and SE sequence (*dashed line*).

Before leaving the topic of BOLD theory it should be pointed out that it is also possible to obtain BOLD sensitivity when using a purely T2-weighted pulse sequence (see also the discussion on T2 contrast below). The reason that the majority of BOLD fMRI studies to date have used pulse sequences that are based on gradient echoes rather than spin echoes can be appreciated by reference to Fig. 8.5. This shows the theoretical effect on the relaxation rate of transverse magnetization (R2=1/T2 for a spin-echo (SE) sequence, and R2*=1/T2* for a gradient-echo (GE) sequence) as a function of the radius of the blood vessels. In both cases the same level of blood deoxygenation has been modelled. It can be seen that the GE sequence (solid line) shows a much larger change in relaxation rate for a given level of deoxygenation than the SE sequence (dashed line), provided the vessel radius is above approximately 8 μm. The origin of this effect lies in the difference in the regimes of characteristic diffusion distances relative to the extent of the field inhomogeneities surrounding vessels of different sizes. Above approximately 8 μm radius the signal dephasing effects of the blood deoxygenation-related field inhomogeneities will be substantially refocused by a SE sequence (leading to small R2 changes), but will continue to dephase in the case of a GE sequence (leading to significant R2* changes). A disadvantage of GE sequences can also be observed in Fig. 8.5, however. This is that GE sequences show signal changes even from very large blood vessels that may not be localized to the active tissue – the so-called draining vein effect (Turner 2002). BOLD signal changes *can* be observed if a SE pulse sequence is employed, but the percentage signal change that is measured is much smaller than in the case of a GE pulse sequence.

8.2.3 Other MR-Accessible Markers of Functional Activity

The description above concentrates on the BOLD effect, since this is the contrast mechanism used in most fMRI examinations. However, it is worth mentioning other physiological and biophysical parameters to which MRI can gain access. None of these other contrast mechanisms is used widely, although each has the prospect of revealing additional functional information, and hence may become clinically relevant.

CBF: Probably the most informative of these additional MRI contrast mechanisms is the measure of CBF. As described in the preceding chapter, there are two principal methods for assessing CBF using MRI: either using an exogenous paramagnetic contrast agent (Ostergaard et al. 1996), or by magnetically labelling the arterial blood itself using specialized RF pulses (Williams et al. 1992; Wong et al. 1999). Both of these methods allow resting levels of perfusion to be measured, although both approaches have certain unresolved methodological issues that limit their interpretation in the clinical setting. One advantage of the non-invasive spin labelling approach, though, is that it can be used to measure dynamic changes in blood flow during neurological stimulation (Kim et al. 1997; Luh et al. 2000). These preliminary results also suggest that perfusion contrast is better localized to the parenchymal tissue and less contaminated by artefacts from draining veins than is BOLD contrast. The main disadvantage of arterial spin labelling is that the contrast-to-noise ratio is very low, despite the fact that the underlying regional CBF changes themselves are quite large (30–100%), with sensitivity down by at least a factor of three relative to BOLD contrast. As a consequence, perfusion fMRI is still only performed in a small number of rather specialist research centres. An example of a perfusion time-course and a perfusion activation map is shown in Fig. 8.6.

CBV: Another physiological correlate of functional activity is that of local changes in CBV. Indeed, the first functional MRI methods used the blood volume change as the basis for the fMRI contrast (Belliveau et al. 1991). The CBV response to neuronal activity is thought to be a purely mechanical response of the cerebral vasculature to increases in CBF, and hence pressure (Buxton et al. 1998; Mandeville et al. 1999). MRI methods to measure CBV have used

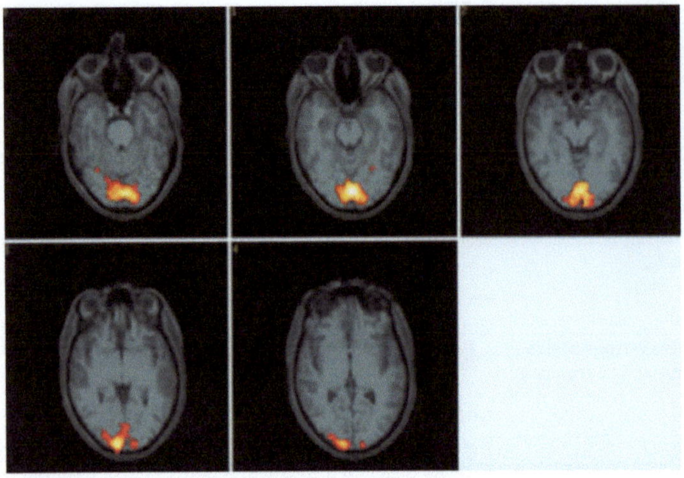

a

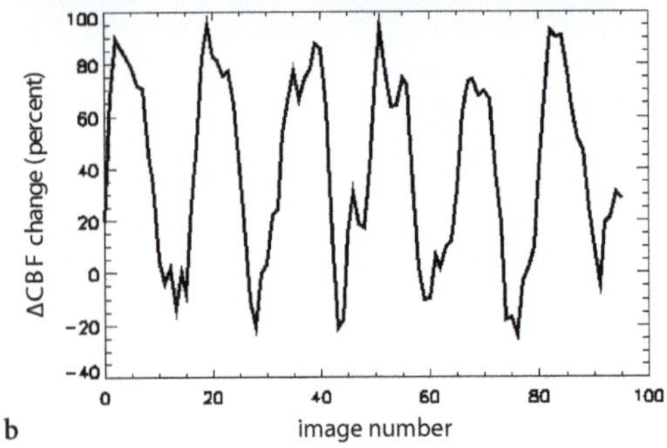

b

Fig. 8.6a,b. Calculated functional activation map and ROI time-course derived from a perfusion-weighted MRI data set collected during alternated periods of visual stimulation and rest. Significant pixels are shown in colour, overlaid on a structural image. The QUIPSS II imaging pulse sequence (WONG et al. 1998) was used to magnetically tag (invert) the arterial blood using a time-course sequence that collected a perfusion-weighted image every 4 s. These images were interleaved with a control pulse sequence in which no inversion was performed. The resulting difference images (temporal resolution 4 s) yield time-course maps of dynamic perfusion change, that can be analysed in a similar way to conventional BOLD fMRI data sets.

exogenous contrast agent injection (e.g. gadolinium-based compounds such as gadopentetate dimeglumine) in order to map blood volume by measuring the passage of a bolus of contrast agent through the tissue of interest (ROSEN et al. 1991). In order to show an fMRI response it is necessary to perform two separate bolus injections, one during stimulus condition A and the other during stimulus condition B. CBV changes can then be calculated from the difference in the CBV maps calculated during conditions A and B, after accounting for any normalization issues. Clearly, this method is cumbersome, since it requires invasive injection procedures, and is also limited to comparison of only a very few stimulus conditions (usually only a single comparison of A and B).

An attractive alternative approach uses long-lasting susceptibility-based exogenous contrast agents that may offer the possibility to map CBV changes dynamically. These iron oxide-based agents have long half lives in the blood (several hours) and so may allow more elaborate CBV-based fMRI to be performed. To date these agents are only permitted for animal use (e.g. MANDEVILLE et al. 1998).

$CMRO_2$: The metabolic rate of consumption of oxygen ($CMRO_2$) is a parameter that is more intimately related to the underlying neuronal activity than either the BOLD or CBF changes. For this reason there have been several attempts to measure $CMRO_2$ using MRI. One approach has recently been proposed by DAVIS et al. (1998) and by HOGE et al. (1999) that allows a determination of the percentage change in $CMRO_2$ during activation, although it does not allow an absolute quantification of $CMRO_2$. The method requires an independent calibration of the confounding effects of CBV in the BOLD response equation (Eq. 2). Since direct dynamic measurement of CBV using MRI is still not possible in humans, the calibration is accomplished by measuring the dynamic CBF response to hypercapnia and then by using the empirical relationship of GRUBB et al. (1974) to infer changes in CBV.

Using this approach, there remain a number of questionable assumptions that are implicit in the determination of $CMRO_2$ change from MRI data. The principal assumption is that Grubb's equation relating changes in CBF and CBV holds for conditions of activation, and that it holds in awake humans (the original empirical relationship was established in anaesthetized monkey brain). Another implicit assumption when fitting to the models used to date is that only the extravascular contribution to $R2^*_{BOLD}$ is modelled. As described in the earlier sections above, this is not strictly true. For now, measurement of $CMRO_2$ change in humans remains very challenging, but may in the future become an important adjunct to fMRI studies, particularly in clinical populations.

T2: There is a long history in the NMR literature of studying the oxygenation dependence of the T2 of blood itself, and indeed debate still exists regarding the precise mechanisms involved in the origin of the phenomenon (SPRINGER 1994; YE and ALLEN 1995). Regardless of the mechanism, the T2 value of blood is dependent on a number of parameters in addition to blood oxygenation, including haematocrit, field strength, and echo time (conventional SE sequence) or echo-to-echo spacing (Carr-Purcell-Meiboom-Gill sequence).

Most current theories of blood T2 (e.g. VAN ZIJL et al. 1998) model the oxygenation dependence as an exchange phenomenon between intracellular and extracellular environments. Empirically, the measurements fit well to the equation:

$$\frac{1}{T2_{blood}} = (1-Hct)\frac{1}{T2_{plasma}} + Hct\frac{1}{T2_{ery}} + \frac{1}{T2_{exch}} \qquad [3]$$

In this equation $T2_{blood}$ is the observed T2 value of the whole blood and $T2_{plasma}$ is the T2 of the plasma compartment alone. $T2_{ery}$ is the T2 of water in the erythrocytes (red blood cells), which depends on the oxygenation fraction of the haemoglobin. $T2_{exch}$ is the term that accounts for exchange of water between the intracellular compartment (i.e. inside the erythrocyte) and the extracellular compartment (i.e. the plasma). The form of this equation is typical for a system that is in fast exchange on the NMR time scale (TE in this case) – for such a system the relaxation rate that is observed is simply the sum of the rates of contributing relaxation processes.

Theory and experiment show that the term ($1/T2_{ery}$) depends linearly on the oxygenation fraction of the haemoglobin, and that the exchange term ($1/T2_{exch}$) depends quadratically on the oxygenation fraction of the haemoglobin, as well as being dependent on the individual's haematocrit. This suggests that blood T2 is able to report on a physiologically meaningful parameter, namely blood oxygenation, if the blood haematocrit can be measured or assumed. Specifically, as the blood oxygenation increases during neuronal stimulation, the T2 value of blood rises, leading to more NMR signal originating from intravascular water spins. In an attempt to utilize this mechanism, van Zijl and colleagues have developed elaborate procedures for calibrating the terms in Eq. 3 such that the blood oxygenation can be estimated from its measured T2 value (VAN ZIJL et al. 1998). Although accurate vascular T2 measurement is very difficult to perform experimentally, and can only really be accomplished in a large draining vein, values have been derived for the change in oxygen extraction fraction that are consistent with literature values (OJA et al. 1999; GOLAY et al. 2001).

8.3 Acquisition Practicalities

8.3.1 Pulse Sequence Selection

Since the GE signal change in response to a change in blood deoxygenation level is significantly larger than for a SE sequence, GE sequences have been used for the majority of BOLD fMRI studies. There are several available pulse sequences that can be applied to fMRI (only a subset of which are discussed in this section). The decision of which to choose depends on such factors as the capability of the available hardware, requirements for spatial and temporal resolution, and the area of the brain that is under study. A review of some of the most commonly encountered pulse sequences is provided below. For most of the sequences a pulse sequence diagram is shown. This is a timing diagram of the events that occur on the three gradient axes (slice select direction G_{sl}, read out direction G_{rd}, and phase encode direction G_{pe}), the radiofrequency pulses (RF), and the data acquisition, controlled by the receiver gate. The purpose of the pulse sequence is to allow the adequate sampling of *k*-space (see Chapter 4 Fast Imaging in this volume for a discussion of *k*-space).

FLASH: The FLASH GE sequence (HAASE et al. 1986) has been used by several groups who do not have access to fast gradient hardware technology. A pulse sequence diagram for the FLASH sequence is shown in Fig. 8.7, along with a map of the way in which *k*-space is sampled for this sequence. Note that each repetition of the pulse sequence acquires only one line of *k*-space, and that *N* repeats must be ac-

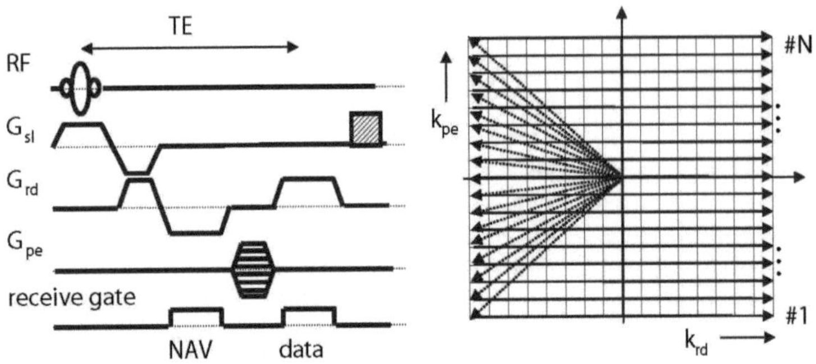

Fig. 8.7. Diagram showing the FLASH pulse sequence, along with the corresponding trajectory through *k*-space. The sequence shown includes a navigator acquisition. The shaded pulse is a spoiler to dephase any remaining transverse magnetization.

quired in order to build up the data for an *N*×*N* image. Also known as the SPGR and FFE sequence, the FLASH sequence is a conventional GE technique that requires 3–6 s per slice to acquire the data. For this reason whole-volume studies are impractical using the FLASH approach, although the method does offer the advantage of having only a low sensitivity to geometric distortion (see below). However, because of the lengthy time of acquisition for each FLASH image the technique is very sensitive to small hardware or physiological instabilities.

EPI: Echo planar imaging (Mansfield 1977) is the most widely used fMRI pulse sequence due to its remarkable speed of acquisition. On modern scanners the whole head can be covered at 4 mm slice thickness in about 3 s (ten slices per second). This enables the experimenter to characterize the haemodynamic response (the time for local flow increases and decreases to occur in the brain in response to brain activity is on the order of 6–8 s), which can yield additional information. EPI can be used to provide either T2* contrast (GE variant) or T2 contrast (SE variant).

Since EPI is so widely used it will be described in some detail here. A pulse sequence for EPI is shown in Fig. 8.8, along with the corresponding *k*-space sampling scheme. The principal difference with respect to the FLASH sequence is the ability of EPI to sample the whole of *k*-space following a single excitation of the slice. Typically, the entire information for an (admittedly low-resolution) image of the slice can be acquired in 40–50 ms. So-called "snap-shot" EPI sequences are limited to acquiring images with a matrix resolution of approximately 64×64 pixels, and on some systems up to 128×128. However, it is possible to use an interleaved version of the basic EPI sequence in which larger image matrix sizes can be achieved (McKinnon 1993). This is at the expense of a decreased temporal resolution, though, since the data for each slice requires the combination of data from multiple excitations of the slice (typically 4–16 excitations).

The major drawback of EPI, aside from its inherently low spatial resolution (usually about 4×4 mm in plane and 4–6 mm slice thickness), is its sensitivity to a number of sources of artefact. The two most prominent issues are those of non-linear geometric distortion and Nyquist ghosting. Geometric distortion occurs principally in the phase encode direction (Jezzard and Balaban 1995), and makes coregistration between EPI and conventionally collected data sets problematic. It is caused by the misrepresentation in the position of pixels that occurs in regions where the magnetic field homogeneity is poor, principally in the frontal and temporal regions of the brain where inherent susceptibility-based distortions are present in the magnetic field. The other prominent image artefact that is encountered with EPI is the phenomenon of Nyquist ghosting. This occurs as a result of the generation of the image from both positive going (left to right) and negative going (right to left) lines in *k*-space (see Fig. 8.8). This is in contrast to almost all other MRI pulse sequences in which every line in *k*-space is collected under the same readout gradient polarity. A number of small imperfections in the scanning process (e.g. scanner hardware imperfections and magnetic field inhomogeneity effects) will lead to a line-to-line modulation in the *k*-space data that, when Fourier-transformed to produce the final image, leads to some of the image signal being displaced by half a field of view (for snapshot EPI – more complex patterns occur for the case of interleaved EPI). This effect is shown in the lower left panel of Fig. 8.8, demonstrating a prominent "ghost" image that is displaced by half the field of view in the phase encode direction of the image. Various correction algorithms have been developed to minimize this artefact (to form the corrected image shown in the lower right panel of Fig. 8.8), but

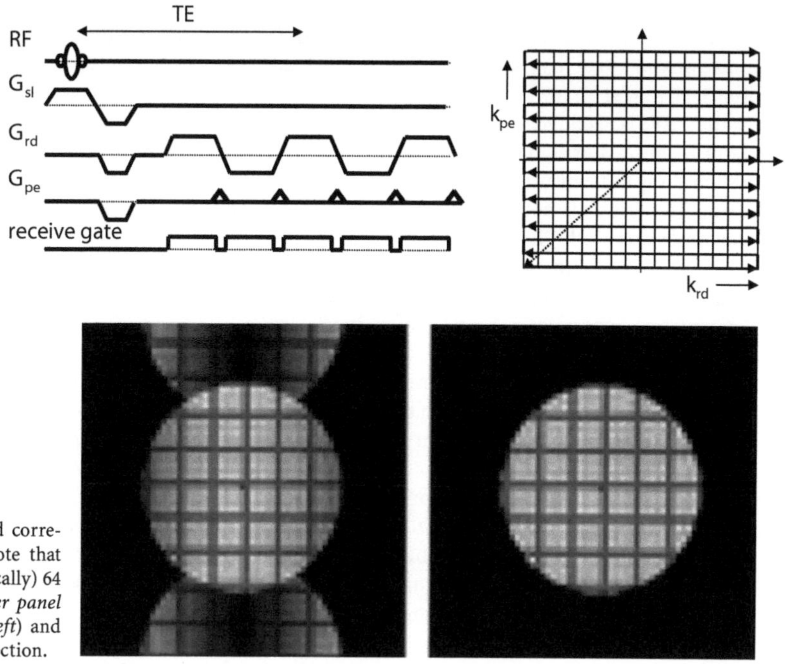

Fig. 8.8. EPI pulse sequence and corresponding *k*-space trajectory. Note that only the first 5 echoes in a (typically) 64 echo train are shown. The *lower panel* shows EPI images with poor (*left*) and good (*right*) Nyquist ghost correction.

in the common situation when the ghost signal impinges on the main image, it is wise to be aware of possible "aliased" fMRI activations that can originate from the ghost and therefore occur half a field of view from their true origin. For example, this has been noted to be a particular problem for "phantom" eye movements (Chen and Zhu 1997).

Spiral: Spiral imaging (Meyer and Macovski 1987) is also increasingly used by fMRI researchers, and is shown in Fig. 8.9. The method is similar to EPI in temporal resolution and in its ability to be run in a GE or SE mode. The artefacts that spiral sequences generate are different to EPI, yielding a local blurring (deterioration in point spread function) rather than geometric distortion in the presence of field inhomogeneity effects. Spiral sequences are also less demanding on the gradient amplifiers, and have therefore been observed to give improved stability.

PRESTO: The PRESTO sequence (Liu et al. 1993) uses echo shifting principles (Moonen et al. 1992) in order to achieve a short TR time without compromising T2* sensitivity. A conventional phase encoding strategy is used, so geometric distortion is minimal with this sequence. Another benefit is that because

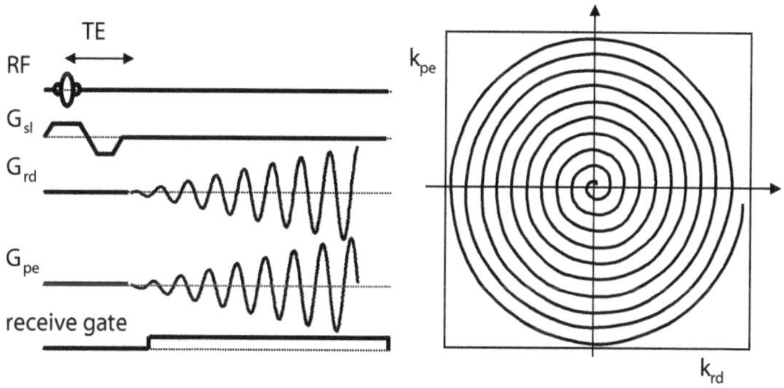

Fig. 8.9. Spiral pulse sequence and *k*-space trajectory.

the sequence can be run in a true 3D mode, it can be made very insensitive to unwanted arterial inflow contamination that can confound the FLASH approach (Duyn et al. 1994). A pulse sequence diagram for the PRESTO sequence is shown in Fig. 8.10. The gradient pulses shown hatched in Fig. 8.10 are used in such a way as to ensure that magnetization excited during TR period *i* is not refocused to form imaging data until the (*i*+1)th TR period. As such, the TE time is equal to 1.5TR (in the sequence shown). This allows adequate GE weighting to be achieved (to give BOLD T2* contrast), but retains a short TR, allowing 3D images to be acquired in a reasonable time.

Spin-Echo BOLD Sequences: As mentioned above, SE sequences generally demonstrate lower BOLD contrast. However, some researchers have used sequences based on SE pulse sequences, either in order to recover some of the signal lost in frontal and temporal regions of the brain, or to quantitatively measure the T2 relaxation time of blood. In the former case a hybrid sequence that combines GE and SE contrast can be used. This is known as an asymmetric spin echo, and is achieved by introducing an asymmetric delay into an otherwise standard SE sequence. A modification of the standard BURST pulse sequence (Hennig and Hodapp 1993; Lowe and Wysong 1993) is one such example. The sequence uses a train of low flip angle RF excitation pulses in the presence of a readout dephasing gradient. These are subsequently refocused as a train of echoes following a 180° pulse. The method is capable of producing "snap-shot" low-resolution images, and has the added benefit of being very quiet (since very few gradient switches are required). The sequence has been applied to fMRI (Jakob et al. 1998) by use of an asymmetric SE approach that provided the T2* BOLD contrast. The BURST sequence has a much lower signal-to-noise ratio than the EPI sequence, but may have applications where a quiet pulse sequence is required (e.g. for auditory activation studies).

8.3.2 Scanner Hardware Requirements

In order to accomplish successful fMRI a scanner that is above all stable and that also offers good signal-to-noise ratio is essential. Further, fast gradient hardware is desirable, since rapid sequences such as EPI provide an increase in the number of independent samples of brain activity, and hence improved statistical confidence in the resulting fMRI maps. Considerations include:

Magnetic Field Strength: Implied within the BOLD equation (Eq. 2) is a dependence of the BOLD relaxation rate that is linear with static magnetic field strength. This is in practice what is observed, although there are a number of qualifying statements to be made. Firstly, Eq. 2 only considers the extravascular spin contribution and, indeed, only for spins surrounding those vessels with a radius above approximately 10 µm. In the case of smaller vessels, and in the case of SE weighted sequences, even higher order dependencies are predicted, making higher field strength all the more attractive. Working against high field, however, is the shorter inherent T2* of the tissue. This attenuates the effect of the change in R2* (i.e., T2*) that accompanies neuronal activation, but has the advantage of suppressing large vein signals. Experimental assessment of these issues indicates that higher field strengths are indeed beneficial (Gati et al. 1997), despite a greater contribution of physiological noise at high field (Kruger and Glover 2001). As a practical guide, a field strength of between 1.5 and 3 T should provide adequate fMRI sensitivity. It should be noted that at very high field (4 T and greater) one encounters increasingly severe RF field homogeneity problems, and severe magnetic susceptibility problems.

Gradient Performance: Fast gradient performance is highly desirable for fMRI studies allowing fast imaging sequences, such as EPI, to be performed.

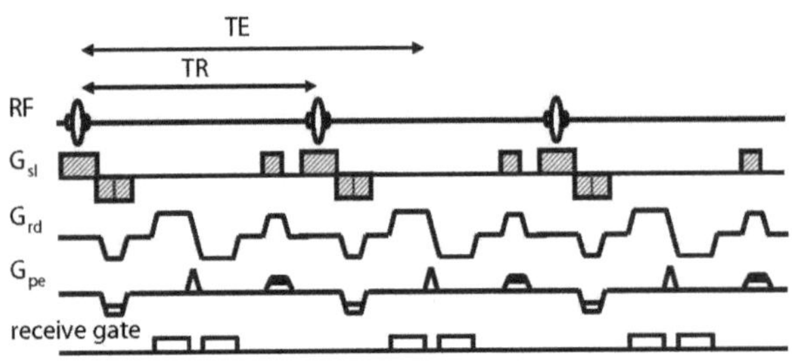

Fig. 8.10. The PRESTO pulse sequence.

Practically, one needs gradient strengths of the order 25 mT/m and gradient slew rates of 150 T/m/s. Lower performance figures than this will perhaps suffice, but fast imaging sequences may become impractical if performance is substantially lower than the above. Related to gradient performance is fast data acquisition and processing capability. As a benchmark figure, a sustainable acquisition rate of ten frames per second in snap-shot EPI mode is desirable.

Stability Requirements: Since fMRI is a subtle effect (0.5–5% signal change typically), it is important to optimize the experiment as much as possible. One critical factor is to ensure that the MRI system hardware is of sufficient signal-to-noise ratio and stability over time that an effect on the order of 0.5% can be detected. It is therefore important to run regular quality assurance tests using a phantom sample that loads the coil in a similar way to the human head. Such data will reveal whether the system has stability problems that should be addressed before fMRI experiments are attempted. A recommended test that can be performed is a pseudo-fMRI experiment in which a phantom sample (e.g. a spherical agar gel phantom) is imaged using an otherwise standard fMRI protocol. One example would be an EPI time-course consisting of 100 volumes, 64×64 pixels, 25 slices, TR/TE/thk=3000 ms/40 ms/5 mm, FOV=24×24 cm. A number of tests can then be performed on each slice of the data, including:

1) *Mean signal variability:* Variability in the time-course of the mean signal from the central 80% of the image. This figure should reflect the transmitter stability and be better than 0.1%.
2) *Signal-to-noise ratio of the individual images:* Signal = mean of central 20% of phantom, Noise = standard deviation of non-ghosted noise region. Ideally the ratio should be more than 250. (Note that a true signal-to-noise measure requires a correction factor of 1.53 (Weisskoff 1996) to account for the Rician nature of noise in magnitude MRI data.)
3) *Level of EPI ghost:* For EPI sequences the ghost should be <2–3% of the main image intensity.
4) *Pixel-by-pixel temporal stability*: For each pixel the temporal standard deviation in intensity is calculated. This is expressed as a percentage of the image mean intensity and should be <0.5%.
5) *Spatial drift test*: A data registration test is useful to assess the drift of the image in the field-of-view throughout the scan. This test can report on problematic gradient coil heating or other instabilities leading to drifts in the B_0 field. The test is best done on the volume data.

8.3.3 The Scanner as a Psychophysical Testing Environment

A key difference between conventional MRI scanning and fMRI is the need for external stimuli to be presented to the subject in the scanner and for response recording to be made from the subject. One principal requirement is the addition of a method of visual stimulus presentation (although many clinical MRI scanners now come equipped with a suitable device designed to minimize patient anxiety). This presentation device needs to be under computer control, and ideally should be capable of being triggered from the scanner. Finally, a comprehensive software package must be provided to control stimulus presentation and scanner synchronization of all stimulus and response events.

8.4 Experimental Design

8.4.1 Block Design Paradigms

The simplest form of fMRI paradigm that can be conducted is known as the block design. This is shown in Fig. 8.11a and consists of blocks of time when the stimulus is present (shown shaded) and blocks of time that act as a control periods. Typically a sustained period of at least 20–30 s forms each stimulus or control period. In some circumstances it is sufficient to use "rest" as the control condition (i.e. subject lying in the scanner "doing nothing"). However, this is a very uncontrolled condition, and often leads to difficulties in interpretation. In such circumstances, it may be necessary to select a control task that replicates many of the stimulus inputs present in the task condition, but excludes a single specific aspect that is the functional processing unit of interest. In addition to the single task period shown in Fig. 8.11a, it is also possible to design paradigms that probe several functional attributes, even in parallel. Such an example is shown in Fig. 8.12 which displays the results of overlapping periods of visual and auditory stimulation, each having a different time course. When analysing the data, the two different time series "signatures" of the visual and auditory stimuli lead to distinguishable activation areas in the brain (coloured yellow–red and green–blue, respectively).

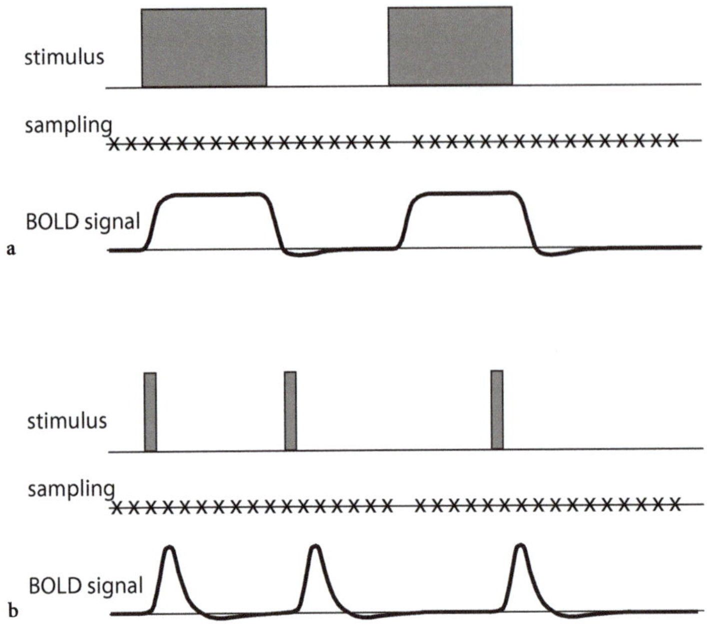

Fig. 8.11a, b. Representation of a block design fMRI paradigm (**a**), and an event-related fMRI paradigm (**b**). For the block design a relatively long (20–30 s) stimulation period is alternated with a control period. For the event-related design a brief stimulus period is used, which can either be periodic or randomized. The crosses indicate the acquisition of volumes of MRI data. The lower curves in each panel indicate the predicted haemodynamic response and are generated by convolving the stimulus input function with a model of the instantaneous haemodynamic response function.

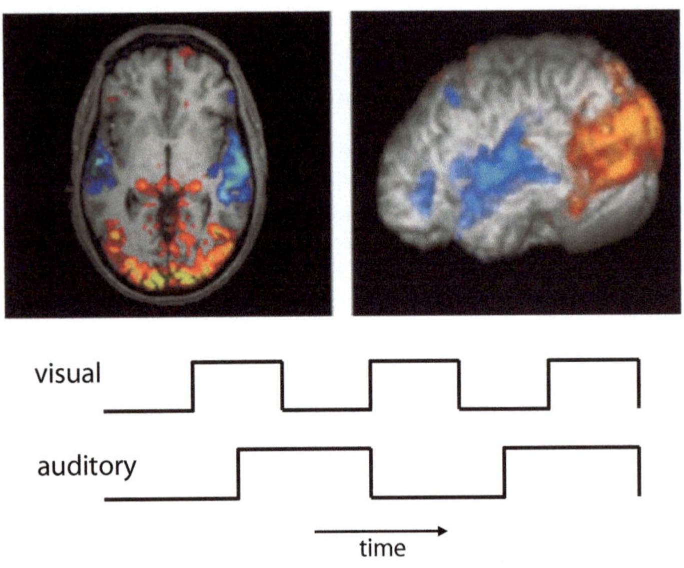

Fig. 8.12. Block design fMRI experiment showing an overlapping paradigm consisting of visual and auditory stimulation epochs. The visual stimulus consisted of a flickering checkerboard (8 Hz frequency) shown for 30 s alternated with 30-s display of a fixation cross. The auditory stimulus consisted of recorded speaking voices for 45 s alternated with 45 s of rest. A combined analysis was applied to reveal the visual (yellow–red) and auditory (green–blue) processing areas of the brain. (Data provided by the FMRIB Centre, University of Oxford, with permission.)

It is also possible to design tasks that modulate a particular functional process, such that it can be detected via a parametric analysis. An example might be to perform sustained periods of motor activity (hand flexion, finger opposition, etc.), but with each stimulus epoch performed at a different level of task difficulty. The analysis of the data then seeks those areas of the brain that show a graded response to the task level.

8.4.2 Event-Related Designs

It is not always appropriate or physiologically feasible to sustain certain stimulus types for an extended period. Such an example might be the application of a brief painful stimulus. Further, there may be a need to introduce an element of unpredictability into the stimulus presentation, for example to avoid confounds of an anticipatory response. In these cases one approach that can be adopted is the use of a so-called "event-related" design (Buckner 1998). This is shown schematically in Fig. 8.11b, in which a series of brief stimuli are presented, perhaps at regular intervals or perhaps at random intervals. It is implicit that a fast imaging sequence be used (2–3 s volume-to-volume interval), since the haemodynamic responses to be characterized are also relatively brief (6–12 s). The data are then analysed for brain areas that show a time-course signature that correlates with the predicted haemodynamic response (also shown in Fig. 8.11b). It should be noted that event-related designs are more sensitive to the details of the haemodynamic response model used (see below) than are block designs. In this sense block designs are more robust, since a sustained cognitive state can be modelled, and hence a sustained (and simple) haemodynamic response can be assumed. In contrast, analysis of event-related designs may produce poor results if an inaccurate haemodynamic response function is assumed. This may be all the more the case if the interval between successive stimuli becomes short, or if widely distributed brain areas are of interest, in which case it may be necessary to model a set of area specific haemodynamic response functions. Nevertheless, event-related designs have proved their use when short-duration stimuli are required.

8.5 Data Analysis Strategies

With the advent of well-packaged analysis programs, and with the introduction of scanners with on-board fMRI analysis, it is becoming less essential to have comprehensive knowledge regarding analytical methods for processing fMRI data. Nevertheless, it should be a high priority to any serious clinician or researcher to appreciate what is being performed within the "black box". Only a brief summary is provided here, but a more lengthy discussion of the details of fMRI data analysis can be found in the book by Jezzard et al. (2001).

8.5.1 Pre-Statistics Procedures

In most fMRI analysis packages a number of steps are first taken to improve the quality of the underlying data, or to otherwise "encourage" the data to conform to the set of assumptions behind a particular statistical model. One important first step is to attempt to correct the time-course data for motion artefacts associated with subject movement. Usually this requires an algorithm that performs a rigid body transformation in order to register successive volumes. Many sites also perform a slice timing correction that attempts to account for the fact that the different slices that comprise a volume are not actually collected simultaneously.

The other principal processing step that is often applied to the data is to perform filtering operations that attempt to improve the conformity of the data to assumptions that are subsequently used during statistical inference. In particular, many packages apply a spatial blurring in order to improve the confidence that the images have a particular point spread function (i.e. a known spatial correlation). Typically the spatial filter that is applied is only marginally wider than the digital (pixel) resolution itself. But in some cases more severe filtering is applied. The advantage of substantial spatial filtering is that the effective signal-to-noise ratio of the data can be significantly improved. However, this is at the expense of blurring the raw data to a lower resolution. A related step that may be applied is to filter the data in the time domain. This is done by selecting the time-course from each pixel in turn and applying a specific filter that suppresses undesirable features in the time series. Typically a band-pass filter is used that suppresses both low temporal fluctuations, that can arise from gradually evolving scanner instabilities or residual effects from subject motion, and high temporal frequencies that may be assumed to be noise (since the haemodynamic response function associated with "real" activations has a certain latency and width).

A number of final pre-statistics procedures may also be applied, such as intensity normalization of each volume (such that the total integrated intensity is the same in each volume). This is appropriate provided that the anticipated brain areas are small relative to the volume of brain covered.

8.5.2 Time-Course Modelling

Once the data have been preprocessed and are ready for final analysis a model of the expected fMRI time-course must be generated (although one can use model-free analysis methods as an alternative). In the case of a simple block design paradigm it may be sufficient simply to model the predicted time-course as a box car function that is "1" during periods of stimulus (or task A) and "0" during rest (or task B). An improvement to this model is to convolve the box car function with an estimate of the instantaneous haemodynamic response function (FRISTON et al. 1994). Such a function represents the response of the MRI signal (and hence vasculature that causes the change in MRI signal) to a brief stimulus event. This approach is used in the field of engineering when one wishes to predict the output signal from a modulating system or device when given an arbitrary input signal. This can be accomplished if one knows the output response function resulting from an instantaneous input signal, and provided one can assume that the modulating system or device acts as a linear system. This latter assumption is not always strictly true in the case of the fMRI signal, but may often be applied regardless, particularly in the case of block stimuli or widely spaced brief stimuli. Examples of the predicted fMRI time-course to a blocked and event-related experimental design are shown in Fig. 8.11a and 8.11b, respectively. Once generated, this time course model can be used as the basis for testing against each pixel time series in the raw fMRI data.

8.5.3 Statistical Inference

The ultimate aim of statistical inference is to identify those pixels whose time-course matches the modelled haemodynamic time-course, and to assign a statistical confidence to this identification, given the level of noise present. The most common approach is to adopt a general linear model (FRISTON et al. 1995), in which the observed data are modelled as:

$$y(t) = \beta * x(t) + c + e \quad [4]$$

where $y(t)$ is the array of observed data (a 1D vector of signal intensities representing a given pixel's time-course); $x(t)$ is the haemodynamic model (also sometimes known as the explanatory variable) describing the expected signal time-course resulting from the stimulus paradigm; β is the parameter estimate for $x(t)$ (in other words it is the scalar that must be multiplied by $x(t)$ in order to fit the data); c is a constant, and represents the signal amplitude during the baseline condition; and e is an error term, that should consist of white Gaussian-distributed random noise if the fit is good. If the paradigm consisted of two different stimuli (for example in the case of the visual and auditory stimulus data set shown in Fig. 8.12) then a second parameter estimate and haemodynamic model can be introduced as $\beta_2 * x_2(t)$. Note also that more sophisticated questions can be asked within this framework by generating new explanatory variables, such as whether the presence of two overlapping stimuli results in an fMRI signal that is greater than the sum of their signals if the stimuli are presented separately.

Once the entire data set has been fitted, one can produce a T statistic for each pixel location, based on the ratio between the size of the parameter estimate (β) and the size of its standard error. Once a T statistic has been calculated one can transform into a P (probability) or Z statistic image. The only remaining step is to set a threshold level at which to accept or reject pixels that pass or fail the statistical test. Typically probability thresholds of $P<0.01$ are selected, after suitable correction has been made for the number of statistical tests that have been performed.

8.6 Spinal Cord fMRI

Advances in the treatments of spinal cord injury and disease have improved outcome in recent years. In addition, active research is currently being undertaken to explore the possibility of promoting axonal regeneration (HORNER and GAGE 2000). The effective use of these treatments will require the accurate monitoring of the anatomical and functional characteristics of the spinal cord within and around the injury site. The application of fMRI to the spinal cord (spinal fMRI) as a non-invasive mapping technique of neural function is therefore potentially of great significance.

One of the earliest studies employed a unilateral hand-closing paradigm at 1.5 T to demonstrate signal change of 4.8% in the ventral grey matter of the ipsilateral seventh cervical cord segment (YOSHIZAWA et al. 1996). Less consistent activation was also noted in the dorsal grey horn and contralateral spinal cord, and was explained by the presence of interneuronal connections.

Subsequently, substantial human spinal fMRI work has been conducted by Stroman et al. They have concentrated on cervical cord imaging and sensory stimulation paradigms. Cervical cord BOLD-related signal changes were initially demonstrated at 3 T (STROMAN et al. 1999) and then at 1.5 T (STROMAN and RYNER 2001; STROMAN et al. 2001b) looking at sensory and motor-related activations. At 1.5 T GE and SE EPI were compared and found to impart similar activation signal changes (about 4–5%) although theoretically GE EPI should be expected to provide much larger signal changes than SE EPI. The authors explained this by alluding to anatomical differences between brain tissue and spinal cord. For example, only small vessels lie within the spinal cord parenchyma and these vessels tend to be radially orientated. The vessel size and orientation would maximize the magnetic field susceptibility gradients and increase the expected BOLD contrast. A further factor is that spinal cord structure, unlike the cerebral cortex, is not tortuous and is more likely to contain homogeneous grey matter and consequently be less susceptible to partial volume effects (Stroman and Ryner 2001).

Studies by Stroman et al. have also demonstrated that there may be a second contrast mechanism that manifests with SE EPI sequences at very short echo times (Stroman et al. 2001a; Stroman et al. 2002a; Stroman et al. 2003). This is because the estimated fractional signal changes during activation in SE EPI fMRI have values of about 2.5% when extrapolated to a TE of zero. This non-zero intercept has been interpreted as perhaps arising from a proton density increase within the extravascular space and has been termed "signal enhancement by extravascular protons" or SEEP. Alternatively, this effect may be related to blood volume increases.

Further work has demonstrated a dermatomal distribution of sensory stimulation (using a cold stimulus) within the cervical cord in a study of 13 healthy volunteers. By using a "clustering" technique that congregates active pixels based upon their intensity time-courses the authors were able to discriminate true activations from false ones (Stroman et al. 2002b). Lumbar spinal fMRI has also been developed in studies using temperature stimulation paradigms and has shown in healthy subjects a relationship between the magnitude of the fMRI response within the dorsal lumbar cord and the degree of noxious stimulation (Stroman et al. 2002c). In patients with spinal cord injuries, fMRI responses have also been demonstrated with lumbar sensory stimulation, even when the patients had no subjective sensations themselves. This activity tends to be localized to the contralateral side of the cord (Stroman et al. 2002c; Stroman et al. 2004).

8.7 Clinical Applications in White Matter Disorders

FMRI has many clinical and research applications. Several examples of its use in helping to understand demyelinating disease and schizophrenia are outlined below. One of its most challenging roles is to explore cortical plasticity in neurological disease.

8.7.1 Cortical Plasticity

Functional improvement is often seen following acute brain injury; however certain aspects of recovery cannot be explained by structural mechanisms such as the resolution of inflammation or oedema. FMRI has presented the opportunity to measure changes relating to interactions at the level of large neuronal populations that follow neural insult (cortical plasticity). The term cortical plasticity has been defined as the "reorganization of distributed patterns of normal task-associated brain activity that accompany action, perception, and cognition and that compensate impaired function resulting from disease or brain injury" (Frackowiak et al. 1997). Plasticity in neuroscience research may also relate to lower levels of neural organization and may include axonal/neuronal mechanisms, for example reflecting changes in sodium channel expression (Waxman 2001) or dendritic arborization (Jones and Schallert 1992), and synaptic mechanisms, for example indicating changes in synaptic density, distribution or strength (Jacobs and Donoghue 1991).

Although the capacity for cortical plasticity is at its greatest during the early years of CNS development, it appears to persist throughout life. The behavioural effects of cortical reorganization following CNS insult may be divided into different categories which describe, for example, *adaptive* and *maladaptive* processes. Adaptive cortical reorganization implies that the redistribution of neural processing in some way contributes to the mechanisms involved in clinical recovery or helps to maintain a degree of clinical function in the presence of structural damage. At least four forms of adaptive plasticity have been suggested (Grafman and Litvan 1999): (1) *homologous area adaptation* – implies that the damaged brain region can be compensated for by transferring the neural operations to other unaffected brain modules (usually in the homologous region of the opposite hemisphere); (2) *cross-modal reassignment*—occurs when cortical modules usually devoted to processing particular sensory inputs, now accept inputs from another sensory modality; (3) *map expansion*—is the enlargement of a functional cortical region in response to frequent stimulus exposure or following adjacent cortical injury; and (4) *compensatory masquerade* – is the novel allocation of a cognitive strategy to perform a task that otherwise would depend on another cognitive process which is now impaired.

However, cortical reorganization may not necessarily contribute to recovery of clinical function. It may also reflect the recruitment of unusual distributed neural networks purely as a 'stress' response to CNS injury implying that it can be *non-adaptive* or *coincidental.*

Indeed, plastic changes in response to injury may also have deleterious behavioural effects resulting in functional loss rather than gain. This form of plasticity is termed *maladaptive* and is, for example, thought to account for phantom limb pain following amputation (Lotze et al. 2001).

8.7.2 Functional MRI in Demyelinating Disease

Several studies have been performed to investigate how the brain possibly adapts to neurological damage in demyelinating disease. These studies have mostly employed experimental paradigms for the visual and the motor systems and can be categorized into those that address (1) clinically isolated syndromes, e.g. optic neuritis, (2) relapsing remitting multiple sclerosis (MS), (3) secondary progressive MS, and (4) primary progressive MS. Further treatment of this subject can be found in Chapter 14 of this book.

8.7.3 Functional MRI in Schizophrenia

Schizophrenia is a debilitating psychiatric disorder characterized by the presence of certain types of 'positive' symptoms such as delusions, hallucinations and thought disorder (Andreasen 1995). These 'positive' symptoms are usually complemented by 'negative' symptoms such as psychomotor retardation and affective flattening. In addition, a significant role for cognitive dysfunction has become increasingly recognized in helping to understand the clinical deficits of schizophrenia. The cognitive deficits are related to but distinct from negative symptoms and appear to significantly influence clinical outcome in schizophrenia (Sharma and Antonova 2003). FMRI has been used to investigate the neural correlates associated with both positive symptoms, negative symptoms and cognitive dysfunction over recent years. Some examples of its contributions are described below.

Auditory hallucinations constitute a prominent feature of positive symptoms and their impact has been explored in several studies. The results have suggested processing abnormalities in primary auditory and association cortices and have also implicated subcortical and limbic structures. Reduced activation in response to auditory stimulation has been found in auditory areas resulting in the concept that auditory hallucinations compete with external auditory stimuli (David et al. 1996; Woodruff et al. 1997).

A novel methodological technique was implemented by Shergill et al. to measure neural activity associated with auditory hallucinations without requiring subjects to signal when the hallucinations occurred. They discovered that auditory hallucinations are associated with activation in a distributed network of cortical and subcortical areas that include the inferior frontal/insular, anterior cingulate, and temporal cortex bilaterally (with greater responses on the right), the right thalamus and inferior colliculus, and the left hippocampus and parahippocampal cortex (Shergill et al. 2000). A further study by the same group investigated the notion of auditory hallucinations as a disorder of the self-monitoring of 'inner speech'. Eight schizophrenic subjects with prominent auditory hallucinations were compared with eight comparison subjects using a paradigm that experimentally varied the generation rate of inner speech. When the rate was increased, the schizophrenia patients showed a relatively attenuated response within the right temporal, parietal, parahippocampal and cerebellar cortices, areas previously implicated in verbal self-monitoring (Shergill et al. 2003).

Abnormalities in the integration of auditory and visual language perception are also felt to correlate with psychotic symptoms. Surguladze et al. (2001) performed three experiments each on seven healthy volunteers and fourteen schizophrenia patients, seven of whom were actively psychotic. The tasks comprised listening to auditory speech, silent lip-reading (visual speech perception) and perception of meaningless lip movements (visual non-speech). Patients overall demonstrated lower activation in temporal regions for the lip-reading task, compared with healthy controls. They also activated fewer posterior (occipitotemporal) and more anterior (frontal, insular and striatal) areas than controls, accounted for largely by the psychotic subgroup. This suggests that schizophrenia patients with psychotic symptoms activate polysensory regions in response to visually ambiguous stimuli (non-speech) (Surguladze et al. 2001).

Investigations into cognitive dysfunction and negative symptoms can be difficult to interpret, especially with studies on working memory. This is because their interpretation can be confounded by impaired working memory function in schizophrenia patients (Sharma 2003). In spite of this, a functional abnormality of the dorsolateral prefrontal cortex (DLPFC) appears to play a significant role in complex cognitive dysfunction. Most studies have demonstrated 'hypofrontality' or reduced activation of the DLPFC in response to complex cognitive tasks when compared with controls (Barch et al. 2001; Barch et al. 2002; MacDonald and Carter 2003; Perlstein et al. 2001; Riehemann et al. 2001). Tasks that do not require complex processing have also demonstrated reduced DLPFC activation in schizophrenia patients relative to controls (Rubia et al. 2001).

Some studies have not observed 'hypofrontality'. Honey et al. controlled for task performance by selecting patients with normal scores on a relatively low-load verbal memory task (Honey et al. 2002). Although no differences were found between schizophrenia patients and controls, the control group exhibited positive correlations between reaction time and the fMRI response within the posterior parietal cortex. This correlation was not found in the schizophrenia group, perhaps implying that 'hypofrontality' occurs only when the ability of the DLPFC to respond to a working memory task is exceeded by the cognitive load.

A few other studies have reported greater DLPFC activation in schizophrenia patients with complex cognitive tasks (Callicott et al. 2000; Manoach et al. 2000; Ramsey et al. 2002). Ramsey et al., in particular, investigated the role of antipsychotic medication and controlled for cognitive performance with a logical reasoning task (Ramsey et al. 2002). Task performance was modestly reduced in the patient group. In patients on medication, the fMRI activity did not differ significantly from controls after correction for task performance. However, in medication-naive patients, the performance-corrected fMRI activity was significantly elevated within the DLPFC. These results point to increased neural recruitment with untreated schizophrenia during logical reasoning. The mixed results presented above indicate that the function(s) of the DLPFC in schizophrenia remain to be elucidated and require further research.

Knowledge about the precise neuropathological and neurophysiological substrates of schizophrenia is also incomplete. Structural findings have included enlargement of the lateral and third ventricles (Daniel et al. 1991; Lawrie and Abukmeil 1998) and reductions in grey and white matter volume and density. Grey matter abnormalities have been found within the limbic system, thalamus, medial frontal, temporal, precuneate, posterior cingulate and insular areas (Andreasen 1997; Gaser et al. 1999; Hulshoff Pol et al. 2001; Wright et al. 2000). White matter abnormalities have been detected in the frontal lobes (Paillere-Martinot et al. 2001), left posterior periventricular area (Sowell et al. 2000), temporal lobes (Sigmundsson et al. 2001) and the corpus callosum (Hulshoff Pol et al. 2004).

It has been proposed that the clinical abnormalities arise from interregional aberrant connectivity or 'disconnectivity' (Friston 1998; Friston and Frith 1995). This hypothesis may explain the symptoms and cognitive deficits in schizophrenia and is generally felt to have some truth, but its precise nature is unknown; for example the spatial scale of the disconnectivity may be present at the synaptic or dendritic level rather than at the level of the cortical region. However, in future, by combining MR measures of function (with fMRI) and of structure (for example, with diffusion tensor imaging) it may be possible to explore the relationships between effective connectivity and anatomical connectivity in schizophrenia and thus contribute to a more complete understanding of its pathophysiology.

8.8 Conclusion

This chapter attempts to describe the principles of functional MRI, and also includes a brief discussion of applications of fMRI to white matter disorders. Conventional fMRI is only able to access haemodynamic, and hence metabolic, information from the grey matter. As such, the information that can be obtained on white matter disorders is derived from the effect that a given disorder has on the participating grey matter networks. Nevertheless, preliminary work has been done to improve our understanding of the evolution and treatment of various white matter disorders, most notably in multiple sclerosis.

One probable evolution that will occur in the field of neuroimaging is the combining of information from several different contrast mechanisms and mo-

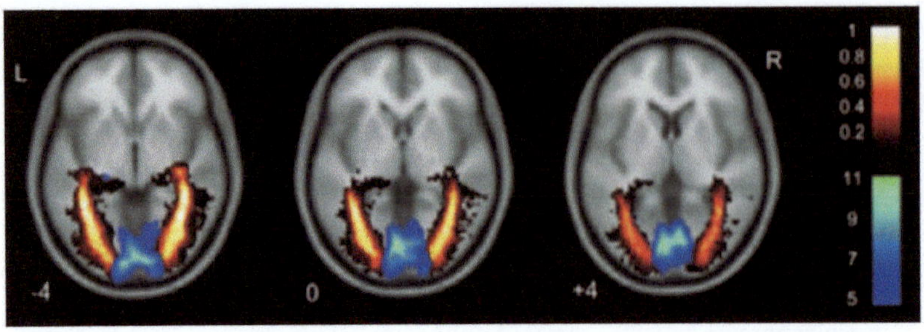

Fig. 8.13. Example of combining fMRI and DTI tractography. Group effects for functional activation and estimated optic radiations are overlaid onto a structural template. The fMRI activity was derived from a one sample **t**-test for 22 subjects with a visual stimulation paradigm. The winter (**blue**) colour scale shows the T scores. The optic radiations were estimated using DTI tractography and are displayed as spatial variability maps which demonstrate the degree of overlap (shown by the hot colour scale) between subjects for the estimated optic radiations. A value of 0.8 indicates 80% overlap between subjects. Greater intersubject overlap is noted towards the cores of the estimated optic radiations. (Reproduced from Toosy et al. 2004, with permission.)

dalities. In the context of MRI contrast it is becoming clear that diffusion-weighted information, and in particular diffusion tractography, will reveal rich information on white matter tracts, and that this information can be combined with standard fMRI contrast of the grey matter processing units. Figure 8.13 shows an example of combined fMRI and diffusion tractography imaging, indicating how structural and functional information can be combined. Beyond MRI there is the prospect of combined electroencephalography (EEG) and fMRI, in order to improve the temporal resolution of the information available. Likewise the spatial resolution of fMRI may be used to constrain the location of sources when analysing magnetoencephalography (MEG) data.

Acknowledgements

P.J. gratefully acknowledges the support of the UK Medical Research Council and the Dunhill Medical Trust. A.T. gratefully acknowledges support from the Brain Research Trust.

References

Andreasen NC (1995) Symptoms, signs, and diagnosis of schizophrenia. Lancet. 346(8973):477–481

Andreasen NC (1997) The role of the thalamus in schizophrenia. Can J Psychiatry 42(1):27–33

Bandettini PA, Wong EC, Hinks RS, Tikofsky RS, Hyde JS (1992) Time course EPI of human brain function during task activation. Magn Reson Med 25(2):390–397

Barch DM, Carter CS, Braver TS, Sabb FW, MacDonald A III, Noll DC, Cohen JD (2001) Selective deficits in prefrontal cortex function in medication-naive patients with schizophrenia. Arch Gen Psychiatry 58(3):280–288

Barch DM, Csernansky JG, Conturo T, Snyder AZ (2002) Working and long-term memory deficits in schizophrenia: is there a common prefrontal mechanism? J Abnorm Psychol 111(3):478–494

Belliveau JW, Kennedy DN Jr, McKinstry RC, Buchbinder BR, Weisskoff RM, Cohen MS, Vevea JM, Brady TJ, Rosen BR (1991) Functional mapping of the human visual cortex by magnetic resonance imaging. Science 254:716–719

Buckner RL (1998) Event-related fMRI and the hemodynamic response. Human Brain Mapping 6:373–377

Buxton RB, Frank LR (1997) A model for the coupling between cerebral blood flow and oxygen metabolism during neural stimulation. J Cereb Blood Flow Metab 17(1):64–72

Buxton RB, Wong EC, Frank LR (1998) Dynamics of blood flow and oxygenation changes during brain activation: the balloon model. Magn Reson Med 39(6):855–864

Callicott JH, Bertolino A, Mattay VS, Langheim FJ, Duyn J, Coppola R, Goldberg TE, Weinberger DR (2000) Physiological dysfunction of the dorsolateral prefrontal cortex in schizophrenia revisited. Cereb Cortex 10(11):1078–1092

Chen W, Zhu XH (1997) Suppression of physiological eye movement artifacts in functional MRI using slab presaturation. Magn Reson Med 38(4):546–550

Daniel DG, Goldberg TE, Gibbons RD, Weinberger DR (1991) Lack of a bimodal distribution of ventricular size in schizophrenia: a Gaussian mixture analysis of 1056 cases and controls. Biol Psychiatry 30(9):887–903

David AS, Woodruff PW, Howard R, Mellers JD, Brammer M, Bullmore E, Wright I, Andrew C, Williams SC (1996) Auditory hallucinations inhibit exogenous activation of auditory association cortex. Neuroreport 7(4):932–936

Davis TL, Kwong KK, Weisskoff RM, Rosen BR (1998) Calibrated functional MRI: mapping the dynamics of oxidative metabolism. Proc Natl Acad Sci U S A 95(4):1834–1839

Duyn JH, Moonen CT, van Yperen GH, de Boer RW, Luyten PR (1994) Inflow versus deoxyhemoglobin effects in BOLD functional MRI using gradient echoes at 1.5 T. NMR Biomed 7(1-2):83–88

Ernst T, Hennig J (1994) Observation of a fast response in functional MR. Magn Reson Med 32(1):146–149

Frackowiak RSJ, Friston KJ, Frith CD, Dolan RJ, Mazziotta JC

(eds) (1997) Human brain function. Academic Press, San Diego
Friston KJ (1998) The disconnection hypothesis. Schizophr Res 30(2):115–125
Friston KJ, Frith CD (1995) Schizophrenia: a disconnection syndrome? Clin Neurosci 3(2):89–97
Friston KJ, Jezzard P, Turner R (1994) Analysis of functional MRI time series. Hum Brain Mapp 1:153–171
Friston K, Holmes A, Worsley K, Poline J-B, Frith C, Frackowiak R (1995) Statistical parametric maps in functional imaging: a general linear approach. Hum Brain Mapp 2:189–210
Gaser C, Volz HP, Kiebel S, Riehemann S, Sauer H (1999) Detecting structural changes in whole brain based on nonlinear deformations—application to schizophrenia research. Neuroimage 10(2):107–113
Gati JS, Menon RS, Ugurbil K, Rutt BK (1997) Experimental determination of the BOLD field strength dependence in vessels and tissue. Magn Reson Med 38(2):296–302
Golay X, Silvennoinen MJ, Zhou J, Clingman CS, Kauppinen RA, Pekar JJ, van Zijl PC (2001) Measurement of tissue oxygen extraction ratios from venous blood T2: increased precision and validation of principle. Magn Reson Med 46(2):282–291
Grafman J, Litvan I (1999) Evidence for four forms of neuroplasticity. In: Grafman J, Christen Y (eds) Neuronal plasticity: building a bridge from the laboratory to the clinic (research and perspectives in neurosciences). Springer, Berlin Heidelberg New York, pp 131–139
Grubb RL Jr, Raichle ME, Eichling JO, Ter-Pogossian MM (1974) The effects of changes in PaCO2 on cerebral blood volume, blood flow, and vascular mean transit time. Stroke 5(5):630–639
Haase A, Frahm J, Matthaei D, Hanicke W Merboldt KD (1986) FLASH imaging: rapid NMR imaging using low flip angles. J Magn Reson 67:217–222
Hennig J, Hodapp M (1993) Burst imaging. MAGMA 1:39–48
Hoge RD, Atkinson J, Gill B, Crelier GR, Marrett S, Pike GB (1999) Linear coupling between cerebral blood flow and oxygen consumption in activated human cortex. Proc Natl Acad Sci U S A 96(16):9403–9408
Honey GD, Bullmore ET, Sharma T (2002) De-coupling of cognitive performance and cerebral functional response during working memory in schizophrenia. Schizophr Res 53(1-2):45–56
Horner PJ, Gage FH (2000) Regenerating the damaged central nervous system. Nature 407(6807):963–970
Hulshoff Pol HE, Schnack HG, Mandl RC, van Haren NE, Koning H, Collins DL, Evans AC, Kahn RS (2001) Focal gray matter density changes in schizophrenia. Arch Gen Psychiatry 58(12):1118–1125
Hulshoff Pol HE, Schnack HG, Mandl RC, Cahn W, Collins DL, Evans AC, Kahn RS (2004) Focal white matter density changes in schizophrenia: reduced inter-hemispheric connectivity. Neuroimage 21(1):27–35
Jacobs KM, Donoghue JP (1991) Reshaping the cortical motor map by unmasking latent intracortical connections. Science 251(4996):944–947
Jakob PM, Schlaug G, Griswold M, Lovblad KO, Thomas R, Ives JR, Matheson JK, Edelman RR (1998) Functional BURST imaging. Magn Reson Med 40(4):614–621
Jezzard P, Balaban RS (1995) Correction for geometric distortion in echo planar images from B0 field variations. Magn Reson Med 34:65–73
Jezzard P, Matthews PM, Smith SM (Eds) (2001) Functional magnetic resonance imaging: an introductory guide. Oxford University Press, Oxford
Jones TA, Schallert T (1992) Overgrowth and pruning of dendrites in adult rats recovering from neocortical damage. Brain Res 581(1):156–160
Kim SG, Tsekos NV, Ashe J (1997) Multi-slice perfusion-based functional MRI using the FAIR technique: comparison of CBF and BOLD effects. NMR Biomed 10(4-5):191–196
Kruger G, Glover GH (2001) Physiological noise in oxygenation-sensitive magnetic resonance imaging. Magn Reson Med 46(4):631–637
Kwong KK, Belliveau JW, Chesler DA, Goldberg IE, Weisskoff RM, Poncelet BP, Kennedy DN, Hoppel BE, Cohen MS, Turner R, et al (1992) Dynamic magnetic resonance imaging of human brain activity during primary sensory stimulation. Proc Natl Acad Sci U S A 89(12):5675–5679
Lawrie SM, Abukmeil SS (1998) Brain abnormality in schizophrenia: a systematic and quantitative review of volumetric magnetic resonance imaging studies. Br J Psychiatry 172:110–120
Liu G, Sobering G, Duyn J, Moonen CTW (1993) A functional MRI technique combining principles of echo-shifting with a train of observations (PRESTO). Magn Reson Med 30:764–768
Logothetis NK, Pauls J, Augath M, Trinath T, Oeltermann A (2001) Neurophysiological investigation of the basis of the fMRI signal. Nature 412(6843):150–157
Lotze M, Flor H, Grodd W, Larbig W, Birbaumer N (2001) Phantom movements and pain: an fMRI study in upper limb amputees. Brain 124(11):2268–2277
Lowe IJ, Wysong RE (1993) DANTE ultrafast imaging sequence (DUFIS). J Magn Reson 101:106–109
Luh WM, Wong EC, Bandettini PA, Ward BD, Hyde JS (2000) Comparison of simultaneously measured perfusion and BOLD signal increases during brain activation with T(1)-based tissue identification. Magn Reson Med 44(1):137–143
MacDonald AW III, Carter CS (2003) Event-related FMRI study of context processing in dorsolateral prefrontal cortex of patients with schizophrenia. J Abnorm Psychol 112(4):689–697
Mandeville JB, Marota JJ, Kosofsky BE, Keltner JR, Weissleder R, Rosen BR, Weisskoff RM (1998) Dynamic functional imaging of relative cerebral blood volume during rat forepaw stimulation. Magn Reson Med 39(4):615–624
Mandeville JB, Marota JJ, Ayata C, Zaharchuk G, Moskowitz MA, Rosen BR, Weisskoff RM (1999) Evidence of a cerebrovascular postarteriole windkessel with delayed compliance. J Cereb Blood Flow Metab 19(6):679–689
Manoach DS, Gollub RL, Benson ES, Searl MM, Goff DC, Halpern E, Saper CB, Rauch SL (2000) Schizophrenic subjects show aberrant fMRI activation of dorsolateral prefrontal cortex and basal ganglia during working memory performance. Biol Psychiatry 48(2):99–109
Mansfield P (1977) Multi-planar image formation using NMR spin echoes. J Phys C 10:L55–L58
McKinnon GC (1993) Ultrafast interleaved gradient-echo-planar imaging on a standard scanner. Magn Reson Med 30(5):609–616
Menon RS, Ogawa S, Hu X, Strupp JP, Anderson P, Ugurbil K (1995) BOLD based functional MRI at 4 Tesla includes a capillary bed contribution: echo-planar imaging correlates

with previous optical imaging using intrinsic signals. Magn Reson Med 33(3):453–459

Meyer CH, Macovski A (1987) Square spiral fast imaging: interleaving and off-resonance effects. Proceedings 6th Society for Magnetic Resonance in Medicine 1:230

Moonen CT, Liu G, van Gelderen P, Sobering G (1992) A fast gradient-recalled MRI technique with increased sensitivity to dynamic susceptibility effects. Magn Reson Med 26(1):184–189

Ogawa S, Lee TM, Nayak AS, Glynn P (1990) Oxygenation-sensitive contrast in magnetic resonance image of rodent brain at high magnetic fields. Magn Reson Med 14(1):68–78

Ogawa S, Tank DW, Menon R, Ellermann JM, Kim SG, Merkle H, Ugurbil K (1992) Intrinsic signal changes accompanying sensory stimulation: functional brain mapping with magnetic resonance imaging. Proc Natl Acad Sci U S A 89(13):5951–5955

Ogawa S, Menon RS, Tank DW, Kim SG, Merkle H, Ellermann JM, Ugurbil K (1993) Functional brain mapping by blood oxygenation level-dependent contrast magnetic resonance imaging. A comparison of signal characteristics with a biophysical model. Biophys J 64(3):803–812

Oja JM, Gillen JS, Kauppinen RA, Kraut M, van Zijl PC (1999) Determination of oxygen extraction ratios by magnetic resonance imaging. J Cereb Blood Flow Metab 19(12):1289–1295

Ostergaard L, Weisskoff RM, Chesler DA, Gyldensted C, Rosen BR (1996) High resolution measurement of cerebral blood flow using intravascular tracer bolus passages. Part I: Mathematical approach and statistical analysis. Magn Reson Med 36(5):715–725

Paillere-Martinot M, Caclin A, Artiges E, Poline JB, Joliot M, Mallet L, Recasens C, Attar-Levy D, Martinot JL (2001) Cerebral gray and white matter reductions and clinical correlates in patients with early onset schizophrenia. Schizophr Res 50(1-2):19–26

Pauling L, Coryell C (1936) The magnetic properties and structure of hemoglobin, oxyhemoglobin and carbon monoxyhemoglobin. Proc Natl Acad Sci U S A 22:210–216

Perlstein WM, Carter CS, Noll DC, Cohen JD (2001) Relation of prefrontal cortex dysfunction to working memory and symptoms in schizophrenia. Am J Psychiatry 158(7):1105–1113

Ramsey NF, Koning HA, Welles P, Cahn W, van der Linden JA, Kahn RS (2002) Excessive recruitment of neural systems subserving logical reasoning in schizophrenia. Brain 125(8):1793–1807

Riehemann S, Volz HP, Stutzer P, Smesny S, Gaser C, Sauer H (2001) Hypofrontality in neuroleptic-naive schizophrenic patients during the Wisconsin Card Sorting Test—a fMRI study. Eur Arch Psychiatry Clin Neurosci 251(2):66–71

Rosen BR, Belliveau JW, Aronen HJ, Kennedy D, Buchbinder BR, Fischman A, Gruber M, Glas J, Weisskoff RM, Cohen MS, et al (1991) Susceptibility contrast imaging of cerebral blood volume: human experience. Magn Reson Med 22(2):293–299

Rubia K, Russell T, Bullmore ET, Soni W, Brammer MJ, Simmons A, Taylor E, Andrew C, Giampietro V, Sharma T (2001) An fMRI study of reduced left prefrontal activation in schizophrenia during normal inhibitory function. Schizophr Res 52(1-2):47–55

Sharma T (2003) Insights and treatment options for psychiatric disorders guided by functional MRI. J Clin Invest 112(1):10–18

Sharma T, Antonova L (2003) Cognitive function in schizophrenia. Deficits, functional consequences, and future treatment. Psychiatr Clin North Am 26(1):25–40

Shergill SS, Brammer MJ, Williams SC, Murray RM, McGuire PK (2000) Mapping auditory hallucinations in schizophrenia using functional magnetic resonance imaging. Arch Gen Psychiatry 57(11):1033–1038

Shergill SS, Brammer MJ, Fukuda R, Williams SC, Murray RM, McGuire PK (2003) Engagement of brain areas implicated in processing inner speech in people with auditory hallucinations. Br J Psychiatry 182:525–531

Sigmundsson T, Suckling J, Maier M, Williams S, Bullmore E, Greenwood K, Fukuda R, Ron M, Toone B (2001) Structural abnormalities in frontal, temporal, and limbic regions and interconnecting white matter tracts in schizophrenic patients with prominent negative symptoms. Am J Psychiatry 158(2):234–243

Sowell ER, Levitt J, Thompson PM, Holmes CJ, Blanton RE, Kornsand DS, Caplan R, McCracken J, Asarnow R, Toga AW (2000) Brain abnormalities in early-onset schizophrenia spectrum disorder observed with statistical parametric mapping of structural magnetic resonance images. Am J Psychiatry 157(9):1475–1484

Springer CS (1994) Bulk magnetic susceptibility frequency shifts in cell suspensions. NMR Biomed 7:198–202

Stroman PW, Ryner LN (2001) Functional MRI of motor and sensory activation in the human spinal cord. Magn Reson Imaging 19(1):27–32

Stroman PW, Nance PW, Ryner LN (1999) BOLD MRI of the human cervical spinal cord at 3 Tesla. Magn Reson Med 42(3):571–576

Stroman PW, Krause V, Frankenstein UN, Malisza KL, Tomanek B (2001a) Spin-echo versus gradient-echo fMRI with short echo times. Magn Reson Imaging 19(6):827–831

Stroman PW, Krause V, Malisza KL, Frankenstein UN, Tomanek B (2001b) Characterization of contrast changes in functional MRI of the human spinal cord at 1.5 T. Magn Reson Imaging 19(6):833–838

Stroman PW, Krause V, Malisza KL, Frankenstein UN, Tomanek B (2002a) Extravascular proton-density changes as a non-BOLD component of contrast in fMRI of the human spinal cord. Magn Reson Med 48(1):122–127

Stroman PW, Krause V, Malisza KL, Frankenstein UN, Tomanek B (2002b) Functional magnetic resonance imaging of the human cervical spinal cord with stimulation of different sensory dermatomes. Magn Reson Imaging 20(1):1–6

Stroman PW, Tomanek B, Krause V, Frankenstein UN, Malisza KL (2002c) Mapping of neuronal function in the healthy and injured human spinal cord with spinal fMRI. Neuroimage 17(4):1854–1860

Stroman PW, Tomanek B, Krause V, Frankenstein UN, Malisza KL (2003) Functional magnetic resonance imaging of the human brain based on signal enhancement by extravascular protons (SEEP fMRI). Magn Reson Med 49(3):433–439

Stroman PW, Kornelsen J, Bergman A, Krause V, Ethans K, Malisza KL, Tomanek B (2004) Noninvasive assessment of the injured human spinal cord by means of functional magnetic resonance imaging. Spinal Cord 42(2):59–66

Surguladze SA, Calvert GA, Brammer MJ, Campbell R, Bullmore ET, Giampietro V, David AS (2001) Audio-visual speech perception in schizophrenia: an fMRI study. Psychiatry Res 106(1):1–14

Thulborn KR, Gisbert A (2001) Clinical applications of mapping neurocognitive processes in the human brain with functional MRI. In: Jezzard P, Matthews PM, Smith SM (eds) Functional magnetic resonance imaging: an introductory guide. Oxford University Press, Oxford, pp 353–382

Thulborn KR, Waterton JC, Matthews PM, Radda GK (1982) Oxygenation dependence of the transverse relaxation time of water protons in whole blood at high field. Biochim Biophys Acta 714(2):265–270

Toosy AT, Ciccarelli O, Parker GJ, Wheeler-Kingshott CA, Miller DH, Thompson AJ (2004) Characterising function-structure relationships in the human visual system with functional MRI and diffusion tensor imaging. Neuroimage 21(4):1452–1463

Turner R (2002) How much cortex can a vein drain? Downstream dilution of activation-related cerebral blood oxygenation changes. Neuroimage 16(4):1062–1067

Turner R, Le Bihan D, Moonen CT, Despres D, Frank J (1991) Echo-planar time course MRI of cat brain oxygenation changes. Magn Reson Med 22(1):159–166

van Zijl PCM, Eleff SM, Ulatowski JA, Oja JME, Ulug AM, Traystman RJ, Kauppinen RA (1998) Quantitative assessment of blood flow, blood volume and blood oxygenation effects in functional magnetic resonance imaging. Nat Med 4(2):159–167

Waxman SG (2001) Acquired channelopathies in nerve injury and MS. Neurology 56(12):1621–1627

Weisskoff RM (1996) Simple measurement of scanner stability for functional NMR imaging of activation in the brain. Magn Reson Med 36:643–645

Williams DS, Detre JA, Leigh JS, Koretsky AP (1992) Magnetic resonance imaging of perfusion using spin inversion of arterial water. Proc Natl Acad Sci U S A 89(1):212–216

Wong EC, Buxton RB, Frank LR (1998) Quantitative imaging of perfusion using a single subtraction (QUIPSS and QUIPSS II). Magn Reson Med 39:702–708

Wong EC, Buxton RB, Frank LR (1999) Quantitative perfusion imaging using arterial spin labeling. Neuroimaging Clin N Am 9(2):333–342

Woodruff PW, Wright IC, Bullmore ET, Brammer M, Howard RJ, Williams SC, Shapleske J, Rossell S, David AS, McGuire PK, Murray RM (1997) Auditory hallucinations and the temporal cortical response to speech in schizophrenia: a functional magnetic resonance imaging study. Am J Psychiatry 154(12):1676–1682

Wright IC, Rabe-Hesketh S, Woodruff PW, David AS, Murray RM, Bullmore ET (2000) Meta-analysis of regional brain volumes in schizophrenia. Am J Psychiatry 157(1):16–25

Ye FQ, Allen PS (1995) Relaxation enhancement of the transverse magnetization of water protons in paramagnetic suspensions of red blood cells. Magn Reson Med 34(5):713–720

Yoshizawa T, Nose T, Moore GJ, Sillerud LO (1996) Functional magnetic resonance imaging of motor activation in the human cervical spinal cord. Neuroimage 4(3):174–182

9 MR Spectroscopy

Robert E. Lenkinski

CONTENTS

9.1 Introduction

Magnetic resonance imaging (MRI) has emerged as the preeminent imaging modality for visualizing neurological diseases in the central nervous system. MRI is a modality that can be used to produce both high resolution anatomically based images, as well as images that reflect a variety of physiological parameters including blood flow, tissue perfusion and water mobility as reflected by diffusion indices. MR spectroscopy (MRS) is a complementary technique that can provide metabolic information that can easily be integrated with MRI. MRS is the more modern version of NMR which over the past five decades has evolved from a technique used in chemistry to determine the structure of molecules to a method with which to probe the metabolism of cells, tissues, intact animals and humans (Allen 1990; Avison et al. 1986; Bernard et al. 1983; Bottomley 1989; Burt and Wyrwicz 1979; Burt et al. 1979; Cerdan and Seelig 1990; Gadian and Radda 1981; Iles et al. 1982; Kuchel 1981; Radda and Taylor 1985; Roberts and Jardetzky 1981; Ruiz-Cabello and Cohen 1993).

The early generations of NMR spectrometers employed room temperature ferromagnetism, and operated at fields between approximately 1 and 2 T, and could accommodate samples that contained less than 1 ml of solution. In the 1970s the development of vertical bore superconducting magnets provided a newer generation of NMR spectrometers that operated at higher fields and could obtain spectra from slightly larger volumes of sample (1–10 ml). As more of these instruments became available, several research groups began to use multinuclear NMR spectroscopy to investigate the bioenergetics and metabolism of cellular suspensions (see for example Evans and Kaplan 1977; Navon et al. 1977a, 1977b) and perfused tissue (see for example Ackerman et al. 1980; Jelicks and Gupta 1989).

Phosphorus-31 NMR spectroscopy was used to study cellular bioenergetics because several important compounds which are involved in cellular energetics, such as adenosine triphosphate (ATP), phosphocreatine (PCR) and inorganic phosphate (Pi), are readily detectable. Carbon-13 NMR spectroscopy could probe metabolism by following isotopically labeled substrates through various metabolic pathways (see for example London 1988). Although proton MRS was used extensively in chemical applications, its use in biological systems where the concentration of the compounds of interest are about 1–10 mM was hampered by the presence of a large background signal arising from water in the sample which could have a concentration approaching 90 *M* in protons. This large difference in signal intensities led to the

R.E. Lenkinski, PhD
Director of Experimental Radiology and 3T Magnetic Resonance Imaging/Spectroscopy Program, Department of Radiology, Beth Israel Deaconess Medical Center; Professor of Radiology, Harvard Medical School, Boston, Massachusetts, USA

development of a variety of techniques that either did not excite the background water signal or suppressed it substantially (see for example Bottomley et al. 1985; Frahm 1989; Frahm et al. 1989. One of the major motivations for employing proton NMR methods is the greater sensitivity of this nucleus as compared to both P-31 and C-13. All other factors being equal, the MR sensitivity scales as the cube of magnetogyric ratio for each nucleus.

The availability of horizontal bore magnets led to the extension of these studies to intact animals (see Chatham and Blackband 2001 for reviews). Since the early 1980s, there has also been an increasing availability of whole-body MR scanners for use in diagnostic imaging. A large number of these MR scanners operate at 1.5 T, a magnetic field that is similar to the magnetic fields employed in the early days of NMR spectroscopy.

The development of spatially localized MRS (Aue 1986; Bolinger and Lenkinski 1992; Narayana and DeLayre 1986) has provided a bridge between metabolism and the anatomic and physiological studies available from MRI. These can now be combined into a single MR examination. In cases where distinct lesions (or lesions) are seen on MR, the MRS can provide metabolic profiles that might aid in the characterization of the lesion(s) and response to treatment. In cases where no distinct lesions are visible on MRI, MRS can provide a non-invasive assessment of the underlying metabolic status of the tissue being studied. This is particularly important in pathologies such as multiple sclerosis (MS) where metabolic alterations in so-called "normal-appearing white matter" may give some insights into the patterns of disease evolution and progression. Because there are several different approaches to acquiring spatially localized MRS, it is more convenient to think of MRS as a family of methods rather than a single technique. The utility and applicability of each technique to a particular kind of neurological disease state depend on a variety of technical and practical factors that are discussed.

In this chapter we review the localization methods currently used in studying white matter disease. In this part of the chapter we discuss the technical and practical factors that determine the applicability of the methods to particular kinds of studies. We also describe the various resonances detected by localized solvent-suppressed proton MRS of the brain in terms of the metabolic and biochemical information that can be derived from an analysis of their concentrations. Finally, we review some of the potential developments that may improve the performance of MRS in the future.

9.2 Spatial Localization

Localization can be achieved in MRS by employing RF gradients, static B_0 gradients, or pulsed spatial gradients (or combinations of these). The technical details of all of these approaches have been described in detail (Aue 1986; Bolinger and Lenkinski 1992; Narayana and DeLayre 1986). The latter methods are similar to those currently employed in MRI. As pointed out above, proton spectroscopy of metabolites presents a problem in that metabolites at millimolar concentrations must be detected in the presence of a background water signal that is present at about 100 molar. For this reason solvent-suppression techniques have been combined with localization schemes to produce spatially localized solvent-suppressed spectra. The T1s of the various proton metabolites are quite long, and the T2s are also quite long permitting the use of methods such as the spin-echo or stimulated-echo sequences. For proton MRS of the brain, localization methods that either preserve the magnetization of only those protons being sampled and destroy the coherence of all of the unwanted spins or pulse sequences where only the spins from the desirable spins are excited, or combinations of these two approaches have found common use.

The unwanted magnetization arises from several sources: the background water signal, and the strong lipid signal arising from fat in the scalp. Regions with high magnetic susceptibility boundaries should be avoided in the excitation schemes. Suppression of the water signal is usually accomplished by 90° frequency-selective excitation of the water followed by dephasing gradients. This process destroys both the Z-magnetization of the water and its XY magnetization. The efficiency of suppression depends on a number of factors including the B1 homogeneity of the 90° frequency-selective excitation of the water (i.e. is this pulse a 90° pulse everywhere within the brain?) and the magnetic field homogeneity across the volume being sampled. The two most commonly used localization methods, STEAM and PRESS, select an orthorhombic volume in space by applying three sequential selective RF pulses in the presence of orthogonal slice-selective gradients. The pulse sequence for PRESS is shown in Fig. 9.1. The stimulated echo (STEAM) sequence (Frahm 1989; Frahm et al. 1989) and PRESS (Bottomley et al. 1985) method can be implemented as single-voxel (i.e. sampling only one region of tissue) or multivoxel methods (by selecting a larger ortho-rhombic volume combined with Fourier phase-encoding methods to produce

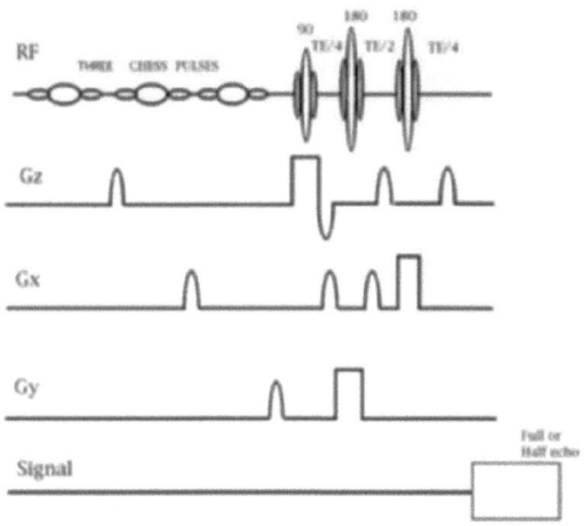

Fig. 9.1. The PRESS pulse sequence shown for a single voxel acquisition. Note the three chemically shift selective (CHESS) pulses each followed by a dephasing gradient that precede the three slice-selective RF pulses.

CSI sequences (Aue 1986; Bolinger and Lenkinski 1992; Narayana and DeLayre 1986)).

Examples of the graphic prescriptions of both single-voxel and multivoxel selections are illustrated in Fig. 9.2. Since only both STEAM and PRESS excite only the spins within the orthorhombic volume, these are examples of methods in which only those protons being sampled are excited, and the other spins are either not excited or destroyed. The advantages of using either of these two spatial preselection methods are that the signal from lipids arising from the scalp is minimized, and the volume over which the B_0 field is adjusted can be restricted to avoid air–tissue boundaries where there may be large variations in the magnetic susceptibility. For reasons associated with instrument performance, such as residual eddy current effects, many of the early reports of proton MRS employed echo delays of 135 or 270 ms. The choice of 135 or 270 ms is made in order to refocus the doublet resonance of the methyl resonance of lactate, which has a value of about 7 Hz for the spin-spin coupling constant to its methenyl proton. As instrumental performance has improved, there has been a larger emphasis placed on acquiring proton spectra at shorter echo delays (20–60 ms). One advantage of these shorter delays is the ability to detect resonances from coupled spin systems (e.g. glutamate, glutamine, inositol) whose apparent T2s are too short to permit detection at longer echo delays.

The STEAM sequence originally provided more precise localization because the slice profiles of the 90° pulses were sharper than those achieved by conventional 180° refocusing pulses (see for example Moonen et al. 1989; Yongbi et al. 1995). The precision of spatial localization was improved in PRESS in two ways. First, the development of so-called digitally-crafted or designer RF pulses has improved the quality of the slice profiles of the 180° pulses (see for example Chan et al. 1992; Conolly et al. 1992; Pauly et al. 1991; Shinnar 1994; Shinnar and Leigh 1989; Shinnar et al. 1989a, 1989b, 1989c; Spielman et al. 1991). Second, slice profiles have been improved through the use of a very selective spatial saturation pulse which can be applied at the six edges of the orthorhombus defined by either STEAM or PRESS spatial preselection (Tran et al. 2000).

In spite of these improvements, STEAM and PRESS may not be ideal methods for performing multivoxel studies of the brain. The requirement of selecting an orthorhombic volume means that major regions of the brain will not fit within this volume on an axial slice (see Fig. 9.2). These deficiencies have led investigators employing spatial presaturation methods to destroy the magnetization from tissues close to air–tissue boundaries where there may be large variations in the magnetic susceptibility. This method of spatial presaturation is often referred to as outer volume suppression (OVS). A popular method with OVS currently being used in the brain by a number of centers is based on the reports of Duyn and Moonen 1993 and Duyn et al. (1993) described at http://www.cc.nih.gov/ldrr/staff/janwydv/index.html. Both a 1.5 T and 3 T version is available for use on gradient-echo scanners. This method employs octagonal spatial presaturation pulses to remove the lipid signal arising from the scalp. It is a multislice sequence, which supports the acquisition of four slices (oblique if desired) in 29 min at a TE of 135 ms. This method acquires 24×24 phase encodes per slice. Processing software is available from Dr. Peter Barker at Johns Hopkins University through an NIH-funded RR facility. An alternate, multislice method without spatial presaturation has been described by Schuff et al. at 1.5 T (Schuff et al. 2001; Wiedermann et al. 2001). In this method the lipid resonance is suppressed with a selective inversion pulse. This method acquires two slices (oblique if desired) in 30 min at a TE of 135 ms. Processing software is also available from this group. The in-plane resolution is determined by 36×36 circularly bounded phase encoding steps across the slice. In both methods, water suppression is achieved through the use of CHESS pulses.

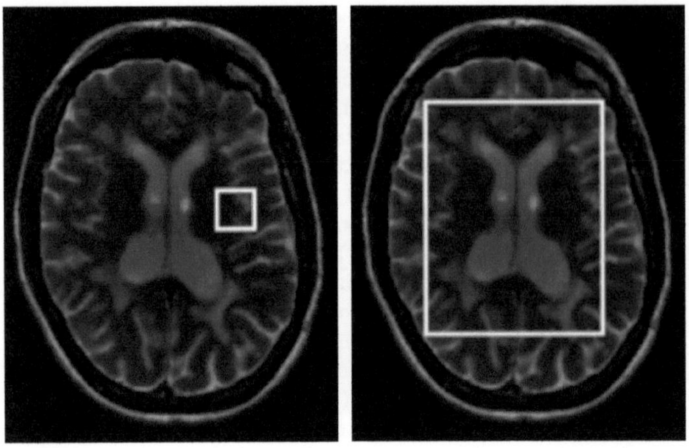

a b

Fig. 9.2a,b. Examples of the graphic prescriptions for a single-voxel and multivoxel sequence. For the single-voxel sequence the volume selected is a cube. For the multivoxel sequence the volume selected is an orthorhombus. Note that the peripheral parts of the brain are not included in this orthorhombus.

9.3 Compounds Detected by MRS in the Human Brain

Examples of proton MR spectra obtained from grey matter and white matter acquired using the PRESS sequence at a TE of 35 ms are shown in Fig. 9.3. The most prominent resonances are labeled on these spectra. We discuss each of these resonances (moving from low to high ppm values in turn). The biochemical basis for interpreting these spectra has been discussed in detail by Ross and Bluml (2001). We briefly review these here.

9.3.1 Lipid/lactate

Lactate is a doublet at 1.3 ppm. It is the end product of glycolysis. In general, lactate can become elevated in the brain in two ways. First, lactate will be produced if the tissue becomes ischemic. Second, it has been shown that lactate can become elevated if there are activated inflammatory cells present. Activated macrophages have been shown to produce high levels of lactate (see Lopez-Villegas et al. 1995).

Lipids can become elevated in some pathologies. In general, most studies have avoided making any interpretations based on these resonances because it is often unclear whether these peaks arise from out-of-voxel contamination, i.e. poor spatial localization.

9.3.2 N-Acetylaspartate

The isolation and identification of N-acetylaspartate (NAA) in the brain of cats was reported by Tallan et al. (1956). Soon after the detection of NAA in proton MRS, Birken and Oldendorf (1989) reviewed the literature regarding NAA' s role in brain biochemistry. In spite of more than 40 years of investigation,

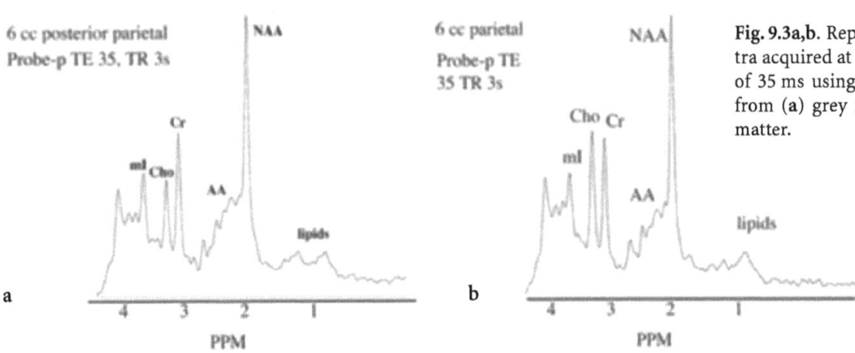

Fig. 9.3a,b. Representative MR spectra acquired at 1.5 T at an echo delay of 35 ms using the PRESS sequence from (a) grey matter and (b) white matter.

the role of NAA in the brain is still somewhat unclear. SIMMONS et al. (1991) reported that NAA was found exclusively in neurons. This and many other observations have led many to conclude that NAA is a neuronal marker. This conclusion was questioned by MARTIN et al. (2001a) who reported MR spectra with little or no NAA in a 3-year-old with developmental deficits. This report was followed by several letters to the editor discussing the role of NAA as a neuronal marker (BARKER 2001; MARTIN et al. 2001b; SULLIVAN et al. 2001).

It is also interesting that there are approximately equal concentrations of NAA in white and grey matter, which raises the issue of whether NAA is a marker of axonal integrity as well. The utility of NAA as an axonal marker is supported by the loss of NAA in many white matter diseases, including leukodystrophies, MS and hypoxic encephalopathy. Since MS is thought to be a disease that affects axons, the level of NAA has been used to monitor axonal viability in white matter lesions of MS and in surrounding normal-appearing white matter.

Several groups have suggested that NAA is a cerebral osmolyte (BASLOW 2002; BASLOW 2003a, 2003b; BLUML et al. 1997). This role proposed for NAA implies that NAA changes might be reversible, an observation that has been made in several human studies, including MS.

9.3.3 Glutamine, Glutamate and γ-Aminobutyric Acid Labeled as Amino Acids or AA in the Spectra

The determination of the concentrations of these compounds using 1H MRS is complicated by the complex spectral appearance of glutamate/glutamine due to J-coupling. There are also other metabolites contributing to the signal at the chemical shift of glutamate/glutamine that makes the accurate and precise determination of their concentrations difficult at 1.5 T. However, there are indications that the use of higher field strengths will improve the quantitation of these compounds (TKAC et al. 2003; UGURBIL et al. 2003). An example of a spectrum obtained at 7 T is shown in Fig. 9.4.

9.3.4 Creatine

The neurobiochemistry of creatine (Cr) has been discussed by ROSS and BLUML (1996, 2001). This resonance is made up of at least two compounds, Cr and PCR, that are in rapid chemical, and enzymatic exchange. The concentration of this compound is estimated to be 8.6 mM in human brain. Many studies employ the level of the Cr peak as an internal standard since the levels of Cr are thought to relatively constant across the brain and do not change in most pathologies. However, caution should be used in cases where there is tissue destruction, since the level of Cr might fall. Also, there has been at least one report where a new human inborn error of Cr biosynthesis was manifested as an absence of cerebral Cr from the proton spectrum, and this deficiency was corrected by dietary administration of Cr (HANEFELD et al. 1993).

9.3.5. Choline(s)

The biochemistry of compounds containing choline (Cho) has been reviewed by MILLER et al. (1991). The Cho resonance arises from the tetramethylamine head group in soluble compounds such as Cho, phosphocholine, glycerophosphocholine, and betaine. In Fig. 9.3, it is clear that there may be different levels of Cho in grey and white matter. ROSS and BLUML (2001) have reported that the concentration of Cho is about 1.6 mM in white matter. During active myelin breakdown, there is thought to be a release of phospholipids leading to an increase of the Cho peak (see for example MATTHEWS et al. 1991).

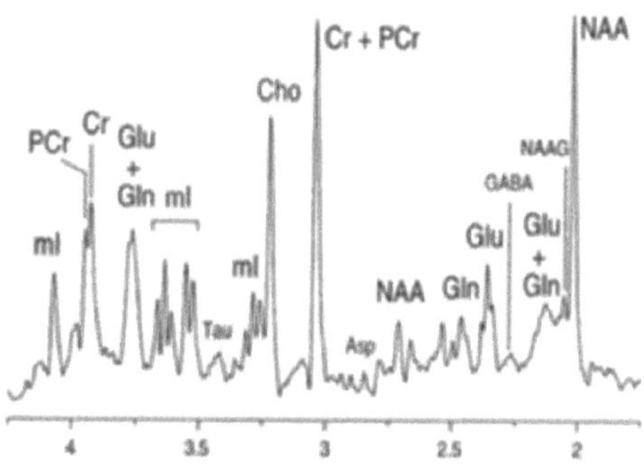

Fig. 9.4. A proton MR spectrum acquired from a dog brain at 9.4 T from a 1 ml volume. Note the separation of all of the peaks allowing the identification of the compounds indicated. Reproduced from Ross and Bluml (1996). The spectrum was collected by Drs. R. Gruetter and I. Tkac at the University of Minnesota.

9.3.6 Myo-Inositol

Myo-inositol (mI) is a simple sugar that has a deceptively simple spectrum at 1.5 T. It has been previously shown that, in the brain, mI is synthesized primarily in glial cells and cannot cross the blood–brain barrier (Brand et al. 1993; Font et al. 1982). For these reasons, mI is considered to be a glial marker, and an increase in its content is believed to represent glial proliferation or an increase in glial cell size. Since both processes may occur in brain inflammation, an increase in mI may be a surrogate marker for inflammation in the brain. Myo-inositol has been suggested as a cerebral osmolyte since 1990. Like Cho, mI has also been labeled as a breakdown product of myelin.

9.4 Quantitation

There is still an ongoing debate on the merits concerning the relative versus absolute quantitation of the compound detected by proton MRS in the brain. One view is that only the determination of absolute concentrations is acceptable. This is based on the observation that the levels of all of the metabolites, including Cr, can change in brain pathologies. The calculation of absolute concentrations requires the correction for many factors including compartmentalization of compounds, correction for T1 and T2 relaxation effects; correction for excitation and reception profiles; determination of the actual, rather than the prescribed, volume sampled both in single-voxel and multivoxel studies; and referencing the results to a known internal or external standard. Several different approaches have been suggested for absolute quantitation (Ernst et al. 1993; Helms 2000; Helms 2001; Hennig et al. 1992; Horska et al. 2002; Knight-Scott et al. 2003; Kreis et al. 1993a, 1993b).

Critics of absolute quantification suggest that it may be impossible to correct for all of these factors, particularly in the presence of pathologies, without making potentially flawed assumptions. For this reason they prefer to report relative concentrations, usually expressed as metabolite to Cr ratios. The potential flaw in this approach is that if the level of Cr is affected by the disease process, the use of ratios themselves might be misleading. There is a common step in both of these approaches, which is fitting the acquired spectra in order to determine the area under each resonance.

There have been a number of approaches suggested for carrying out this step in the brain. These various approaches, applied to processing and fitting spectral data, were recently reviewed in a special issue of *NMR in Biomedicine* (vol. 14(4), 2001) devoted to spectral quantitation (for reviews see Mierisova and Ala-Korpela 2001; Provencher 2001; Vanhamme et al. 2001; Zandt et al. 2001). A method that appears to be gaining wide acceptance is LC-Model that we employ routinely to automatically fit CSI data sets obtained from the brain. The version of LC-Model that we employ is similar to that described by McLean et al. (2000, 2001). An example of the results of a fit of LC-Model to a spectrum obtained at 3 T from a normal volunteer is shown in Fig. 9.5. Note that the output of LC-Model includes both relative and absolute concentrations of the various compounds detected.

9.5 Applications to White Matter Disease

The applications of MRS to study white matter disease has been reviewed by Filippi (2001) and Rudkin and Arnold (2002).

9.5.1 HIV

MRS of HIV has recently been reviewed by Boska et al. (2004) and Rudkin and Arnold (2002). We also reviewed this area in 1998 (Cecil and Lenkinski 1998). A common finding in all of the MR spectroscopy studies on HIV infection of the brain is the reduced level of NAA in the intermediate to later stages of disease. This finding is consistent with the pathological evidence of neuronal loss reported in HIV-1-infected patients at intermediate or late stages of disease.

Another common finding, although not present in all of the MRS studies, is the increase in Cho/Cr ratio (Chang et al. 1999; Chong et al. 1993; English et al. 1997; Jarvik et al. 1993; Laubenberger et al. 1996; Meyerhoff et al. 1993, 1994, 1999; Paley et al. 1995; Salvan et al. 1997; Tracey et al. 1996). The significance of the elevation in Cho/Cr ratio remains uncertain. A possible interpretation for this increase in HIV-1-infected patients is that the

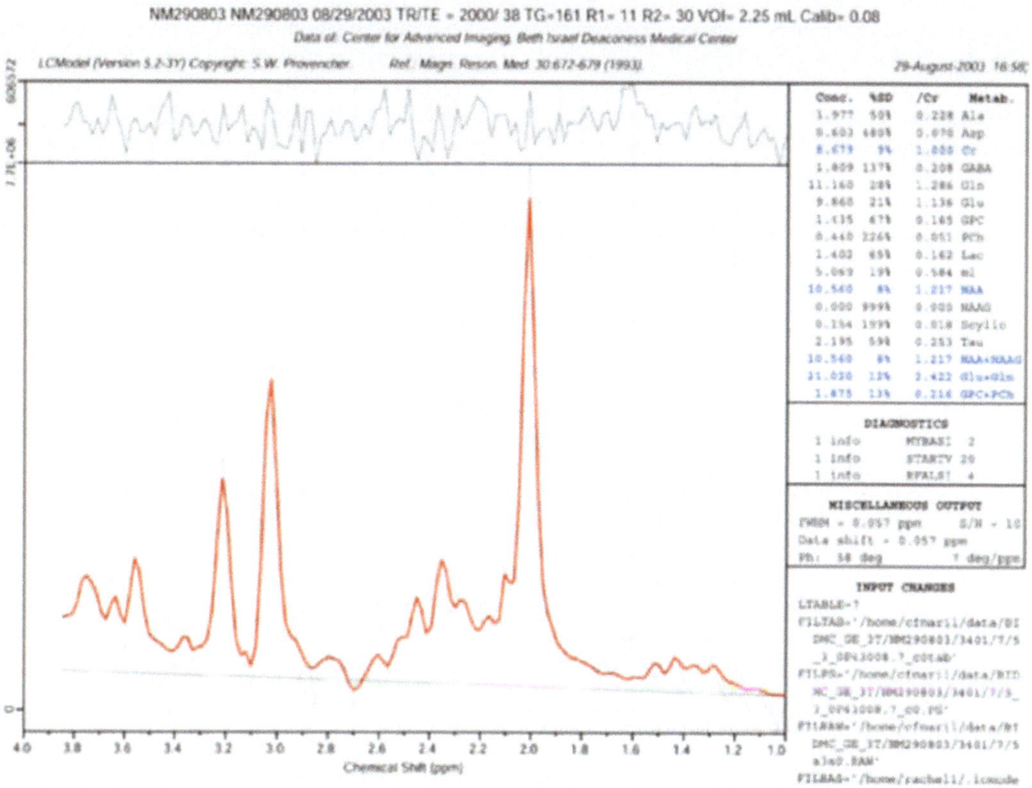

Fig. 9.5. An example of the output of LC-Model fitting of a spectrum obtained at 3 T from a normal volunteer using PRESS at TE 35 ms. Note that LC-Model provides both the relative and absolute concentrations of the compounds listed on the right.

increased Cho may not directly arise from changes in neurons but may result from metabolic alterations in glial cells. An alternate interpretation is that the increase in Cho/Cr ratio is a result of more cellular material being present in the volume of interest, perhaps as a result of increases in microglial cells and the presence of macrophages. Both of these explanations for the increase in Cho/Cr ratio are consistent with the neuropathological finding of inflammatory infiltrates in the brains of HIV-infected patients. An additional source of an increased Cho/Cr ratio may be as a result of breakdown in myelin. Choline phosphoglycerides contribute 11.2% of myelin lipids, with phosphatidylcholine being the most abundant. Therefore, as myelin damage occurs, free Cho may be released, increasing the Cho resonance detected by MR spectroscopy. This explanation for the increase in the Cho/Cr ratio is consistent with the neuropathological finding of white matter abnormalities in the brain of HIV-1-infected patients.

There is an emerging consensus that there is an increase in the mI resonance in HIV (Chang et al. 1999; Laubenberger et al. 1996; Lopez-Villegas et al. 1997; von Giesen et al. 2001). Brand et al. (1993) have shown that mI is produced exclusively in glial cell and not in neurons. This observation has led to the view that mI is a marker for gliosis. The possibility that the elevation of mI may precede the loss of NAA has previously been suggested for patients with Down syndrome, although the interpretation of the increased mI in this pathology might be different. Increased mI has been reported in Alzheimer's disease, in which there is evidence for gliosis. Additional support for the use of mI as a marker for gliosis comes from studies of MS. Bitsch et al. (1999) showed that increases in both Cho and mI corresponded to glial proliferation on histology in MS plaques. Helms et al. (2000) found elevated mI in chronic but not acute MS lesions. This finding was interpreted in terms of gliosis in the chronic lesions. These results, taken together with our own observation that the mI increases in white matter before any NAA loss, indicate that this metabolite may be a valuable early indicator for gliosis in the pathogenesis of HIV.

There also been several reports that have correlated spectral abnormalities with other indicators of disease progression (Chang et al. 1999; Chong et al. 1993; Jarvik et al. 1993; Lopez-Villegas et al. 1997; Meyerhoff et al. 1993, 1994, 1999). Some of these spectral alterations have been shown to reverse in response to therapy (Chang et al. 1999; Stankoff et al. 2001; Vion-Dury et al. 1995).

Several groups have suggested that there are distinct patterns of spectral abnormalities that occur as the disease progresses (Cecil and Lenkinski 1998; Salvan et al. 1997). We have proposed a model for the time-course of spectral alterations during disease progression (Cecil and Lenkinski 1998). This model fits with both literature observations of mI changes during the progression of disease and the model for immunopathogenesis of HIV-associated dementia (HAD). The ability of MRS to provide separate indices of inflammation (mI) and neuronal damage (NAA) may provide the capability to identify patients who have HAD which may reverse on treatment and which patients will not improve. This important step can potentially lead to individual optimized treatment effectiveness. There have been several papers in the literature (see for example McGuire and Marder 2000; Pulliam et al. 2001) which have suggested that there are new opportunities for developing therapies based on targets identified through an improved understanding of the immunopathogenesis and pathogenesis of HAD. Since proton MRS can monitor the course of disease progression it can provide a sensitive method for the early detection of HIV migration for the monitoring of the response to novel therapies in individual patients.

9.3.2 Progressive Multifocal Leukoencephalopathy

Progressive multifocal leukoencephalopathy (PML) is a demyelinating disease of the CNS caused by the polyomavirus JC (JCV) which occurs in the context of severe immunosuppression, such as in patients with AIDS, hematological malignancies, and in organ transplant recipients. There is no specific treatment for PML and the outcome is fatal in about 50% of HIV-positive (HIV+) patients with PML, despite the availability of highly active antiretroviral therapy (HAART) (Clifford et al. 1999). Indeed, contrast enhancement of PML lesions on MRI is not a very sensitive method to evaluate intraparenchymal inflammation, and it can only be detected in approximately 20% of PML cases (Chang et al. 1997). In addition, distinction between active and chronic lesions is impossible by MRI. On the other hand, ^{1}H-MRS has shown promise in the study of the metabolic alterations associated with PML. Cross-sectional studies have shown a typical ^{1}H-MRS pattern in PML lesions, including a decreases NAA/Cr ratio consistent with axonal compromise, increased Cho/Cr ratio, indicating cell membrane breakdown and turnover, and occasional elevation of lipid/lactate and mI (Chang et al. 1995, 1997; Iranzo et al. 1999; Simone et al. 1998). In one study, the two patients who had the longest survival showed the highest mI, consistent with increased glial activity and inflammation in PML lesions (Chang et al. 1997). These data suggest that ^{1}H-MRS may be an ideal tool to measure the inflammatory component of PML lesions over time.

9.5.3 Multiple Sclerosis

MS is a demyelinating disease with the preservation of axonal integrity. For convenience we will discuss the findings of MRS in acute and chronic lesions and normal-appearing white and grey matter, respectively.

Acute lesions: One of the complicating technical factors is that unless the lesion is quite large the voxel chosen for MRS might contain a substantial amount of normal-appearing white matter. Hyperacutely, lesions display increased mI (Davie et al. 1994; Narayana et al. 1998), lipid, lactate and Cho (Davie et al. 1994; De Stefano et al. 1995). These lesions show decreases in Cr (De Stefano et al. 1995) followed by subsequent reductions in NAA (Davie et al. 1994; Ferguson et al. 1997; Husted et al. 1994; Miller et al. 1991; Trapp et al. 1998). The decrease in the level of Cr calls into question the utility of using metabolite ratios in this situation. One of the interesting findings is the observation that these reductions in NAA may reverse (Arnold et al. 1992) as the plaque evolves. The MR spectrum of an acute, highly inflammatory, plaque such as seen in tumefactive MS, can be very similar to that seen for some tumors (Butteriss et al. 2003; Law et al. 2002; Saindane et al. 2002). Thus, caution should be employed in attempting to use MRS for making differential diagnoses between these two kinds of brain lesions.

Chronic Plaques: For chronic lesions, i.e. those visible as hyperintense lesions on T2-weighted scans, most reports have focused on decreases in NAA. This is based on the observations that the levels of the other compounds detected by MRS return back to normal values over time. Several groups have made important interpretations based on the levels of NAA in chronic lesions. For example, Falini et al. (1998) reported that chronic lesions from patients with benign MS have much higher NAA levels than the chronic lesions from patients with secondary progressive MS, suggesting a greater recovery of NAA in acute lesions from less-disabled MS patients.

Normal-Appearing White Matter: There has been a consistent pattern observed in MS patients where the levels of NAA are decreased in so-called NAWM (Filippi et al. 1999). Decreased NAA levels are found in patients with established MS from the early phases of the disease (Arnold et al. 1992). This decrease is interpreted in terms of axonal loss in NAWM. Recently, Gonen et al. (2000) reported a method to determine whole-brain NAA in an effort to find a global index of NAA loss which might provide a better correlation with disability than more conventional indices, such as lesion volume or lesional NAA levels (Filippi et al. 2003; Gonen et al. 2002).

Grey Matter in MS: Although MS is thought to be a disease that affects white matter, there have been a number of recent reports that have indicated reduced NAA in regions that are in primarily grey matter (Adalsteinsson et al. 2003; Chard et al. 2002; Cifelli et al. 2002; Sarchielli et al. 2002). Adalsteinsson et al. (2003) have suggested that the NAA levels in grey matter may help explain the more severe clinical symptoms in patients with the more aggressive forms of MS.

9.5.4 Alzheimer's Dementia

Decreased NAA and increased mI have been reported in the occipital, temporal, parietal, and frontal regions of patients with AD, even at the early stages of the disease (for a recent review see Valenzuela and Sachdev 2001). Similar metabolite changes are being reported in the mild cognitive impairment prodrome and in the medial temporal lobe.

9.5.5 Other White Matter diseases

The MRS of leukoencephalopathies, leukodystrophies, Canavan's disease and vascular dementias has been reviewed by Filippi (2001).

9.6 Summary and Future Directions

MRS of white matter disease can detect a number of compounds that provide biochemical insight about the underlying metabolic basis for each of the pathologies discussed above. In spite of the great interest in proton MRS, there are still gaps in the understanding of the biochemistry of each of the compounds detected in the spectra. For example, the precise function of NAA is not completely understood. This is evidenced by the debates about its role as a neuronal marker. Also, over the past decade the techniques for acquiring localized spectra have improved substantially. However, most of the methods are mainly slice-selective 2D methods. Generalizing these methods to 3D, whole-brain methods are either too time-consuming or too prone to artifacts. For example, using a low number of phase encoding steps in the slice direction can lead to a poor point spread function. An approach to solving this problem has been reported by Gonen et al. (1997, 1998) in which slice-encoding is achieved using the Hadamard method. This method gives much sharper slice profiles than the Fourier encoding for a small number of encoding steps.

There are high-speed MRSI methods based on either echo-planar methods (see for example Posse et al. 1994 and Posse et al. 1995) or spiral acquisitions (see for example Adalsteinsson et al. 1998). These methods are capable of acquiring spectral data in relatively short scan times but are usually acquired at relatively high bandwidths that may limit their signal-to-noise. The combination of these methods with higher field strength such as 3 or 4 T may overcome these deficiencies.

References

Ackerman JJ, Bore PJ, Gadian DG, Grove TH, Radda GK (1980) NMR studies of metabolism in perfused organs. Philos Trans R Soc Lond B Biol Sci 289:425–436

Adalsteinsson E, Irarrazabal P, Topp S, Meyer C, Macovski A, Spielman DM (1998) Volumetric spectroscopic imaging with spiral-based k-space trajectories. Magn Reson Med 39:889–898
Adalsteinsson E, Langer-Gould A, Homer RJ, et al (2003) Grey matter-N-acetyl aspartate deficits in secondary progressive but not relapsing-remitting multiple sclerosis. Am J Neuroradiol 24:1941–1945
Allen PS (1990) In vivo nuclear-magnetic-resonance spectroscopy applied to medicine. J Can Assoc Radiol 41:39–44
Arnold DL, Matthews PM, Francis GS, Oconnor J, Antel JP (1992) Proton magnetic-resonance spectroscopic imaging for metabolic characterization of demyelinating plaques. Ann Neurol 31:235–241
Aue WP (1986) Localization methods for in vivo nuclear magnetic resonance spectroscopy. Rev Magn Reson Med 1:21–72
Avison MJ, Hetherington HP, Shulman RG (1986) Applications of NMR to studies of tissue metabolism. Annu Rev Biophys Biophysical Chem 15:377–402
Barker PB (2001) N-acetyl aspartate – a neuronal marker? Ann Neurol 49:423–424
Baslow MH (2002) Evidence supporting a role for N-acetyl-L-aspartate as a molecular water pump in myelinated neurons in the central nervous system – an analytical review. Neurochem Int 40:295–300
Baslow MH (2003a) Brain N-acetylaspartate as a molecular water pump and its role in the etiology of Canavan disease – a mechanistic explanation. J Mol Neurosci 21:185–189
Baslow MH (2003b) N-acetylaspartate in the vertebrate brain: metabolism and function. Neurochem Res 28:941–953
Bernard M, Canioni P, Cozzone PJ (1983) P-31 nuclear magnetic-resonance study of cellular metabolism in vivo. Biochimie 65:449–470
Birken DL, Oldendorf WH (1989) N-acetyl-L-aspartic acid – a literature-review of a compound prominent in H-1-NMR spectroscopic studies of brain. Neurosci Biobehav Rev 13:23–31
Bitsch A, Bruhn H, Vougioukas V, et al (1999) Inflammatory CNS demyelination: histopathologic correlation with in vivo quantitative proton MR spectroscopy. Am J Neuroradiol 20:1619–1627
Bolinger L, Lenkinski RE (1992) Localization in clinical NMR spectroscopy. In: Berliner LJ, Reuben J (eds) Biological magnetic resonance. Plenum Press, New York, pp 1–53
Boska MD, Mosley RL, Nawab M, et al (2004) Advances in neuroimaging for HIV-1 associated neurological dysfunction: clues to the diagnosis, pathogenesis and therapeutic monitoring. Curr HIV Res 2:61–78
Bottomley PA (1989) Human in vivo NMR spectroscopy in diagnostic medicine: clinical tool or research probe? Radiology 170:1–15
Bottomley PA, Edelstein WA, Foster TH, Adams WA (1985) In vivo solvent-suppressed localized hydrogen nuclear magnetic resonance spectroscopy: a window to metabolism? Proc Natl Acad Sci U S A 82:2148–2152
Bluml S, McComb JG, Ross BD (1997) Differentiation between cortical atrophy and hydrocephalus using 1H MRS. Magn Reson Med 37:395–403
Brand A, Richterlandsberg C, Leibfritz D (1993) Multinuclear NMR-studies on the energy-metabolism of glial and neuronal cells. Dev Neurosci 15:289–298
Burt CT, Wyrwicz AM (1979) P-31 nuclear magnetic resonance observations in biological systems .1. Intact tissue. Trends Biochem Sci 4:244–246
Burt CT, Cohen SM, Barany M (1979) Analysis of intact tissue with P-31 NMR. Annu Rev Biophys Bioeng 8:1–25
Butteriss DJA, Ismail A, Ellison DW, Birchall D (2003) Use of serial proton magnetic resonance spectroscopy to differentiate low grade glioma from tumefactive plaque in a patient with multiple sclerosis. Br J Radiol 76:662–665
Cecil KM, Lenkinski RE (1998) Proton MR spectroscopy in inflammatory and infectious brain disorders. Neuroimaging Clin N Am 8:863–880
Cerdan S, Seelig J (1990) NMR studies of metabolism. Annu Rev Biophys Biophysical Chem 19:43–67
Chan F, Pauly J, Macovski A (1992) Effects of RF amplifier distortion on selective excitation and their correction by prewarping. Magn Reson Med 23:224–238
Chang L, Ernst T, Aronow H, et al (1995) Proton spectroscopy in progressive multifocal leukoencephalopathy. Neurology 45:A444
Chang L, Ernst T, Tornatore C, et al (1997) Metabolite abnormalities in progressive multifocal leukoencephalopathy by proton magnetic resonance spectroscopy. Neurology 48:836–845
Chang L, Ernst T, Leonido-Yee M, et al (1999) Highly active antiretroviral therapy reverses brain metabolite abnormalities in mild HIV dementia. Neurology 53:782–789
Chang L, Ernst T, Leonido-Yee M, Walot I, Singer E (1999) Cerebral metabolite abnormalities correlate with clinical severity of HIV-1 cognitive motor complex. Neurology 52:100–108
Chard DT, Griffin CM, McLean MA, et al (2002) Brain metabolite changes in cortical grey and normal-appearing white matter in clinically early relapsing-remitting multiple sclerosis. Brain 125:2342–2352
Chatham JC, Blackband SJ (2001) Nuclear magnetic resonance spectroscopy and imaging in animal research. ILAR J 42:189–208
Chong WK, Sweeney B, Wilkinson ID, et al (1993) Proton spectroscopy of the brain in HIV infection: correlation with clinical, immunologic, and MR imaging findings. Radiology 188:119–124
Cifelli A, Arridge M, Jezzard P, Esiri MM, Palace J, Matthews PM (2002) Thalamic neurodegeneration in multiple sclerosis. Ann Neurol 52:650–653
Clifford DB, Yiannoutsos C, Glicksman M, et al (1999) HAART improves prognosis in HIV-associated progressive multifocal leukoencephalopathy. Neurology 52:623–625
Conolly S, Pauly J, Nishimura D, Macovski A (1992) Two-dimensional selective adiabatic pulses. Magn Reson Med 24:302–313
Davie CA, Hawkins CP, Barker GJ, et al (1994) Serial proton magnetic resonance spectroscopy in acute multiple sclerosis lesions. Brain 117 (Pt 1):49–58
De Stefano N, Matthews PM, Antel JP, Preul M, Francis G, Arnold DL (1995) Chemical pathology of acute demyelinating lesions and its correlation with disability. Ann Neurol 38:901–909
Duyn JH, Moonen CTW (1993) Fast proton spectroscopic imaging of human brain using multiple spin-echoes. Magn Reson Med 30:409–414
Duyn JH, Gillen J, Sobering G, Vanzijl PCM, Moonen CTW (1993) Multisection proton MR spectroscopic imaging of the brain. Radiology 188:277–282
English CD, Kaufman MJ, Worth JL, et al (1997) Elevated fron-

tal lobe cytosolic choline levels in minimal or mild AIDS dementia complex patients: a proton magnetic resonance spectroscopy study. Biol Psychiatry 41:500–502

Evans FE, Kaplan NO (1977) 31P nuclear magnetic resonance studies of HeLa cells. Proc Natl Acad Sci U S A 74:4909–4913

Falini A, Calabrese G, Filippi M, et al (1998) Benign versus secondary-progressive multiple sclerosis: the potential role of proton MR spectroscopy in defining the nature of disability. Am J Neuroradiol 19:223–229

Ferguson B, Matyszak MK, Esiri MM, Perry VH (1997) Axonal damage in acute multiple sclerosis lesions. Brain 120:393–399

Filippi M (2001) In-vivo tissue characterization of multiple sclerosis and other white matter diseases using magnetic resonance based techniques. J Neurol 248:1019–1029

Filippi M, Tortorella C, Bozzali M (1999) Normal-appearing white matter changes in multiple sclerosis: the contribution of magnetic resonance techniques. Mult Scler 5:273–282

Filippi M, Bozzali M, Rovaris M, et al (2003) Evidence for widespread axonal damage at the earliest clinical stage of multiple sclerosis. Brain 126:433–437

Font C, Garia-Campos M, Hansen AJ, Siemkowicz E, Gjedde A (1982) Simultaneous diffusion of inositol and mannitol in the rat brain (in Spanish). Rev Esp Fisiol 38:317–319

Frahm J, Bruhn H, Gyngell ML, Merboldt KD, Hanicke W, Sauter R (1989) Localized proton NMR spectroscopy in different regions of the human brain in vivo. Relaxation times and concentrations of cerebral metabolites. Magn Reson Med 11:47–63

Frahm J, Michaelis T, Merboldt KD, et al (1989) Localized NMR spectroscopy in vivo. Progress and problems. NMR Biomed 2:188–195

Gadian DG, Radda GK (1981) NMR studies of tissue metabolism. Annu Rev Biochem 50:69–83

Gonen O, AriasMendoza F, Goelman G (1997) 3D localized in vivo H-1 spectroscopy of human brain by using a hybrid of 1D-Hadamard with 2D chemical shift imaging. Magn Reson Med 37:644–650

Gonen O, Murdoch JB, Stoyanova R, Goelman G (1998) 3D multivoxel proton spectroscopy of human brain using a hybrid of 8th-order Hadamard encoding with 2D chemical shift imaging. Magn Reson Med 39:34–40

Gonen O, Catalaa I, Babb JS, et al (2000) Total brain N-acetylaspartate—a new measure of disease load in MS. Neurology 54:15–19

Gonen O, Moriarty DM, Li BSY, et al (2002) Relapsing-remitting multiple sclerosis and whole-brain N-acetylaspartate measurement: evidence for different clinical cohorts—initial observations. Radiology 225:261–268

Hanefeld F, Holzbach U, Kruse B, Wilichowski E, Christen HJ, Frahm J (1993) Diffuse white matter disease in three children: an encephalopathy with unique features on magnetic resonance imaging and proton magnetic resonance spectroscopy. Neuropediatrics 24:244–248

Helms G (2000) A precise and user-independent quantification technique for regional comparison of single volume proton MR spectroscopy of the human brain. NMR Biomed 13:398–406

Helms G (2001) Volume correction for edema in single-volume proton MR spectroscopy of contrast-enhancing multiple sclerosis lesions. Magn Reson Med 46:256–263

Helms G, Stawiarz L, Kivisakk P, Link H (2000) Regression analysis of metabolite concentrations estimated from localized proton MR spectra of active and chronic multiple sclerosis lesions. Magn Reson Med 43:102–110

Hennig J, Pfister H, Ernst T, Ott D (1992) Direct absolute quantification of metabolites in the human brain with in vivo localized proton spectroscopy. NMR Biomed 5:193–199

Horska A, Calhoun VD, Bradshaw DH, Barker PB (2002) Rapid method for correction of CSF partial volume in quantitative proton MR spectroscopic imaging. Magn Reson Med 48:555–558

Husted CA, Goodin DS, Hugg JW, et al (1994) Biochemical alterations in multiple-sclerosis lesions and normal-appearing white matter detected by in vivo P-31 and H-1 spectroscopic imaging. Ann Neurol 36:157–165

Iles RA, Stevens AN, Griffiths JR (1982) NMR-studies of metabolites in living tissue. Prog Nucl Magn Reson Spectrosc 15:49

Iranzo A, Moreno A, Pujol J, et al (1999) Proton magnetic resonance spectroscopy pattern of progressive multifocal leukoencephalopathy in AIDS. J Neurol Neurosurg Psychiatry 66:520–523

Jarvik JG, Lenkinski RE, Grossman RI, Gomori JM, Schnall MD, Frank I (1993) Proton MR spectroscopy of HIV-infected patients: characterization of abnormalities with imaging and clinical correlation. Radiology 186:739–744

Jelicks LA, Gupta RK (1989) Multinuclear NMR studies of the Langendorff perfused rat heart. J Biol Chem 264:15230–15235

Knight-Scott J, Haley AP, Rossmiller SR, et al (2003) Molality as a unit of measure for expressing H-1 MRS brain metabolite concentrations in vivo. Magn Reson Imaging 21:787–797

Kreis R, Ernst T, Ross BD (1993a) Absolute quantitation of water and metabolites in the human brain. 2. Metabolite concentrations. J Magn Reson B 102:9–19

Kreis R, Ernst T, Ross BD (1993b) Development of the human brain—in vivo quantification of metabolite and water content with proton magnetic resonance spectroscopy. Magn Reson Med 30:424–437

Kuchel PW (1981) Nuclear magnetic resonance of biological samples. Crit Rev Anal Chem 12:155–231

Laubenberger J, Haussinger D, Bayer S, et al (1996) HIV-related metabolic abnormalities in the brain: depiction with proton MR spectroscopy with short echo times. Radiology 199:805–810

Law M, Meltzer DE, Cha S (2002) Spectroscopic magnetic resonance imaging of a tumefactive demyelinating lesion. Neuroradiology 44:986–989

London RE (1988) C-13 labelling in studies of metabolic-regulation. Prog Nucl Magn Reson Spectrosc 20:337–383

Lopez-Villegas D, Lenkinski RE, Wehrli SL, Ho WZ, Douglas SD (1995) Lactate production by human monocytes/macrophages determined by proton MR spectroscopy. Magn Reson Med 34:32–38

Lopez-Villegas D, Lenkinski RE, Frank I (1997) Biochemical changes in the frontal lobe of HIV-infected individuals detected by magnetic resonance spectroscopy. Proc Natl Acad Sci U S A 94:9854–9859

Martin E, Capone A, Schneider J, Hennig J, Thiel T (2001a) Absence of N-Acetylaspartate in the human brain: impact on neurospectroscopy? Ann Neurol 49:518–521

Martin E, Thiel T, Capone A, Hennig J, Schneider J (2001b) N-Acetylaspartate: usefulness as an indicator of viable neuronal tissue – reply. Ann Neurol 50:824–825

Matthews PM, Francis G, Antel J, Arnold DL (1991) Proton

magnetic resonance spectroscopy for metabolic characterization of plaques in multiple sclerosis. Neurology 41:1251–1256
McGuire D, Marder K (2000) Pharmacological frontiers in the treatment of AIDS dementia. J Psychopharmacol 14:251–257
McLean MA, Woermann FG, Barker GJ, Duncan JS (2000) Quantitative analysis of short echo time H-1-MRSI of cerebral grey and white matter. Magn Reson Med 44:401–411
McLean MA, Woermann FG, Simister RJ, Barker GJ, Duncan JS (2001) In vivo short echo time H-1-magnetic resonance spectroscopic imaging (MRSI) of the temporal lobes. Neuroimage 14:501–509
Meyerhoff DJ, MacKay S, Bachman L, et al (1993) Reduced brain N-acetylaspartate suggests neuronal loss in cognitively impaired human immunodeficiency virus-seropositive individuals: in vivo 1H magnetic resonance spectroscopic imaging. Neurology 43:509–515
Meyerhoff DJ, MacKay S, Poole N, Dillon WP, Weiner MW, Fein G (1994) N-acetylaspartate reductions measured by 1H MRSI in cognitively impaired HIV-seropositive individuals. Magn Reson Imaging 12:653–659
Meyerhoff DJ, Bloomer C, Cardenas V, Norman D, Weiner MW, Fein G (1999) Elevated subcortical choline metabolites in cognitively and clinically asymptomatic HIV+ patients. Neurology 52:995–1003
Mierisova S, Ala-Korpela M (2001) MR spectroscopy quantitation: a review of frequency domain methods. NMR Biomed 14:247–259
Miller BL (1991) A review of chemical issues in H-1-NMR spectroscopy—N-acetyl-L-aspartate, creatine and choline. NMR Biomed 4:47–52
Miller DH, Austin SJ, Connelly A, Youl BD, Gadian DG, McDonald WI (1991) Proton magnetic resonance spectroscopy of an acute and chronic lesion in multiple sclerosis. Lancet 337:58–59
Moonen CT, von Kienlin M, van Zijl PC, et al (1989) Comparison of single-shot localization methods (STEAM and PRESS) for in vivo proton NMR spectroscopy. NMR Biomed 2:201–208
Narayana PA, DeLayre JL (1986) Localization methods in NMR. In: Partain CL, Price RR, Patton JA, Kulkarni MV, James AE (eds) Magnetic resonance imaging. WB Saunders, Philadelphia, pp 1609–1630
Narayana PA, Doyle TJ, Lai D, Wolinsky JS (1998) Serial proton magnetic resonance spectroscopic imaging, contrast-enhanced magnetic resonance imaging, and quantitative lesion volumetry in multiple sclerosis. Ann Neurol 43:56–71
Navon G, Ogawa S, Shulman RG, Yamane T (1977a) High-resolution 31P nuclear magnetic resonance studies of metabolism in aerobic Escherichia coli cells. Proc Natl Acad Sci U S A 74:888–891
Navon G, Ogawa S, Shulman RG, Yamane T (1977b) 31P nuclear magnetic resonance studies of Ehrlich ascites tumor cells. Proc Natl Acad Sci U S A 74:87–91
Paley M, Wilkinson ID, Hall-Craggs MA, Chong WK, Chinn RJ, Harrison MJ (1995) Short echo time proton spectroscopy of the brain in HIV infection/AIDS. Magn Reson Imaging 13:871–875
Pauly J, Leroux P, Nishimura D, Macovski A (1991) Parameter relations for the Shinnar-Leroux selective excitation pulse design algorithm. IEEE Trans Med Imaging 10:53–65
Posse S, Decarli C, Lebihan D (1994) 3-Dimensional echo-planar MR spectroscopic imaging at short echo times in the human brain. Radiology 192:733–738
Posse S, Tedeschi G, Risinger R, Ogg R, Lebihan D (1995) High-speed H-1 spectroscopic imaging in human brain by echo-planar spatial-spectral encoding. Magn Reson Med 33:34–40
Provencher SW (2001) Automatic quantitation of localized in vivo H-1 spectra with LCModel. NMR Biomed 14:260–264
Pulliam L, Irwin I, Kusdra L, Rempel H, Flitter WD, Garland WA (2001) CPI-1189 attenuates effects of suspected neurotoxins associated with AIDS dementia: a possible role for ERK activation. Brain Res 893:95–103
Radda GK, Taylor DJ (1985) Applications of nuclear magnetic-resonance spectroscopy in pathology. Int Rev Exp Pathol 27:1–58
Roberts JKM, Jardetzky O (1981) Monitoring of cellular-metabolism by NMR. Biochim Biophys Acta 639:53–76
Ross BD, Bluml S (1996) New aspects of brain physiology. NMR Biomed 9:279–296
Ross B, Bluml S (2001) Magnetic resonance spectroscopy of the human brain. Anat Rec 265:54–84
Rudkin TM, Arnold DL (2002) MR spectroscopy and the biochemical basis of neurological disease. In: Atals SW (ed) Magnetic , 2nd edn. Lippincott Williams and Wilkins, Philadelphia
Ruiz-Cabello J, Cohen JS (1993) NMR and the study of pathological state in cells and tissues. Int Rev Cytol 145:1–63
Saindane AM, Cha S, Law M, Xue X, Knopp EA, Zagzag D (2002) Proton MR spectroscopy of tumefactive demyelinating lesions. Am J Neuroradiol 23:1378–1386
Salvan AM, Vion-Dury J, Confort-Gouny S, Nicoli F, Lamoureux S, Cozzone PJ (1997) Brain proton magnetic resonance spectroscopy in HIV-related encephalopathy: identification of evolving metabolic patterns in relation to dementia and therapy. AIDS Res Hum Retroviruses 13:1055–1066
Sarchielli P, Presciutti O, Tarducci R, et al (2002) Localized H-1 magnetic resonance spectroscopy in mainly cortical grey matter of patients with multiple sclerosis. J Neurol 249:902–910
Schuff N, Ezekiel F, Gamst AC, et al (2001) Region and tissue differences of metabolites in normally aged brain using multislice 1H magnetic resonance spectroscopic imaging. Magn Reson Med 45:899–907
Shinnar M (1994) Reduced power selective excitation radio frequency pulses. Magn Reson Med 32:658–660
Shinnar M, Leigh JS (1989) The application of spinors to pulse synthesis and analysis. Magn Reson Med 12:93–98
Shinnar M, Bolinger L, Leigh JS (1989a) The synthesis of soft pulses with a specified frequency response. Magn Reson Med 12:88–92
Shinnar M, Bolinger L, Leigh JS (1989b) The use of finite impulse response filters in pulse design. Magn Reson Med 12:81–87
Shinnar M, Eleff S, Subramanian H, Leigh JS (1989c) The synthesis of pulse sequences yielding arbitrary magnetization vectors. Magn Reson Med 12:74–80
Simmons ML, Frondoza CG, Coyle JT (1991) Immunocytochemical localization of N-acetyl-aspartate with monoclonal antibodies. Neuroscience 45:37–45
Simone IL, Federico F, Tortorella C, et al (1998) Localised H-1-MR spectroscopy for metabolic characterisation of diffuse and focal brain lesions in patients infected with HIV. J Neurol Neurosurg Psychiatry 64:516–523

Spielman D, Pauly J, Macovski A, Enzmann D (1991) Spectroscopic imaging with multidimensional pulses for excitation: SIMPLE. Magn Reson Med 19:67–84

Stankoff B, Tourbah A, Suarez S, et al (2001) Clinical and spectroscopic improvement in HIV-associated cognitive impairment. Neurology 56:112–115

Sullivan EV, Adalsteinsson E, Spielman DM, Hurd RE, Pfefferbaum A (2001) N-acetylaspartate—a marker of neuronal integrity. Ann Neurol 50:823

Tallan HH, Moore S, Stein WH (1956) N-acetyl-L-aspartic acid in brain. J Biol Chem 219:257–264

Tkac I, Rao R, Georgieff MK, Gruetter R (2003) Developmental and regional changes in the neurochemical profile of the rat brain determined by in vivo 1H NMR spectroscopy. Magn Reson Med 50:24–32

Tracey I, Carr CA, Guimaraes AR, Worth JL, Navia BA, Gonzalez RG (1996) Brain choline-containing compounds are elevated in HIV-positive patients before the onset of AIDS dementia complex: a proton magnetic resonance spectroscopic study. Neurology 46:783–788

Tran TKC, Vigneron DB, Sailasuta N, et al (2000) Very selective suppression pulses for clinical MRSI studies of brain and prostate cancer. Magn Reson Med 43:23–33

Trapp BD, Peterson J, Ransohoff RM, Rudick R, Mork S, Bo L (1998) Axonal transection in the lesions of multiple sclerosis. New Engl J Med 338:278–285

Ugurbil K, Adriany G, Andersen P, et al (2003) Ultrahigh field magnetic resonance imaging and spectroscopy. Magn Reson Imaging 21:1263–1281

Valenzuela MJ, Sachdev P (2001) Magnetic resonance spectroscopy in AD. Neurology 56:592–598

Vanhamme L, Sundin T, Van Hecke P, Van Huffel S (2001) MR spectroscopy quantitation: a review of time-domain methods. NMR Biomed 14:233–246

Vion-Dury J, Nicoli F, Salvan AM, Confort-Gouny S, Dhiver C, Cozzone PJ (1995) Reversal of brain metabolic alterations with zidovudine detected by proton localised magnetic resonance spectroscopy (letter). Lancet 345:60–61

von Giesen HJ, Wittsack HJ, Wenserski F, Koller H, Hefter H, Arendt G (2001) Basal ganglia metabolite abnormalities in minor motor disorders associated with human immunodeficiency virus type 1. Arch Neurol 58:1281–1286

Wiedermann D, Schuff N, Matson GB, et al (2001) Short echo time multislice proton magnetic resonance spectroscopic imaging in human brain: metabolite distributions and reliability. Magn Reson Imaging 19:1073–1080

Yongbi NM, Payne GS, Collins DJ, Leach MO (1995) Quantification of signal selection efficiency, extra volume suppression and contamination for ISIS, STEAM and PRESS localized 1H NMR spectroscopy using an EEC localization test object. Phys Med Biol 40:1293–1303

Zandt H, van der Graaf M, Heerschap A (2001) Common processing of in vivo MR spectra. NMR Biomed 14:224–232

10 Molecular Imaging and High-Field MRI in Multiple Sclerosis

ALAYAR KANGARLU

CONTENTS

10.1 Molecular Imaging

Considering the early success of contrast-based imaging techniques it is essential to understand the basis for molecular imaging (MI). While all imaging modalities have distinct capabilities in visualizing inner structure and function of biological tissues, no single technique has all the desirable characteristics of specificity, sensitivity and resolution. As far as MRI is concerned, there is a fundamental barrier against directly accessing a small number of molecules at field strengths below 10 Tesla (T) at room temperature. The physical basis of the obstacle against MRI access to individual molecular events is discussed in the following sections. The minute magnetic dipole of the individual hydrogen protons necessitates an observation of magnetization of a large ensemble or amplification to the MRI signal in order to detect a small group of molecules. Since magnetization is directly proportional to the magnetic field, i.e., magnetic flux density, there is a relationship between field strength and the signal to noise ratio (SNR) obtained from a specific voxel. Within a specific magnetic field, the image contrast to noise ratio (CNR) can be manipulated using paramagnetic contrast agents. These contrast agents usually have one or more unpaired electrons. This assigns a high magnetic susceptibility to these contrast agents which enables them to generate strong positive, i.e., T1 shortening, or negative, i.e., T2 shortening, contrast generating attributes. This is not signal amplification but a contrast augmentation. This artificial contrast will greatly enhance the focusing power of MRI for small area observations. This technique is taken one step further by conjugating these agents with specialized macromolecules. These macromolecules possess biochemical properties that enable them to distinguish a particular biological process. Contrast agents can be designed to reach and build up at a specific pathological site by passive or active targeting mechanisms (LI and BEDNARSKI 2002; BADDANOV 2002). In passive targeting, the probe can be a radiolabeled ligand, substrate, antibody, or cytokine. In active MI, the probes are capable of being activated by a particular RF pulse and extracellular proteases, among others, for targeted delivery and interrogation of a desired site. In both cases, however, pathophysiologically guided contrast agents are made to accumulate at a specific site and enhance visualization.

In general, there are two mechanisms through which image contrast at molecular level can be achieved. One way is to probe endogenously expressed proteins using contrast agents. The second approach for contrast rendering at molecular level is by using reporter genes that could be transfected

A. KANGARLU, PhD
Head of MRI Physics and Assistant Professor of Clinical Neuroscience, Columbia University College of Physicians and Surgeons and New York State Psychiatric Institute, 1051 Riverside Drive, Unit 74, New York, NY 10032, USA

to enable expression (LUKER et al. 2002; RAY et al. 2004). MRI application in the visualization of endogenous expression has been very limited to date. Such a technique would be very powerful as it would enable diagnosis and staging for many neuropathologic conditions. In addition, the potential now exists for using imaging and therapeutic agents synergistically to mutually optimize their performance to enable monitoring and therapy by imaging. This could eventually lead into MI capable of identifying pre-disease conditions during which therapy could be more effective. In active MI, reporter genes interrogating specific intracellular events require that an exogenous contrast reagent is attached to them (GILLIES 2002). These reagents will detect the presence of gene products and intracellular processes. The challenges include overcoming the blood–brain barrier (BBB) to get the imaging probes to their targets. For MRI, a challenge is to devise techniques to produce good SNR and CNR for target concentrations which are in the micro- to picomolar range.

10.1.1 Biomarkers

Pathological events involve molecules whose MR signals are too small to detect directly. The difficulty of enhancing the resolution of imaging to visualize the molecular events is primarily due to the energy gap of the spin groups. Because of the minute energy difference between the spin dipole moments parallel to and opposing the main magnetic field, the excess protons that participate in the spin flipping dynamics as a result of RF excitation are a tiny fraction of molecular density. Approximately one part per million (1 ppm) of the total protons are magnetically accessible for each 1 T of magnetic field. As such, there are two possible ways of enhancing the MR signal to access molecular events, invasive and noninvasive. High magnetic field is a noninvasive method and targeted contrast agents are the invasive method for enhancing molecular signal. The ability of high field in enhancing the resolution of MR images (see Figs. 10.1 and 10.2) has been described in this article in the context of the performance of an 8-T whole body MR scanner. The existence of contrast agents or biomarkers can cause positive (T1 shortening groups such as Gd-DTPA) and negative (T2 shortening groups of ultra-small superparamagnetic iron oxide or USPIO macromolecules coated with dextran) signal modulation. In making them relevant to pathology studies they must be targeted to pathology sites. The biochemistry of biomarker design has been analyzed in many review articles (LI and BEDNARSKI 2002; ALLEN et al. 2004; FLOYD and MCSHANE 2004). In short, their sensitivity must

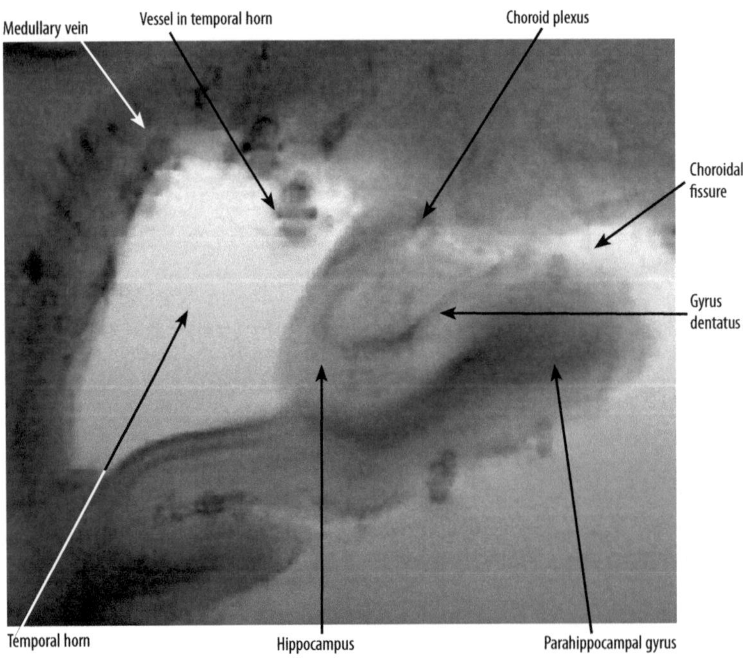

Fig. 10.1. A 2D gradient echo image of a coronal hippocampal section of a human brain imaged ex vivo at 8 T. The image was acquired with TR/TE of 500/30 ms, FOV=15 cm, 1024×1024, with 150-µm in-plane resolution and a slice thickness of 1 mm. The resolution of the T2* image is sufficient to visualize many hippocampal subfields, such as granule cell layer of gyrus dentatus, vestigial hippocampal sulcus, and some layers of the CA1

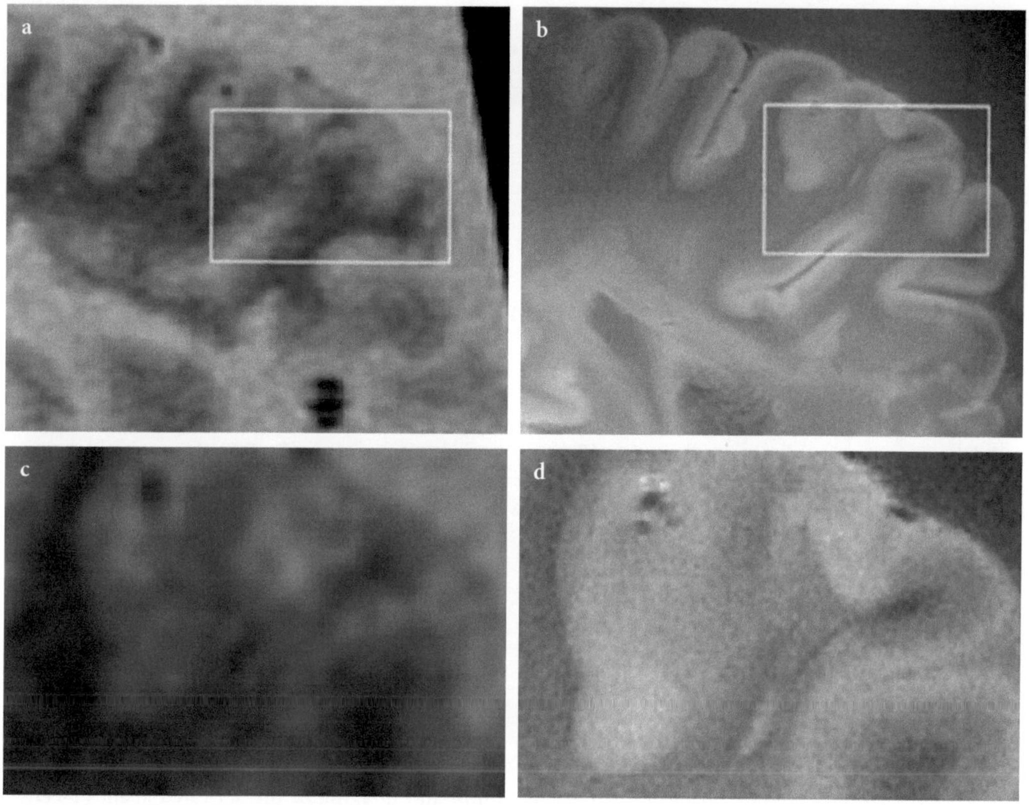

Fig. 10.2a–d. MR images of whole brain slices of an MS patient. **a** A 1.5-T FLAIR T2 acquired with a 256×256 matrix. **b** An 8-T GRE with a 1024×1024 matrix and 150-μm resolution. As is evident, the SNR in the 1.5-T case was not sufficient for larger matrix size. **c** Magnified view of the inset in (**a**). **d** Magnified view of the inset in **b**

be such that a tolerable amount could be delivered to the target site. As such, targeted contrast agents possessing the combined properties of pathology detection and signal amplification have found a vital role to play in imaging based diagnosis and therapy.

10.1.1.1
Natural Biomarkers

Present MR techniques used for MS studies and to assess disease burden include MR spectroscopy (MRS) measurements identifying decreased *N*-acetyl aspartate (NAA), choline/NAA ratio, and creatine/NAA ratio. Other techniques include comparative brainstem analysis and probes of plaque demyelination, thalamic neuronal loss on MR images, tissue characterization by fMRI, MRI morphometry, cortical thickness, etc. The use of these natural biomarkers in multiple sclerosis (MS) has shown potential for the quantification of abnormal accumulation of metabolites (Pan et al. 1996). Proton MRS studies have shown enhancement of these metabolites which might enable early detection and assessment of therapy.

10.1.1.2
Passive Targeting

It is possible to use the body's natural defense mechanisms for passively targeting pathology. Gd-chelate, iron oxide particles and all other blood pool agents are of this type and are handled by phagocytic cells removing these foreign particles from the body. Macrophages are among the most important components of the immune defense system and play a major role in clearance of particulate contrast media such as USPIO. The use of USPIO in achieving cellular imaging at 1.5 T has been reported (Oweida et al. 2004).

10.1.1.3 Active Targeting

Contrast agents have shown great success in detecting the breakdown of BBB and visualization of blood vessels. This has raised the hope of them being used as guided carriers with molecular accuracy (Bulte et al. 2004). The success of T1 and T2 contrast agents encouraged researchers to work to overcome the limitation of their site inspecificity. In the absence of selective localization of contrast agents in a specific region of the body their application will be restricted to the detection of permeable blood vessels. Within the past 10 years a wide range of research has demonstrated the ability to achieve targeting of pathology and delivery of contrast agents to their sites (Pirko et al. 2004). Efforts towards this goal have taken two distinct paths. On the one hand gadolinium contrast agents are developed for targeted imaging (Allen and MacRenaris 2004; Shahbazi-Gahrouei et al. 2001). On another front, iron oxide-based contrast agents such as USPIOs are developed for various pathology and delivery mechanism (Anderson et al. 2004; Arbab et al. 2004; Zelivyanskaya et al. 2003; Wood et al. 2004; Stoll et al. 2004; Artemov et al. 2003; Beckmann et al. 2003; Bendszus and Stoll 2003). This is combined with advances in coating of iron oxide nanoparticles of various sizes and the technology to increase their blood half-lives. In particular, in MS and cancer, their potential (Anderson et al. 2004; Weissleder 2002; Ray et al. 2004) to play a significant role in their diagnosis has already been demonstrated. Iron-oxide complexes whose size is within 10–100 nm are usually referred to as USPIOs. The coatings of these nanoparticles are designed to provide them with colloidal properties. The origin of iron oxide complexes as contrast agents refers back to when monocrystalline iron oxide nanoparticles, or MIONs, were first developed for this purpose (Weissleder et al. 1990). Each particle comprises about 1000 atoms of iron in a crystalline form wrapped with dextrin. When the dextrin is cross-linked, the particles are called CLIONS (cross-linked iron oxide nanoparticles).

Access to the brain at the cellular level is difficult. However, sampling biological events in the brain at molecular level would greatly enhance understanding of the neurodegenerative diseases. These diseases could be characterized as genomic disorders. Considering the progress in MI, degenerative diseases could potentially be directly imaged. This possibility is due to the availability to tag proteins involved in MS, Alzheimer disease (AD) and Huntington disease (HD). The common feature among these diseases is their sensitivity to their amino acid packing order within the structure of the protein. In the case of damage or replacement of an amino acid within the protein structure the stability of the protein structure will be lost. This is the hallmark of these neurological diseases. Protemonomics study of the amino acids and the implications of their replacement in protein structure provide the basis for the development of techniques for tracking the activity site of the protein.

Design of various MI contrast agents or biomarkers is based on the difference between structure and function of the amino acid responsible for disability of the protein. In this regard, animal models play a critical role in the study of various neurological diseases. For MS, the most widely used animal model, experimental autoimmune encephalomyelitis (EAE), has been used for the delivery and imaging of demyelination sites (Ahrens et al. 1998; Dousset et al. 1999). In targeted EAE imaging studies T-cell or macrophages are magnetically labeled by tagging activated lymphocytes, which are the disease-inducing agent in the mouse model. The spinal cord and the brain images are shown to be affected immediately on clinical manifestation of the disease (Anderson et al. 2004). The significance of these studies is the demonstration of the feasibility and imaging of the activated agent (T-cells). Considering that these agents (T-cells) are the cause of EAE, this technique will provide insight into the mechanism of the disease process. Furthermore, Anderson et al. (2004) have demonstrated that cells are immunologically comparable to unlabeled active lymphocytes and the labeling technique has achieved the important objective of supply a large enough population of iron oxide (SPIO)/transfection agent to enable their in vivo MR detection. The high resolution images acquired with this technique in the mouse is a significant step forward in tagging, site-specific delivery, and imaging a group of cells directly involved in etiology of EAE.

In cancer, in vivo staging of brain tumors is the goal of MI. Here, differences in the genomic profiles of various brain tumor subtypes are used as the basis for targeted imaging. This will eventually lead to the development of a specific and more effective therapy (Gutin 2002; Tropres et al. 2004).

Incorporation of this approach to imaging will allow in vivo study of the biology of these diseases, MS, AD, HD and cancer, with the ability to acquire information on the structure and function at the cellular and molecular level. Such tools will help develop significant advances in treatment.

10.1.2 Technical Issues of MRI in MI

10.1.2.1 Animal Studies

As noted, EAE is an animal model inducing inflammatory and demyelinating disease of the central nervous system (CNS). It is the widely accepted model for MS (Alvord et al. 1984). Genetically susceptible animal species are injected with proteins derived from the CNS in order to induce the disease. These proteins include proteolipid protein (PLP), myelin basic protein (MBP), and synthetic peptides emulsified in Freund's adjuvant (CFA).

Histologically, EAE is characterized by a mononuclear cell infiltrate affecting the white matter by inducing demyelination. The white matter lesions are inflicted by T-cells, B-cells, and macrophages infiltrates. In addition, compromised BBB and edema are the primary characteristics of EAE lesions. In mice, the spinal cord is more extensively affected than the brain. Progression of the disease is accompanied by demyelination and axonal loss. The form taken by the two subtypes of the disease, acute or relapsing-remitting, is dependent upon the specific mouse model. As with other inflammatory processes, direct visualization by MRI is performed using techniques that are sensitive to edema and changes in diffusion, and contrast agents may be used to identify regions of BBB breakdown.

The challenges in direct visualization of myelin abnormalities in acute EAE are due to their spread far outside the MR-visible inflammatory lesions. This microdemyelination within normal appearing white matter (NAWM) could amount to an extensive cumulative loss of myelin proteins. Studies in acute EAE have shown that MR-visible demyelinated regions only account for less than a third of the immunocytochemically detected decrease in myelin protein expression (Kawczak et al. 1998). Thus, along with visible areas of demyelination a majority of abnormalities will manifest in more diffuse micro-demyelination. This is demonstrated by the decreased staining in normal appearing white matter. To probe these microscopic abnormalities one must resort to techniques with microscopic resolution. This is truer in small animal models due to small lesion sizes. As such, high resolution is necessary to delineate EAE lesions and techniques in this area have not been extensively developed in vivo. EAE lesions have been visualized in the spinal cord using T2*-weighted MR microscopy (MRM) and diffusion-weighted imaging (DWI) (Ahrens et al. 1998). Ex vivo MR studies in the rat spinal cord (Lanens et al. 1994) and mouse spinal cord (Ahrens et al. 1998) show hyperintensities in white matter and meninges with T2 or T2* weighting that correspond to demyelinated inflammatory lesions on histology. Demyelination, remyelination, inflammation and edema are not specifically distinguished, though decreased diffusion anisotropy has been demonstrated in lesions as well, indicating loss of structural order in the white matter. Loss of order may be due to edema, myelin loss and or axonal loss. The gray-white matter boundary is ill-defined in the presence of lesion in both the mouse and rat. Inflammatory lesions may progress to a wide area of the white matter in advanced disease.

There are few in vivo routine and high resolution MRI studies of EAE in the mouse (Floris et al. 2004). Contrast enhancement of lesions from the brain parenchyma has been seen in T1- and T2-weighted images in diseased mice and rats (Rausch et al. 2003). Other reports have shown that USPIO-enhanced images have detected EAE lesions with high sensitivity (Dousset et al. 1999). In these studies T2-weighted images and gadolinium-enhanced T1-weighted images showed poor sensitivity. Confirmation of the USPIO findings by histologic examination showing macrophages at the same sites as found by USPIO-enhanced images has validated specificity of this technique. Different aspects of iron based contrast are the subject of other studies to enhance its ability to identify lesions in the EAE mouse brain (Xu et al. 1998). USPIO and MION examine issues such as prolongation of blood half-life. These particles must both have a high blood half-life and be able to cross the disrupted BBB areas in EAE lesions. MION enhanced lesion conspicuity at areas of BBB disruption and enabled lesion detection has not been possible without contrast. In MRI corresponding to inflammatory and demyelinating lesions on histology, hypointense and hyperintense (possible T1 shortening or phase shift) areas have been seen.

10.1.2.2 Human Studies

Recent MRI studies on MS patients have also revealed subtle abnormalities of the central nervous system in NAWM, which is difficult for routine imaging to detect. These abnormalities involve microdemyelination and widespread membrane turnover that could precede the formation of inflammatory lesions (Pan et al. 1996). Furthermore, the inflammatory cells, T-cells, B-cells and macrophages penetrate the CNS via an elusive mechanism whose understanding is an important step in unraveling the basis of the onset and progression of demyelination and forging therapeutic methods. MRI studies of MS have been able to measure myelin loss, and efforts to correlate that with the clinical manifestation of the disease have scored mixed results. What routine MRI lacks is the ability to monitor directly the pathologic processes in order to find the one specific for demyelination. In this regard, it appears that routine MRI techniques have reached a level of maturity for clinical MS studies. A wide range of well-optimized sequences have been brought into the clinical care of patients with MS. While these techniques have improved the quality of images and have accelerated the acquisition, the main contrast mechanisms of MR appear to be unable to definitively detect lesion evolution and determine disease subtype. Also, within the past decade the limits of SNR have been reached by the ever-improving technology incorporated in the new MRI scanners. This has led to a search for external agents to sensitize pathology for MR visualization. Among all the existing contrast enhanced imaging techniques for molecular detection of diseases MRI has many unique attributes. It has a better penetration depth than optical imaging, non-ionizing radiation in contrast to nuclear medicine and superior resolution versus PET and SPECT. As such, enhancement of MRI capabilities will play an important role in making MR-based MI a reality for pathophysiology studies and study of function in the brain of patients with MS.

10.1.2.2.1 Imaging Time

Compared to optical imaging and PET, MR images take longer to acquire. This difficulty, however, will be alleviated through many fast imaging techniques. Parallel imaging is one such technique in which multiple surface coils are used as arrays and their independent images are used to construct the final image. It has been shown that acceleration factors of up to 10 could be achieved, which proportionally reduces the imaging time (Pruesseman et al. 1999; Sodickson and Manning 1997). In addition, ultra-short echo time sequences, fast imaging sequences with innovative k-space filling techniques, and faster switching gradients will help reduce the acquisition time for MR studies to within ranges of other imaging techniques.

10.1.2.2.2 Contrast

The MR signal from biological tissues carries useful information. This is largely due to the sensitivity of the proton resonance to its environment and the massive number of excess ^{1}H protons for generation of bulk magnetization per imaging voxel. The contrast in MRI is the difference in SNR between two adjacent tissues. As such, if adjacent biological tissues produce nearly the same SNR the contrast will be poor. This condition does exist in the case of certain diseases. For the diseases in which structural or functional modification of the tissues has little MR implication the technique will not detect the pathology very sensitively. Contrast agents are used in these situations to deliver artificial contrast to the affected areas. As T1 contrast agents, macromolecules with the lanthanide ion gadolinium incorporated in their molecular structure have found many applications in detecting breakdown of the BBB. The paramagnetic field of these ions due to their unpaired electrons creates a fluctuating local magnetic field which enhances the relaxation of water protons. The coupling of these dipole–dipole interactions in tissue magnetization causes a decrease in T1. The characteristic relaxivity of these agents is proportional to the sixth power of the inverse of the distance. The theoretical basis of relaxivity caused by paramagnetic contrast agents is formulated by Solomon-Bloembergen-Morgan equations. Paramagnetic enhancement of nuclear relaxation rates is a function of magnetic field. In general there are longitudinal and transverse relaxation rate enhancements caused by contact and dipolar electron–nucleus interactions. The lanthanides need to be chelated for safety and to achieve maximum water proton relaxivity. This achieves optimization of the water exchange rate and rotational correlation time. Lanthanides and transition metal ions like iron are suitable for use as contrast agents due to their relatively large magnetic moments and unpaired electrons. They are, however, toxic for use with human subjects. As such, appropriate ligands or chelates are used to cloak the metal ions and screen their toxicity.

10.1.2.2.3 Limits of Detection

There are a number of ways in which MRI can characterize structure and function of biological tissues. Relaxation mechanisms and tissue density are the primary ways that tissues are probed structurally.

Physiological information acquired in MRI can be divided into two categories. A class of functional investigations of the brain involves MRS which detects metabolite concentrations. Another class of physiological measurements relies on the paramagnetic properties of blood. Here, perfusion, blood volume, blood flow, and the permeability of capillaries are accessible to MR experiments. These quantities are indirect measures of physiological events of the vasculature. The first order events are the blood magnetic properties which are directly assessed by MRI. Natural variation in the paramagnetic state of blood or blood oxygenation level dependence (BOLD) acts as an inherent contrast mechanism for blood/functional measurements. This is proven to be insufficient for the study of biological events at cellular or molecular level. As such, external agents are used to manipulate the CNR. This does not amplify the signal beyond the limits set by the magnetic field strength. The augmentation of the image is due to the rapid recovery of transverse magnetization as a result of the presence of large magnetic dipole of paramagnetic or superparamagnetic molecules. Accordingly, a measure of maximum detectable MR signal for medical scanners must be found in order to evaluate the limitations of MRI for attaining molecular and cellular resolution.

In order to gain insight into how contrast agents will enhance visualization of pathology one needs to know the fundamental SNR of MR signal from biological tissues. The limit of detection of routine MRI is a function of the magnetic field strength. This subject is analyzed at length in the next section. But as far as SNR effect on the feasibility of MI is concerned the following argument aims at understanding the fundamental limits against attaining imaging with molecular/cellular scale resolution.

To this end, an account of the resolution necessary for endogenous-contrast-based imaging is needed. The resolution of typical images acquired at 1.5 T for medical diagnosis has 1×1 mm^2 with 5-mm slice thickness. As such the voxels represented on medical images have a volume of 5 ml. It is conceivable that the highest-field magnets feasible for human studies will operate at a field of 10 T. This will reduce the voxel size to about 50 nl. Considering the typical volume of human cell of about 1 nl there is a 100-fold deficit in endogenous resolution to attain cellular sensitivity. It must be noted, however, that susceptibility effects are capable of projecting the dephasing and signal loss beyond cellular dimensions. This does not amount to the amplification of the signal beyond the limits set by the magnetic field strength. This limit is governed by the Boltzmann distribution of the magnetic dipoles parallel and antiparallel with the static field. Based on these principles, at a field of 10 T, which is presently the limit for human magnets, only 10 protons for every million protons will participate in MR signal formation. In the absence of a photonic technique a large number of spins are required to make up a signal large enough to be detected by human MR scanners. As such, endogenous-contrast-based whole body imaging is unable to achieve single molecule detection. Thus, a significant augmentation of MR signal is required to overcome the fundamental limits against realization of human imaging at molecular level. Among various approaches the signal enhancement offered by MI is the most realistic and feasible.

10.1.3 State of the Art in MI of Animal Models in MS

EAE in rodents has been the workhorse of technique development for MS imaging research. While a valuable model, it has not been fully explored due to the difficulties involved with the techniques. It is conceivable that removal of these obstacles will greatly enhance the contribution this valuable tool could make to technique development of demyelination imaging. MI is one such approach for dealing with the technical difficulties of imaging EAE, and researchers have began exploring targeted imaging by using labeled T-cells for imaging in EAE mice (de Laquintane et al. 2002; Corot et al. 2004; Anderson et al. 2004).

In recent studies on EAE mice it has been shown that the labeled lymphocytes in the new lesion enable lesion visualization in addition to their own detection ('t Hart et al. 2004). This is based on the presence of cells bearing contrast that are specific to a lesion site. MR visualization of EAE lesions in the cord, both directly, and indirectly, has been reported in the live mouse (Anderson et al. 2004) (Fig. 10.3). Considering the inflammatory processes, MRI can directly visualize EAE lesions using methods that are particularly sensitive to edema and changes in diffusion. Due to the general difficulty of detecting microscopic changes, contrast agents with the ability to cross a damaged BBB have also been used. Active targeting is now becoming available, beginning with a detection scheme based on cellular imaging of labeled cells in the lesion (Fig. 10.4).

The contrast from SPIO in the lymphocytes produces both a stronger effect and a larger area of hypointensity than the actual area containing the labeled cells, known as the blooming effect, from the

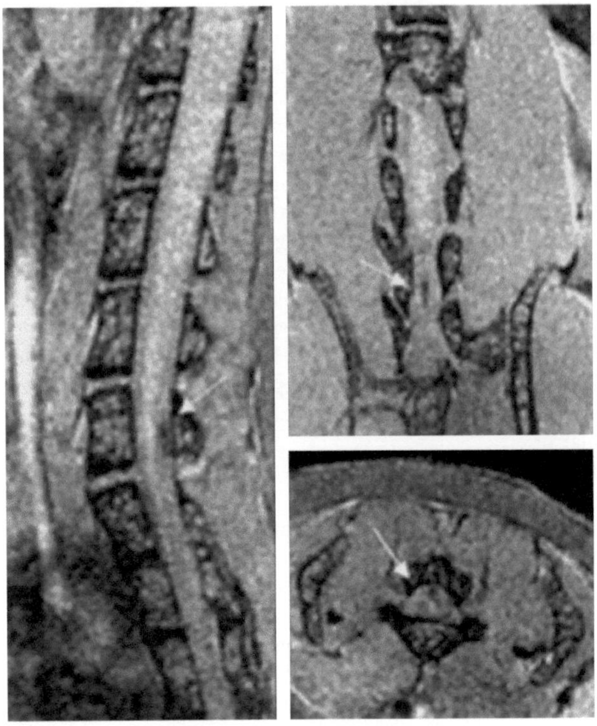

Fig. 10.3. MR image at 7 T of the spinal cord of a live EAE mouse with systemic injection of labeled T-lymphocytes. The spinal cord was imaged at 100 µm isotropic resolution with a 3D fast gradient echo sequence, TR/TE=22 ms/3.3 ms. The hypointense lesion (*arrows*) is shown in three planes and indicates the localized presence of iron labeled, activated T-lymphocytes. (Images courtesy of Stasia Anderson)

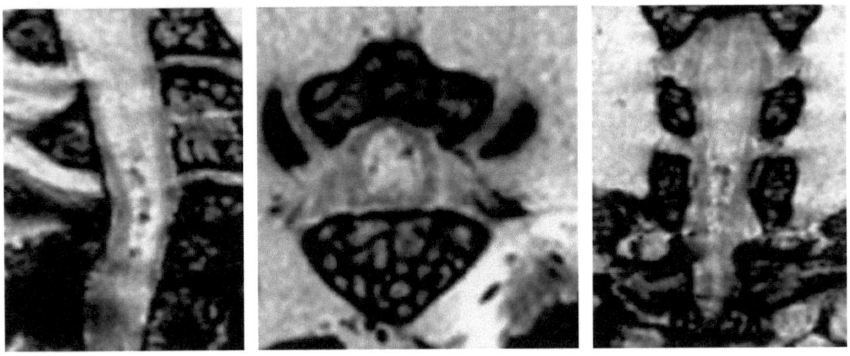

Fig. 10.4. Microscopic ex vivo 7-T MR images in an EAE mouse. EAE was induced by intravenous infusion of FE-PLL-labeled T cells and administration of pertussis. Clinical score 1.5. 3D coronal spin echo images were acquired with 30×30×46 μm^3. The spinal cord images show hypointense white matter and nerve roots. The hypointense spots indicate site of cellular infiltrates. (Images courtesy of Stasia Anderson)

iron susceptibility artifact. In such images (Figs. 10.3 and 10.4) the lesion of about 100 µm in diameter appeared ~160 µm in the image. This is a moderate effect compared to images in which there is a large concentration of iron, due to the relatively low iron load in the cells, and this somewhat low level is advantageous because the end result is an effect that is visible but does not obscure the anatomy.

The effect of the contrast in these cells has potentially further-reaching utility in time than the T-cell detection. It has been shown (Anderson et al. 2004) that when the spinal cord is imaged early in the disease course at the onset of symptoms, direct images from active T-cell infiltration can be acquired (Fig. 10.3). These images are specific to T-cell migration. Such a technique allows the measurement of the time evolution of the later stages of the disease, in which T-cells can die and macrophages can pick up T-cells as well as the label. In such a situation the lesion would remain hypointense on MR with less specificity for a particular type of cell, but still specific to the presence of a lesion.

These targeted EAE imaging studies indicate that the labeling method improves the chances of visualizing the trafficking of these cells on MR, while not interfering with the functioning of the T-cell, B-cell or macrophages. A complex preparation process in magnetic labeling techniques is involved in which the cells are transfected with iron oxides and then stored in endosomes in the cytoplasm (Anderson et al. 2004). Generally, in choosing or designing how the cells will be transfected with a contrast agent one has to consider the efficiency coupled with potential effects on the cell based on where and how the agent will be stored in the cell. The small volume of cytosol in T-cells has to accommodate the iron tag. This makes their interaction with the surfaces rather frequent and significantly affects their function. For T-cells in particular it has been shown to be important to transfect with more iron. It is also important to limit effects on the surface activation, which is to be controlled by the activation mechanism of the cell. These requirements have been met by ferumoxide-poly-L-lysine (FE-PLL) complex (Anderson et al. 2004).

Presently, work is being done on improving the efficiency of the targeting molecules in binding to the target (Arbab et al. 2004). Activatable agents are being designed with two internal modes. The "on" mode is assigned to the condition of high contrast and the "off" mode represents low contrast enhancement. These agents will be capable of responding to a specific physiological or metabolic event that will cause them to switch from one mode to another. The switching mechanism of these agents is based on the mechanism of signal modulation by paramagnetic properties (Allen et al. 2004). The switching mechanism depends on the molecular structure of the agent. Mechanisms such as chemical exchange are at work for activation of Gd agents, while USPIOs use switching processes by dipolar coupling-induced anisotropy enhancement, which causes decreased T2. This technology has demonstrated great potential in enabling in vivo monitoring of lesion formation and activity. However, it has to overcome the barriers summarized in this article along the complex path to development of ideal labeling agents for cellular and molecular imaging of MS.

10.2 High-Field MRI

Challenges to MRI becoming a complete diagnostic tool are multidimensional. It is clear that routine MRI within a short time has scored remarkable achievements in the diagnosis and treatment of MS. The ability to visualize areas of demyelination in the brains of patients with MS by MRI has enabled the systematic examination of some aspects of the development of the "MS plaques". In particular, MRI has enabled monitoring of lesion load, which is unique information attainable only by MRI (Grossman and McGowan 1998). Nevertheless, the lesion load has not shown a strong correlation with clinical manifestation of MS. Particularly, the fact remains that presently no imaging modality can detect the main event of the lesion formation in MS, i.e., T-lymphocyte migration through the BBB. Recently, using high resolution microscopic MRI, we have shown that plaques are centered on the microvasculature in the white matter of MS patients' brains (Kangarlu et al. 2002). This offers unique information accessible in vivo which contains clues on the vascular injury and possibly axonal implication in the disease. An understanding of the details of these events will permit the definition of therapeutic strategies and evaluation of their efficacy by MRI. High-field (HF) MRI may possess such capability. It is, however, confronting a number of challenges before becoming a tool with the ability to offer accurate diagnosis consistent with clinical measures of the disease. These challenges include high magnetic susceptibility, RF inhomogeneity, dielectric resonances, RF penetration effects and RF coil design (Figs. 10.5 and 10.6). In the absence of a viable remedy for these artifacts, signal intensity variations across the head will significantly compromise the information content of HF MR images.

We will describe the merits and challenges of the process of developing in vivo magnetic resonance microscopy (MRM) as a method for routine study of patients with MS. Such an imaging technique could be used to study the rate of BBB breakdown in acutely relapsing (AR), primary progressive (PP), and active secondary progressive (ASP) MS and its difference from that seen in patients with inactive secondary progressive (ISP) disease. Since it has been established that the migration of lymphocytes obtained from AR and ASP is higher than those obtained from ISP, an opportunity exists to establish such a correlation through MRM. Considering that relapses of MS occur regularly, as is evident from

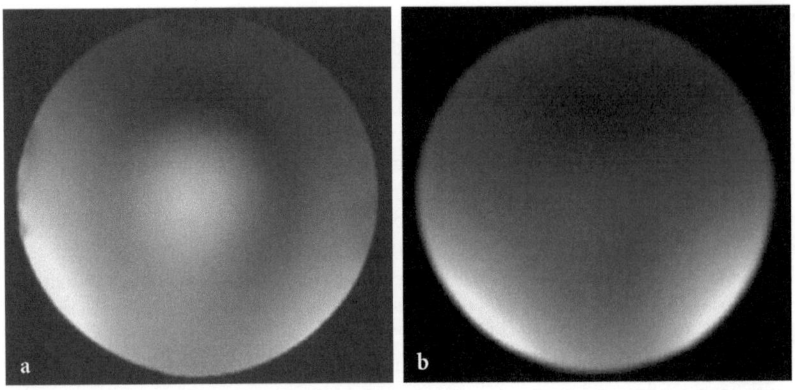

Fig. 10.5a,b. Image of a spherical phantom filled with saline. Both images are gradient echo axial slices with TR=700 ms, TE=11 ms with the same RF power level. Image (**a**) was acquired with a standard quadrature mode while image (**b**) was acquired with two-port transmit/receive with variable amplitude and phase difference between the two ports. Notice the vastly improved homogeneity in the image on the right. The bright center of (**a**) is completely eliminated in (**b**) as a result of the phase variation on the two ports independently

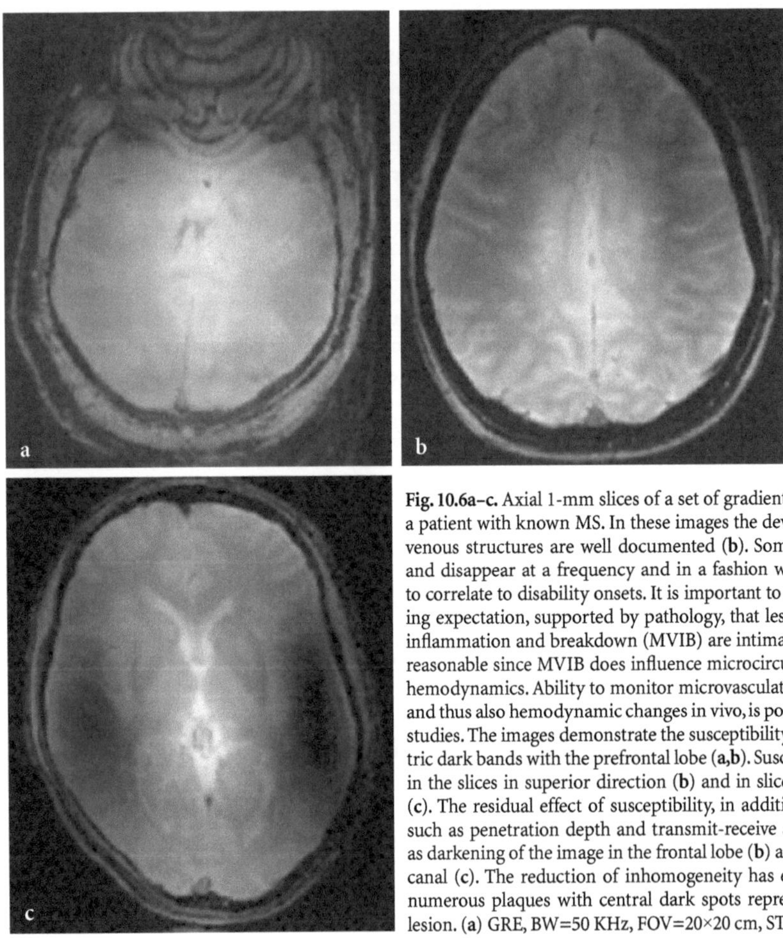

Fig. 10.6a–c. Axial 1-mm slices of a set of gradient echo images taken at 8 T from a patient with known MS. In these images the development of MS plaques along venous structures are well documented (**b**). Some of these plaques will appear and disappear at a frequency and in a fashion which diagnostic imaging is yet to correlate to disability onsets. It is important to note that there is a long-standing expectation, supported by pathology, that lesion activity and microvascular inflammation and breakdown (MVIB) are intimately related. This expectation is reasonable since MVIB does influence microcirculation and, as a result, cerebral hemodynamics. Ability to monitor microvasculature changes and inflammation, and thus also hemodynamic changes in vivo, is possible using such HF MRI in MS studies. The images demonstrate the susceptibility artifact in the form of concentric dark bands with the prefrontal lobe (**a,b**). Susceptibility is much less dramatic in the slices in superior direction (**b**) and in slices above the semicircular canal (**c**). The residual effect of susceptibility, in addition to other high-field artifacts such as penetration depth and transmit-receive asymmetry, are still observable as darkening of the image in the frontal lobe (**b**) and slices above the semicircular canal (**c**). The reduction of inhomogeneity has enabled better depiction of the numerous plaques with central dark spots representing central vessels of each lesion. (**a**) GRE, BW=50 KHz, FOV=20×20 cm, ST=1 mm, TR=500 ms, TE=7ms

MRI, but only a small fraction of such exacerbations become manifest clinically, the role of: (a) cortical gray matter (CGM) lesions, and (b) comparison of the microscopic structure of white matter plaques, with and without microvasculature involvement, with clinical disability could help reveal the immunological origin of MS. Drugs under investigation for their efficacy could be examined for their ability to modify the MRM profile, and a favorable effect on MRM imaging CGM and microvasculature of white matter plaques could become an important measure of efficacy. In this regard, the effect of interferon, for instance, would be more objectively quantified with MRM.

10.2.1 State of the Art in MR Research in MS

Insofar as the MR assessment of MS is concerned, it has become evident that loss of myelin does not always equal loss of function. Sensitivity of MRI to loss of myelin and its relative insensitivity to changes in axonal function present a challenge to this imaging modality. This is particularly notable since it has become evident that lesions as seen on conventional MRI do not correlate well with the presence or absence of neurological function. This is in spite of the fact that MR imaging and spectroscopy at 1.5 T has permitted some examination of the evolution of the plaques of MS and provided some understanding of the pathogenesis of this disorder that was previously impossible (Filippi et al. 2000). But, although significant advances have been made in this regard, it is becoming increasingly clear that MRI at 1.5 T has limitations in defining all of the pathological events in the brain. Specifically, the total disease burden does not seem to correlate with clinical disability. Even though MR spectroscopy (MRS) (Helms et al. 1999) has identified decreased *N*-acetyl aspartate (NAA) in NAWM in patients with early relapsing-remitting MS, it has not been able to offer a consistent predictor of disability and quality of life for MS patients (de Stefano et al. 1999; Davie et al. 1997). Decreased levels of NAA, a marker for axons, however, implicate axonal dysfunction in MS. Furthermore, it has been known that MS patients suffer severe disability during which time MR detects no new lesions (Leary et al. 1999). While BBB disruption is related to MS disease activity, it can only be assessed with contrast-enhanced MRI. Even then, direct observation of the internal structure of the enhanced plaques is difficult. Various techniques, such as Gd-DTPA enhanced MRI, MRS and magnetization transfer (MT) have demonstrated (Leary et al. 1999) promising potential to provide evidence for activity of MS lesions through correlation with enhancement (Horsfield et al. 2000). In many studies, indications such as decreased magnetization transfer ratio (MTR) in NAWM of MS patients support the suggestion that there are inherent changes in NAWM. These observations may point to the possibility that internal changes in NAWM beyond the reach of conventional MRI could cause the disability. Conventional imaging, as such, is incapable of detecting any changes in the affected areas of impaired axonal function. A non-invasive measure of disease activity in MS has not yet been established.

10.2.2 High Field

In search of novel MRI techniques with the ability to probe the internal machinery of brain tissues, a number of basic MR parameters could be considered. Magnetic field (B0) is one parameter known to set a fundamental limit on the SNR, which in turn determines the resolution (Chen et al. 1986; Ugurbil et al. 1993). The gradient strength and novel RF coil designs also play an important role in this regard. We will highlight the role of high magnetic field in MRI in improving MS diagnosis and treatment. Both advantages and challenges involved in applying HF MRI for human subjects will be analyzed.

The nature of the tissues and the etiology of MS are the two most important factors to be considered for the assessment of the opportunities that HF MR will offer. The work employing 7-T and 8-T whole- body human scanners has shown that this technology is indeed feasible (see Fig. 10.6) and offers many advantages in imaging (Burgess et al. 1999; Ugurbil et al. 2003). It has also been shown that neither RF energy of common sequences nor the gradient slew rate poses a safety hazard at field strengths up to 8 T (Kangarlu and Robitaille 2000). It is known that gradient echo (GRE) is the most sensitive sequence for the detection of paramagnetic molecules such as iron and this effect is amplified at higher fields (see Fig.10.2). GRE at HF will provide a simple and sensitive tool that is available for the detection of BBB implications within the lesions. The ultra high-resolution images (30–50 μm in-plane resolution) of brain samples of newly deceased MS patients

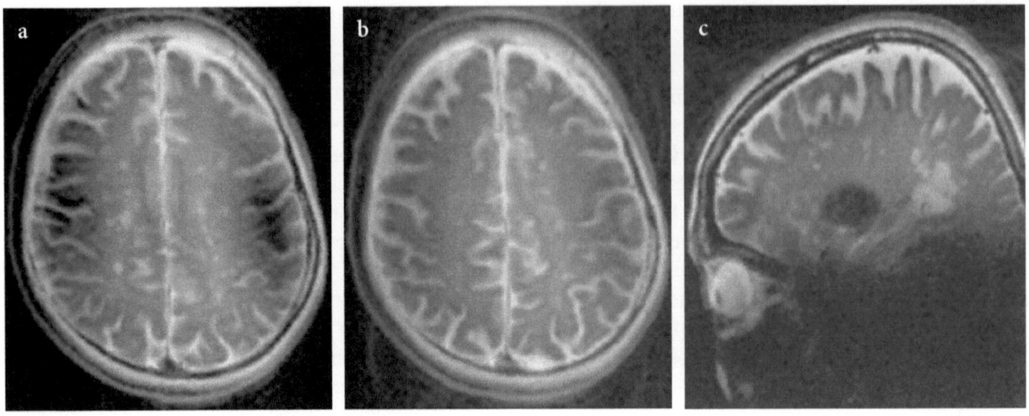

Fig. 10.7a–c. Rapid acquisition with relaxation enhancement (RARE) images in axial plane (**a**,**b**) and sagittal plane (**c**) from a patient with MS. All images are acquired with reduced RF inhomogeneity. The image reveals the ability of spin-echo based images to suppress susceptibility artifacts. These images demonstrate some reminiscence of the susceptibility (**a**) and coil RF profile (**c**). The susceptibility of the semicircular canals is much reduced in (**a**) in a superior direction but still visible. The residual effect of the susceptibility, in addition to other high-field artifacts, is less prominent. In these spin-echo based images the susceptibility and RF inhomogeneity are reduced to the point of allowing detection of the many plaques with central dark spots representing central vessels of each lesion. Acquisition parameters are as follows; RARE, BW=70 KHz, FOV=18×18 cm, ST=2 mm, TR=3 ms, TE=22 ms, matrix=512×512, PW=6 ms

using GRE, SE (see Figs. 10.7 and 10.8) and DWI at 8 T have also proven to be promising sequences in visualizing cortical microanatomy (Kangarlu et al. 2004). For the first time, multilaminar structures have been identified in the CGM and CGM plaques are clearly seen (Fig. 10.8). These CGM plaques are not observed in routine clinical imaging at 1.5 T. The work, to date, has demonstrated that MR scanners at such high fields are capable of developing MRM techniques for in vivo application for human neuroimaging. MRM could produce results that would correlate the clinical deficit with presence or absence of different types of lesions. Development of in vivo human MRM with a 10–100 µm resolution will amount to the next quantum leap in medical imaging. Our images with a 30–50 µm resolution (see Fig. 10.8), have revealed the power of detecting CGM lesions with remarkable contrast. In vivo human MRM will be the precursor to in vivo human cellular imaging. The technical issues in achieving in vivo MRM are presented below.

10.2.3 SNR

Is SNR relevant to the enhancement of MR capabilities in achieving specificity in MS studies? With the advent of whole body HF MR up to 8 T, unprecedented improvement in SNR was achieved in human subjects (Figs. 10.6 and 10.7). Histopathologic findings have implicated axonal injury in the early stages of the disease (Trapp et al. 1999). This fact is confirmed by MRS in a qualitative way. The pathogenesis of the axonal changes in NAWM will be better defined using HF MRI. In our work, we have shown, using HF MRI, that abnormalities can be detected in NAWM of brains of patients with early relapsing-remitting disease that previously were only seen by pathologic techniques (Kangarlu et al. 2004). Further, experiments with techniques such as MTR at lower fields indicate that such abnormalities can be correlated with future occurrence of progressive disease. The primary MRI techniques used in visualization of the neuroinflammation associated with MS and acute EAE are T2 weighting, T1 weighting, MT, and DWI. The integrity of the BBB has also been examined using gadolinium(III)-diethyltriaminepentaacetic acid (Gd-DTPA). In addition, MRS has been utilized to demonstrate a decrease in NAA and choline levels in NAWM of MS patients and has offered a way of probing possible non-focal magnetically hidden lesion activity. Determination of activities in NAWM would be significant for the detection of microdemyelination (Pan et al. 1996). Decreased levels of NAA, a marker for axons, implicates axonal loss or dysfunction in MS (Arnold 1999). MRI has been able to detect changes in these areas of impaired

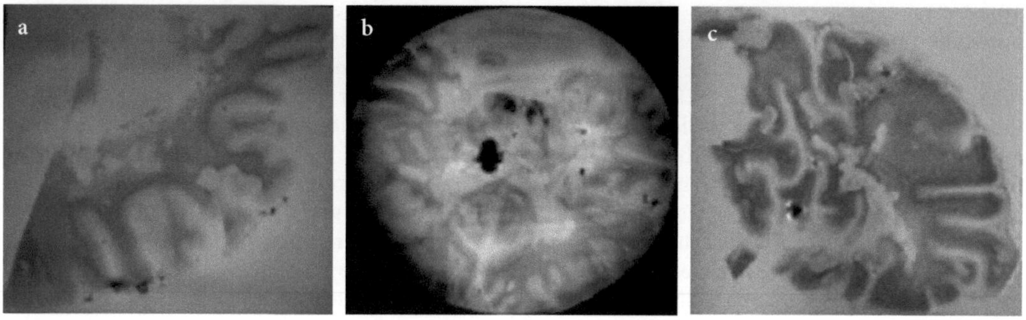

Fig. 10.8a–c. Brain samples imaged with gradient echo (GRE) or diffusion weighted imaging (DWI) in pieces (**a,c**) and whole (**b**) within a container filled with distilled water. Slices are taken from a patient with known MS. The in-plane resolutions are 150 μm (**a,b**) and 300 μm (**c**) and demonstrate susceptibility artifact in the form of concentric dark bands with prefrontal lobe (**a,b**). In these images many artifacts, including dielectric resonance, bulk susceptibility, and inductive coupling with the head have been reduced. Reduction of artifacts has also improved visualization of the many plaques. Acquisition parameters are as follows: **a** GRE, BW=70 KHz, FOV=15.0×15.0 cm, TR=700 ms, TE=11.0 ms, matrix=1024×1024, PW=4 ms; **b** GRE, BW=70 KHz, FOV=15.0×15.0 cm, ST=5.0 mm, TR=700 ms, TE=11.0 ms, matrix=1024×1024, PW=4 ms; **c** DWI, BW=50 K, FOV=15.0×15.0 cm, TR=1088 ms, TE=67.8 s, matrix=512×512, PW=4 ms

axonal function. At higher fields, MR SNR increases, making it more sensitive to changes in axonal function through spectroscopy and other techniques such as MT and diffusion. Accordingly, through SNR it may be possible to establish a correlation between axonal loss in NAWM and lesions with presence or absence of neurological function. MR imaging and spectroscopy at lower field strengths have permitted examination of the evolution of the plaques of multiple sclerosis and provided some clues regarding the pathogenesis of this disorder (Arnold 1999). Although significant advances have been made in this regard, it is becoming increasingly clear that HF MRI is needed to define such parameters as the total disease burden and its correlation with clinical disability. In particular, some inherently low SNR sequences such as EPI and its derivatives like DWI and DTI will become possible to implement at higher resolutions. Considering the nature of diffusion (Cercignani et al. 2001) and its sensitivity to sub-voxel events, more basic information on the pathology of inflammation and neurodegeneration becomes available. DTI imaging has shown potential for offering correlation with disability in patients with RR and SP MS (Cercignani et al. 2001). This further reinforces the expectation that HF MRI could make diffusion-based techniques such as DWI and DTI a potent candidate for probing structural information at the microscopic level (Kangarlu et al. 2002; Basser and Pierpaoli 1996).

In addition, HF MRI is capable of examining hypothesis driven experiments in murine model EAE and directly applying the developed technique to humans within the same system. The SNR at high field is affected by the inherent inhomogeneity of RF distribution (see Fig. 10.6). The characteristic central brightness of these images creates a higher SNR within the deep tissues compared to peripheral tissues (Fig. 10.3). In fact, this effect, also know as dielectric resonance phenomenon (Fig. 10.1), presents a challenge to generating a uniform image. The relatively lower peripheral SNR will particularly hinder cerebral cortex studies (Figs. 10.6 and 10.7).

Depiction of microvascular veins and their position with respect to the lesions (see Figs. 10.6–10.8), new and old, is another way that high SNR and susceptibility based contrast could be utilized for MS studies. BOLD contrast has long been recognized as a mechanism for visualization of veins (Cho 1992), and field-dependent BOLD venography has been demonstrated (Reichenbach et al. 1998, 2001). We have exploited this promising mechanism at 8 T (Kangarlu et al. 2002; Burgess et al. 1999) as well as the utility of paramagnetic deoxyhemoglobin in blood for BBB studies in visualizing microvasculatures within MS plaques (Kangarlu et al. 2004). Even though relevance of blood vessels and formation of plaques around them had been addressed previously (Schelling), it had never been observed in vivo. The clear central vein depiction on some plaques by 8-T MRI (Kangarlu et al. 2002) suggests possible inflammation and breakdown of vessel walls that could be used in distinguishing active plaques from dormant ones.

10.2.4 Susceptibility

It has become clear that various MR parameters by themselves will not match the challenges of in vivo microscopy. SNR, relaxation times, chemical exchange mechanisms and diffusion play an important role in defining the image contrast, specificity, and sensitivity to microscopic events. But the short history of MR has shown that interdependence of these parameters will, in spite of initial challenges, inevitably point in the direction that MR evolution has taken, namely a steady increase in magnetic field. As the field increases, there is a proportional increase in the magnetic susceptibility that would enhance MR sensitivity to paramagnetic elements within the body. The susceptibility increase causes a loss of signal on the microscopic and macroscopic scale, the former enhancing MR capabilities and the latter presenting a fundamental challenge for imaging of areas in the near proximity of large cavities such as brain tissues near air interfaces such as the sinuses and mastoids (see Fig. 10.3c). In these areas of the head, magnetic susceptibility discontinuity calls for innovative techniques to suppress the local field inhomogeneities. There have been sequences proposed including GESEPI and z-shim with various degrees of success (Yang et al. 1999; Glover 1999). The impact of susceptibility induced relaxation accelerations to time scales of 1 ms makes it quite challenging to recover the signal losses without a combination of hardware, RF coil, and pulse sequence improvements as human in vivo imaging marches towards 10 T (Gelman 1999; Vymazal et al. 1996; Duewell et al. 1996). The ultimate barrier to achieving microscopic resolution for in vivo imaging is being unable to harness SNR lost to susceptibility and diffusion. In addition, the Boltzmann distribution governing the size of signal from the voxel compounded by the blurring effect of motion convinced the MR community that without resort to simultaneous detection of signal by a number of detectors in parallel valuable signal will be lost to the slow imaging acquisition governed by the serial Fourier phase encoding scheme. HF MRI should be more sensitive to some contrast agents (Tanimoto 2001). T2* contrast agents should be very effective at high field.

10.2.5 RF Penetration

The RF frequency (ω_0) used for spin excitation increases with field strength. The electrodynamic properties of the tissues will vary proportional to ω_0. This includes an increase in tissue conductivity which enhances the RF absorption, requiring higher power for implementation of the same pulse sequences. Considering the heterogeneous nature of biological tissues the RF power will be absorbed nonuniformly (Gandhi et al. 1979). A number of other factors, i.e., head position and size, affect the extent of nonuniform distribution of RF (Durney et al. 1986). Furthermore, the image quality, SNR and penetration depth are intimately related to the coil design and dimensions. For volume head coils optimization of image quality is largely a function of the coil design, and the filling factor effect is maximized by constructing the smallest coil for any particular application. Smaller coils and phase array coils with their surface-like characteristic offer higher SNR. TEM designs are relatively larger and prone to inductive coupling between struts, which creates deep field focusing. This compensates for RF penetration effects, but at the same time causes safety concerns due to the high RF requirements compared to a 1.5-T MR system. Consequently, HF MRI causes more deep RF focal heating than at lower field strengths (Leussler 1999; Singerman 1997; Ibrahim 1999). As such, better understanding of the RF power deposition, penetration depth and innovative coil designs are required for better quality and safe human imaging. In order to better manage RF requirements of HF MRI, new techniques such as parallel excitation and detection of induced EMF within each coil element of a multi-element RF coil with ability to independently control the amplitude and phase of each port are necessary (Ibrahim 1999). This will allow RF-intense pulse sequences such as fast spin echo, RARE, and MDEFT (modified driven equilibrium Fourier transform) to be used for clinical HF applications. Moreover, this will allow many beneficial sequences for MS studies such as inverse recovery and magnetization transfer contrast (MTC) techniques to be used.

10.2.6 RF Coil Design

For scanners with magnetic fields above 7 T the imaging in MRI studies are difficult to perform without a new coil design called transverse electromagnetic (TEM) resonators (Roschman 1988; Vaughan 1994). Imaging at 7 and 8 T was made possible due to the construction of such resonators for use in humans and animals for fields ≥7.0 T (Baertline 1999). In spite of the inherent artifacts at high field (Figs. 10.1–10.3), the

TEM resonator has provided an alternative to birdcage design for HF MRI. With TEM coils, however, due to the increasing wavelike behavior of the RF within the subjects of a high dielectric constant, incorporation of a parallel transmit and receive (pT/R) function at high field offers an opportunity to reduce acquisition time and enhance homogeneity.

For low-γ nuclei, i.e., 31P and 13C, with field strengths up to 10 T, the existing birdcage coil design will suffice (Hayes et al. 1985). It has been shown that driving this coil in quadrature for low-γ nuclei frequencies provides improved SNR and improved homogeneity compared to similar designs such as the Alderman-Grant coil (Hayes et al. 1985). Unfortunately, at high fields the head-size birdcage resonators with their lumped-element structure do not lend themselves to operations beyond 300 MHz frequency range even in the presence of radiation shields. Furthermore, the B1 field of the RF wave generated by birdcage coils is inherently inhomogeneous. The need for the ability to evaluate large volumes of the brain without loss of image quality drives the intense research in RF coil design. As was pointed out earlier, high-field coils operating at B0>3T produce head images with bright centers and lower SNR at the peripheries. This makes study of the cerebral cortical pathology difficult (see Fig. 10.2). In our work on the CGM in MS brain samples, since the study was conducted in the whole brain sample (Fig. 10.4), variation of image quality was addressed through the design of a special TEM coil and acquisition of images using optimized sequences for enhanced homogeneity (Kangarlu et al. 2004). Such provisions are difficult to apply for in vivo studies, making high B1 field inhomogeneity within the head a severe challenge (Ibrahim 2001; Collins et al. 2001). It is conceivable that for the studies of deep tissues the dielectric resonance effect provides higher SNR within these tissues enabling depiction of finer structures. Application of independently phase adjusted parallel imaging and phased array techniques (Ibrahim 1999; Griswold et al. 2000) will alleviate this condition and could lead to improved SNR distribution across the entire body parts at high field.

10.2.7 Gradients and Receivers

Gradient coils for high-field systems have already been successfully constructed and many improvements in their design and drive systems have been achieved (Chronik et al. 2000). Availability of slew rates up to 1000 T/m/s is the long-term goal, safety issues permitting. Already, manufactures are delivering head scanners with 600 T/m/s slew rates. The integration of 3 T within clinical settings has been greatly accelerated following the demonstration of safe exposure of human subjects to fields of up to 8 T (Kangarlu et al. 1999; Schenck 2000). These systems are equipped with the hardware and software to perform basic and clinical scans as well as research quality MRS, fMRI, and DTI fiber tracking. A typical head-only scanner appropriate for MS studies would have gradient hardware of a 36-cm I.D. asymmetric gradient coil capable of imaging at 50–80 mT/m with slew rates of 500–700 T/m/s at a duty cycle of about 70%. Such system will allow a 1-mm slice thickness considering the SNR available at 3 T and will also be capable of executing single shot EPI at a sustained rate of 10–20 images/second. The RF power in state of the art systems should be within a 15- to 30-kW range. Considering the new developments in parallel imaging, independent RF preamp channels will enable lower RF power deposition and will provide more homogeneous and faster acquisition. Consequently an 8-RF channel technology for transmitting and receiving would greatly enhance a high resolution MR scanner for MS studies. Such systems must contain software that is designed for PC platforms to enable researchers to benefit from the Unix/Linux open environment and ancillary software development, particularly in image post processing.

Using gradient capabilities of 30–50 mT/m, a slew rate of 150 T/m/s and RF power of about 2.5 kW we have acquired high quality images from the human head at 8 T using TEM resonators driven in single drive, quadrature and 4-port drive mode. In Fig. 10.3, such images are shown indicating improvement in image homogeneity. It is also possible to use the TEM resonator for parallel imaging using different struts as an independent transmitter/receiver. Nonetheless, it is inevitable that new coil designs such as phase array and microstrip design will be added to the RF coil collection of HF MR researchers. We have investigated the possibility of multiport drive on TEM and others have done similar work at 7 T (Ibrahim 1999; Collins 2003). This is expected to further improve the homogeneity of RF distribution as has already been demonstrated using FDTD calculations.

10.2.8 Relaxation Effects

The relaxation mechanisms based on which contrast is generated in MRI are field-dependent. Prolongation and convergence of T1 with B0 creates a situation that makes acquisition of T1-weighted images at very high field more challenging. T1W images have been acquired at 4 T, 7 T and 8 T using MDEFT (Ugurbil et al. 1999; Norris et al. 1999). A simple comparison was made between 3 T and 8 T T1-weighted MDEFT images indicating an eight-fold increase in CNR at 8 T (Norris et al. 1999). This indicates that SNR combined with relaxation effects are responsible for such high CNR. Such CNR will play an important role in characterizing gray matter (GM)/white matter (WM) contrast and consequently rendering the exploration of WM and GM at microscopic level more readily possible. These results are significant in the context of MS imaging. An at least threefold increase in SNR and eightfold increase in CNR at 8 T compared to 3 T point to the necessity for making HF MRI work if the microstructures of WM and GM are to become accessible by MR. By making microscopic MRI more viable, all aspects of the technique such as SNR, relaxation and paramagnetic susceptibility properties of biological tissues appear to have arrived at a critical stage as human MRI marches on towards 400 MHz. Ability, for instance, to acquire high resolution T1-weighted images in a short time is an important area of using the high SNR of HF MRI for microstructure visualization in MS. Relaxation effects have also been used through exogenous agents with relaxation modifying properties to generate enhanced contrast in regions of interest such as areas where BBB are compromised. As discussed earlier, capabilities of MRI combined with the conspicuity of new contrast agents such as SPIO have raised hopes of making targeted molecular imaging possible (Frank et al. 2002). A number of developments in novel MR signal amplifiers such as SPIOs have taken place in the past few years which have facilitated their delivery and tolerance. In this regard, approaches based on enzyme-mediated polymerization of paramagnetic substrates into oligomers of higher magnetic relaxivity (Bogdanov et al. 2002) have proved to be particularly promising.

10.2.9
Ultra-High-Resolution MRI

The advent of 8-T whole body MRI made acquisition of high resolution images of the human head with an in-plane resolution of 100 μm possible. A TEM resonator was used to acquire the GRE images from the human head of normal subjects. Serial acquisitions of such images require an average of 15 min. Though at the limit of clinically accepted time, its implementation triggered an intense HF MR activity within the community. Various technological innovations such as parallel imaging (Pruessmann et al. 1998; Sodickson 1999) have been reported since the first 8-T human head images were acquired that present a realistic opportunity for reducing the acquisition times to 2–4 min. Images acquired at this resolution and within 2 min will produce up to half a gigabyte of unprocessed information from a human head. Acquisition of a 2000×2000 matrix image with a field of view of 20 cm, slice thickness of 1 mm, and flip angle=45° could be TR=750 ms, TE=17 ms, receiver bandwidth=69.4 kHz. Such techniques will allow MRI signal to be acquired from a 0.02-mm^3 or 20-nl voxel. The capability of in-vivo acquisition from such a minute volume from the human head begins a new era for high resolution study of pathology such as MS. Combined with susceptibility contrast and parallel imaging, there is the possibility of a ten-fold increase in in-plane resolution relative to the conventional 256×256 images obtained with a 20-cm field of view and a 5-mm slice thickness within a clinically acceptable time. Furthermore, the higher resolution images could be acquired with adequate image quality using new technologies including phased array coil design and parallel imaging. Human head images with a 1k×1k matrix at 8 T reveal numerous small venous structures throughout the image plane and provide reasonable delineation between gray and white matter (see Fig. 10.6). The elevated SNR observed in HF MRI could be utilized to acquire images with a level of resolution approaching the histological level under in vivo conditions. These images represent a significant advance in our ability to examine small anatomical features with noninvasive imaging methods.

10.2.10
New Technologies in MS Imaging

Plaques in MS patients are mostly seen in the white matter. Involvement of gray matter does not lend itself to in vivo detection. The white matter lesions appear in an unpredictable shape, size, and distribution (Trapp et al. 1999). Ability to distinguish the plaques into new and old or active and inactive is important. The newer plaques are identified with inflammation and are producing fat debris due to lipid breakdown. The chronic plaques are mostly characterized with gliosis. The MRI manifestation of these two mechanisms has been difficult.

Histological studies (LUMSDEN 1970) have found that newer plaques are associated with veins but routine MRI has just been unable to demonstrate this pathogenesis of the plaque in vivo. HF MRI seems to be able to study this vasocentral characteristic of MRI-visible plaques. In order to enhance MRI capability toward in vivo histology, plaques must be distinguished in terms of age, activity, and possibly response to therapeutic techniques based on pathogenic mechanisms. These capabilities would require that MRI features sensitive to MS plaques be probed at the microscopic level. Events at this level are macrophage infiltration, edema, myelin swelling, lymphocyte infiltration and endothelial cell activation (LASSMANN et al. 1998). It is difficult for any MR-based technique to target any one or more of these mechanisms. The relaxation effects associated with edema and diffusion manifestation of myelin swelling have been and are subject to imaging exploitation.

10.2.11
HF MRI of MS

The major challenge in achieving the goals summarized above is to enhance MRI specificity for characteristics of individual lesions. The ability to visualize the internal structure of lesions would put MRI on the path to producing distinct contrast for those lesions sharing a particular histopathologic type. The 8-T MRI depiction of WM plaques with their central microvessel was the first step in that direction (see Fig. 10.7). As plaques in WM have been mostly observed for diagnostic and therapeutic purposes in MS, the involvement of GM has received little attention in MRI. Our depiction of CGM lesions in brain samples (Figs. 10.2–10.4), has provided an opportunity for their detection and monitoring in vivo. Through the use of HF MRI it could be feasible to interrogate each plaque based on its structural characteristics and association with CGM lesions as classified by KIDD et al. (1999). Assuming that the technological issues listed above are met then HF MRI could proceed in further expanding its capabilities for classification and probing of MS plaques by developing fMRI, DTI, and quantitative MRS. Imaging at 8 T has detected multiple cortical lesions that are not evident by conventional imaging at 1.5 T (Fig. 10.6–10.8). Lesions are visualized using gradient echo, spin echo, and diffusion-weighted images (Figs. 10.7 and 10.8). The high quality images at 8 T allow for the identification of the different types of cortical lesions previously described at histology (KIDD et al.). Such imaging tools, once applied to in vivo detection of CGM pathology, would allow development of techniques to study whether CGM is a primary event or alternately a consequence of the overwhelming white matter pathology. Furthermore, determination of the contribution and sequence of CGM and WM events could be correlated to disabilities. Such imaging capabilities have not been available in multiple sclerosis to date.

10.2.12
Other MRI Methods

One other approach would be the use of dynamic contrast enhanced (DCE) MRI using SPIO contrast media to quantitatively assess the microvessels within the plaques. These contrast agents will help susceptibility enhanced contrast between the microvessels and the brain tissues, which will make these vessels more visible in anatomical images. In addition, perfusion fMRI studies based on the DCE techniques will demonstrate the activity and the extent of BBB breakdown within the plaques. Using computer processing of the imaging data and a relatively simple two-compartment kinetic model, it is possible to non-invasively assay the relative blood volume, microvascular endothelial leakiness, and the interstitial volume of any solid tumor. DCE MRI and its capability in quantifying the permeability of microvessels in the brain at high field will offer an additional tool in characterizing plaque activity and classification. Considering these combined capabilities, HF MRI could offer a powerful predictor of disability and measure of drug efficacy. Using HF MRI and SPIO contrast agents, therapeutic responses could be more accurately detected. Optimization of techniques such as DTI and DCE MRI would complement the high resolution anatomical depiction of MS abnormalities and should lead to an even greater future benefit from diagnostic imaging in MS.

10.3
Conclusion

Observation of the evolution of inflammation will be greatly assisted by targeted MI. Considering that ultra-high-field MRI is producing images whose quality is comparable to histology, and the ability to image regions comparable to cell size, combined with biochemical techniques of attaching molecules with affinity for pathologic cells, MI appears to be poised to add a powerful tool to our diagnostic capabilities. The 8-T MR images have shown histologic quality. These images possess ultra-high resolution capable of visualizing microanatomic details. MI is capable of monitoring the cell trafficking. With regard to MS etiology, this aspect of MI offers the ability of directing cells to a specific target in the body. A wide range of cellular processes such as macrophage infiltration into CNS, leukocyte role in inflammatory diseases, and hematopoietic stem cell targeting have and will become available for imaging. These novel imaging strategies may provide methods for detecting early inflammatory events, at the cellular level, before the consequences of inflammation become macroscopically detectable by traditional imaging techniques. This would amount to a strategic transition in diagnostic imaging modalities. Such a transition could usher in the era of a functional and physiological approach versus the present conventional anatomic approach.

On another front, the need for possible extrapolation of animal results to human subjects necessitates that all possible enhancements that could be achieved be exploited in human scanners as well. Currently, whole body research scanners operate at 9.4 T. There are plans for construction of a few neuroimaging centers equipped with 3-T, 7-T, 9.4-T and 11.7-T MR systems for human clinical trials. Other scanners include 11.7-T and 14-T units for primate studies, and an up to 17-T MR scanner for rodent studies. Imaging centers are growing in number and size. Centers typically have 30–50 members, with some larger MR research units employing up to 200 researchers. The prospect of fruitful research in MR, and particularly in active areas such as MI, has brought biologists, physicists, engineers, and chemists into collaborative projects. These multidisciplinary efforts have given rise to innovative techniques such as MI. With higher field strength and more complex imaging techniques it is inevitable that targeted MR MI will accelerate its expansion to other areas of in vivo physiology imaging. MI is not restricted by the same limitations as other functional imaging techniques. The ability to probe cellular events and monitor their spatiotemporal evolution unrestricted by the time frame of fMRI is looming in many laboratories.

References

Ahrens ET, Laidlaw DH, Readhead C, Brosnan CF, Fraser SE, Jacobs RE (1998) MR microscopy of transgenic mice that spontaneously acquire EAE. Magn Reson Med 40:119

Allen MJ, MacRenaris KW, Venkatasubramanian PN, Meade TJ (2004)Cellular delivery of MRI contrast agents. Chem Biol 11:301-307

Alvord EC Jr, Kies MW, Suckling AJ (1984) Experimental encephalomyelitis: a useful model for multiple sclerosis. Liss, New York

Anderson SA, Shukaliak-Quandt J, Jordan EK, Arbab AS, Martin R, McFarland H, Frank JA (2004) Magnetic resonance imaging of labeled T-cells in a mouse model of multiple sclerosis. Ann Neurol 55:654-659

Arbab AS, Yocum GT, Kalish H, Jordan EK, Anderson SA, Khakoo AY, Read EJ, Frank JA (2004) Efficient magnetic cell labeling with protamine sulfate complexed to ferumoxides for cellular MRI. Blood 104:1217-1223

Arnold DL (1999) Magnetic resonance spectroscopy: imaging axonal damage in MS. J Neuroimmunol 98:2-6

Artemov D, Mori N, Okollie B, Bhujwalla ZM (2003) MR molecular imaging of the Her-2/neu receptor in breast cancer cells using targeted iron oxide nanoparticles. Magn Reson Med 49:403-408

Basser PJ, Pierpaoli C (1996) Microstructural features measured using diffusion tensor imaging. J Magn Reson B 111:209-219

Beckmann N, Falk R, Zurbrugg S, Dawson J, Engelhardt P (2003) Macrophage infiltration into the rat knee detected by MRI in a model of antigen-induced arthritis. Magn Reson Med 49:1047-1055

Bendszus M, Stoll G (2003) Caught in the act: in vivo mapping of macrophage infiltration in nerve injury by magnetic resonance imaging. J Neurosci 23:10892-10896

Bogdanov A Jr, Matuszewski L, Bremer C, Petrovsky A, Weissleder R (2002) Oligomerization of paramagnetic substrates result in signal amplification and can be used for MR imaging of molecular targets. Mol Imaging 1:16-23

Bourekas EC, Christoforidis GA, Abduljalil AM, Kangarlu A, Chakeres DW, Spigos DG, Robitaille PM (1999) High resolution MRI of the deep gray nuclei at 8 tesla. J Comput Assist Tomogr 23:867-874

Bulte JW, Arbab AS, Douglas T, Frank JA (2004) Preparation of magnetically labeled cells for cell tracking by magnetic resonance imaging. Methods Enzymol 386:275-299

Burgess RE, Yu Y, Christoforidis GA, Bourekas EC, Chakeres DW, Spigos D, Kangarlu A, Abduljalil AM, Robitaille PM (1999) Human leptomeningeal and cortical vascular anatomy of the cerebral cortex at 8 Tesla. J Comput Assist Tomogr 23:850-856

Cercignani M, Inglese M, Pagani E, Comi G, Filippi M (2001) Mean diffusivity and fractional anisotropy histograms of patients with multiple sclerosis. AJNR Am J Neuroradiol 22:952-958

Chen CN, Sank VJ, Cohen SM, Hoult DI (1986) The field dependence of NMR imaging. I. Laboratory assessment of signal-to-noise ratio and power deposition. Magn Reson Med 3:722-729

Chronik BA, Alejski A, Rutt BK (2000) Design and fabrication of a three-axis edge ROU head and neck gradient coil. Magn Reson Med 44:955-963

Collins CM, Smith MB (2001) Signal-to-noise ratio and

absorbed power as functions of main magnetic field strength, and definition of "90°" RF pulse for the head in the birdcage coil. Magn Reson Med 45:684-691

Corot C, Petry KG, Trivedi R, Saleh A, Jonkmanns C, Le Bas JF, Blezer E, Rausch M, Brochet B, Foster-Gareau P, Baleriaux D, Gaillard S, Dousset V (2004) Macrophage imaging in central nervous system and in carotid atherosclerotic plaque using ultrasmall superparamagnetic iron oxide in magnetic resonance imaging. Invest Radiol 39:619-625

Davie CA, Barker GJ, Thompson AJ, Tofts PS, McDonald WI, Miller DH (1997) 1H magnetic resonance spectroscopy of chronic cerebral white matter lesions and normal appearing white matter in multiple sclerosis, J Neurol Neurosurg Psychiatry 63:736-742

De Laquintane BD, Dousset V, Solanilla A, Petry KG, Ripoche J (2002) Iron particle labeling of haematopoietic progenitor cells: an in vitro study. Biosci Rep 22:549-554

De Stefano N, Narayanan S, Matthews PM, Francis GS, Antel JP, Arnold DL (1999) In vivo evidence for axonal dysfunction remote from focal cerebral demyelination of the type seen in multiple sclerosis. Brain 122:1933-1939

Dousset V, Ballarino L, Delalande C, Coussemacq M, Canioni P, Petry KG, Caille JM (1999) Comparison of ultrasmall particles of iron oxide (USPIO)-enhanced T2-weighted, conventional T2-weighted, and gadolinium-enhanced T1-weighted MR images in rats with experimental autoimmune encephalomyelitis. AJNR Am J Neuroradiol 20:223-227

Duewell S, Wolff SD, Wen H, Balaban RS, Jezzard P (1996) MR imaging contrast in human brain tissue: assessment and optimization at 4 T. Radiology 199:780-786

Filippi, M, Tortorella C, Rovaris M, Bozzali M, Possa F, Sormani M P, Iannucci G, Comi G (2000) Changes in the normal appearing brain tissue and cognitive impairment in multiple sclerosis. J Neurol Neurosurg Psychiatry 68:157-161

Floris S, Blezer EL, Schreibelt G, Dopp E, van der Pol SM, Schadee-Eestermans IL, Nicolay K, Dijkstra CD, de Vries HE (2004) Blood-brain barrier permeability and monocyte infiltration in experimental allergic encephalomyelitis: a quantitative MRI study. Brain 127:616-627

Floyd E, McShane TM (2004) Development and use of biomarkers in oncology drug development. Toxicol Pathol 32 [Suppl 1]:106-115

Frank JA, Zywicke H, Jordan EK, Mitchell J, Lewis BK, Miller B, Bryant LH Jr, Bulte JWM (2002) Magnetic intracellular labeling of mammalian cells by combining (FDA-approved) superparamagnetic iron oxide MR contrast agents and commonly used transfection agents. Acad Radiol 9 [Suppl 2]:S484-S487

Gandhi OP, Hagmann MJ, D'Andrea JA (1979) Partbody and multibody effects on absorption of radio frequency electromagnetic energy by animals and by models of man. Radio Sci 14:15-22

Gillis RJ (2002) In vivo molecular imaging. J Cell Biochem [Suppl] 39:231-238

Glover GH (1999) 3D z-shim method for reduction of susceptibility effects in BOLD fMRI 3D z-shim method for reduction of susceptibility effects in BOLD fMRI. Magn Reson Med 42:290-299

Griswold MA, Jakob PM, Nittka M, Goldfarb JW, Haase A (2000) Partially parallel imaging with localized sensitivities (PILS). Magn Reson Med 44:602-609

Grossman RI, McGowan JC (1998) Perspectives on multiple sclerosis. AJNR Am J Neuroradiol 19:1251-1265

Gutin PH (2002) The potential value of iron oxide nanoparticles in brain tumor treatment. AJNR Am J Neuroradiol 23:505

Hayes CE, Edelstein WA, Schenk JF, Mueller OM, Eash M (1985) An efficient, highly homogeneous radiofrequency coil for whole-body NMR imaging at 1.5T. J Magn Reson 63:622-628

Helms G, Stawiarz L, Kivisakk P, Fredrikson S, Hillert J, Link H (1999) Quantitative proton MRS of cerebral multiple sclerosis lesions: regression analysis of metabolite concentrations. Proceedings of International Society of Magnetic Resonance in Medicine , Philadelphia, p 43

Horsfield MA, Rocca MA, Cercignani M, Filippi M (2000) Activity revealed in MRI of multiple sclerosis without contrast agent - a preliminary report. Magn Reson Imaging 18:139-142

Kangarlu A, Robitaille PM (2000) Biological effects and health implications in magnetic resonance imaging. Concept Magn Reson 12:321-359

Kangarlu A, Abduljalil AM, Norris DG, Schwartzbauer C, Robitaille PM (1999) Human RARE imaging at 8 tesla:RF intense imaging without SAR violation. Magn Reson Mater Phys Biol Med (MAGMA) 9:81-84

Kangarlu A, Rammohan KW, Bourekas EC, Chakeres DW (2002) In-vivo microscopic imaging of multiple sclerosis with high filed MRI. In: Filippi M, Comi G (eds) New frontiers of MR-based techniques in MS. Springer, Berlin Heidelberg New York

Kangarlu A, Rammohan KW, Bourekas EC, RayChaudhry A (2004) Imaging of cortical lesions in multiple sclerosis. Proceedings of 12th Meeting of the International Society of Magnetic Resonance in Medicine, Kyoto

Kawczak JA, Mathisen PM, Drazba JA, Fuss B, Macklin WB, Tuohy VK (1998) Digitized image analysis reveals diffuse abnormalities in normal-appearing white matter during acute experimental autoimmune encephalomyelitis. J Neurosci Res 54:364-372

Kidd D, Barkhof F, McConnell R, Algra PR, Allen IV, Revesz T (1999) Cortical lesions in multiple sclerosis. Brain 122:17-26

Lanens D, Van der Linden A, Gerrits PO, 's-Gravenmade EJ (1994) In vitro NMR micro imaging of the spinal cord of chronic relapsing EAE rats. Magn Reson Imaging 12:469

Lassmann H, Raine CS, Antel J, Prineas JW (1998) Immunopathology of multiple sclerosis: report on an international meeting held at the Institute of Neurology of the University of Vienna. J Neuroimmunol 86:213-217

Leary SM, Silver NC, Stevenson VL, Barker GJ, Miller DH, Thompson AJ (1999) Magnetization transfer of normal appearing white matter in primary progressive multiple sclerosis. Multiple Sclerosis 5:313-316

Li KC, Bednarski MD (2002) Vascular-targeted molecular imaging using functionalized polymerized vesicles. J Magn Reson Imaging 16:388-393

Luker GD, Sharma V, Pica CM, Dahlheimer JL, Li W, Ochesky J, Ryan CE, Piwnica-Worms H, Piwnica-Worms D (2002) Noninvasive imaging of protein-protein interactions in living animals. Proc Natl Acad Sci USA 99:6961-6966

Lumsden CE (1970) The neuropathology of multiple sclerosis: multiple sclerosis and other demyelinating diseases. In: Vinken P, Bruyn GW (eds) Handbook of clinical neurology, vol 9. North Holland, Amsterdam, pp 217-309

Moffat BA, Reddy GR, McConville P, Hall DE, Chenevert TL,

Kopelman RR, Philbert M, Weissleder R, Rehemtulla A, Ross BD (2003) A novel polyacrylamide magnetic nanoparticle contrast agent for molecular imaging using MRI. Mol Imaging 2:324-232

Moore A, Basilion J, Chiocca AE, Weissleder R (1998) Measuring transferin receptor gene expression by NMR imaging. Biochim Biophys Acta 1402:239-249

Morawski AM, Winter PM, Crowder KC, Caruthers SD, Fuhrhop RW, Scott MJ, Robertson JD, Abendschein DR, Lanza GM, Wickline SA (2004) Targeted nanoparticles for quantitative imaging of sparse molecular epitopes with MRI. Magn Reson Med 51:480-486

Norris DG, Kangarlu A, Abduljalil A, Schwartzbauer C, Robitaille PM (1999) Human MDEFT imaging at 8 tesla. Magn Reson Mater Phys Biol Med (MAGMA) 9:92-96

Oweida AJ, Dunn EA, Foster PJ (2004) Cellular imaging at 1.5 T: detecting cells in neuroinflammation using active labeling with superparamagnetic iron oxide. Mol Imaging 3:85-95

Pan JW, Hetherington HP, Vaughan JT, Mitchell G, Pohost GM, Whitaker JN (1996) Evaluation of multiple sclerosis by 1H spectroscopic imaging at 4.1 T. Magn Reson Med 36:72-77

Pirko I, Johnson A, Ciric B, Gamez J, Macura SI, Pease LR, Rodriguez M (2004) In vivo magnetic resonance imaging of immune cells in the central nervous system with superparamagnetic antibodies. FASEB J 18:179-182

Pomper MG (2002) Can small animal imaging accelerate drug development? J Cell Biochem [Suppl] 39:211-220

Pruessmann KP, Weiger M, Scheidegger MB, Boesiger P (1999) SENSE: sensitivity encoding for fast MRI. Magn Reson Med 42:952-962

Rausch M, Hiestand P, Baumann D, Cannet C, Rudin M (2003) MRI-based monitoring of inflammation and tissue damage in acute and chronic relapsing EAE. Magn Reson Med 50:309-314

Ray P, De A, Min JJ, Tsien RY, Gambhir SS (2004) Imaging tri-fusion multimodality reporter gene expression in living subjects. Cancer Res 64:1323-1330

Reichenbach JR, Essig M, Haacke EM, Lee BC, Przetak C, Kaiser WA, Schad LR (1998) High-resolution venography of the brain using magnetic resonance imaging. Magn Reson Mater Phys Biol Med (MAGMA) 6:62-69

Reichenbach JR, Jonetz-Mentzel L, Fitzek C, Haacke EM, Kido DK, Lee BC, Kaiser WA (2001) High resolution blood oxygen-level dependent MR venography (HRBV): a new technique. Neuroradiology 43:364-369

Schellenberger EA, Bogdanov A Jr, Hogemann D, Tait J, Weissleder R, Josephson L (2002) Annexin V-CLIO: a nanoparticle for detecting apoptosis by MRI. Mol Imaging 1:102-107

Schenck JF (2000) Safety of strong, static magnetic fields. Magn Reson Imaging 12:2-19

Shahbazi-Gahrouei D, Williams M, Rizvi S, Allen BJ (2001) In vivo studies of Gd-DTPA-monoclonal antibody and Gd-porphyrins: potential magnetic resonance imaging contrast agents for melanoma. J Magn Reson Imaging 14:169-174

Sodickson DK, Manning WJ (1997) Simultaneous acquisition of spatial harmonics (SMASH): fast imaging with radiofrequency coil arrays. Magn Reson Med 38:591-603

Stoll G, Wesemeier C, Gold R, Solymosi L, Toyka KV, Bendszus M (2004) In vivo monitoring of macrophage infiltration in experimental autoimmune neuritis by magnetic resonance imaging. J Neuroimmunol 149:142-146

't Hart BA, Vogels J, Bauer J, Brok HP, Blezer E (2004) Non-invasive measurement of brain damage in a primate model of multiple sclerosis. Trends Mol Med 10:85-91

Thulborn KR, Waterton JC, Matthews PM, Radda GK (1982) Oxygenation dependence of the transverse relaxation time of water protons in whole blood at high field. Biochim Biophys Acta 714:265-270

Trapp BD, Bo L, Mork S, Chang A (1999) Pathogenesis of tissue injury in MS lesions. J Neuroimmunol 98:49-56

Tropres I, Lamalle L, Peoc'h M, Farion R, Usson Y, Decorps M, Remy C (2004) In vivo assessment of tumoral angiogenesis. Magn Reson Med 51:533-541

Ugurbil K, Garwood M, Ellermann J, Hendrich K, Hinke R, Hu X, Kim SG, Menon R, Merkle H, Ogawa S et al (1993) Imaging at high magnetic fields: initial experiences at 4 T. Magn Reson Q 9:259-277

Ugurbil K, Hu X, Chen W, Zhu X-H, Kim S-G, Georgopoulos A (1999) Functional mapping in the human brain using high magnetic fields. Philos Trans R Soc Lond B Biol Sci 354:1195-1213

Ugurbil K, Adriany G, Andersen P, Chen W, Garwood M, Gruetter R, Henry P, Kim SG, Lieu H, Tkac I, Vaughan T, van de Moortele PF, Yacoub E, Zhu XH (2003) Ultrahigh field magnetic resonance imaging and spectroscopy. Magn Reson Imaging 21:1263-1281

Vymazal J, Brooks RA, Baumgarner C, Tran V, Katz D, Bulte JW, Bauminger R, di Chiro G (1996) The relation between brain iron and NMR relaxation times: an in vitro study. Magn Reson Med 35:56-61

Weissleder R (2002) Scaling down imaging: molecular mapping of cancer in mice. Nat Rev Cancer 2:11-18

Weissleder R, Elizondo G, Wittenberg J, Rabito CA, Bengele HH, Josephson L (1990) Ultrasmall superparamagnetic iron oxide: characterization of a new class of contrast agents for MR imaging. Radiology 175:489-493

Wood JC, Fassler JD, Meade T (2004) Mimicking liver iron overload using liposomal ferritin preparations. Magn Reson Med 51:607-611

Xu S, Jordan EK, Brocke S, Bulte JW, Quigley L, Tresser N, Ostuni JL, Yang Y, McFarland HF, Frank JA (1998) Study of relapsing-remitting experimental allergic encephalomyelitis SJL mouse model using MION-46L enhanced in vivo MRI: early histopathological correlation. J Neurosci Res 52:549-558

Yang QX, Smith MB, Briggs RW, Rycyna RE (1999) Microimaging at 14 tesla using GESEPI for removal of magnetic susceptibility artifacts in T2*-weighted image contrast. J Magn Reson 141:1-6

Zelivyanskaya ML, Nelson JA, Poluektova L, Uberti M, Mellon M, Gendelman HE, Boska MD (2003) Tracking superparamagnetic iron oxide labeled monocytes in brain by high-field magnetic resonance imaging. J Neurosci Res 73:284-295

Disorders of Myelination

11 MR Imaging of Brain Development

Charles Raybaud

CONTENTS

C. Raybaud, MD FRCPC
Division Head of Neuroradiology, The Hospital for Sick Children, 555 University Avenue, Toronto, Ontario, Canada M5G 1X8

11.1 The Factors of Early Brain Development

The brain development corresponds to morphological and maturational changes, which result from the histogenesis, synaptogenesis and myelination.

11.1.1 The Morphological Changes

The morphological changes include two main phenomena: the first one is the global process leading the neuroepithelium from the embryonal epiblast to an essentially recognizable brain; the second consists of the cellular development and organization, with the changes in brain weight and surface configuration (that is the developing sulcation).

The steps leading from the midline epiblast to the central nervous system (embryonic period) are outside the scope of this chapter. Briefly, they include the neurulation (differentiation of the neuroectoderm, and formation of the neural tube), the formation of the cerebral vesicles with the specific development of the anterior neural plate (forebrain) and of the rhombencephalon (hindbrain), the opening of the 4th ventricle together with the formation of the leptomeninges and of the dura. From the end (week 7) of the embryonic period, the neuroepithelial cells proliferate and, till midgestation (week 20), build up the cerebral cortex together with the telencephalic commissures. This cellular proliferation, along with migration and differentiation, accounts for the increase in brain weight during the embryonic and early fetal stages.

During the second half of gestation, the neuronal migration is achieved, and a significant number (30%–50%) of neurons are actually bound to disappear by apoptosis, as part of the organization of the brain. From then on, and during infancy, the cortical synaptogenesis develops tremendously, peaking at 2 years (Huttenlocher 1990), with the concomitant development of the fiber network, the increase of the metabolic activity that becomes mostly aerobic (and is therefore accompanied with an increase of the vascularity), the enormous development of the supporting cells, mostly the astrocytes, and of course, mostly after birth but beginning already in the fetus, the mass production of myelin by the oligodendrocytes. While the brain weighs approximately 80 g at 20 weeks of gestation, it weighs 350 g at birth at 40 weeks (a fourfold increase in 4.5 months), 1000 g at 1 year (threefold increase in 12 months), and 1400 g at 18 years (40% increase in nearly two decades). This early increase in volume concerns the cortex more than the subcortical white matter (Hüppi et al. 1998a), with an important tangential growth of the cortical plate, at least in the higher mammals, and therefore a cortical folding resulting in the species-specific sulcal/gyral pattern.

11.1.2 The Internal Appearance

The internal appearance of the parenchyma (that is the tissular organization of the cellular layers within the cortical mantle) also evolves according to the stages of histogenesis (Fees-Higgins and Larroche 1987), mostly during the fetal period and the first 2 post-natal years. The histogenetic processes include the proliferation, the differentiation and the migration of the cells toward their anatomical destination, and their organization. Because myelin is made of lipids, the maturation also leads to a significant change of the physical-chemical composition of the brain: the fatty myelin replaces the water, and some of its components modify the relaxivity of the water protons. The medical consequence of this is that, as MRI reflects the physical-chemical status of the brain, the orderly changes of the maturation will be reflected in the MR images, allowing a direct evaluation of normal development, as well as of the diseases that affect these processes.

All neural cells originate from common neural stem cells. These proliferate in the germinal matrices (McConnell 1995). Two different germinal matrices exist in the cerebral hemispheres (Lavdas et al. 1999; Letinic and Rakic 2001; Nadarajah and Parnavelas 2002). The germinal matrix of the mantle lines the ventricular wall under the white matter of the hemispheres, lateral to the basal ganglia; it produces the cells for the cortical plate, namely the pyramidal neurons and the astrocytes. The germinal matrix of the ganglionic eminence covers the surface of the basal ganglia; it produces the interneurons for both the cortical plate and the basal ganglia. Seemingly parts of both matrices may produce the oligodendrocytes for the white matter tracts to be myelinated. The germinal matrices are the sites of the cellular proliferation. There are two stages in this proliferation, depending on the type of division (McConnell 1995; Rakic 1995). The initial one is the stage of symmetrical division, in which a stem cell produces two identical stem cells. The second stage is of asymmetrical division, in which a stem cell produces another stem cell and a differentiated cell. The number of division cycles probably accounts for the differences of neural development between lower and higher mammals (Rakic 1995; Caviness et al. 1995). It is estimated that there are approximately 30–35 cycles of divisions in the primates, against 7–11 in the rodents. If one cycle fails, the pool of brain cells is theoretically cut by 50%. In the very early stage of development, the germinal matrix of the mantle produces early, transient neurons to form a primary cortical preplate (or plexiform layer), which serves as an organizer for the coming cortical plate (Meyer et al. 2000; Xie et al. 2002).

There are basically four types of brain cells: the pyramidal neurons, the astrocytes, the interneurons and the oligodendrocytes.

- The *pyramidal neurons* represent 80% of the neuronal population of the cortex. They are glutamatergic excitatory cells. They originate from the germinal matrix of the cerebral mantle lateral to the ganglionic eminence, deep to the future white matter. They migrate radially toward the brain surface (Sidman and Rakic 1973), settling within the pre-existing preplate to form the cortical plate (Meyer et al. 2000). In the process, the preplate is split in two layers. The superficial layer forms the (future) molecular layer (or layer 1) with its transient Cajal-Retzius cells (CRCs). The deep layer forms the transient subplate (Kostovic and Rakic 1990) which eventually attenuates during the second half of gestation to disappear about birth. The migration of the pyramidal neurons is conducted by specialized guiding cells, the radial glia (Sidman and Rakic 1973) from which they actually differentiate even during the migration (Tamamaki et al. 2001). This migration process is also under the control of the CRCs (Marin-Padilla 1998), which stop the neurons before they reach the brain surface. Therefore, in the successive waves of migration, young neurons pass the older ones to be stopped only before the molecular layer and as a consequence, the oldest neurons form the deep layers (5 and 6) of the cortex, the youngest ones, the superficial layers (2 and 3): this is called the "inside-out process". The migration of the forebrain pyramidal neurons continues until mid-gestation (20–23 weeks). After that no neurons are produced in the brain, except in the hippocampal dentate gyrus (granule cells) and in the olfactory bulbs (Barres 1999).

- The *astrocytes* are glial cells. They support the neurons, being interposed between the vessels and the neurons. They also assist the neuronal function, especially in the management of the neurotransmitters. They are initially produced together with the neurons in the germinal matrix of the mantle, and constitute the radial glia which guides the neurons toward the surface. Recent studies have shown that in fact, the neuron is produced by the radial glia and still differentiating while separating from it (Tamamaki et al. 2001). After the end of the neuronal migration, the cells of the radial glial become the cortical astrocytes. Other astrocytes keep being produced by the germinal matrix until it disappears, especially for the superficial cortical layers (Gressens et al. 1992). In contrast with neurons, astrocytes do die and form during the whole life by division of pre-existing astrocytes.
- The *interneurons* are GABAergic inhibitory neurons, making up 20% of the cortical neuronal population. They originate from the germinal matrix of the ganglionic eminence over the future basal ganglia. From there, some migrate toward the cortex, while others move toward the basal ganglia and the thalamus (Lavdas et al. 1999; Zhu et al. 1999; Letinic and Rakic 2001; Nadarajah and Parnavalas 2002). Their migration to the cortex is not well understood yet. They seem first to follow the fibers toward the cortex, then migrate inward to the germinal matrix of the mantle, where they get "messages" to be assigned a final position into the cortex, which they reach by outward migration.
- The *oligodendrocytes* remain the most mysterious cells of the central nervous system, although they have been extensively studied (Baumann and Pham-Dinh 2001). It is not even clear whether they represent a single or multiple different lineages (Baumann and Pham Dinh 2001). Their best known role is the mass production of myelin, which has been extensively documented (Yakovlev and Lecours 1966; Holms 1986; Brody et al. 1987; Kinney et al. 1988). Myelin facilitates the conduction of the potentials along the axons, and the extensive myelination of the white matter is a characteristics of the development of the young brain during the end of gestation and the first years after birth. While the normal turn-over of the myelin components has been evaluated (in the range of several months to a year), the turn-over of the oligodendrocytes themselves is unknown. They seem to originate in restricted ventral or laterobasal areas of the prosencephalon (Bauman and Pham-Dinh 2001). They proliferate (myelination gliosis) and migrate toward the axonal fascicles when they are still in the progenitor stage. As dysmyelinating diseases often present with quite specific fascicular patterns (van der Knaap et al. 1991), it seems likely that the position of the oligodendrocytes is genetically defined.

After completion of the cortical plate, synaptogenesis develops intensively, especially after birth and during the first 2 years of life (Huttenlocher 1990). This means a tremendous expansion of the fibers network, and particularly of the axons. It has been demonstrated that the subplate, the transient subcortical remnant of the primary preplate (Kostovic and Rakic 1990) acts as a waiting zone for the axons approaching the cortex before the cortical organization is ready. This concerns the thalamo-cortical fibers, the association fibers as well as the commissural fibers (Kostovic and Rakic 1990; Super et al. 1998). In the hippocampus, this role of waiting zone may be played by the superficial molecular layer (Super et al. 1998). Synaptogenesis induces a significant increase of the needs of oxygen, with the subsequent development of an adapted vascularity (Raybaud 1990) and blood flow. The enormous development of the axons and dendrites, with their species-specific organization and attachments are likely to be responsible for the shaping of a species-specific cortical sulcal/gyral pattern (van Essen 1997). It makes up the white matter, which in mature humans represents 50% of the volume of the hemispheres (this does not take the intracortical fibers into account).

The synaptogenesis is also accompanied by the development of myelination. As stated above, the myelination has been extensively studied over the past decades, histologically and chemically. It develops according to a well defined program, roughly said from the cord to the hemispheres, the sensory structures before the motor before the associative ones (Yakovlev and Lecours 1966), and in the hemisphere, from the back to the front. In fact things are more complex. The primary systems (sensory-motor, auditory, visual, and the hippocampi) are myelinated first. In each system, the myelination of the fibers proceeds toward the cortex. The associative areas myelinate last, especially the anterior frontal and the anterior temporal cortices. Central myelination occurs in the portions of the basal ganglia adjacent to the posterior limbs of the internal capsules (PLICs). Together with the brainstem, this area appears already well developed even before birth.

On MR imaging, the demonstration of the myelination processes depends on two phenomena. The first is the depiction of the precursors of myelin. These precursors, cholesterol and specially galactocerebrosides, have a strong magnetization transfer effect (Fralix et al. 1991; Koenig 1991; Kucharczyk et al. 1994), and as such appear early on T1 imaging as a bright signal. The second is the replacement of water by the fatty myelin. The brain of fetus and neonates contains approximately 90% water; in the adult it drops to 70% in the white matter, and to 85% in the cortex after completion of the myelination. As the water is dark on T1 and bright on T2, the myelination reverses the white matter appearance to bright on T1 and dark on T2.

11.2 MR Imaging: Technical Considerations

11.2.1 Problems in Imaging Infants (Premature or Term-Born)

Conventional T1 and T2 sequences are used in neonates as in mature children or adults. T1 imaging includes spin-echo (SE) or gradient-echo (GE) imaging, and T2 imaging, spin-echo (SE) or turbo-spin-echo (TSE) sequences. These are more heavily T2-weighted sequences, and show "more" myelination than standard SE. Inversion-recovery (IR) sequences are heavily T1 weighted and yield superb images of the maturation of the brain (Christophe et al. 1990).

It was observed from the outset that the relaxation times in infants were different from those in adults (Holland et al. 1986); as they are strongly dependent on the stage of the maturation, MR imaging can be used to evaluate the progresses of myelination in normal and diseased brains (Barkovich et al. 1988; Bird et al. 1989; Christophe et al. 1990; van der Knaap and Valk 1990; Girard et al. 1991; Martin et al. 1991; Sie et al. 1997; Barkovich 1998), to a degree that no other imaging modality had permitted before. This evolving normality should be taken into account to appreciate disease. But another consequence of this maturation process is that in the first months of life, the design of the sequences should be adapted to the physical-chemical status, that is the degree of maturation, of the cerebral tissue. Typically, when designing a T2w SE sequence, the TR is chosen to be three times longer than the calculated T1 in order to eliminate all T1 contamination effect (Kastler et al. 2001). In adults, at 1.5 T, the calculated T1 is approximately 750 ms: the TR of the T2w sequence should therefore be around 2250 ms, with a TE of about 90 ms. In neonates, depending on the part of the brain examined, the calculated T1 is around 3000 ms (personal data); this correlates with the high content of free water. Consequently, the TR of the T2w SE sequence should be set around 10,000 ms. In normal SE sequences, this would lead to too long an acquisition time, but it can be achieved in a couple of minutes with TSE techniques (although TSE yield images slightly different from standard SE, the myelination appearing "more advanced"). Also, as the T2 value is longer in infants than in adults, the TE should be prolonged at 120 ms to obtain as much T2 effect as possible, while keeping enough signal. In a similar way, in a T1w sequence, the TR having only to be maintained below the calculated T1 (Kastler et al. 2001), it can be chosen longer for neonates than for mature children, resulting in a better signal-to-noise ratio.

Another sequence routinely used in mature patients is the FLAIR sequence. It is a T2w sequence in which the signal of the free water has been suppressed by a 2200 ms pulse. The FLAIR images seem somewhat confusing in the first months and years (Fig. 11.1), but they can also be understood from the changing composition of the parenchyma (Ashikaga et al. 1999; Murakami et al. 1999). In the heavily hydrated neonatal brain, the signal of the white matter is canceled as well, so that it appears dark, and therefore looks the same as on T1 imaging. But as the myelination proceeds, the signal increases quickly and the white matter becomes fully bright by 4 or 5 months. Later, as on regular T2w images, the signal decreases progressively, but over a much longer span of time (up until 4 years of age).

To summarize, as the different types of sequences represent different factors of the physical-chemical composition of the brain, they evolve at their own pace which does not necessarily reflect the histology. As a consequence, the infantile brain appears mature at about 12 months on T1 images (when the magnetization transfer effect is predominant); at about

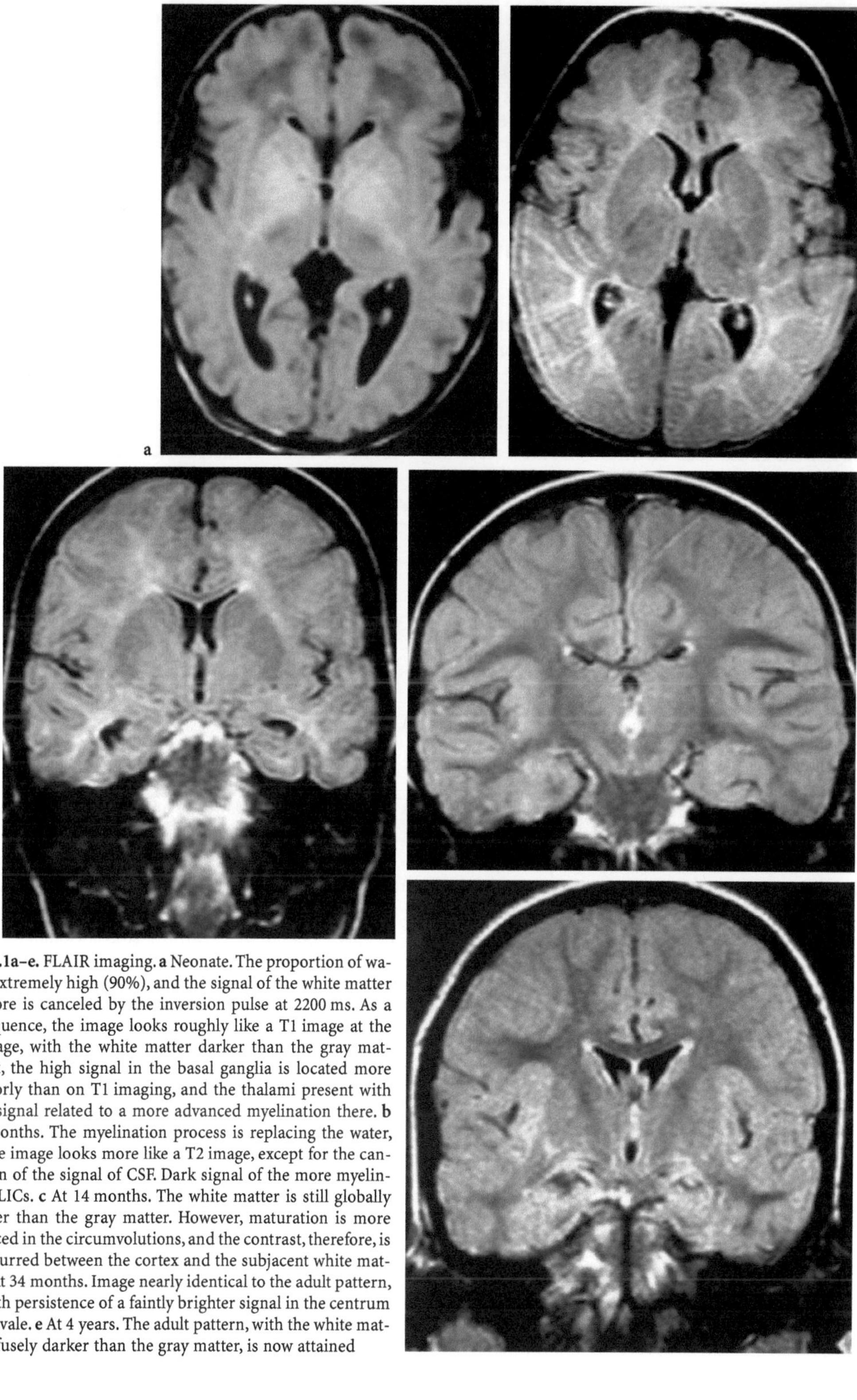

Fig. 11.1a–e. FLAIR imaging. **a** Neonate. The proportion of water is extremely high (90%), and the signal of the white matter therefore is canceled by the inversion pulse at 2200 ms. As a consequence, the image looks roughly like a T1 image at the same age, with the white matter darker than the gray matter. Yet, the high signal in the basal ganglia is located more anteriorly than on T1 imaging, and the thalami present with a low signal related to a more advanced myelination there. **b** At 7 months. The myelination process is replacing the water, and the image looks more like a T2 image, except for the cancelation of the signal of CSF. Dark signal of the more myelinated PLICs. **c** At 14 months. The white matter is still globally brighter than the gray matter. However, maturation is more advanced in the circumvolutions, and the contrast, therefore, is now blurred between the cortex and the subjacent white matter. **d** At 34 months. Image nearly identical to the adult pattern, but with persistence of a faintly brighter signal in the centrum semi-ovale. **e** At 4 years. The adult pattern, with the white matter diffusely darker than the gray matter, is now attained

2 years on T2 images (where the loss of signal due to the accumulation of myelin predominates); and at about 4 years on FLAIR images. These three patterns remain consistent in normal patients; they may diverge in disease, and should therefore be read accordingly.

11.2.2
Limits of MR Imaging of the Developing Brain

Even adapted to the developing brain, these approaches present two types of insufficiencies. The first is that the clinical images obtained from MR are not quantitative images similar to those of the X-ray scanner, but images of which the contrast results from the relative signals of the various structures under examination. As each structure matures according to its own timetable and pace, a given one may seem myelinating in the late fetus because nothing else is myelinated, but less myelinated months later because the rest of the brain then becomes more mature more quickly. To compensate for this, semi-quantitative imaging using relaxometry (images made with absolute relaxation time measurements) can be used, but they are time consuming and therefore not ethically acceptable in clinical conditions. Thus the milestones of maturation used by most correspond to patterns produced at a given time by the relative myelination of the most significant structures of the brain (Barkovich et al. 1988; Bird et al. 1989).

The second insufficiency of MR imaging regarding myelination is that it shows a so-called mature pattern while the brain is still developing: one year (T1), two years (T2), four years (FLAIR), whereas we know from histology that the myelination process is not completed until the end of adolescence. This means that a normal mature appearance may correspond to a maturation which is not complete. Sequences sensitive to the late maturational changes have still to be developed and clinically evaluated (Steen et al. 1997). Also, the term "myelination delay", commonly used in clinical practice, should be avoided unless successive studies have shown an improvement. And even if this is the case, the "normal" stage attained may be only the myelination stage of the age of 2 or 4 years.

A last point is important to keep in mind when reading the brain development through the MR signals. This point is that the signal intensity of the brain tissue reflects the myelination in normal subjects only. In a diseased brain, a low T1, high T2 signal may reflect absence of, or poor, myelination, but it may also mean a de-myelination. Beyond the myelination status, it may express edema, or gliosis, or even a focal dysplasia of the brain tissue.

11.2.3
Special Problems of MR Imaging in Fetuses

Imaging fetuses is possible only at and after mid-pregnancy. The main reason for this is the size of the fetal brain (approximately 50 mm diameter at that stage), which yields little signal in the abdominal cavity (abdominal volume and especially fat volume) and allows only a poor imaging definition, the size of the voxels being disproportionate to the size of the brain. Another problem, at any time, is motion: the fetus moves with the mother's organs, following respiration; this effect is diminished when the head is incarcerated in the pelvis. The fetus himself has his/her own motion, as a whole or when sucking, moving limbs, etc. Other motion artifacts result from the moving fluids and gas of the bowels, and from the flowing blood in moving aorta and vena cava. The magnetic field homogeneity is altered, and the signal received from the fetal brain uneven. Sedating the mother (and therefore the fetus) does not seem to improve things significantly, and may be unacceptable for the parents.

Therefore the imaging technique should compensate for these difficulties. Imaging equipment is important, especially the abdominal coil, as much as possible multiple and in phase array, to get a more homogeneous signal. The most dramatic improvement has been brought about by the introduction of ultrafast, "snapshot" single-slice T2 imaging, making it possible to minimize motion effects. Yet this ultrafast imaging, when used post-natally, is of suboptimal quality as compared with the conventional, adapted T2 sequences. But it allows a fairly good depiction of the fetal brain anatomy at as early as 18 weeks. For T1 imaging, only conventional GE sequences are available; they last a couple of minutes, and are therefore more often altered by the motion artifacts. They are still needed for proper identification of the tissues, as a complement to T2 imaging. Fat saturation reduces the loss of signal in the fat. Slices should be as thin as possible, and the fastest acquisition time compatible with the diagnostic needs should be obtained when defining the sequences.

Other sequences are not used routinely. Angio MR can be used, but without contrast agent (time of flight, TOF), to avoid any risk regarding toxicity. DWI and MR spectroscopy are potentially useful; they are still under evaluation and not used routinely.

11.3 MR Imaging of the Brain in Fetuses and Prematures

The main anatomic features of the evolving fetal brain have been relatively well established (Fees-Higgins and Larroche 1987; Girard et al. 1995; van der Knaap et al. 1996; Battin and Rutherford 2002). The brain is essentially complete by mid-gestation (20 weeks), but it is still very simple. The migration of the neurons to the cortex is achieved, the anterior posterior development of the corpus callosum is completed, but the brain is small (about 5 cm) and smooth.

There are two ways of calculating the age of a fetus: from the time of conception, which is often uncertain, and from the time of the last period, which is more easy to identify. By convention, the mode of dating used by obstetricians, based on the last period, is used here. In theory at least, the gestational age is 2 weeks less.

11.3.1 Gross Morphology of the Fetal and Premature Brain

The sylvian pits are largely open with exposed insula at 20 weeks (Fig. 11.2), then the operculation of the adjacent lobes progressively encloses it. Around it, the gyration is just appearing: parieto-occipital fissure (present at 20 weeks), calcarine fissure (ap-

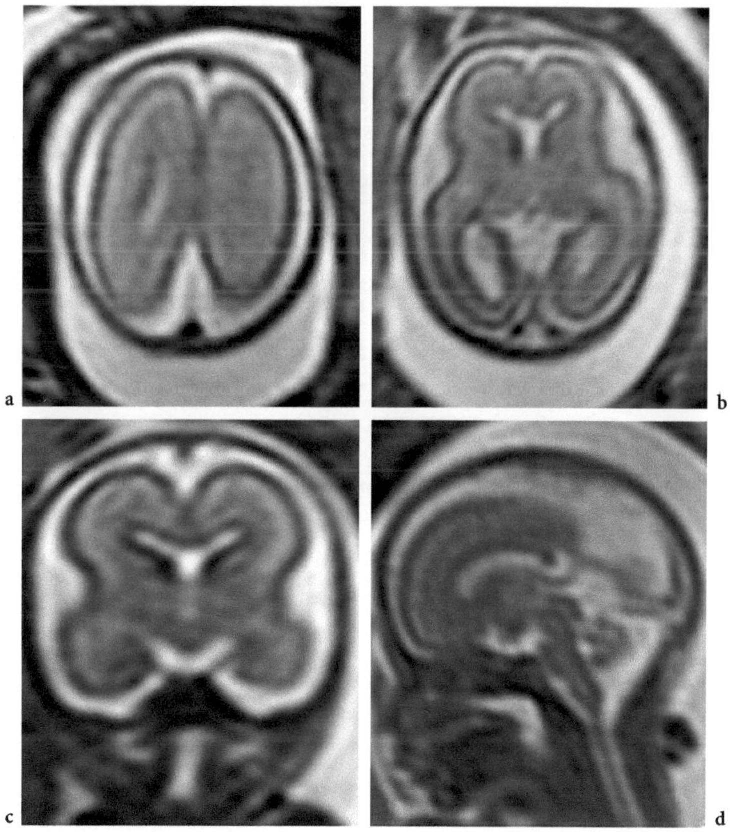

Fig. 11.2a–d. Fetus, 20 weeks. **a** T2 axial, centrum semi-ovale. Smooth cortex. Within the mantle, from the ventricle to the periphery: germinal matrix of the mantle, adjacent to the ventricle (dark, on the *right side*); subcortical zone/migrating glia layer (intermediate signal); subplate (brighter); smooth cortical ribbon; wide pericerebral fluid spaces; calvarium. **b** T2 axial, basal ganglia. Ventricular pseudo-dilatation (colpocephaly, fetal "hydrocephalus"), relative to the still under-developed mantle. Darker cluster of the germinal matrix of the ganglionic eminence over the heads of the caudates. The signal of the basal ganglia is brighter than that of the cortex, and about identical to that of the subventricular zone. **c** T2 coronal. **d** T2 sagittal, midline. In the normal posterior fossa (the tentorium facing the inion), the vermis looks small. Wide interparietal subarachnoid spaces

pearing by 24 weeks, achieved and Y-shaped by 28 weeks), calloso-marginal sulcus (28 weeks), central sulcus (apparent by 24 weeks, achieved by 35 weeks) with the pre- and post-central sulci (from 26 to 35 weeks), and the superior temporal sulcus (clearly demarcated from its anterior to its posterior end by 28 weeks). These sulci, very shallow at the beginning, become progressively deeper as the gyri develop, until after birth (van de Knaap et al. 1996). Up to the last weeks, these sulci are linear (Fig. 11.4), and devoid of tertiary branching. It is only during the last weeks before term, when the cortex comes to abut against the vault, that the sulcal pattern becomes more complex, and then difficult to analyze precisely because of the packing against the bone (Fig. 11.7).

The lateral ventricles are less than 10 mm at the atrium at mid-gestation (Fig. 11.2 and 11.3), with a slight reduction toward birth (7.5 mm). The apparent fetal "hydrocephalus", also called colpocephaly, is only in relation to the brain mantle thickness. The width of the lateral ventricles remains almost constant, whereas the brain is building up around them. But as the brain is growing in every direction, the length of the ventricles also increases. From the beginning, the ventricular segments (frontal, temporal horns, body, atrium, 3rd ventricle, 4th ventricle, even commonly the aqueduct) are clearly rec-

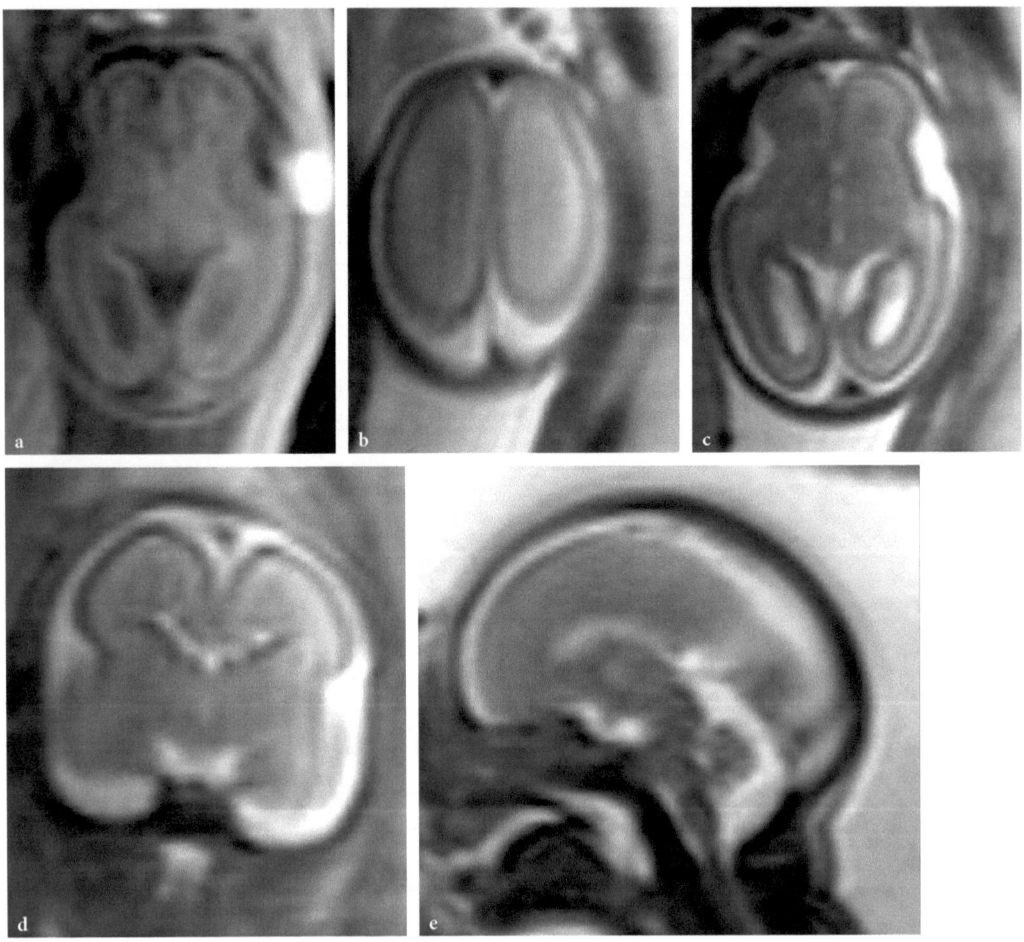

Fig. 11.3a–e. Fetus, 24 weeks. **a** T1 axial, basal ganglia. Morphology still similar to that of 20 weeks. The grey matter structures (cortex, germinal matrix, basal ganglia, subventricular zone/ migrating glia layer) have a brighter signal than that the subplate subjacent to the cortex. **b** T2 axial, centrum semi-ovale. Smooth cortex. **c** T2 axial, basal ganglia. Similar to the 20-week brain. **d** T2 coronal, 3rd ventricle. Early operculation of the sylvian fissure. **e** T2 sagittal, midline. Faint appearance of the main vermian sulci

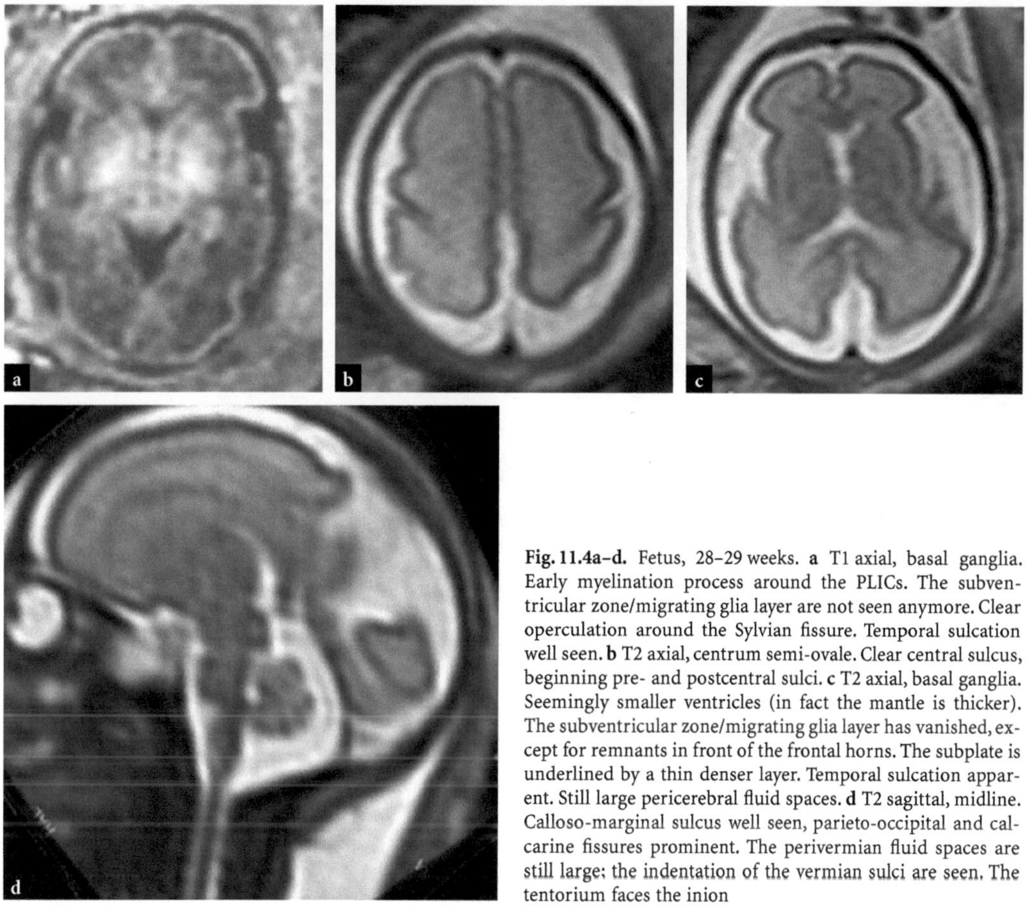

Fig. 11.4a–d. Fetus, 28–29 weeks. **a** T1 axial, basal ganglia. Early myelination process around the PLICs. The subventricular zone/migrating glia layer are not seen anymore. Clear operculation around the Sylvian fissure. Temporal sulcation well seen. **b** T2 axial, centrum semi-ovale. Clear central sulcus, beginning pre- and postcentral sulci. **c** T2 axial, basal ganglia. Seemingly smaller ventricles (in fact the mantle is thicker). The subventricular zone/migrating glia layer has vanished, except for remnants in front of the frontal horns. The subplate is underlined by a thin denser layer. Temporal sulcation apparent. Still large pericerebral fluid spaces. **d** T2 sagittal, midline. Calloso-marginal sulcus well seen, parieto-occipital and calcarine fissures prominent. The perivermian fluid spaces are still large; the indentation of the vermian sulci are seen. The tentorium faces the inion

ognizable. In between the frontal horns, the cavum septi pellucidi is relatively large, sometimes slightly bulging. The corpus callosum (and on occasion the hippocampal commissure as well) is better depicted on the coronal cuts. The peri-cerebral subarachnoid fluid spaces are large and conspicuous in the early pregnancy; they progressively attenuate until 32 weeks, when the cortex comes to abut the vault (Figs. 11.2–11.7).

The cerebellum is disproportionately small in relation to the size of the posterior fossa at about 20 weeks, but grows significantly to nearly fill it at term (Figs. 11.2–11.8), but keeps a clearly demarcated cisterna magna. The limits of the posterior fossa, and especially the insertion of the tentorium facing the inion, are always evident. At 20 weeks (at best) or slightly later, only the main cerebellar fissures are seen on the sagittal cut of the vermis. The other vermian sulci become apparent as the vermis enlarge. It should be noted that not seeing the vermian sulci does not mean that they are not present, but simply that they are blurred by the partial volume effects, since even 2 mm cuts are still exceedingly thick as compared with the structures studied. The brainstem is also well depicted with its three segments, midbrain, pons and medulla (Figs. 11.2–11.8).

11.3.2 The Intrinsic Anatomy of the Fetal and Premature Brain

In the fetus, or in the premature, the brain is a clearly multilayered structure. This results from the fact that the histogenesis is not yet achieved, even though the neuronal migration is practically complete by 20 weeks. Cellular proliferation goes on until term, in both germinal matrices (mantle and ganglionic eminence), to produce astrocytes and oligodendrocytes.

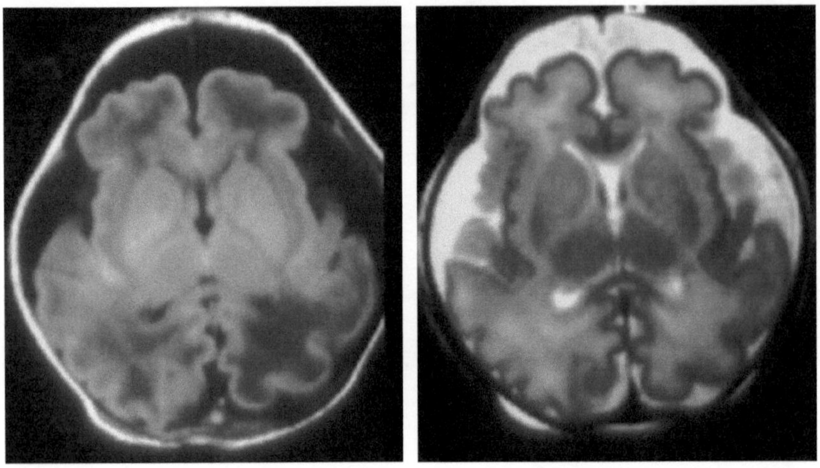

a b

Fig. 11.5a,b. Premature baby, 30 weeks. Ex utero imaging with conventional, age-adapted MR sequences: the image definition and contrast are much better than with in utero imaging. **a** T1 axial, basal ganglia. Clear contrast between the grey and the white matter, even in the PLICs. At least on the *right*, the subplate is clearly seen as a denser subcortical layer. Residues of the subventricular zone/migrating glia layer in front of the frontal horns. Early myelination process apparent in the posterior lentiform nuclei and anterior-lateral thalami, as well as in the primary acoustic cortices in the posterior insular areas. No myelination seen in the PLICs. **b** T2 axial, basal ganglia. Clearly established sulcation, globally. Well advanced perisylvian operculation. The subplate is clearly seen in the frontal lobes. A denser appearance of the corpus callosum and fornices reflects a early myelination in respect to the rest of the white matter. Large pericerebral subarachnoid and perhaps, subdural fluid spaces

These cells constitute a transient, highly cellular layer located around the ventricles in the deeper portion of the white matter (Figs. 11.2–11.4). This so-called layer of migrating glial cells (Childs et al. 1998), however, stays away from the cortex, from which it is separated by the (also) transient neuronal layer of the subplate (Figs. 11.2–11.8). All these structures develop and then disappear at different times, giving the cerebral mantle different appearances at different stages of development. In addition, in the last gestational trimester, the myelination is clearly beginning to appear mostly in the deep central structures (Figs. 11.4–11.8).

The germinal matrix lining of the ventricular wall is present until term, mostly from the ganglionic eminence (Fig. 11.7). In relation to the whole brain, it is more prominent at the beginning, then it disappears nearly completely around term. It is highly cellular, and therefore clearly seen as a dark T2, bright T1 periventricular band; on T1 however it tends to blend with the adjacent highly cellular subventricular zone. The germinal matrix appears thicker over the basal ganglia (ganglionic eminence) than along the white matter. Germinal matrix hemorrhages developing in the premature typically affect the ganglionic eminence, but more modern studies in premature babies using MR imaging rather than US or X-CT demonstrate that the germinal matrix of the mantle, along the ventricles, is also affected. When the germinal matrix of the mantle, lining the white matter, shows discontinuities on fetal MR imaging, a destructive process (infection and/or periventricular leukomalacia) should be suspected.

Until week 28, the dense subventricular zone is seen deep in the white matter, extending to the periphery only to about midway between the germinal matrix and the cortex (Figs. 11.2–11.4). It is generally considered that it contains the differentiating and migrating glial cells, but recent evidence indicates that it is a mixture of a deeper fiber rich zone, of the subventricular cellular zone and migrating glia layer, and of the future white matter (Kostovic et al. 2002). On T1 imaging, it tends to fuse with the image of the germinal matrix. On T2, it is identified by a denser line that separates it from the subplate. The image of this intermediate layer "dissolves" between weeks 28 and 30, but leaves behind a few remnants persisting until term, especially in front of the frontal horns (Figs. 11.4–11.8).

After the disappearance of the subventricular layer, the sub-cortical layer of the transient subplate is better demonstrated against the underlying white matter, as a high T1, low T2 band subjacent to the cortex (Fig. 11.5 to 11.8). Its inner limit is commonly marked

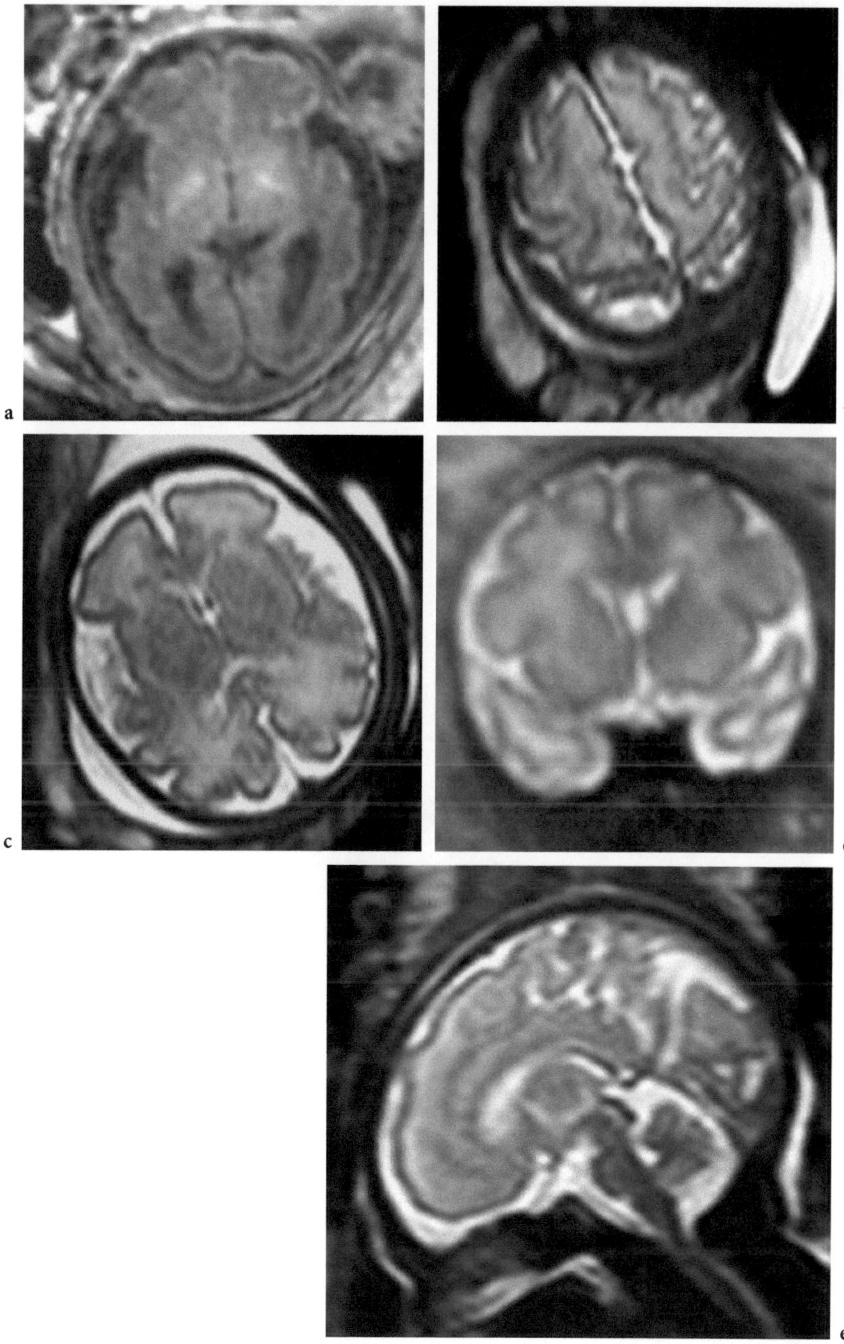

Fig. 11.6a–e. Fetus, 32–33 weeks. **a** T1 axial, basal ganglia. Clearly seen bright signal of myelination in process in and around the PLICs. The cortex is well convoluted, the pericerebral spaces still large. **b** T2 axial, centrum semi-ovale. Essentially complete sulcation pattern, even if the sulci are still shallow. **c** T2 axial, basal ganglia. Clearly delineated subplate. Subventricular residue adjacent to the frontal horns. The thalami are darker, together with the myelinating proximal optic radiations. **d** T2 coronal. Clearly sulcated cortex. **e** T2 sagittal, midline. The vermis is larger and now fills the posterior fossa better. Vermian sulci clearly apparent. Sylvian aqueduct well seen. Well developed medial hemispheric sulcal pattern. Dark, already well myelinated brainstem

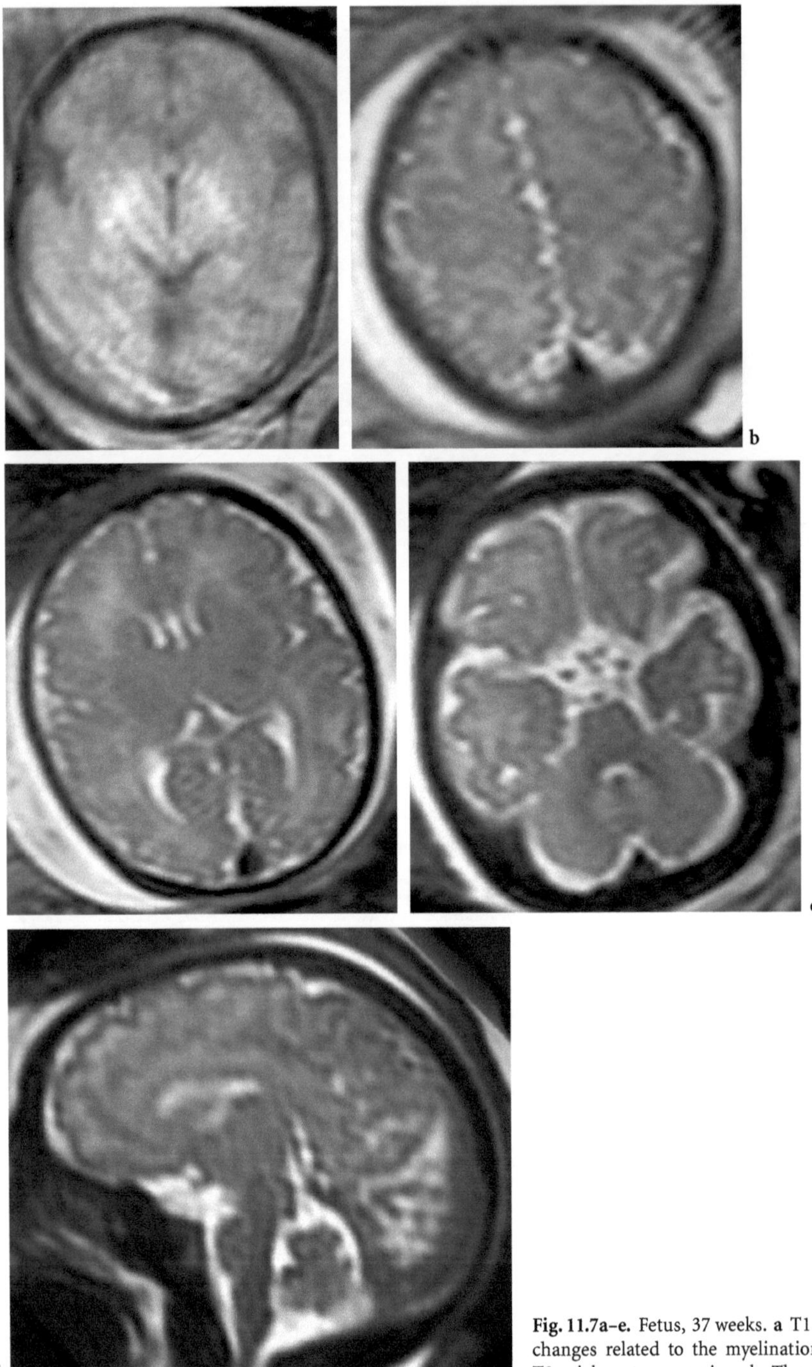

a b c d e

Fig. 11.7a–e. Fetus, 37 weeks. **a** T1 axial, basal ganglia. Clear changes related to the myelination process in the PLICs. **b** T2 axial, centrum semi-ovale. The sulcation is well developed, the cortex is poorly seen because it is now thin in relation to the mantle, and quite convoluted. The pericerebral fluid spaces are not large anymore. **c** T2 axial, basal ganglia. Focally, the dark cluster of the germinal matrix of the ganglionic eminence persists at the level of the foramen of Monro. The optic radiations are seen lining the ventricular atria, against the non-myelinated, adjacent white matter. The subplate can still be recognized as a subcortical blurring. Discrete areas of myelination in the basal ganglia and thalami adjacent to the unmyelinated PLICs [(compare with (**a**)]. **d** T2 axial, posterior fossa. Myelination apparent in the tegmentum pontis and the adjacent brachia pontis. The cerebellum now almost fills the posterior fossa. **e** T2 sagittal, midline by a T2 denser line. This layer persists until term. Its signal is related to the composition of its extracellular matrix rather than to the cellular density (Kostovic et al. 2002). It is the subcortical remnant of the primary preplate (or plexiform layer) that has been divided by the developing cortical plate (Kostovic and Rakic 1990). It is an extremely important structure as it serves as a transient relay for the in-coming fibers of the corona radiata (thalamo-cortical fibers), of the association paths, and of the commissures (Kostovic and Rakic 1990; Super et al. 1998; Xie et al. 2002). This role in controlling the connectivity of the cortex may be compromised by the occurrence of subcortical injuries.

The cortical ribbon is already close to its final thickness (1–3 mm for most of the cortical areas) at mid-gestation, but because of the developing connections (intracortical fibers, thalamo-cortical fibers, association and commissural fibers), it will not be fully organized until birth. It is clearly identified as a bright T1, dark T2 ribbon lining the periphery of the brain. Because it grows tangentially more than the spheric volume of the brain would allow, it progressively develops indentations corresponding to the sulci (Figs. 11.2–11.8). As the brain grows and presses against the vault, it becomes less and less easy to see, and it seems thinner in relation to the globally increased brain size.

The basal ganglia and thalamus form a mass of dense cellularity, brighter on T1 and darker on T2, overlaid by the germinal matrix of the ganglionic eminence, already at 20 weeks (Fig. 11.2). After 30–32 weeks, the T1 signal increases in and around the PLICs (Figs. 11.4–11.8), reflecting the myelination process that develops early in this area that includes the cortico-spinal tract and the adjoining portions of the basal ganglia and thalami, the optic tracts, as well as in the brainstem. This pre-myelination high signal extends toward the central cortex in the last weeks before term.

11.4 MR Imaging of the Brain in Term-Born Infants

Many publications have been devoted to imaging of the development of the brain in the first months of life (Barkovich et al. 1988; Bird et al. 1989; Christophe et al. 1990; van der Knaap and Valk 1990; Girard et al. 1991; Martin et al. 1991; Sie et al. 1997; Barkovich 1998). In children born at term, the brain anatomy is essentially complete. Yet the corpus callosum is thinner than it will be later, not so much due to lack of fibers but because being markedly myelinated, it reaches its final size only after maturation is completed. In the posterior fossa, the neuronal proliferation in the cerebellum continues until the end of the second year, and only then does the cerebellum present its "final" appearance.

From a general point of view, however, most of the changes occurring in the first 2 years are related to myelination. As specified earlier in this chapter, two essential phenomena are responsible for producing the contrast of the MR images. The first is the magnetization transfer effect induced by the precursors of the myelin, which shortens the relaxation time T1 and results in a bright signal on T1w images. The second is the substitution of the achieved myelin to the water, which leads to a general loss of signal and shortens the relaxation time T2, and therefore results in a dark signal on T2w images. The T1 and the T2 images therefore bring different information at this stage. T1 images basically depict the early stages of the myelination processes, while T2 images show the "completed" myelination. Therefore there is an "appearance delay" between the T1 and the T2 images, the changes on T1 being more precocious than on T2, roughly by 4 months. Histologically, this myelination process develops itself according to a precisely determined timetable, both in the cortex, in the white matter, in the central area (gray nuclei and capsules), in the brainstem and in the cerebellum.

11.4.1 The Brain at Term

11.4.1.1 T1 Imaging

At birth, the white matter appears globally darker than the cortex. However, different areas in each structure may show a different appearance. Areas of higher signal are more mature than areas of lower signal.

In the cerebral cortex, four areas have a higher signal than the surrounding structures: the pericentral (peri-rolandic, sensory-motor) cortex, the medial occipital cortex centered on the calcarine fissure (primary visual cortex), the posterior insular temporal area (primary auditory cortex), and the temporo-mesial structures (hippocampus). These are the primary cortical areas, the oldest phylogenetic cortical struc-

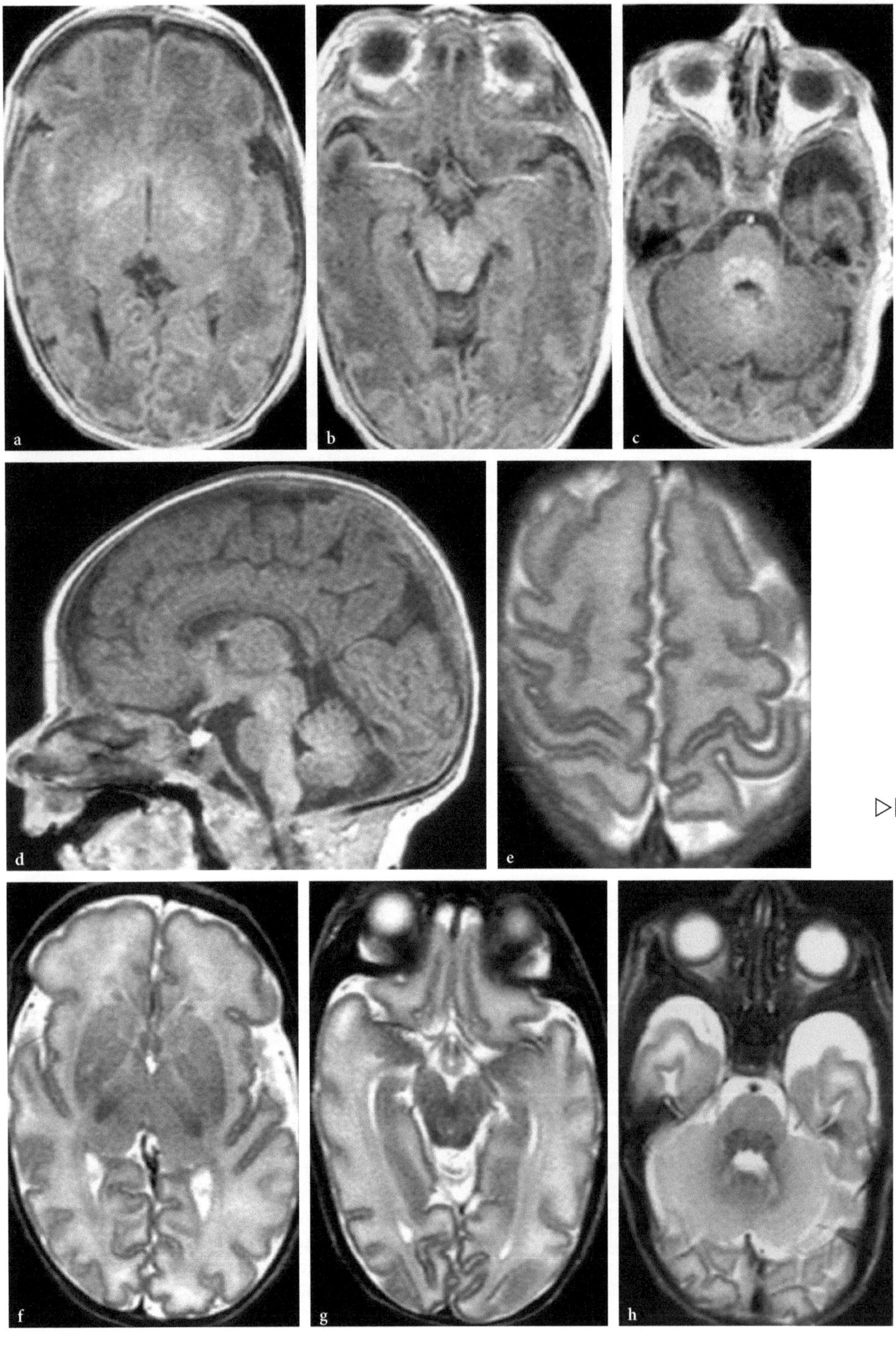
a
b
c
d
e
f
g
h

▷▷

tures, already present in rudimentary mammals such as the shrew (Romer and Parsons 1977).

In the subcortical white matter, a diffuse higher signal is seen below the central area, more consistent centrally and more diluted peripherally; it corresponds to the cortico-spinal tract. Some higher signal is also seen lining the ventricular atria, fitting the distribution of the optic radiations.

In the central brain, there is a conspicuous high signal centered on the PLICs, and involving the adjacent portions of the lentiform nuclei and the ventrolateral portions of the thalami. In the same area, the anterior commissure and the anterior optic pathways (optic nerves, chiasm, tracts) also show some higher signal.

Fig. 11.8a–i. Premature baby, 37 weeks. Ex utero imaging (compare with Fig. 11.6). **a** T1 axial, basal ganglia. Myelination in process in the portions of the basal ganglia and thalami adjacent to the PLICs, which themselves appear not yet to myelinate. **b** T1 axial, midbrain. Clearly brighter signal of the colliculi. **c** T1 axial, pons. Clear myelination process in the tegmentum pontis. **d** T1 sagittal midline. Clear myelination process of the midbrain, tegmentum pontis, medulla. Strong high signal of the pituitary gland against the globally lower signal of the (only partially myelinated) brain. **e** T2 axial, centrum semi-ovale. Clearly well developed sulcation. **f** T2 axial, basal ganglia. The subplate can still be identified, as well as the remnants of the subventricular zone/migrating glia layer in front of the frontal horns. Clear myelination of the posterior-lateral thalami, and of the rest of the basal ganglia to a lesser degree, but the adjacent PLICs remain apparently not, or only poorly, myelinated. Early myelination of the optic radiations clearly apparent. **g** T2 axial, midbrain. Global myelination, more advanced in the colliculi. **h** T2 axial, pons. Fascicular and nuclear myelination in the tegmentum pontis. **i** T2 sagittal, midline. Well developed sulcation of the medial cortex. Nuclear/fascicular partial myelination of the brainstem and deep vermian white matter. Clear vermian sulcation

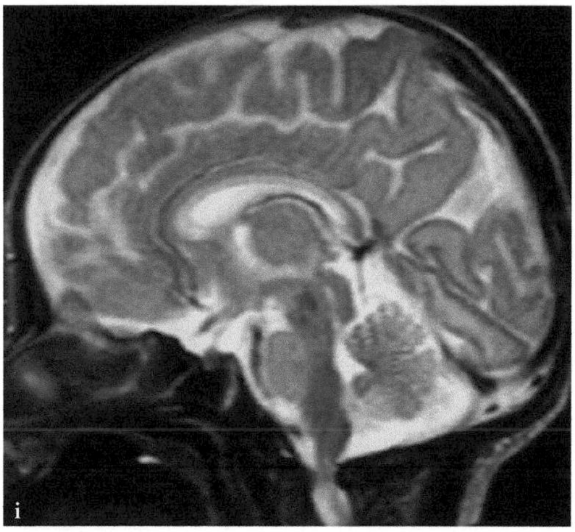

In the posterior fossa, the tegmentum (posterior segment) of the brainstem has a higher signal than the anterior pons, as well as the adjacent white matter of the cerebellum. The colliculi are also brighter.

It is worthwhile noting that at this age, the pituitary gland appears exceedingly bright on cerebral imaging. In fact, it has the normal signal of the soft tissue, but it is the brain that has an unusually low signal, to which the imaging windows are adjusted. This contrast between the pituitary gland and the brain eventually disappears as the brain becomes myelinated.

11.4.1.2
T2 Imaging

The images at this stage are nearly, but not exactly, the reverse of the T1 images. Globally, the white matter is brighter than the cortex.

Within the cortex, areas of lower signal (more mature) are found again in the sensory-motor area, the primary motor area, the primary auditory area, and the hippocampus.

In the white matter, areas of faint, decreased signal are seen in the location of the cortico-spinal tracts, but typically not at the level of the optic radiations. An area of lower signal may be observed at some distance in front of the lower part of the frontal horns. This does not reflect myelination, but rather a remnant of the cellular subventricular band.

In the central forebrain, a minute dark fascicle is inconstantly observed in the postero-lateral portion of the PLICs. Dark spots are also seen in the adjacent thalami.

In the brainstem, the tegmentum is darker than the anterior brainstem. The colliculi also appear more mature, as well as the cerebellar white matter surrounding the cerebellar dentate nuclei.

11.4.2
The Brain at 4 Months

11.4.2.1
T1 Imaging

Four months is an important time to evaluate myelination as typically at this stage the diffuse increase of signal of the white matter matches the signal of the cortex, globally with a loss of the contrast between the two. The primary bundles of white matter have progressively taken a more mature appearance, from the center to the periphery toward their corresponding cortex.

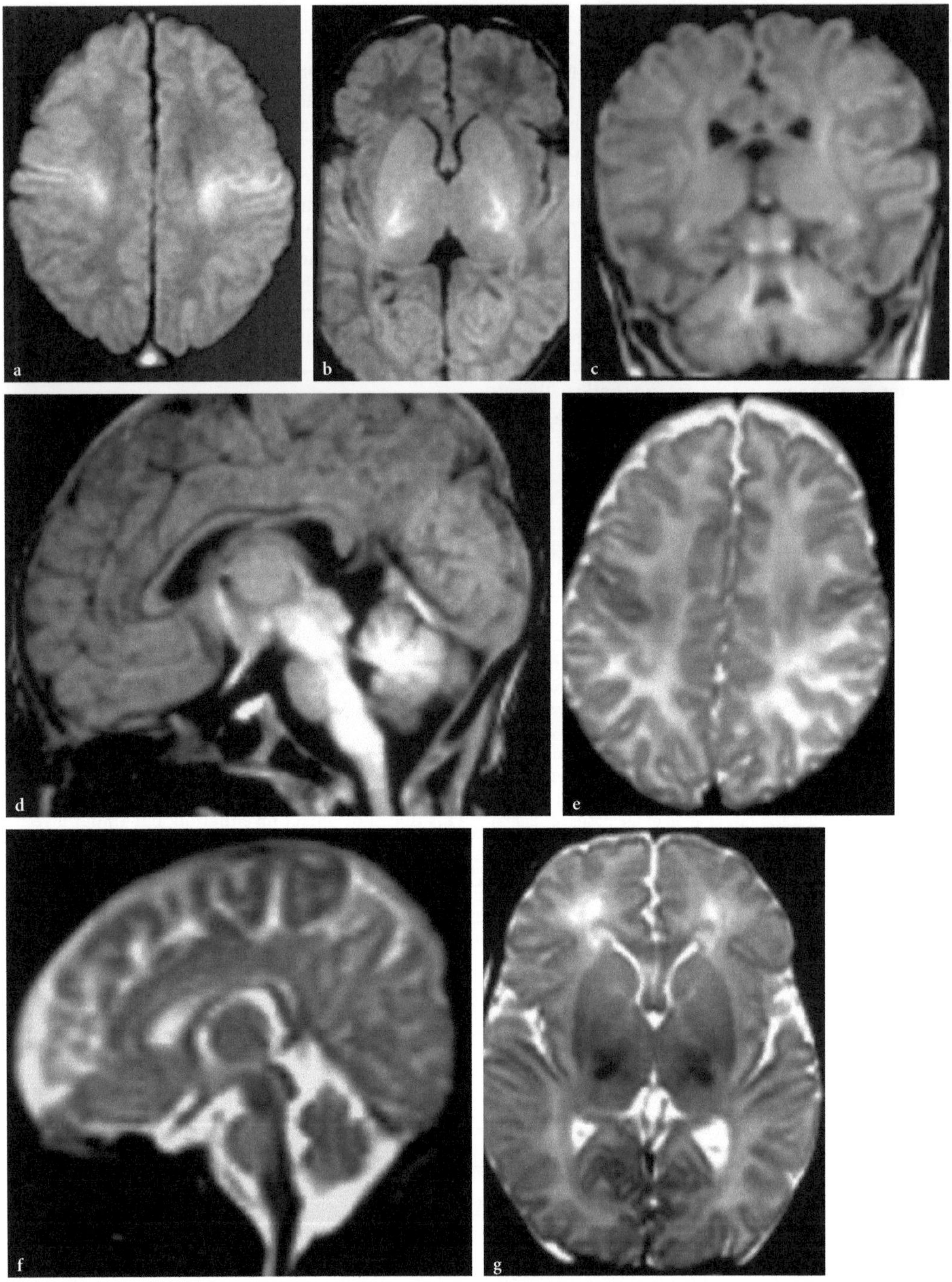

Fig. 11.9a–g. Term neonate. **a** T1 axial, centrum semi-ovale. White matter clearly darker than the cortex. Myelination in process of the peri-central cortices and of the subjacent bundles of cortico-subcortical fibers. **b** T1 axial, basal ganglia. White matter darker than the cortex and the basal ganglia. Bright signal of the myelination process in the whole area surrounding the PLICs, and to a lesser degree of the optic radiations. **c** T1 coronal, thalami. Myelination in process of the corticospinal bundles (centrum semi-ovale on each side), the optic radiations (lateral to the temporal horns), the colliculi, and of the deep cerebellar white matter. **d** T1 sagittal, midline. Myelination in process of the hypothalamic structures and optic chiasm, the midbrain, tegmentum pontis, medulla and cerebellar white matter. **e** T2 axial, centrum semi-ovale. Darker myelination signal of the cortex in the vicinity of the central sulcus, and more faintly, of the subjacent white matter. **f** T2 axial, basal ganglia. Myelination of the lateral portions of the thalami, the posterior putamina to a lesser degree, as well as of a clearly demarcated fascicle in the posterior lateral part of the PLICs. **g** T2 sagittal, midline. Strong myelination signal of the fornix and optic chiasm, the midbrain, the tegmentum pontis (and perhaps the anterior pes pontis), and of the medulla

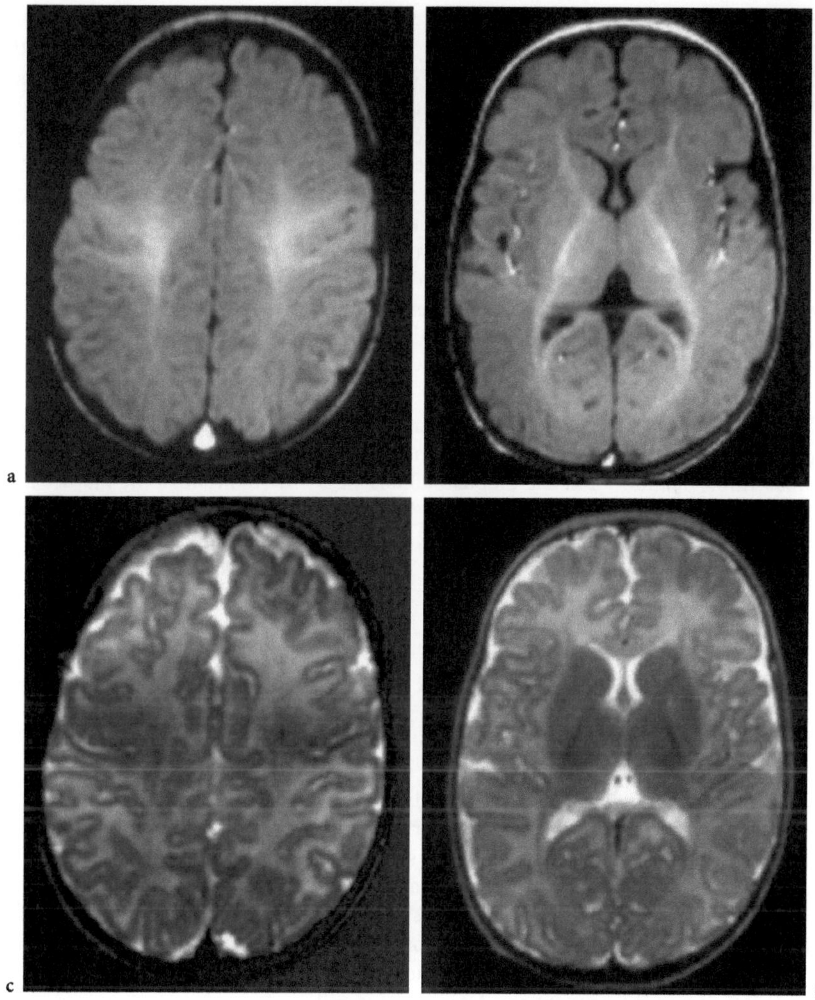

Fig. 11.10a–d. A 4-month-old infant. **a** T1 axial centrum semi-ovale. The signal is now practically even between the gray and the white matter. There is clearly myelination in process, however, in the white matter subjacent to the central sensory-motor area, and probably also along a longitudinal tract that could be the superior longitudinal fasciculus. **b** T1 axial, basal ganglia. Loss of contrast between the gray and white matter, except for the internal capsules (anterior and posterior limbs) and portions of the corona radiata such as the thalamo-frontal fibers, or the optic radiations. The internal capsule is now brighter than the adjacent lentiform nuclei and thalami. **c** T2 axial, centrum semi-ovale. Pattern similar to that of the neonate. The contrast is still strong between the cortex and the white matter, except in the area subjacent to the central cortex. **d** T2 axial, basal ganglia. Still similar to the neonatal pattern but the PLICs are now clearly and globally myelinated, and also the anterior limbs, the optic radiations and faintly, the thalamo-frontal fibers

Within the cortex, the areas of previously higher contrast are now even. Over this ground of increased signal, the contrast of the basal ganglia is also lost. But the capsules form a striking pattern of high signal corresponding to the whole internal capsules (anterior and posterior limbs) with its radiations. In the white matter, they extend toward the fronto-central cortex as the cortico-spinal tract, which is now brighter than the cortex; the optic radiations from the lateral geniculate bodies to the inner occipital cortex; and anteriorly, the thalamo-frontal segment of the corona radiata. The posterior corpus callosum also appears brighter.

In the posterior fossa, the brainstem is diffusely brighter with "hotspots" corresponding to the main fascicles. The whole cerebellar white matter is bright.

11.4.2.2 T2 Imaging

In contrast to T1 imaging, little change appears on T2 between birth and four months. The cortex still shows a lower signal in the primary areas. In the white matter, the corticospinal tract is still faint, but on the contrary, the optic radiations are clearly demarcated. This is an important landmark: poorly defined optic radiations at this stage indicate that oligodendrocytes have been damaged, even if a fully fledged picture of periventricular leukomalacia is not observed.

The myelination of the PLICs is more advanced, but still well circumscribed. In the basal ganglia some difference appears between the striatum and the thalamus (more mature), and the globus pallidus (less mature). Little change is apparent in the brainstem and cerebellum.

11.4.3 The Brain from 8 to 12 Months

11.4.3.1 T1 Imaging

At this stage, an obvious maturation gradient is observed between the posterior and the anterior part of the hemispheres. The posterior part looks like fully mature: bright signal of the white matter against the lower signal of the cortex, but the cortical-subcortical junction is still blurred. The thalami are now brighter than the basal ganglia. The more anterior, fronto-temporal part of the hemispheres by contrast is still similar to what it was at 4 months.

In the posterior fossa, the fully mature appearance is now attained.

The adult appearance is reached at about 12 months, with a diffusely bright signal of the white matter, brighter than the cortex and the central grey nuclei; the adult pattern of signal gradient between the striatum, globus pallidus and thalamic nuclei is present.

11.4.3.2 T2 Imaging

From 6 to 8 months, the cortex is still darker than the white matter, but this becomes attenuated. The basal ganglia and thalami also appear darker, but not as much as the internal capsule with its radiations toward the frontal lobes, the fronto-central areas, and the visual cortices. The posterior corpus callosum appears clearly darker than the centrum semi-ovale. The posterior fossa is still incompletely myelinated.

But from 8 to 10 months, and later, the signal of the white matter globally equates the signal of the gray matter, in the cortex or in the central grey nuclei, giving the brain a blurry, contrastless appearance. Surprisingly, the corpus callosum and the internal capsules are much darker than the adjacent white matter. The posterior fossa looks almost mature.

11.4.4 The Brain at 18–24 Months

At 18 months, the mature appearance is completed on T1, and almost reached on T2. The white matter is darker than the gray matter, but the centrum semi-ovale is still diffusely brighter in its central portion, the subcortical arcuate fibers being clearly darker. The final "adult" appearance is reached at 2 years, with the exception of the terminal area, which is the deep white matter lateral and at a distance from the ventricular atria, which remains slightly brighter than the surrounding white matter until adulthood.

11.5 MR Morphometry, Diffusion, and Spectroscopy

11.5.1 Morphometry

As the normal developing brain grows, and as any injury will affect this growth in a perhaps unapparent fashion, quantitative volumetry has been developed in healthy and diseased infants, and can be used as a predictor of outcome. Volumetry is achieved by segmentation methods (Hüppi et al. 1998a). It has been shown in presumably normal premature babies (Hüppi et al. 1998a) that at between 29 and 41 weeks, the total volume of the brain is increased 2.7-fold; and that most of this increase is due to the increase of volume of the folding cortical white matter, of which the part in the brain volume increases from 35% at 29 weeks, to 50% at term, in relative terms, and is multiplied four-fold in absolute terms.

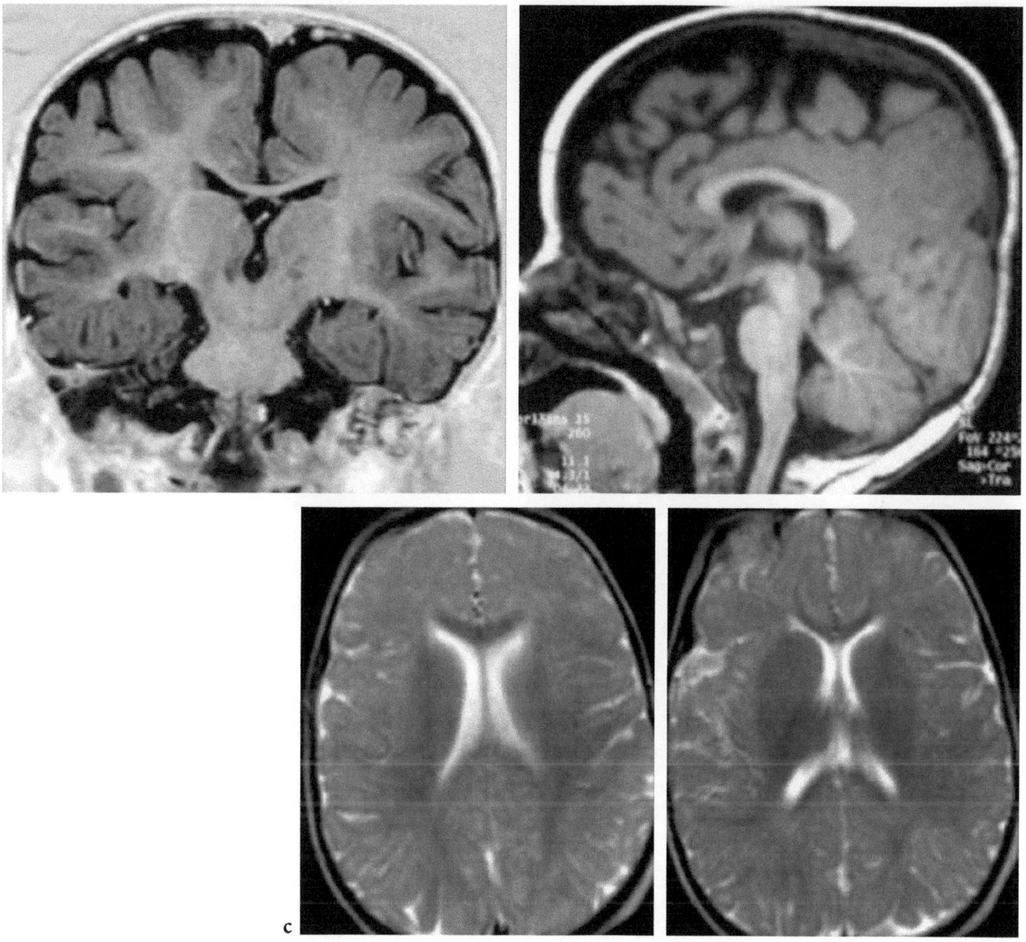

Fig. 11.11a–d. An 18-month-old infant. **a** T1 coronal, thalami (IR). The signal of the white matter now is approaching the adult pattern, globally brighter than the cortex except in the peripheral white matter close to the cortex (arcuate fibers mostly). **b** T1 sagittal, midline. The anterior portions of the brainstem now appear brighter than the tegmentum. The corpus callosum looks fully myelinated. **c** T2 axial, ventricular bodies. Loss of the previous contrast between the white and the grey matter, with a blurry appearance related to the even signals. The corpus callosum, however, appears darker, more myelinated. **d** T2 axial, basal ganglia. Poor grey/white contrast, diffusely, except for a stronger myelination of the PLICs and of the corpus callosum

11.5.2 Diffusion Imaging

Beside the usual T1 and T2 parameters, other methods have been developed to approach brain maturation. Diffusion imaging (DWI) has been shown to be promising (LeBihan et al. 1986). In contrast to conventional MRI, it is not based on relaxation times, but capitalizes on the influence of the structure on the brownian motion of the free water protons. When these protons are in a free space, that is free to move in any direction, there is a loss of the resonant signal (proton dephasing), while this resonant signal is better preserved when the motion is restricted to smaller spaces (less proton dephasing). This apparent motion can be quantified by calculating the apparent diffusion coefficient (ADC), restituted as a map. The intracranial water is located in the CSF spaces, where it moves freely; within the cells, where its motion is hampered by the numerous cytoplasmic organelles; and in the extracellular spaces, where motion is dependent on the space allowed by the volume of the cells. It is this last water sector that is studied in DWI, together with some of the water crossing the cellular membranes. In the normal mature brain, the extracellular sector represents about 20% of cerebral

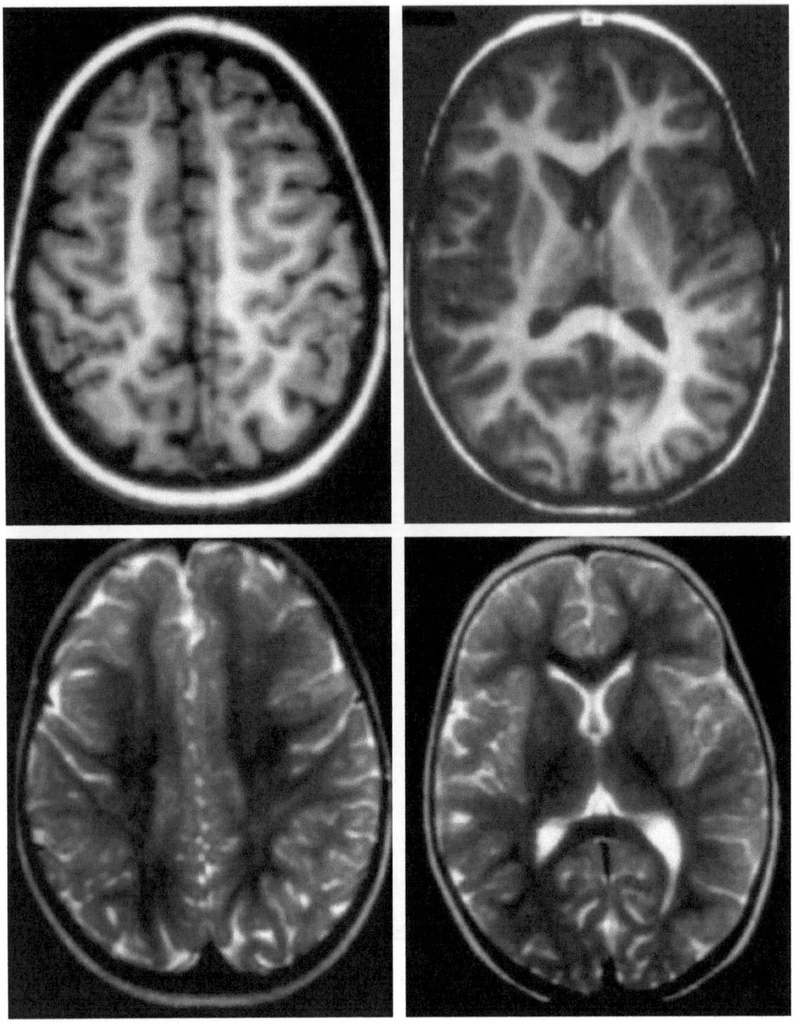

Fig. 11.12a–d. An 18-month-old infant. **a,b** T1, axials; **c,d** T2, axials. The adult pattern is practically reached at this stage, on T1 and T2 imaging. Some faintly higher T2-signal areas are acceptable after 2 years in the centrum semi-ovale, and in the deep white matter lateral to the atria (zona terminalis) up to adolescence

volume. Because of the particular organization of the brain, another factor can also be evaluated, which is the anisotropy: the brain contains fibers organized in bundles, so that the motion of the water protons is more restricted in the directions perpendicular to the fibers than in the direction parallel to them. The higher the anisotropy coefficient, the more packed the fibers. It is also possible to identify the direction of the less restricted motion in a given voxel, giving the direction of the fibers, and therefore to reconstruct the organization of the fibers; this is the basis of tractography by diffusion tensor imaging (DTI) (Pierpaoli et al. 1996).

Studies have shown that ADC is high in the immature white matter, and decreases progressively until the age of 6 months when adult values are reached. This is explained in part by the development of the myelination but as the reduction begins before myelination starts, it is likely that other factors also interact, probably the glial multiplication of astrocytes and oligodendrocytes (myelination gliosis) that would limit the extracellular spaces (Wimberger et al. 1995). The anisotropy also increases early, partly explained by the myelination, but also by the multiplication in a parallel fashion of the axons and the dendrites. Therefore this increase expresses the organization of the bundles of white matter.

The ADC decreases also in the gray matter during maturation (multiplication of fibers), but the anisotropy does not change (no fascicular organization within the cortex).

11.5.3 Spectroscopy

Finally, as the maturation of the brain is accompanied by tremendous metabolic changes, MR spectroscopy is also a means to approach it. In clinical settings, proton MRS can bring useful information about the relative amounts of *N*-acetyl aspartate (NAA) (marker of the neuronal function, but also oligodendroglial marker in the immature brain), choline (cell membrane turnover, including the myelin which is a stack of oligodendrocytic membrane), creatine (high energy products), lactate (anaerobic metabolism), myo-inositol (glial marker), and glutamate–glutamine (neurotransmitters, and intermediate form of the metabolism of the amino-acids). Typically, two types of spectra are used, with long and short echo times, either in a single-voxel technique (restricted to a portion of the tissue), or according to the chemical shift imaging (CSI) technique exploring a whole slice of brain.

Using the single-voxel technique, it has been shown that in the fetus, from 30 to 40 weeks, NAA increases significantly, together with myo-inositol and creatine (Heershap et al. 2003). This trend continues after birth, as the concentration of NAA in the newborn is 50% of that in the adult. The evaluation of the metabolites, however, can only be relative: increased NAA in relation to choline and creatine. Because of myelination, the choline peak is high in the developing brain, and then decreases in relation to creatine, together with myo-inositol. Actually, this pattern varies from place to place in the brain and at a given place, at its own pace as the brain matures. The use of spectroscopy is also hampered by the difficulty to get absolute values.

11.6 Imaging, Development, and Brain Disease

In the first half of gestation, there is no clear-cut separation between the inborn and the acquired disorders, part of the morphologic consequences depending on the timing of the insult rather than on its mechanism. For instance, polymicrogyria, which is a disorder of the cortical development characterized by the accumulation of too many overly small gyri with a (typically) four-layered cortex, and fused molecular layer, may be observed in families (then of genetic origin), after infections by the cytomegalovirus in the early stages of pregnancy, and seemingly as well, as a consequence of fetal anoxia. On the contrary, as the brain is considered as constitutionally achieved after 23 weeks, any later interference is considered a scarring process more than a malformation, even if the difference, in individual cases, may sometimes be academic.

11.6.1 The Early Gross Brain Malformations

From the time of the development of the neural plate, the malformations may be classified according the developmental stage that failed:

- Failure of neurulation: the neural tube stays open (myelomeningocele), and mechanically, the development of the rhombencephalon (hindbrain) and of the prosencephalon (forebrain) are altered, resulting in a Chiari 2 deformity (McLone and Knepper 1989). This is both a genetic and an environmental (folic acid deficiency) disorder.
- Failure of development of the anterior neural plate. This primordium of the forebrain also gives rise to the face, to the vault and to the anterior cephalic soft tissues. When the process fails, the brain (holoprosencephaly) as well as the face (cyclopia, hypotelorism) are affected (Couly and Le Douarin 1987). Several genes have been invoked, as well as cholesterol and toxic factors such as veratrin, an alkaloid from *Veratrum californicum.*
- Failure of development of the roof of the rhombencephalon: it normally produces the vermis superiorly, and the foramen of Magendie inferiorly. An arrested development produces the typical Dandy-Walker malformation, or one of its minor forms (Raybaud 1982).
- Failure of commissuration: the crossing of the commissural fibers results from the complex involvement of tissular (guiding/repulsing molecules, fasciculating factors), cellular (glial sling, glial wedge, indusium griseum, meninges) and genetic influence to go through the inner wall of the hemispheres, cross the midline and enter the opposite side. Disorders of these processes result in the various types of complete, partial and dissociated commissural anomalies (Raybaud and Girard 1998).

11.6.2
The Malformations of Cortical Development

The development of the cortical plate goes through the stages of proliferation, differentiation, migration, and organization. Each of these steps may be defective, leading to specific malformations (Barkovich et al. 2001):

- Proliferation: if one cycle of division fails, 50% of cells are missing. Microcephaly (three standard deviations or more below normal, commonly with simplified gyral pattern) is usually due to a genetic defect.
- Differentiation: in the process of migration from the mantle germinal matrix to the cortical plate, pyramidal neurons differentiate from the guiding radial glia. If the process fails, abnormally differentiated cells are produced, with abnormal migration and poor segregation between the cortex and the white matter. This constitutes the group of the focal cortical dysplasias, the hemimegalencephalies and the tuberous sclerosis complex.
- Normal neurons may fail to migrate properly, forming masses or layers of abnormally located normal grey matter: they are called heterotopias, either nodular (periventricular, subcortical) or laminar, with a normal ("band heterotopia", "double-cortex") or a simplified (agyria-pachygyria) cortical pattern. Laminar heterotopias are clearly genetic as some of the nodular heterotopias.
- The neurons may migrate normally to the cortex but may not get organized properly: this results in the so-called polymicrogyria, which may be due to genetic, infectious, metabolic, and probably anoxic disorders.
- The schizencephaly ("cleft brain") is a uni- or bilateral focal failure of development of the cortical mantle, resulting in clefts lined with a polymicrogyric cortex that is continuous, inwards, with the ependyma. This is rarely familial, more often acquired (cytomegalovirus, toxoplasmosis), or idiopathic.

11.6.3
Destructive Lesions and the Developing Brain

Specific fetal or neonatal pathologies may interfere with development. In fetuses and prematures, hemorrhages in the germinal matrix may not only induce hydrocephalus; they also destroy the source of oligodendrocytes, possibly compromising forever myelination of the brain. Also in prematures, peri-ventricular leukomalacia may destroy the para-ventricular white matter (resulting in posterior enlargement of the lateral ventricles), but also, in milder cases, may only reduce the population of the late astrocytes, and above all that of the more vulnerable oligodendrocytes. It may also reduce connectivity in prematures (Hüppi et al. 1998b). In the term neonate, anoxia produces specific lesions in the most active parts of the brain, the basal ganglia and thalami (status marmoratus), as well as in the cortex, especially in the deepest part of the sulci, often predominantly in the central sensory motor areas.

Other pathologies have specific developmental consequences. Fetal brain viral infections almost constantly produce microcephaly as well as myelination defects. Ischemia produces different effects depending on the degree of development: in the last trimester of pregnancy, it produces a cavitation with complete detersion of the necrosed tissue, without scar formation. In mature brains, it produces a conventional astrocytic scar. In intermediate stages, it produces the intermediate picture of the multi-cystic encephalomalacia. In all cases, as a portion of the cortex is destroyed, the corresponding white matter fibers are missing, reducing the size of the whole hemisphere and restricting its connectivity. The association and commissural fibers that should have connected with the destroyed area tend to connect with the surrounding preserved cortical margins, creating abnormal neuronal circuits that are thought to explain the high rate of epileptogenicity of these lesions. The ipsilateral half of the brainstem may also be atrophic, as well as the contra-lateral cerebellar hemisphere. Even in older children, longstanding thalamic tumors, especially thalamic germinomas, are associated not with an increased, but with a reduced volume of the hemisphere, because of the reduced number of thalamo-cortical and cortico-thalamic fibers of the corona radiata. In the infant, chronic anoxia-hypoxia such as that produced by arteriovenous steal effects (vein of Galen aneurysm, dural fistula of the torcular) commonly produces atrophy, with sub-cortical calcifications of uncertain mechanism.

In contrast, the potential of the infantile brain to massively produce connections has a positive effect on recovery from any focal cerebral injury: the contrast between the size of the destructive lesions and the relative mildness of the symptomatology is often striking, at least for the perinatal and the infantile injuries. Also, the prognosis of hydrocephalus and its response to its treatment varies significantly depending on the maturational stage. Hydrocephalus in utero is usually devastating, perhaps because of the destruction of the periventricular germinal matrices. By contrast, early post-natal mechanical hydrocephalus (without associated destructive lesions) often present impressive recoveries, the initially excessively thinned brain mantle being able to re-grow to a normal thickness in a matter a few months. This could be explained by the ability of the neurons to re-grow axons, of which the path-finding is not yet impeded by the accumulation of interstitial astrocytes. In older children, massive hydrocephalus never recovers to such a degree.

Globally, the most sensitive cells of the brain seem to be the oligodendrocytes, which are not only vulnerable to anoxia, but also to immune related disorders, and to specific infections. The mechanism allowing the recovery, or not, of the oligodendrocytic pool is to date poorly understood. Non-myelination (or insufficient myelination) is a common result of varied diseases: periventricular leukomalacia, of which the "milder forms" are those in which only the oligodendrocytes are affected, with no cystic necrosis, as well as hydrocephalus, fetal infections. Malnutrition in late pregnancy and early postnatal period has also been shown to compromise myelination. Leukoencephalopathies are common in mitochondrial cytopathies (Chabrol and Raybaud 2002). Obviously, the metabolic diseases affecting specifically the enzymes related to the metabolism, maintenance and degradation of the myelin ("dysmyelinating" diseases) are genetic diseases concerning the oligodendrocyte. Immune-related, inflammatory disorders may induce demyelination, either acutely (acute disseminated encephalomyelitis or ADEM) or in a more protracted way (group of the scleroses), the oligodendrocyte itself being better preserved in the former, less in the latter. Finally, the oligodendrocyte may be the specific target of particular viruses, like the papova/JCV in the progressive multifocal leukoencephalopathy (PML). Finally, vasculopathies in the elderly may also lead to a demyelination (Binswanger disease). All taken together, the disorders affecting the oligodendrocytes, and therefore the myelin, are among the most common neurological disorders in the child, the adult, and the elderly, because of the multiple ways pathologies may alter them.

11.7 Conclusions

MR imaging is the first imaging modality to be able to demonstrate the morphological and structural changes in the maturing brain, in the fetus, and in the term-born infant. The fetal brain cellularity first and later, the mass production on myelin with its effects on T1 and the T2, produce age-specific images that make it possible to evaluate the course of brain maturation. This evaluation has opened new diagnostic avenues, since the sensitivity of the oligodendrocytes to injury, as well as the involvement of myelin in numerous pathologic processes, make the evaluation of maturation an essential element of the imaging approach to the pathology. However, there are a few restrictions to be remembered. T1 and T2 images reflect two different things, not necessarily parallel, and should be used as such. Conventional MR images are composite, non-quantitative images, reflecting only the myelination of diverse areas relative to others: it is therefore a biased picture during the entire course of development. This image is technology-dependent, and pictures are not necessarily exactly comparable from one center to the other. Also, MR imaging is blind to the development, and to slight myelin anomalies, that occur after infancy. Finally, the signal in the images equates to the degree of myelination only in normal subjects, as a "high T2", or a "low T1" signal are not specific, reflecting only the relative concentration of myelin and water, regardless of the mechanism, be it for example an increase of water (edema), or a loss of axons (hence also of myelin). Nevertheless, bearing these restrictions in mind not to "over-read" the images, MRI is an efficient tool, that has allowed a completely new view of brain pathologies in the fetus and the developing infant.

References

Ashikaga R, Araki Y, Ono Y, Nishimura Y, Ishida O (1999) Appearance of normal brain maturation on fluid attenuated inversion-recovery (FLAIR) MR images. AJNR 20:427-431

Barkovich AJ (1998) MR of the normal neonatal brain: assessment of deep structures. AJNR 19:1397-1403

Barkovich AJ, Kjos BO, Jackson DE Jr, Norman D (1988) Normal maturation of the neonatal and infant brain: MR imaging at 1.5T. Radiology 166:173-180

Barkovich AJ, Kuzniecky RI, Jckson GD, Guerrini R, Dobyns WB (2001) Classification system for malformations of cortical development. Update 2001. Neurology 57:2168-2178

Barres BA (1999) A new role for glia: generation of neurons. Cell 97:667-670

Battin M, Rutherford MA (2002) Magnetic resonance imaging of the brain in preterm infants: 24 weeks' gestation to term. In: Rutherford M (ed) MRI of the neonatal brain. Saunders, London, pp 25-49

Baumann N, Pham-Dinh D (2001) Biology of oligodendrocyte and myelin in the mammalian central nervous system. Physiol Rev 81:871-927

Bird C, Hedberg M, Drayer BP et al (1989) MR assessment of myelination in infants and children: usefulness of marker sites. AJNR 10:731-740
Brody BA, Kinney HC, Kloman AS, Gilles FH (1987) Sequence of central nervous system myelination in human infancy. I. An autopsy study of myelination. J Neuropathol Exp Neurol 46:283-301
Caviness VS, Takahashi T, Nowakowski RS (1995) Numbers, time and neocortical neurogenesis: a general developmental and evotionary model. Trends Neurosci 18:379-383
Chabrol B, Raybaud C (2002) Inborn and acquired mitochondrial leucodystrophies. In: Desnuelles C, di Mauro S (eds) Mitochondrial disorders. Springer, Berlin Heidelberg New York, pp 221-229
Childs AM, Ramenghi LA, Evans DJ, Ridgeway J, Saysell M, Martinez D, Arthur R, Tanner S, Levine MI (1998) MR features of developing periventricular white matter in preterm infants: evidence of glial cell migration. AJNR 19:971-976
Christophe C, Muller MF, Balériaux D et al (1990) Mapping of normal brain maturation in infants on phase-sensitive inversion-recovery images. Neuroradiology 32:173-178
Couly GF, Le Douarin NM (1987) Mapping of the early neural primordium in Quail-chick chimeras. II. The prosencephalic neural plate and neural folds: implications for the genesis of cephalic human congenital abnormalities. Dev Biol 120:198-214
Fees-Higgins A, Larroche JC (1987) Development of the human fetal brain. An anatomical atlas. INSERM/Masson, Paris
Fralix TA, Ceckler TL, Wolff SD et al (1991) Lipid bilayer and water proton magnetization transfer: effect of cholesterol. Magn Reson Med 18:214-223
Girard N, Raybaud C, du Lac P (1991) MRI study of brain myelination. J Neuroradiol 18:320-332
Girard N, Raybaud C, Poncet M (1995) In vivo MR study of brain mayuration in normal fetuses. AJNR 16:407-413
Gressens P, Richelme C, Kadhim HJ, Gadisseux JF, Evrard P (1992) The germinative zone produces the most cortical astrocytes after neuronal migration in the developing mammalian brain. Biol Neonate 61:4-24
Heershap A, Kok RD, van den Berg PP (2003) Antenatal proton MR spectroscopy of the human brain in vivo. Childs Nerv Syst 19:418-421
Holland BA, Haas DK, Norman D, Brant-Zawadski M, Newton TH (1986) MRI of normal brain maturation. AJNR 7:201-208
Holms GL (1986) Morphological and physiological maturation of the brain in the neonate and young child. J Clin Neurophysiol 3:209-238
Hüppi PS, Warfield S, Kikinis R, Barnes PD, Zientara GP, Jolesz FA, Tsuji MK, Volpe JJ (1998a) Quantitative magnetic resonance imaging of brain development in premature and mature newborns. Ann Neurol 43:224-235
Hüppi PS, Maier SE, Peled S, Zientara GP, Barnes PD, Jolesz FA, Volpe JJ (1998b) Microstructural development of human newborn cerebral white matter assessed in vivo by diffusion tensor magnetic resonance imaging. Pediatr Res44:584-590
Huttenlocher PR (1990) Morphometric study of human cebral cortex development. Neuropsychologia 28:517-527
Kastler B, Vetter D, Patay Z, Germain P (2001) Comprendre l'IRM, 4th edn. Masson, Paris
Kinney HC, Brody BA, Kloman AS, Gilles FH (1988) Sequence of central nervous system myelination in human infancy. II. Patterns of myelination in autopsied infants. J Neuropathol Exp Neurol 47:217-234
Koenig SH (1991) Cholesterol of myelin is the determinant of gray-white contrast in MRI of the brain. Magn Reson Med 20:285-291
Kostovic I, Rakic P (1990) Developmental history of the transient subplate zone in the visual and somatosensory cortex of the macaque monkey and human brain. J Comp Neurol 297:441-470
Kostocic I, Judas M, Rados M, Hrabac P (2002) Laminar organization of the human fetal cerebrum revealed by histochemical markers and magnetic resonance imaging. Cerebral Cortex12:536-544
Kucharczyk W, MacDonald P, Stanisz G, Henkelman RM (1994) Relaxivity and magnetization transfer of white matter lipids at MR imaging: importance of cerebrosides and pH. Radiology 192:521-529
Lavdas AA, Grigoriou M, Pachnis V, Parnavelas JG (1999) The medial ganglionic eminence gives rise to a population of early neurons in the developing cerebral cortex. J Neurosci 99:7881-7888
Le Bihan, D, Breton E, Lallemand D, Grenier P, Cabanis E, Laval-Jeantet M (1986) MR imaging of intravoxel incoherent motion: applications to diffusion and perfusion in neurologic disorders. Radiology 161:401-407
Letinic K, Rakic P (2001) Telencephalic origin of human thalamic GABAergic neurons. Nature Neurosci 4:931-936
Marin-Padilla M (1998) Cajal-Retzius cells and the development of the neocortex. Trends Neurosci 21:64-71
Martin E, Krassnitzer S, Kaelin P, Boesch C (1991) MR imaging of the brainstem: normal postnatal development. Neuroradiology 33:391-395
McConnell SK (1995) Constructing the cerebral cortex: neurogenesis and fate determination. Neuron 15:761-768
McLone DG, Knepper PA (1989) The cause of Chiari II malformation. A unified theory. Pediatr Neurosci 15:1-12
Meyer G, Schaaps JP, Moreau L, Goffinet AM (2000) Embryonic and early fetal development of the human neocortex J Neurosci 20:1858-1868
Murakami JW, Weinberger E, Shaw DWW (1999) Normal myelination of the pediatric brain imaged with fluid attenuated inversion-recovery (FLAIR) MR imaging. AJNR 20:1406-1411
Nadarajh B, Parnavelas JG (2002) Modes of neuronal migration in the developing cerebral cortex. Nature Rev Neurosci 3:423-432
Pierpaoli C, Jezzard P, Basser P, Barnett A, di Chiro G (1996) Diffusion tensor MR imaging of the human brain. Radiology 201:637-648
Rakic P (1995) A small step for the cell, a giant leap for mankind: a hypothesis of neocortical expansion during evolutiobn. Trends Neurosci 18:383-338
Raybaud C (1982) Cystic malformations of the posterior fossa. Abnormalities of the development of the roof of the 4th ventricle and adjacent meningeal structures. J Neuroradiol 9:103-133
Raybaud C (1990) Development of the arterial supply to the brain tissue. In: Lasjaunias P, Berenstein A (eds) Surgical neuro-angiography. 3. Functional vascular anatomy of brain, spinal cord and spine. Springer, Berlin Heidelberg New York, pp 1-13
Raybaud C, Girard N (1998) Etude anatomique par IRM des

agénésies commissurales télencéphaliques. Corrélations cliniques et interpétation morphogénétique. Neurochirurgie (Paris) 44 [Suppl 1]:38-60

Romer AS, Parsons TS (1977) The vertebrate body, 5th edn. Saunders, Philadelphia

Sidman RL, Rakic P (1973) Neuronal migration, with special reference to developing human brain: a review. Brain Res 62:1-35

Sie LTL, van der Knaap MS, van Wezl-Meijler G, Valk J (1997) MRI assessment of myelination of motor and sensory pathways in the brain of preterm and term-born infants. Neuropediatrics 28:97-105

Steen RG, Ogg RJ, Reddick WE, Kingsley PB (1997) Age-related changes in the pediatric brain: quantitative MR evidence of maturational changes during adolescence. AJNR 18:819-828

Super H, Soriano E, Uylings HB (1998) The functions of the preplate in development and evolution of the neocortex and hippocampus. Brain Res Rev 27:40-64

Tamamaki N, Nakamura K, Okamoto K, Kaneko T (2001) Radial glia is a progenitor of neocortical neurons in the developing cerebral cortex. Neurosci Res 41:51-60

Van der Knaap MS, Valk J (1990) MR imaging of the various stages of normal myelination during the first year of life. Neuroradiology 31:459-470

Van der Knaap MS, Valk J, de Neeling N, Nauta JJP (1991) Pattern recognition in magnetic resonance imaging of white matter disorders in children and young adults. Neuroradiology 33:478-493

Van der Knaap MS, van Wezel-Meijler G, Barth PG, Barkhof F, Ader HJ, Valk J (1996) Normal gyration and sulcation in preterm and term neonates: appearance on MR images. Radiology 200:389-396

Van Essen D (1997) A tension-based theory of morphogenesis and compact wiring in the central nervous system. Nature 385:313-318

Wimberger DM, Roberts TP, Barkovich AJ et al (1995) Identification of "premyelination" by diffusion weighted MRI. J Comput Assist Tomogr 19:28-33

Xie Y, Skinner, Landry C, Handley V, Schonmann V, Jacobs E, Fisher R, Campagnoni A (2002) Influence of the embryonic preplate on the organization of the cerebral cortex: a targeted ablation model. J Neurosci 22:8981-8991

Yakovlev PI, Lecours AR (1966) The myelinogenic cycles of regional maturation of the brain. In: Minkovski A (ed) Regional development of the brain in early life. Blackwell, Oxford, UK, pp 3-70

Zhu Y, Li HS, Zhou L, Wu JY, Rao Y (1999) Cellular and molecular guidance of GABAergic neuronal migration from an extracortical origin to the neocortex. Neuron 23:473-485

12 Imaging of Inherited and Acquired Metabolic Brain Disorders

Mauricio Castillo

CONTENTS

12.1 Predominantly White Matter Disorders with Increased Head Size

12.1.1 Alexander Disease

This is a very rare disorder also called fibrinoid leukodystrophy (van der Knaap et al. 2001). Recently, a heterozygous dominant mutation in the glial fibrillary acidic protein has been described. There is no identifiable biochemical defect. Histologic examination shows Rosenthal fibers in the brain, ependyma and pia. It is thought that intracellular deposition of these fibers lead to abnormal functioning of the oligodendrocytes. Arbitrarily it has been divided into infantile, juvenile and adult forms. Macrocephaly is typical and the manifestations include progressive spastic quadriparesis and intellectual failure leading to death (generally all patients die by their teenage years). It generally presents in infancy or adolescence and death occurs as early as 3–10 years after diagnosis. Treatment is only palliative. The disease begins in the frontal regions and then extends posteriorly, and is seen as areas of high T2 signal intensity (Fig. 12.1). The subcortical u-fibers are initially spared but rapidly become affected. The basal ganglia may also appear swollen initially. Although contrast enhancement was, in the past, thought to be rare, it is now known that it occurs in most patients early in the course of the disease. This contrast enhancement

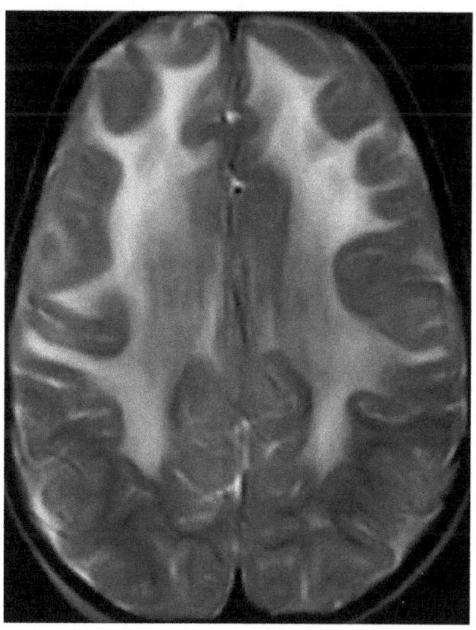

Fig. 12.1. Alexander disease. Axial T2-weighted image shows abnormal hyperintensity in the deep and superficial white matter of the frontal lobes in a symmetrical distribution. (Case courtesy of A. Rossi, Genoa, Italy)

M. Castillo, MD, FACR
Professor and Chief of Neuroradiology, University of North Carolina School of Medicine, Chapel Hill, NC 27599, USA

may involve all the areas of abnormal white matter including the basal ganglia. In the end-stage disease, brain cysts may form. This cystic leukomalacia may also show contrast enhancement.

12.1.2 Canavan Disease

Canavan disease (spongiform leukoencephalopathy) is more common in Ashkenazi Jews, and patients generally die 2–3 years after diagnosis (McAdams et al. 1990). Many patients with macrocephaly and imaging findings identical to those of Canavan disease probably have "van der Knaap disease" (van der Knaap et al. 1999). In patients with van der Knaap disease the clinical course is milder and generally only the white matter is diffusely affected. In this disorder, subcortical cysts may be present. Canavan disease is a very rare disorder and is characterized by a deficiency of the enzyme N-acetylaspartylase [which deacetylates *N*-acetyl aspartate (NAA) to acetate and aspartate], and therefore proton MR spectroscopy shows markedly elevated NAA (Fig. 12.2a). This enzyme is expressed in oligodendrocytes and is involved with the synthesis of myelin lipids. The accumulation of NAA is toxic to the brain and results in myelin splitting (Brismar et al. 1990a). Histologically, there is extensive vacuolization (spongy degeneration) of the brain with increased water content. Canavan disease is autosomal recessive and the gene encoding for acetylaspartylase is located on chromosome 17. Canavan disease generally begins during the first 6 months of life but there are also congenital and juvenile forms of the disease. Most patients die during the first decade of life. There is no effective treatment available. Canavan disease involves all of the white matter in a diffuse fashion including the sub-cortical U-fibers (Fig. 12.2b). In addition, the globi pallidi and thalami are nearly always affected (they show high T2 signal). Much of the affected white and gray matter also show restricted diffusion on diffusion-weighted imaging. No contrast enhancement is present. As the disease progresses, the size of the head begins to decrease.

Another disease that needs to be included in the differential diagnosis of Canavan disease is Cree leukoencephalopathy. The imaging findings are identical to those of Canavan but Cree has been reported only in northern Quebec and Manitoba in Canada (Alorayni et al. 1999). Patients with congenital muscular dystrophy of the merosin-deficient type may also present with diffuse increased T2 signal intensity in the brain (Fig. 12.2c). These patients, however, have near normal psychomotor development (compared to those with Canavan disease), have muscle weakness of early onset and may have seizures. In both of the previously mentioned disorders, the head size is not enlarged. Diffuse white matter involvement may also be seen in the rare "vanishing brain syndrome" (Fig. 12.2d).

12.1.3 Krabbe Disease

This is also a very rare disorder, although in the author's experience it is perhaps somewhat more common than Alexander and Canavan diseases. It is also called globoid cell leukodystrophy. It is a lysosomal disorder characterized by a deficiency of the enzyme galactocerebroside beta galactosidase, and is inherited as an autosomal recessive trait (Hittmair et al. 1994). The enzymatic defect blocks the degradation of beta galactocerebroside, which is a critical component of the myelin sheaths. The presence of end products such as psychosine is toxic to the oligodendrocytes. The diagnosis is confirmed by establishing the levels of leukocyte lysosomal beta galactosidase (Choi and Enzmann 1993). Krabbe disease generally affects infants and young children, and most patients are diagnosed between the 3rd and 6th month of life (one of the earliest leukodystrophies). The head is initially large and then becomes small (at presentation most patients are microcephalic). CT may show increased density in the thalami but, since this study is nowadays seldom obtained for patients suspected of having leukodystrophies, this finding is not commonly observed (Finelli et al. 1994). MRI shows increased signal intensity around the ventricles in a non-specific pattern (Hittmair et al. 1994). High T2 signal may also be seen in the pyramidal tracts and in the medial aspect of the cerebellar hemispheres. In the late onset variant, the splenium of the corpus callosum may be involved. Atrophy ensues in most patients, particularly late in the disease. The brain abnormalities generally do not show contrast enhancement. Krabbe disease may result in hypertrophy of the cranial and spinal nerves (simulating the findings seen in Guillain-Barrè syndrome) (Lee et al. 1995). These large nerves may show contrast enhancement. Bone marrow transplantation may be helpful in the treatment of the disease. Diffusion tensor imaging may be the best way to evaluate these patients. Tensor imaging shows more abnormalities than T2 weighted imaging and provides a quanti-

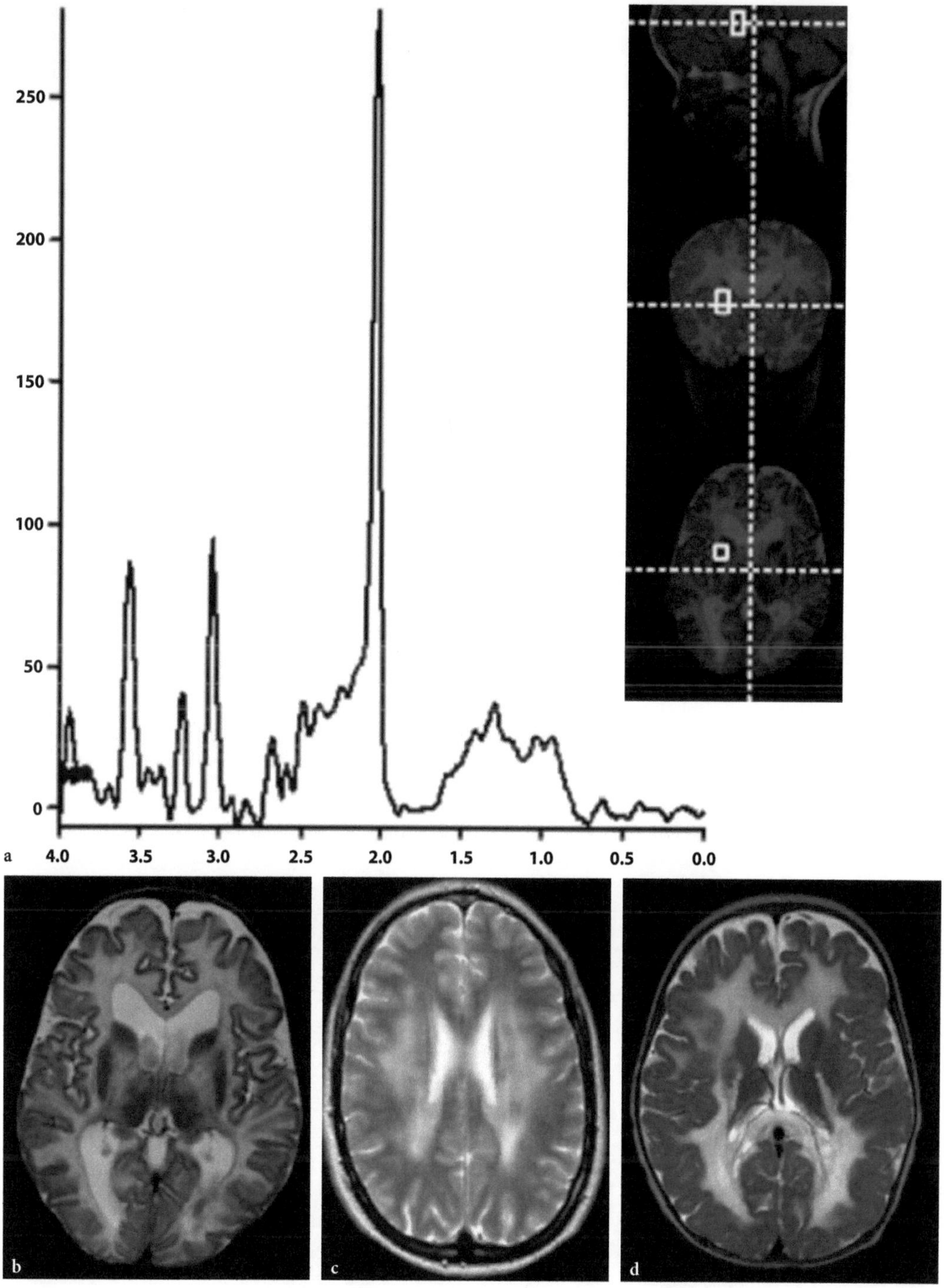

Fig. 12.2a–d. Canavan disease and mimics. **a** Long echo time MR spectroscopy obtained from the white matter shows that the peak of *N*-acetyl aspartate (2.0 ppm) is markedly elevated. **b** Axial T2-weighted image in the same child shows diffuse abnormal hyperintensities throughout the white matter and also in the globi pallidi and thalami. **c** In a child with merosin-deficient muscular dystrophy, axial T2-weighted image shows abnormal signal intensity from the white matter at the level of corona radiata. **d** In this child with the vanishing brain syndrome, there is abnormal T2 hyperintensity in all of the white matter

tative measurement of the severity of the disease, making it an optimal way to study the response to therapy.

12.1.4 Mucopolysaccharidoses

This group of disorders also affects the white and the gray matters, and is included here because children may also present with an enlarged head (in reality the diagnosis is well established in most patients by the time of imaging evaluation). They are not true leukodystrophies, but glycosaminoglycans are deposited along the perivascular spaces, leading to focal changes mostly in the periventricular white matter. These compounds are also accumulated inside the cells and are toxic to them. The mucopolysaccharidoses may be considered as disorders of lysosomes (Johnson et al. 1984). Initially there is macrocephaly but progression of these disorders eventually results in brain atrophy. All are inherited in an autosomal recessive fashion, except for Hunter's disease which is x-linked. The most common mucopolysaccharidoses are Hurler, Morquio, Hunter, while the least common are Sanfilippo and Maroteaux-Lamy disease. The life span of these patients is variable, but is now improved with the availability of bone marrow transplantation and replacement with recombinant human enzyme (L-iduronidase). The skull is thick and there is dolichocephaly and a thick and somewhat keel-shaped frontal bone (these are prominent features in Hurler disease). Expansion of the skull may lead to multiple cranial nerve deficits. Ventricular dilatation with or without increased intracranial pressure is common (Kumar et al. 1987). It is often very difficult to tell whether there is increased intracranial pressure due to the ventricular dilatation. The white matter may show abnormal T2 signal intensity and may contain multiple dilated peri-vascular spaces (Fig. 12.3). It is not clear if these peri-vascular spaces are dilated by the glycosaminoglycans or are part of the spectrum of the communicating hydrocephalus. In the author's experience, their signal intensity is identical to that of cerebrospinal fluid in all MR imaging sequences, including FLAIR and DWI. The presence of multiple dilated peri-vascular spaces involving the corpus callosum is typical of the mucopolysaccharidoses (in tuberous sclerosis there are multiple dilated perivascular spaces, but they almost never involve the corpus callosum and, when they do, they are few and isolated). The cortical sulci may be prominent due to brain atrophy, and occasionally one or more arachnoid cysts are presumably present secondary to the deposition of glycosaminoglycans in the meninges. Little correlation, however, has been seen by the author between the patient's clinical deficits and the imaging findings, that is, the brain may be severely involved but the patient may have only mild clinical manifestations of the disease.

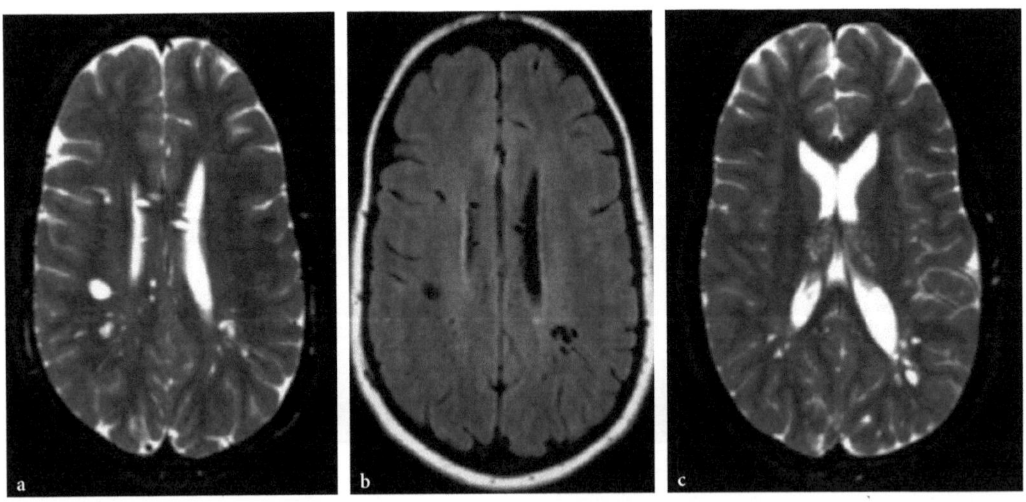

Fig. 12.3a–c. Hunter disease. **a** Axial T2-weighted image shows dilated perivascular spaces in the posterior periventricular white matter. **b** Corresponding FLAIR image shows that the lesions are isointense to the cerebrospinal fluid. **c** There are also dilated perivascular spaces in the peri-trigonal white matter and in the thalami

12.2 Predominantly White Matter Disorders with Normal Head Size

12.2.1 Adrenoleukodystrophy

Adrenoleukodystrophy (ALD) is the most important peroxisomal disorder and one of the most common primary white matter disorders in children. The most common type of these disorders is inherited as an x-linked recessive trait (Xq28) and thus it is only seen in males (JENSEN et al. 1990). The neonatal form of ALD is inherited as an autosomal recessive trait and is very rare. Other types of the disease include the adrenomyeloneuropathy that affects older individuals and the presymptomatic ALD, in which the genetic defect is present but imaging and clinical abnormalities are nearly absent. The affected gene in x-linked ALD encodes for the formation of coenzymes derived from the fatty acids within the peroxisomes. This leads to impaired oxidation of fatty acids and their accumulation, which is detrimental to the formation and stabilization of myelin, resulting in active demyelination and inflammation. Very long chain fatty acids are not correctly metabolized and become elevated in serum and other tissues. The defect is at the level of the lignoceroyl coenzyme A ligase. X-linked ALD occurs in boys of 3–10 years of age and a vegetative state or death may occur as soon as 2 years after the diagnosis (SNYDER et al. 1991). The most common clinical symptoms are sensorineural hearing loss (90%), pyramidal tract symptoms (50%), visual deficits (40%), behavioral abnormalities (33%) and seizures (6%). All patients will become vegetative within 5 years of diagnosis. The only hope for cure is early bone marrow transplantation.

In 80% of cases, CT and MRI show abnormalities in the white matter of the occipital regions, also involving the splenium of the corpus callosum and extending anteriorly (Fig. 12.4a). The location of the abnormalities closely correlates with the symptoms (LOES et al. 1994). Early in the disorder, only the corticospinal tracts and/or the medial lemnisci may be affected (MELHEM et al. 1996) (Fig. 12.4b). The anterior border of these abnormalities may enhance after contrast administration and this finding implies breakdown of the blood–brain barrier due to active demyelination and inflammation (Fig. 12.4c). Pathologically, the following changes are seen in ALD: zone A (inner zone) corresponds to scar and gliosis and shows no contrast enhancement and high T2 signal; zone B (middle zone) corresponds to inflammation and demyelination with axonal preservation and shows contrast enhancement and high T2 signal intensity; and zone C (outer zone) which has active destruction of myelin but no inflammation. This latter zone is very thin and is not clearly visualized.

Proton MR spectroscopy obtained at the level of the disease front (zones B and C) shows significant elevation of the choline secondary to the presence of inflammatory cells. On MR spectroscopy, NAA (a neuronal marker) is decreased, and lactate and lipids (from cellular breakdown) may be elevated (RAJNANAYAGAM et al. 1996, 1997) (Fig. 12.4d). Peaks between 0.9–2.4 may be seen and are believed to be related to the presence of the very long chain fatty acids. Patients with an inflammatory component have a more rapid and severe course and a worse prognosis. Diffusion-weighted images may show restriction of water diffusion early in the course of the disease (Fig. 12.4e,f). ALD rarely begins in the frontal regions. In the chronic stage of the disease, dystrophic calcifications may be seen in the white matter (BARKOVICH et al. 1994). This finding is not only unusual, but it is seldom seen, because CT is no longer commonly obtained in ALD patients.

12.2.2 Metachromatic Leukodystrophy

Metachromatic leukodystrophy (MLD) is a lysosomal disorder that is characterized by a deficiency in arylsulfatase A (or one of its cofactors) and accumulation of sulfatides that are toxic to the white matter (KIM et al. 1997). There is lack of breakdown and reutilization of myelin and the sulfatides impair the function of macrophages and Schwann cells. The presence of sulfatides in urine and deficient arylsulfatase A in leukocytes confirms the diagnosis. It is the most common leukodystrophy and is inherited as an autosomal recessive trait. There is gene mutation in chromosome 22 but this is not present in all patients. Most patients become symptomatic between 1–3 years of age (late infantile form). There is a less common juvenile form in which the patients generally present between 5–7 years of age. Death occurs 1–4 years after diagnosis. Bone marrow transplantation has been tried with varying degrees of success. On imaging studies, the white matter is diffusely affected but the subcortical u-fibers are spared (KIM et al. 1997). The pattern of involvement is periventricular, bilateral and symmetrical ('butterfly' pattern) (Fig. 12.5a). The areas of high T2 signal inten-

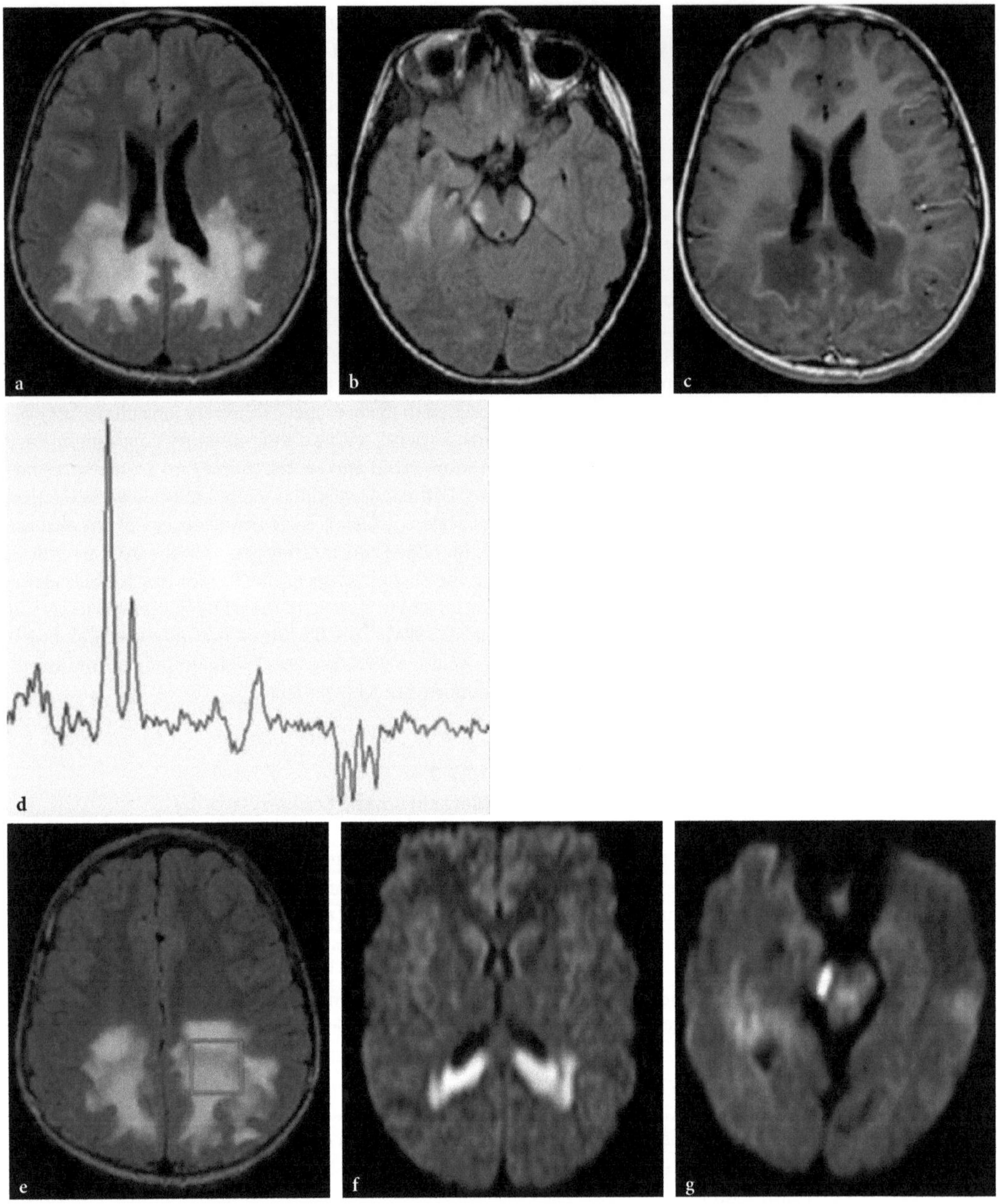

Fig. 12.4a–g. X-linked adrenoleukodystrophy. **a** Axial FLAIR image shows increased abnormal signal intensity in the occipitoparietal white matter and crossing the callosal splenium. **b** In the same patient, a FLAIR image shows symmetrical hyperintensities in the region of the lateral lemnisci. **c** Post contrast T1-weighted image at same level as (**a**) shows enhancement of the periphery of the lesions. **d** MR spectroscopy study obtained with an echo time of 135 ms shows very low NAA, high choline and presence of lactate. **e** Axial FLAIR image shows location of the voxel used for the MR spectroscopy study shown in (**d**). **f** In a different patient, axial trace diffusion-weighted image shows increased signal intensity in the peri-trigonal white matter and in the splenium of the corpus callosum. **g** In the same patient, there is restricted water diffusion in the region of the right lateral lemniscus

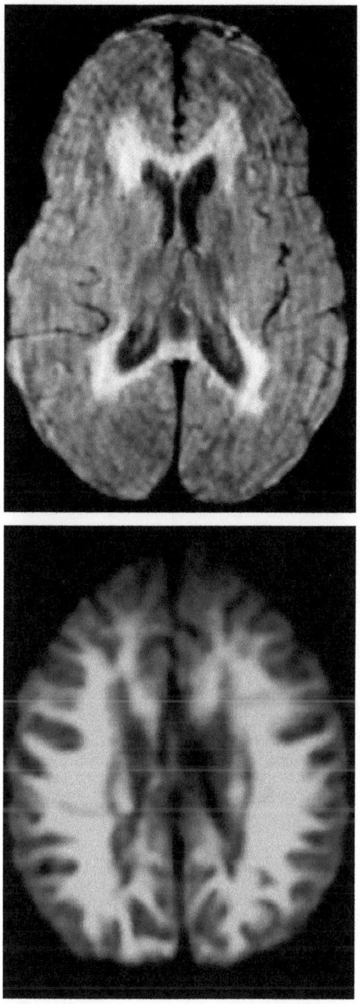

a

b

Fig. 12.5a,b. Metachromatic leukodystrophy. **a** Axial FLAIR image shows non-specific symmetrical periventricular abnormal high signal intensity. **b** In a different patient, axial trace diffusion-weighted image shows abnormal high signal intensity throughout the white matter

sity may also be somewhat patchy in appearance. There is no contrast enhancement and the areas of abnormal T2 signal also show abnormal diffusion (Fig. 12.5b). The medial regions of the cerebellum may be involved early in the course of the disease. Eventually all of the brain (including corpus callosum and brainstem) become involved and atrophy ensues (Stillman et al. 1994).

12.3 Predominantly White Matter Disorders with Small Head Size

12.3.1 Pelizaeus-Merzbacher Disease

Pelizaeus-Merzbacher disease (PMD) is an x-linked disorder (classic form) that is characterized by the lack of myelin specific lipids leading to abnormal function of the oligodendrocytes and hypomyelination. It belongs to the group of disorders called 'sudanophilic' leukodystrophies (Silverstein et al. 1990). PMD presents very early in life. All of the patients seen by the author presented with abnormal eye movements and cerebral palsy-like symptoms. The patients also show developmental delay, seizures, spasticity and all die a few years after the initial diagnosis (Silverstein et al. 1990). The white matter never forms normally due to a defect of the gene that encodes for a 'proteolipid' protein, which is essential for the development of myelin. On histology, the white matter has a "tigroid" appearance (van der Knaap and Valk 1989). On imaging studies, the white matter is diffusely abnormal and the brain retains an in utero appearance (the abnormalities may be so diffuse and symmetrical that at first glance the studies may even be interpreted as normal) (Fig. 12.6a,b). There is lack of mature myelin throughout most of the white matter. In the later stages of the disease, the basal ganglia may be dark due to increased iron deposition. The cerebellum may be small and eventually the brain shows atrophy.

Trichothiodystrophy deserves to be briefly mentioned here because the brain may show abnormalities similar to those seen in PMD on MRI. These patients have ectodermal defects such as brittle hair and abnormal dental enamel (Wetzburger et al. 1998). In addition to the usual neurological findings seen in most white matter disorders, patients with trichothiodystrophy have a peripheral neuropathy and abnormal hearing. This disease is extremely rare.

12.4 Osmotic Myelinolysis

Osmotic myelinolysis is an acute demyelinating disorder most often seen 2–3 days after the rapid correction of hyponatremia (<15 mmol/L), but may also occur in hypernatremic states or even in the

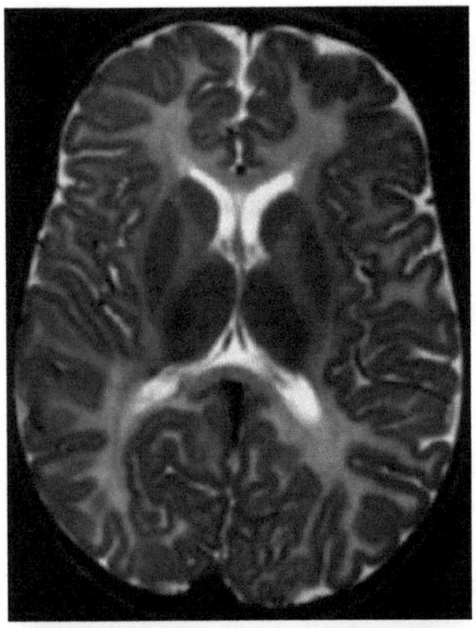

a

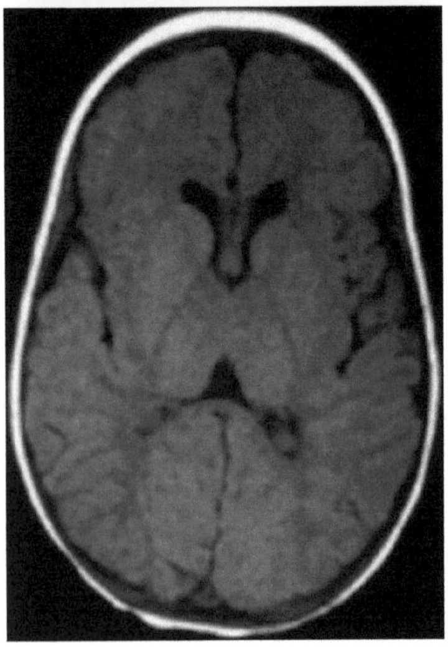

b

Fig. 12.6a,b. Pelizaeus-Merzbacher disease. **a** Axial T2-weighted image at 3 years of age shows diffuse lack of myelination. **b** In a different patient, a T1-weighted image shows diffusely low signal intensity from the white matter indicating lack of mature myelin

absence of sodium concentration abnormalities (Ho et al. 1993). It is possible that rapid influx of water into the cells associated with sodium alterations results in their damage. The neurological symptoms of hyponatremia may be divided as follows: early stage (anorexia, nausea, vomiting, muscle spasm and weakness), advanced stage (impaired responses to verbal commands and pain, bizarre behavior, hallucinations, obtundation, respiratory distress) and severe stage (decortication, bradycardia, hyper- or hypotension, altered temperature regulation, seizures, respiratory arrest and coma).

Most patients with osmotic myelinolysis are chronic alcoholics, have extensive burns, sepsis, Hodgkin disease, or other malignancies. Osmotic myelinolysis has a high mortality rate, but currently many patients survive. On imaging, most patients show abnormalities in the pontomedullary junction (called 'central pontine myelinolysis' or CPM for short) (Sztencel et al. 1983). Histologically, CPM shows acute demyelination (particularly of the pontine transverse fibers), with preservation of the neurons and axons. Patients with CPM present with lethargy, cranial nerve abnormalities, problems in swallowing, and may progress to quadriparesis, including a 'lock in' syndrome.

Imaging studies are reported as normal in up to 85% of patients with the clinical syndrome of CPM. MRI shows an area of high T2 signal centered in the lower pons (Korogie et al. 1993; Price et al. 1987) (Fig. 12.7). Sometimes the lesion has a triangular appearance on axial images with its apex located in the midline and pointing forward (pontine infarcts may be triangular-shaped, but the lesion is nearly always off midline and its apex points posteriorly). In most patients, CPM has a nonspecific appearance and involves the entire cross section of the brainstem. The lesion is devoid of mass effect and contrast enhancement. Although the cerebellar cortex is affected commonly, this finding is not usually appreciated on MRI. In 10% of patients, the supratentorial gray matter structures that are surrounded

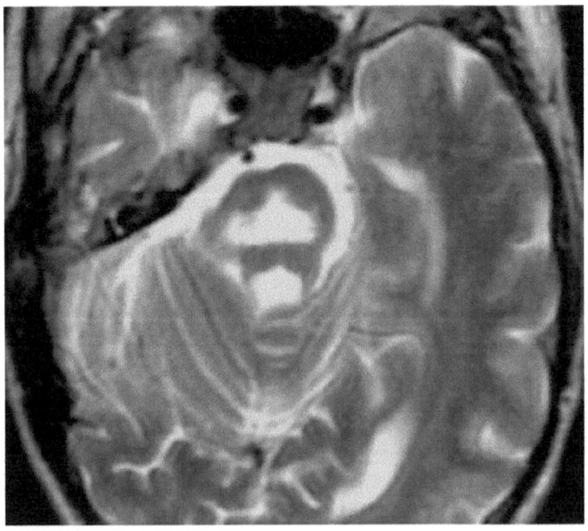

Fig. 12.7. Central pontine myelinolysis. Axial T2-weighted image shows a triangular-shaped area of abnormal high signal intensity in the mid pons

by white matter may be affected (extrapontine myelinolysis). The regions most commonly affected are the lentiform nuclei and the thalami. Occasionally, supratentorial white matter structures such as the internal capsule and corpus callosum may be involved. When the patients survive, a slow and gradual decrease in the size of the lesions is noted on follow-up studies, but their lesion does not resolve completely (Rosenbloom et al. 1984).

12.5 Predominantly Gray Matter Disorders

12.5.1 Effects of Liver Failure and Parenteral Nutrition

It is well known that hepatic insufficiency will lead to abnormalities on brain MR imaging. T1 weighted images show increased signal intensity in the caudate nucleus, tectum (particularly the inferior colliculi), globus pallidus, putamen, subthalamic nucleus, red nucleus, adenohypophysis, and substantia nigra (Etsuo et al. 1991). The abnormalities are bilateral, symmetrical, and of homogenous signal intensity; there are no corresponding abnormalities on T2 weighted images and CT scans are normal. The MR imaging findings are believed to be due to increased amounts of manganese (Mn) and other factors leading to shortening of the relaxation time. Increased plasma levels of Mn may be found in chronic liver failure, patients receiving long-term parenteral nutrition, and occupational toxicity (Krieger et al. 1995). Nearly 95% of Mn is excreted in bile. Manganese is involved in some enzymatic cell cycles, including superoxide dismutase and glutamine synthetase. Manganese reaches the brain by way of erythrocytes and plasma. Transferrin and albumin are its carriers in plasma. The half-life of blood Mn is 10–42 days, but when it reaches the brain it may remain there for prolonged periods of time. Astrocytes have specific transport systems for Mn. Manganese is neurotoxic and results in striatal dopamine depletion, NMDA excitotoxicity, and oxidative stress (Krieger et al. 1995). Thus, Mn may play a role in the development of hepatic encephalopathy that is clinically characterized by pyramidal and extrapyramidal dysfunction, brisk tendon reflexes, and tremors. The concentration of Mn in the pallidus of cirrhotic patients is three-fold higher compared to controls (Pomier-Layrargues et al. 1995). The frequency of MR imaging abnormalities in the brain of cirrhotic patients is approximately 73% (Pomier-Layrargues et al. 1995).

Long-term total parenteral nutrition results in increased T1 signal intensity in the same regions. These solutions are rich in Mn and lead to development of neurological symptoms. Once the parenteral nutrition is discontinued, the MR abnormalities may reverse to normal (Fell et al. 1996). The amount of time required for these abnormalities to resolve is not clear, but most do within 1 year after cessation of parenteral nutrition (Mirowitz and Westrich 1992). T1 hyperintensity in the adenohypophysis and dorsal brainstem due to total parenteral nutrition may revert to normal 4 months after treatment is discontinued (Okamoto et al. 1998). Similar findings are noted in patients following liver transplantation (Krieger et al. 1995). Although the clinical and imaging abnormalities are reversible in adults, its long-term effect on the child's brain is not known.

Other MR techniques may be more sensitive to the effects of liver disease on the brain than just imaging. Magnetization transfer contrast ratios are abnormal not only in the previously named brain regions but also in the white matter (Iwasa et al. 1999). With liver failure there is an increased proliferation of Alzheimer type II astrocytes in the affected brain regions. The etiology for the proliferation of these cells may be hyperammonemia. These cells are characterized by cytoplasmic hypertrophy and increased water content. This relatively large amount of water may decrease magnetization transfer by virtue of protein dilution. Repeated episodes of hepatic failure may lead to the development of acquired (non-Wilsonian) hepatocerebral degeneration. The clinical symptoms are permanent and death commonly follows. By imaging, these patients no longer show the typical T1 hyperintensities in the basal ganglia described above for chronic hepatic encephalopathy. Patients with acquired hepatocerebral degeneration show increased T2 signal intensity, particularly in the middle cerebral peduncles (Lee et al. 1998). These zones correspond to spongiform myelinolytic changes, most likely the sequelae of ischemia. These changes are not secondary to osmotic myelinolysis.

12.5.2 Bilirubin Encephalopathy

Kernicterus is now a rare disorder and most cases are the result of isoimmunization to Rh factor or from ABO blood group incompatibility. As such, it is almost always a disease of neonates (Rorke 1998).

Later in life, most cases are due to genetic, hematologic, or liver diseases, such as defects of glucose-6-phosphate-dehydrogenase, Crigler-Najjar disease, Gilbert disease and in rare cases secondary to breast feeding or severe sepsis. In kernicterus, the liver is unable to conjugate bilirubin. The enzyme uridine-diphosphate glucuronyl transferase does not function well and albumin-bound (insoluble) bilirubin cannot be deconjugated into bilirubin diglucuronide or "water soluble" bilirubin. Initially the child appears hypotonic, then he/she becomes hypertonic, and after approximately 1 week the hypotonia returns. On gross brain examination, there is yellow staining of the globus pallidus, mammillary bodies, subthalamic nuclei, and the indusium griseum. In the brainstem, the substantia nigra and some of the cranial nerve nuclei may be involved (Rorke 1998).

The histological findings are identical to those caused by hypoxia and/or hypoglycemia and reflect tissue necrosis. Surrounding inflammatory changes are common. MR imaging has been used to evaluate mostly the sequelae of kernicterus (Erbetta et al. 1998). During the chronic stage there is increased T2 signal intensity in the globus pallidus and in the cerebellar dentate nucleus. These structures are also atrophic (Fig. 12.8). Acutely, babies with kernicterus may show increased T1 signal intensity in the basal ganglia without corresponding T2 weighted abnormalities. I believe that this finding is probably related to acute hepatic insufficiency and may be similar to that seen in adults with chronic liver disease.

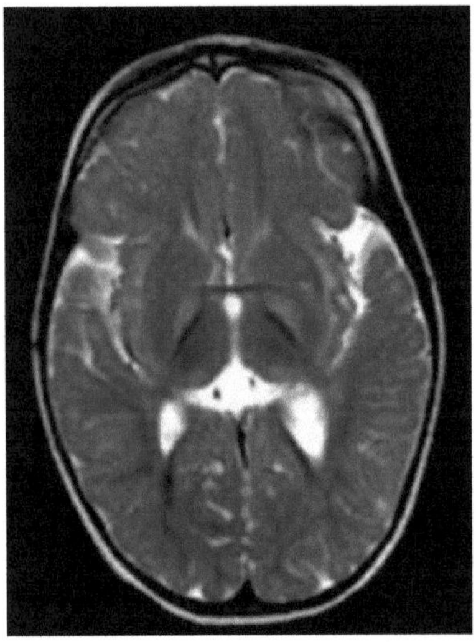

Fig. 12.8. Effects of liver failure. Axial T1-weighted image shows increased symmetrical signal intensity in the lentiform nuclei

12.5.3 Wilson Disease

Wilson disease is a genetic disorder of copper metabolism that is characterized by failure to incorporate copper into ceruloplasmin in the liver, failure to excrete copper by the liver into the bile, and toxic accumulation of copper in multiple organs (Albernaz et al. 1997). The defect has been mapped on chromosome 13 q14.3. In addition, concentrations of other heavy metals such as zinc, iron, silver, and aluminum are also increased. The genetic defect is localized to 13q 14.3 and several mutations have been described (Albernaz et al. 1997). Most children present with hepatic failure while most adults present with neurological symptoms. Accumulation of copper within Descemet's membrane results in the Kayser-Fleischer rings. Accumulation of copper in the lens results in the rare "sunflower" cataracts. Pathologically there is cell loss and cavitation in the lentiform nucleus. Copper concentration at these sites is markedly increased. Other regions involved include the thalamus, subthalamus, red nucleus, substantia nigra, dentate nucleus, and the brainstem. Microscopically, these regions contain large cells with small nuclei (termed Opalski cells) and these are thought to be typical for Wilson disease. Similar to effects of other liver disorders on the brain Alzheimer type II cells are also found in the affect areas. The brain is diffusely atrophic.

MR imaging shows abnormalities even in absence of clinical neurological findings. The paramagnetic effects of copper are visible by MR imaging only in untreated patients (Magalhaes et al. 1994). Basal ganglia lesions are most often bilateral and symmetrical. The putamina shows striking increase in T2 signal intensity (Fig. 12.9a). This is present to a lesser degree in other deep gray matter structures. Thalamic lesions are often present but typically spare the dorsomedial nuclei. White matter tracts including the dentatothalamic, corticospinal, and pontocerebellar tracts are commonly involved. The claustrum may show high T2 signal intensity. The midbrain is bright on T2 weighted images with relative sparing of its deep nuclei giving rise to the so-called Panda sign (Albernaz et al. 1997) (Fig. 12.9b). Although it seems attractive to postulate that high copper concentrations are responsible for the MR imaging findings, this is probably not true. Copper results in T1 and T2 shortening, thus the imaging findings in Wilson disease are probably secondary to spongy degeneration, cavitation, neuronal loss, and reactive astrocytosis. There is a correlation between the clinical and MR

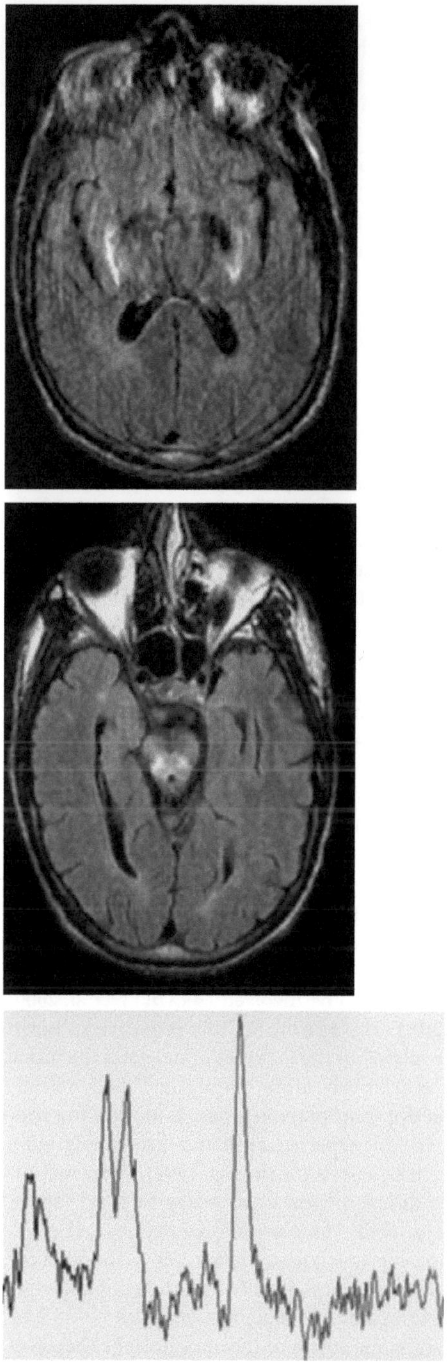

a

b

c

Fig. 12.9a–c. Wilson disease. **a** Axial FLAIR image shows low signal intensity from the globi pallidi and abnormal high signal intensity from the lateral putamina. **b** In the same patient, there is abnormal high signal intensity in the peri-aqueductal region in the midbrain. **c** Long echo time MR spectroscopy shows mildly decreased *N*-acetyl aspartate

imaging findings. An abnormal appearing striatum correlates with pseudoparkinsonism, an abnormal dentatothalamic tract with cerebellar signs, and an abnormal pontocerebellar tract with pseudoparkinsonism. The presence of portosystemic shunting may correlate with abnormalities seen in the globus pallidus. The abnormal T2 signal intensity may improve after copper trapping therapy (King et al. 1996). Contrast enhancement is rare but may be seen when patients are receiving treatment with penicillamine. Positron emission tomography shows diffusely reduced glucose metabolism particularly marked in the caudate nucleus, frontoparietal cortex, and lentiform nucleus (van Wassenaer-van Hall et al. 1996; Engelbrecht et al. 1995). These findings correlate with the severity of the disease and may be reversed following adequate therapy (Hawkins et al. 1987).

12.5.4 Disorders of Iron Metabolism That May Involve the Brain

Although the disorders involving iron metabolism are relatively common (particularly those related to iron deficiencies), their effects on the CNS are few. It is well known that anemia related to chronic and debilitating disorders such as AIDS may result in a spine that appears hypointense on T1 weighted MR imaging. This is presumably due to a compensatory mechanism that leads to storage of iron in the bone marrow. The presence of iron results in a diffuse hypointense appearance of the bone marrow (Kuwert et al. 1992).

Disorders of iron overload are less common than anemias, but occasionally give rise to interesting, albeit uncommon, imaging findings. Iron overload occurs when the iron-binding capacity of transferrin is exceeded or when an increased catabolism of erythrocytes leads to accumulation of iron in the reticuloendothelial and organ cells. Patients with hereditary hemochromatosis have an increased iron intestinal absorption. In the brain, iron is deposited in the pituitary gland and may give rise to abnormal and low endocrine functions. In these patients adenohypophysis may appear as an area of very low or no signal in both T1 and T2 weighted images (Cordato et al. 1998). In a recent article, a ratio of the signal intensity of the pituitary gland to fat was correlated with gland function (Geremia et al. 1989). These authors found that reductions in this ratio correlated with hypogonadotropic hypogonadism and higher ferritin levels. In addition, in these patients the liver is damaged and the brain may show findings related to chronic hepatic encephalopathy. African iron overload (Bantu siderosis) is due to increased ingestion of iron and also may lead to liver failure. Juvenile hemochromatosis is nearly identical to the hereditary type but manifests earlier in life and most patients die young due to heart failure (Sparacia et al. 1999). Transfusional siderosis occurs only after chronic and repeated whole blood transfusions and is more commonly seen in cancer patients and individuals with sickle cell anemia. Aceruloplasminemia is different from Wilson disease (see above) in that ceruloplasmin is completely absent, not just low (Sparacia et al. 2000). Ceruloplasmin has ferroxidase action that is partly responsible for the release of iron from many cells. In the absence of ceruloplasmin, iron accumulates in the basal ganglia and dentate nuclei of the cerebellum, and gives rise to progressive extrapyramidal signs, cerebellar ataxia, and eventually dementia.

Hallervorden-Spatz disease (HS) and Friedreich's ataxia are also related to iron overload and degenerative brain disease. Little is known about the biochemical abnormalities of HS but it has been linked to an abnormality in chromosome 20p12.3-p13. Large amounts of iron are deposited in the globus pallidus and pars reticulata of the substantia nigra (Sparacia et al. 2000). Iron deposition leads to axonal swelling and decreased myelin thickness. Microscopy demonstrates the presence of abnormal, spherical bodies that contain superoxide dismutase and are believed to be typical for HS. Eventually, these regions of the brain are destroyed. Patients with HS demonstrate dystonia, muscle rigidity, hyperreflexia, and choreoathetosis. Mental retardation is variable and death occurs 1–2 years after the diagnosis. Because laboratory findings are non-specific, the combination of clinical symptoms and imaging findings are used to establish a diagnosis. The findings on CT scanning are non-specific and MR is the imaging method of choice. Initially, only hypointensity (more pronounced on T2 than on T1 weighted sequences) is seen in the globus pallidus. When gliosis ensues, the globus pallidus becomes hyperintense on T2 weighted images but remains surrounded by hypointensity. This represents the so-called eye of the tiger sign and is said to be characteristic for HS.

Friedreich's ataxia (FA) is a rare autosomal recessive disorder. It is part of the hereditary ataxic syndromes and will be discussed here because of its possible relation to abnormal iron metabolism. In 97% of patients it is caused by an abnormality located in chromosome 9, which encodes a protein called frataxin which has been localized in the mitochondria, although its function is unknown (Berg et al. 2000). Increased iron deposition is found in the heart, liver and spleen in a pattern consistent with a mitochondrial location. There is iron accumulation, mitochondrial respiratory chain dysfunction and mitochondrial DNA depletion. The spinal cord is pathologically atrophic with damaged white matter tracts. The lumbar and sacral nerves are also atrophic. The cerebellar cortex and the brainstem may also show atrophy. Atrophy of the gray matter in the central sulcus is occasionally evident on gross and imaging examinations.

12.5.5 Hypoglycemia and Hyperglycemia

Most cerebral insults due to hypoglycemia occur in young children. Oxygen and glucose are the major substrates needed for normal brain metabolism and absence of either of both leads to significant injury. Hypoglycemia uncommonly affects the neonatal brain, which is normally fairly resistant to it. Acute symptoms of hypoglycemia include jitteriness, seizures, and vomiting (Hermann et al. 2000). Hypoglycemia is diagnosed when the whole blood glucose concentration falls below 20 mg/dl in preterm babies, 30 mg/dl in term babies, and 45 mg/dl in adults. Sequelae of hypoglycemia are mental retardation, spasticity, visual abnormalities, and microcephaly. In neonates, hypoglycemia leads to diffuse edema and infarctions. Typically, the occipital regions are affected more severely but the basal ganglia may also be involved (Bradley et al. 2000) (Fig. 12.10). The reason for this is not clear, but it may be related to the fact that in neonates the visual cortex is relatively more mature and metabolically more active than other regions, as during the neonatal period it experiences intense axonal migration and synaptogenesis (Spar et al. 1994). Other reasons include diffuse hypoxia secondary to heart failure, loss of cerebral vascular autoregulation, and excitatory toxicity (Aslan and Dinc 1997). Although the gray matter is especially affected, the occipital white matter and posterior thalamus may also be injured. Chronically, the cortex of the occipital lobes becomes thin, malacia develops, and these findings correlate with visual abnormalities. In adults, hypoglycemia may also induce occipital infarctions in addition to infarctions elsewhere (which are generally multiple), laminar necrosis, and transient imaging abnormalities.

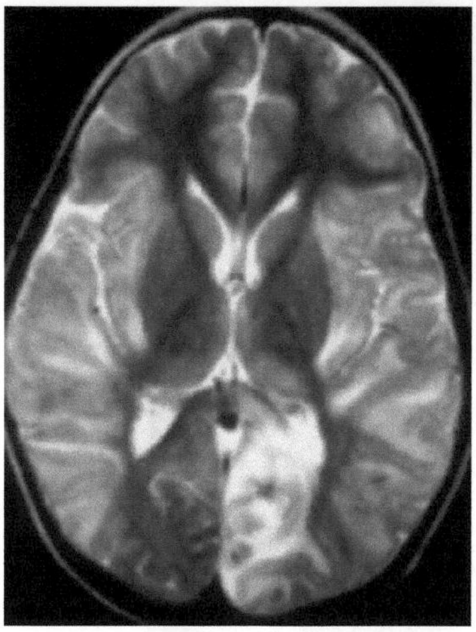

Fig. 12.10. Hypoglycemia. Axial T2-weighted image shows infarctions in the territories of both middle and the left posterior cerebral arteries

Hyperglycemia also has adverse affects on the CNS. Hyperglycemia may lead to increases in cerebral lactic acid, which may damage the brain primarily or worsen the outcome of patients with underlying infarctions. A typical manifestation, and at times the initial one, of hyperglycemia is hemichorea-hemiballism (HH). The clinical manifestation of HH are random and fast jerking motion in the distal extremities (chorea) and violent flinging and kicking, mainly involving the proximal joints (ballismus) (Kinnala et al. 1999). In these patients, CT shows high density conforming to one lentiform nucleus and the head of the ipsilateral caudate nucleus (Fig. 12.11a). These regions are of increased signal intensity on MR T1 weighted images, and T2 weighted images are normal or show only slightly high T2 signal intensity (Fig. 12.11b,c). Occasionally, the ipsilateral cerebral peduncle may also show T1 hyperintensity in its anteromedial region (Kinnala et al. 1999). Hemorrhage and/or calcifications have not been reported in HH and the findings are thought to be due to the presence of gemistocytes. MR spectroscopy obtained from the region of T1 signal intensity abnormality demonstrates elevated lactic acid and decreased creatine. These features have been interpreted as being due to depletion of energy leading to neuronal malfunction. Although the above described MR abnormalities are fairly typical for HH, they have also been noted in a patient with lupus erythematosus and chorea (Barkovich et al. 1998).

12.6 Disorders Affecting Gray and White Matter

12.6.1 Mitochondrial Disorders

Mitochondrial encephalopathies are relatively rare disorders involving a defect in the oxidative respira-

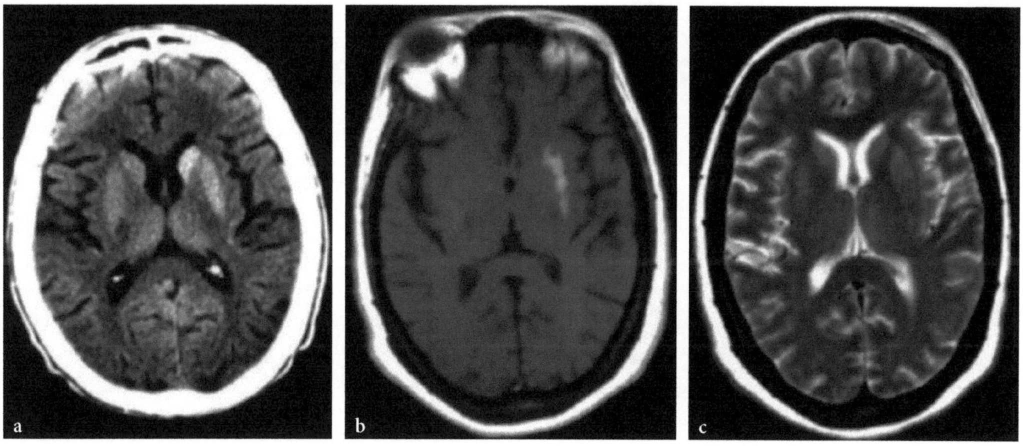

Fig. 12.11a–c. Hemiballismus, hemichorea in hyperglycemia. **a** Axial CT image shows increased density in the left basal ganglia. **b** In a different patient, axial T1-weighted image shows increased signal intensity in the left putamen. **c** Corresponding T2-weighted image shows subtle high signal intensity in the same location

tory mechanism (usually due to impaired production of adenosine triphosphate) that leads to accumulation of lactic acid. Lactic acid may then be detected in serum or in the CSF on laboratory studies or by proton MR spectroscopy (Shan et al. 1998). Although most patients begin to have symptoms during childhood, some may present when they are adults. Most mitochondrial disorders affect the skeletal muscles and brain and as such most present with weakness and seizures (due to ischemia) (Kashihara et al. 1998). Mitochondrial disorders and organic acidurias share many biochemical and clinical features. The most common mitochondrial disease is MELAS (mitochondrial myopathy, encephalopathy, lactic acidosis, and strokes) that results in large non-territorial cerebral infarctions (including the basal ganglia and thalami) (Castillo et al. 1995) (Fig. 12.12). It more commonly manifests during the second decade of life, and strokes are the result of impaired function of the muscle in the walls of cerebral arteries. Pathologically there is spongy degeneration, neuronal loss, gliosis, and microcystic liquefaction in the affected regions.

MERFF is characterized by myoclonic epilepsy and its imaging findings are identical to those described for MELAS. Leigh disease (subacute necrotizing encephalomyelopathy) is due to pyruvate and cytochrome C oxidase deficiencies (Allard et al. 1988). This disease is usually diagnosed during the first year of life. It produces abnormalities in the basal ganglia,

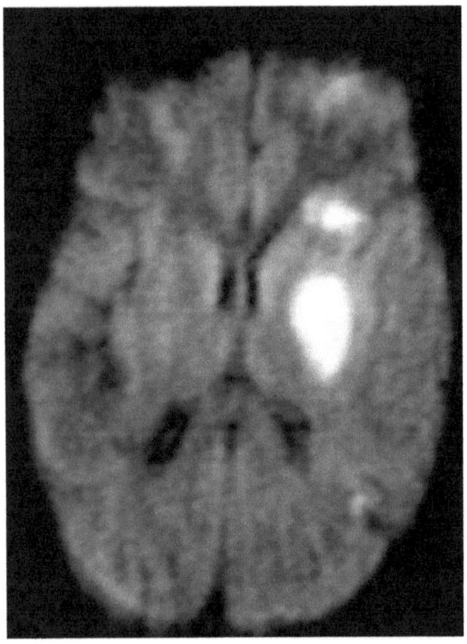

Fig. 12.12. Mitochondriopathy of the MELAS type. Axial trace diffusion-weighted image shows acute infarction confined mostly to the left lentiform nucleus

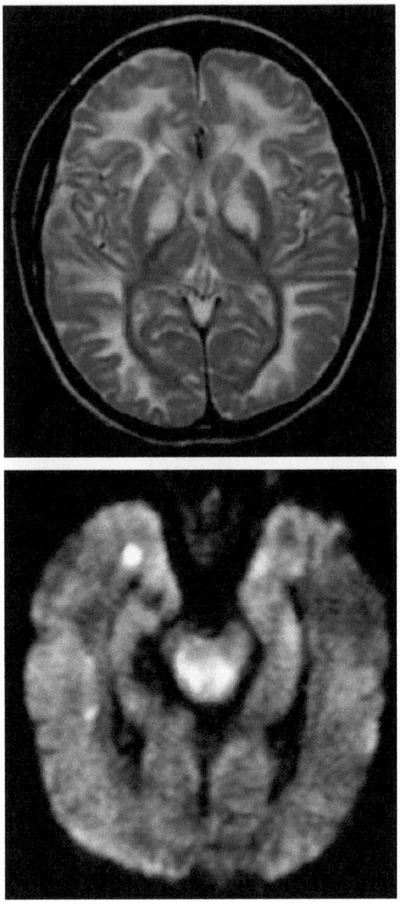

a

b

Fig. 12.13a,b. Mitochondriopathy of the Leigh type. **a** Axial T2-weighted image shows abnormal high signal intensity in all of the white matter and in the medial lentiform nuclei and thalami. **b** In the same patient, axial trace diffusion-weighted image shows increased signal intensity in the peri-aqueductal region of the midbrain

the periaqueductal gray matter, and the subcortical white matter (Kim et al. 1996) (Fig. 12.13a,b).

Kearns-Sayre syndrome is characterized by abnormalities in the basal ganglia and in the white matter (which are extensive) (Medina et al. 1990). The typical clinical findings in these patients are ophthalmoplegia and cardiac conduction abnormalities. Pathologically there is capillary proliferation, necrosis, vacuolization, and demyelination of the affected areas. The MR imaging findings are extensive and include involvement of all deep gray matter structures (high T2 signal intensity) and extensive increased T2 signal in the white matter.

12.6.2 Amino Acidurias

Although amino acid disorders are not true leukodystrophies, they affect predominantly the white matter. In these disorders there is an abnormal formation of proteolipids that are needed to form normal myelin. The most common disorders in this group are: phenylketonuria (PKU) (non-specific white matter changes and atrophy on MR imaging), maple syrup disease (white matter and basal ganglia shows high T2 signal on MR imaging), homocystinuria (strokes and arterial occlusions on MRI and MRA respectively), and glutaric (dilated sylvian fissures and increased T2 signal in the basal ganglia and thalami), methylmalonic, and propionic acidurias (both show increased T2 signal in the deep gray matter structures and hemispheric white matter) (Paltiel et al. 1987; Demange et al. 1989; Shaw et al. 1991; Brismar et al. 1990b; Ruano et al. 1998; Brismar and Ozand 1995; Hald et al. 1991). Because of the neonatal screening for PKU mandated by law, this disorder is no longer as severe as it used to be. Patients with PKU are promptly started with a special diet and the imaging findings are mild (Paltiel et al. 1987). Glutaric aciduria type 1 (type 2 is very rare) is the one that classically results in cyst formation in the regions of the sylvian fissures (some believe that these are arachnoid cysts while others believe that they are the reflection of underlying temporal lobe hypoplasia), white matter abnormalities, and basal ganglia abnormalities (Brismar et al. 1990b; Ruano et al. 1998) (Fig. 12.14a,b). Methylmalonic acidemia results in extensive white matter abnormalities and characteristically high T2 signal intensity in the globi pallidi (Brismar and Ozand 1995; Hald et al. 1991). The findings in propionic aciduria are similar to those seen in methylmalonic aciduria (Brismar and Ozand 1995). Many of these disorders will show a dramatic improvement on MRI after a few weeks of treatment. The myelination milestones are delayed in all of these disorders. Proton MR spectroscopy generally shows several peaks between 1.5 and 2.5 parts per million (ppm) which are thought to represent abnormal accumulation of amino acids and low NAA. In my opinion, it is extremely difficult to suggest these diagnoses based on imaging findings.

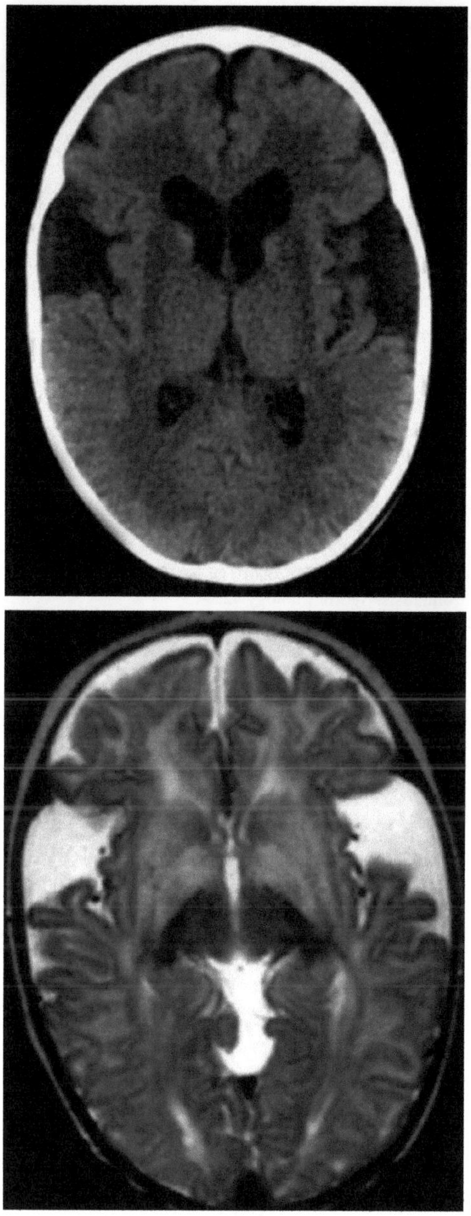

a

b

Fig. 12.14a,b. Glutaric aciduria type 1. **a** Axial CT shows prominent sylvian fissures and low density from the periventricular white matter and putamina. **b** Axial T2-weighted image in a different patient shows wide sylvian fissures and high signal intensity in the white matter and basal ganglia bilaterally

References

Albernaz VS, Castillo M, Mukherji SK, Siatkowski RM, Naidich TP (1997) Facies to remember, number 11, part I: the challenge. Int J Neuroradiol 3:206-217

Allard JC, Tilak S, Carter AP (1988) CT and MR of MELAS syndrome. AJNR 9:1234-1238

Alorayni IA, Patenaude YG, O'Gorman AM, Black DN, Meagher-Villemure K (1999) Cree leukoencephalopathy: neuroimaging findings. Radiol 213: 400-406

Andreula CF, De Blasi R, Carella A (1991) CT and MR studies of methylmalonic acidemia. AJNR Am J Neuroradiol 12:410-412

Aslan Y, Dinc H (1997) MR findings of neonatal hypoglycemia. AJNR Am J Neuroradiol 18:994-995

Barkovich AJ, Ferreiro DM, Bass N, Boyer R (1994) Involvement of the pontomedullary corticospinal tracts: a useful finding in the diagnosis of X-linked adrenoleukodystrophy. AJNR Am J Neuroradiol 15:1767-1771

Barkovich AJ, Ali FA, Rowley HA, Bass N (1998) Imaging patterns of neonatal hypoglycemia. AJNR Am J Neuroradiol 19:523-528

Berg D, Hoggenmuller U, Hofmann E, Fischer R, Kraus M, Scheurlen M, Becker G (2000) The basal ganglia in haemochromatosis. Neuroradiology 42:9-13

Bradley JL, Blake JC, Chamberlain S, Thomas PK, Cooper JM, Schapira AHV (2000) Clinical, biochemical and molecular genetic correlations in Freidreich's ataxia. Hum Mol Genet 9:275-282

Brismar J, Ozand PT (1995) CT and MR of the brain in glutaric acidemia type I: a review of 59 published cases and a report of 5 new patients. AJNR Am J Neuroradiol 16:675-683

Brismar J, Brismar G, Gascon G, Ozand P (1990a) Canavan disease: CT and MR imaging of the brain. AJNR Am J Neuroradiol 11:805-810

Brismar J, Aqueel A, Brismar G, Coates R, Gascon G, Ozand P (1990b) Maple syrup urine disease: findings on CT and MR scans of the brain in 10 infants. AJNR Am J Neuroradiol 11:1219-1228

Castillo M, Kwock, Green C (1995) MELAS syndrome: imaging and proton MR spectroscopic findings. AJNR Am J Neuroradiol 16:233-239

Choi S, Enzmann DR (1993) Infantile Krabbe disease: complementary CT and MR findings. AJNR Am J Neuroradiol 14:1164-1666

Cordato DJ, Fulham MJ, Yiannikas C (1998) Pretreatment and posttreatment positron emission tomographic scan imaging in a 20-year-old patient with Wilson's disease. Mov Disord 13:162-166

Demange P, Pham Gia H, Kalifa G, Sellier N (1989) MR of Kearns-Sayre syndrome. AJNR 10[5 Suppl]:S91

Engelbrecht V, Schlaug G, Hefter H, Kahn T, Modder U (1995) MRI of the brain in Wilson disease: T2 signal loss under therapy. J Comput Assist Tomogr 19:635-638

Erbetta A, Ciceri E, Chiapparini L, Botteon G, Erba A, Nardocci N, Savoiardo M (1998) Magnetic resonance imaging findings in bilirubin encephalopathy. Int J Neuroradiol 4:161-164

Etsuo I, Shinichi H, Narumi Y, Fujita M, Kuriyama K, Kadota T, Kuroda T (1991) Portal-systemic encephalopathy: presence of basal ganglia lesions with high signal intensity on MR images. Radiology 179:551-555

Fell JME, Reynolds AP, Meadows N, Khan K, Long SG, Quaghebeur G, Taylor WJ, Milla PJ (1996) Manganese toxicity in children receiving long-term parenteral nutrition. Lancet 347:1218-1221

Finelli DA, Tarr RW, Sawyer RN, Horwitz SJ (1994) Deceptively normal MR in early infantile Krabbe disease. AJNR Am J Neuroradiol 15:167-171

Gebarski SS, Gabrielsen TO, Knake JE, Latack JT (1983) Cerebral CT findings in methylmalonic acid propionic acidemas. AJNR Am J Neuroradiol 4:955-957

Geremia GK, Mccluney K, Adler S, Charletta D, Hoile R, Huckman M, Ramsey R (1989) The magnetic-resonance hypointense spine of AIDS. AJNR Am J Neuroradiol 10:880-881

Hald JK, Nakstad PH, Skjeldal, Stromme P (1991) Bilateral arachnoid cysts of the temporal fossa in four children with glutaric aciduria type I. AJNR Am J Neuroradiol 12:407-409

Hawkins RA, Mazziotta JC, Phelps ME (1987) Wilson's disease studied with FDG and positron emission tomography. Neurology 37:1707-1711

Hermann W, Reuter M, Barthel H, Dietrich J, Georgi P, Wagner A (2000) Diagnosis of Hallervorden-Spatz disease using MRI, I-123-beta-CIT-SPECT and I-123-IBZM-SPECT. Eur Neurol 43:187-188

Hittmair K, Wimberger D, Wiesbauer P, Zehetmayer M, Budka H (1994) Early infantile form of Krabbe disease with optic hypertrophy: serial MR examinations and autopsy correlation. AJNR Am J Neuroradiol 15:1454-1458

Ho VB, Fitz CR, Yoder CC, Geyer CA (1993) Resolving MR features in osmotic myelinolysis (central pontine and extrapontine myelinolysis). AJNR Am J Neuroradiol 14:163-167

Inoue Y, Fukuda T, Takashima S, Ochi H, Onoyama Y, Kusuda S, Matsuoka O, Murata R (1983) Adrenoleukodystrophy: new CT findings. AJNR Am J Neuroradiol 4:951-954

Iwasa M, Kinosada Y, Nakatsuka A, Watanabe S, Adachi Y (1999) Magnetization transfer contrast of various regions of the brain in liver cirrhosis. AJNR Am J Neuroradiol 20:652-654

Jensen ME, Sawyer RW, Braun IF, Rizzo WB (1990) MR Imaging appearance of childhood adrenoleukodystrophy with auditory, visual, and motor pathway involvement. Radiographics 10:53-66

Johnson MA, Desai S, Hugh-Jones K, Starer F (1984) Magnetic resonance imaging of the brain in Hurler syndrome. AJNR Am J Neuroradiol 5:816-819

Kashihara K, Nakashima S, Kohira I, Shohmori T, Fujiwara Y, Kuroda S (1998) Hyperintense basal ganglia on T1-weighted MR images in a patient with central nervous system lupus and chorea. AJNR Am J Neuroradiol 19:284-286

Kim IO, Kim JH, Kim WS, Hwang YS, Yeon KM, Hang MC (1996) Mitochondrial myopathy-encephalopathy-lactic acidosis and strokelike episodes (MELAS) syndrome: CT and MR findings in seven children. AJR 166:641-645

Kim TS, Kim IO, Kim WS, Choi YS, Lee JY, Kim OW, Yeon KM, Kim KJ, Hwang YS (1997) MR of childhood metachromatic leukodystrophy. AJNR Am J Neuroradiol 18:733-738

King AD, Walshe JM, Kendall BE, Chinn RJS, Paley MNJ, Wilkinson ID, Halligan S, Hall-Craggs MA (1996) Cranial MR imaging in Wilson's disease. AJR 167:1579-1584

Kinnala A, Rikalainen H, Lapinleimu H, Parkkola R, Kormano M, Kero P (1999) Cerebral magnetic resonance imaging and ultrasonography findings after neonatal hypoglycemia. Pediatrics 103:724-729

Korogi Y, Takahashi M, Shinzato J, Sakamoto Y, Mitsuzaki K,

Hirai T, Yoshizumi (1993) MR findings in two presumed cases of mild central pontine myelinolysis. AJNR Am J Neuroradiol 14:651-654
Krieger D, Krieger S, Jansen O, Gass P, Theilmann L, Lichtnecker H (1995) Manganese and chronic hepatic encephalopathy. Lancet 346:270-274
Kumar AJ, Rosenbaum AE, Naidu S, Wener L, Citrin CM, Lindenberg R, Kim WS, Zinreich SJ, Molliver ME, Mayberg HS, Moser HW (1987) Adrenoleukodystrophy: correlating MR imaging with CT. Radiol 165:495-504
Kuwert T, Hefter H, Scholz D, Mitz M, Weiss P, Arendt G et al (1992) Regional cerebral glucose consumption measured by positron emission tomography in patients with Wilson's disease. Eur J Nucl Med 19:96-101
Lee C, Dineen TE, Brack M, Kirsch JE, Runge VM (1995) The muccopolysaccharidoses: characterization by cranial MR imaging. AJNR Am J Neuroradiol 16:1402-1403
Lee J, Lacomis D, Comu S, Jacobsohn J, Kanal E (1998) Acquired hepatocerebral degeneration: MR and pathologic findings. AJNR Am J Neuroradiol 19:485-487
Loes DJ, Hite S, Moser H, Stillman AE, Shapiro E, Lockman L, Latchaw RE, Krivit W (1994) Adrenoleukodystrophy: a scoring method for brain MR observations. AJNR Am J Neuroradiol 15:1761-1776
Magalhaes ACA, Caramelli P, Menezes JR, Lo LS, Bacheschi LA, Barbosa ER, Rosemberg LA (1994) Wilson's disease: MRI with clinical correlation. Neuroradiology 36:97-100
McAdams HP, Geyer CA, Done SL, Deigh D, Mitchell M, Ghaed VN (1990) CT and MR imaging of Canavan disease. AJNR Am J Neuroradiol 11:397-399
Medina L, Chi TL, DeVivo DC, Hilal SK (1990) MR findings in patients with subacute necrotizing encephalomyelopathy (Leigh syndrome): correlation with biochemical defect. AJNR Am J Neuroradiol 11:379-384
Melhem ER, Breiter SN, Ulug AM, Raymond GV, Moser HW (1996) Improved tissue characterization in adrenoleukodystrophy using magnetization transfer imaging. AJR 166:689-695
Mirowitz SA, Westrich TJ (1992) Basal ganglial signal intensity alterations: reversal after discontinuation of parenteral manganese administration. Radiology 185:535-536
Okamoto K, Ito J, Furusawa T, Sakai K, Tokiguchi S (1998) Reversible hyperintensity of the anterior pituitary gland on T1-weighted MR images in a patient receiving temporary parenteral nutrition. AJNR Am J Neuroradiol 19:1287-1289
Paltiel HJ, O'Gorman AM, Meagher-Villemure K, Rosenblatt B, Silver K, Watters GV (1987) Subacute necrotizing encephalomyelopathy (Leigh disease): CT study. Radiology 162:115-118
Pomier-Layrargues G, Spahr L, Butterworth RF (1995) Increased manganese concentrations in pallidum of cirrhotic patients. Lancet 345:735
Price DB, Kramer J, Hotson GC, Loh JP (1987) Central pontine myelinolysis: report of a case with distinctive appearance on MR imaging. AJNR Am J Neuroradiol 8:576-577
Rajanayagam V, Grad J, Krivit W, Loes DJ, Lockman L, Shapiro E, Balthazor M, Aeppli D, Stillman AE (1996) Proton MR spectroscopy of childhood adrenoleukodystrophy. AJNR Am J Neuroradiol 17:1013-1024
Rajanayagam V, Balthazor M, Shapiro E, Krivit W, Lockman L, Stillman AE (1997) Proton MR spectroscopy and neuropsychological testing in adrenoleukodystrophy. AJNR Am J Neuroradiol 18:1909-1914
Rorke L (1998) Neuropathologic findings in bilirubin encephalopathy (Kernicterus). Int J Neuroradiol 4:165-170
Rosenbloom S, Buchholz D, Kumar AJ, Kaplan RA, Moses H 3d, Rosenbaum AE (1984) Evolution of central pontine myelinolysis on CT. AJNR Am J Neuroradiol 5:110-112
Ross BD, Jacobson S, Villamil F, Korula J, Kreis R, Ernst T, Shonk T, Moats RA (1994) Subclinical hepatic encephalopathy: proton MR spectroscopic abnormalities. Radiology 193:457-463
Ruano MM, Castillo M, Thompson JE (1998) MR imaging in a patient with homocystinuria. AJR 171:1147-1149
Shan DE, Ho DMT, Chang C, Pan HC, Teng MMH (1998) Hemichorea-hemiballism: an explanation for MR signal changes. AJNR Am J Neuroradiol 19:863-870
Shaw DW, Maravilla KR, Weinberger E, Garretson J, Trahms CM, Scott CR (1991) MR imaging of phenylketonuria. AJNR Am J Neuroradiol 12:403-406
Silverstein AM, Hirsch DK, Trobe JD, Gebarski SS (1990) MR imaging of the brain in five members of a family with Pelizaeus-Merzbacher disease. AJNR Am J Neuroradiol 11:495-499
Snyder RD, King JN, Keck GM, Orrison WW (1991) MR imaging of the spinal cord in 23 subjects with ALD-AMN complex. AJNR Am J Neuroradiol 12:1095-1098
Spar JA, Lewine JD, Orrison WW Jr (1994) Neonatal hypoglycemia: CT and MR findings. AJNR Am J Neuroradiol 15:1477-1478
Sparacia G, Midiri M, D'Angelo P, Lagalla R (1999) Magnetic resonance imaging of the pituitary gland in patients with secondary hypogonadism due to transfusional hemochromatosis. Magma 8:87-90
Sparacia G, Iaia A, Banco A, D'Angelo P, Lagalla R (2000) Transfusional hemochromatosis: quantitative relation of MR imaging pituitary signal intensity reduction to hypogonadotropic hypogonadism. Radiology 215:818-823
Stillman AE, Krivit W, Shapiro E, Lockman L, Latchaw RE (1994) Serial MR after bone marrow transplantation in two patients with metachromatic leukodystrophy. AJNR Am J Neuroradiol 15:1929-1932
Sztencel J, Baleriaux D, Borenstein S, Brunko E, Zegers de Beyl D (1983) Central pontine myelinolysis: correlation between CT and electrophysiologic data. AJNR Am J Neuroradiol 4:529-530
Van der Knaap MS, Valk J (1989) The reflection of histology in MR imaging of Pelizaeus-Merzbacher disease. AJNR Am J Neuroradiol 18:99-103
Van der Knaap MS, Breiter SN, Naidu S, Hart AAM, Valk J (1999) Defining and categorizing leukoencephalopathies of unknown origin: MR imaging approach. Radiology 213:121-133
Van der Knaap MS, Naidu S, Breiter SN et al (2001) Alexander disease: diagnosis with MR imaging. AJNR Am J Neuroradiol 22:541-552
Van Wassenaer-van Hall HN, van den Heuvel AG, Algra A, Hoogenraad TU, Mali WPTM (1996) Wilson disease: findings at MR imaging and CT of the brain with clinical correlation. Radiology 198:531-536
Vanhanen SL, Raininko R, Santavuori P (1994) Early differential diagnosis of infantile neuronal ceroid lipofuscinosis, Rett syndrome, and Krabbe disease by CT and MR. AJNR Am J Neuroradiol 15:1443-1453
Wetzburger CL, Van Regemorter N, Szliwowski HB, Abramowicz MJ, van Bogaert P (1998) Gray matter heterotopia and acute necrotizing encephalopathy in trichothiodystrophy. Pediatr Neurol 19:392-394

13 Proton MR Spectroscopy in Metabolic Disorders of the Central Nervous System

NICOLA DE STEFANO and MARZIA MORTILLA

CONTENTS

13.1 Introduction

The advent of magnetic resonance (MR) imaging (MRI) has revolutionized the clinical approach to the evaluation of the metabolic disorders affecting the cerebral white matter and has contributed significantly to the expansion of these diseases. The clinical importance of MRI in the management of patients with metabolic disorders lies in its great sensitivity for detecting brain white matter lesions. However, in these disorders the detected lesions can be due to a variety of pathological processes and can be associated with many different types of myelin abnormality (demyelinization, hypomyelinization, myelin rarefaction, etc.) (KOLODNY 1993).

On clinical grounds, the diagnostic work-up of a given metabolic disease is particularly challenging. This is due to both extreme variability of the clinical picture and heterogeneity of the underlying pathology. Unfortunately, the white matter lesions detected on MRI are often not characteristic enough to allow the diagnosis of these complex disorders (VAN DER KNAAP et al. 1991). Lack of specificity of conventional MRI and its limitations in analyzing the nature of the lesions can account, at least in part, for the significant amount of patients with focal or diffuse white matter pathology that cannot fit the criteria for any defined disorder (VAN DER KNAAP et al. 1991; SCHIFFMANN and VAN DER KNAAP 2004).

In recent years, nonconventional MR techniques have been used to complement conventional MRI and overcome some of its limitations. Among these, MR spectroscopy (MRS) techniques have proven to offer additional information and have been particularly useful in patients with metabolic disorders as they can simultaneously provide chemical-pathological correlates of changes occurring within and outside visible MRI lesions. Thus, an expanding number of research groups have been using single-voxel proton MRS and multivoxel MR spectroscopic imaging (MRSI) in vivo to study patients with metabolic disorders involving the cerebral white matter (ARNOLD and MATTHEWS 1996; DE STEFANO et al. 2000b; VAN DER KNAAP 2001). These MRS techniques have demonstrated to increase diagnostic accuracy and the understanding of the evolution of pathology in many leukoencephalopathies. However, the increasing use of proton MRS techniques in white matter diseases also has revealed that most of the metabolic changes detected in these disorders are not disease-specific.

Metabolic changes of several white matter pathologies as detected by proton MRS techniques and their clinical interpretation are reported below. As mentioned before, the group of white matter diseases with inherited or acquired metabolic abnormalities is very heterogeneous and includes pathologies with different pathogenesis. Here, we will simply give an overview on MRS changes of the most frequently studied metabolic disorders affecting the cerebral white matter.

13.2 Proton MRS Changes in Demyelinating and Dysmyelinating Diseases

Myelinogenesis is a complex process that can be altered by various hereditary metabolic defects result-

N. DE STEFANO, MD, PhD
Associate Professor, Department of Neurology and Behavioral Sciences, University of Siena, Viale Bracci 2, 53100 Siena, Italy
M. MORTILLA, MD
Department of Radiology, Children Hospital Anna Meyer, Florence, Italy

ing in disorders that are generically grouped under the term of leukodystrophies. This congenital failure in myelinogenesis is comprehensive of several mechanisms of myelin disruption such as hypomyelination, demyelination, myelin rarefaction, etc., and is due to very different genetic and biochemical abnormalities, most of which are still undefined (Kolodny 1993).

Proton MR spectra of the normal human brain at long echo time reveal four major resonances: a large signal from N-acetyl groups [mainly *N*-acetyl aspartate (NAA)], a smaller resonance from choline-containing phospholipids (Cho), a resonance from creatine and phosphocreatine (Cr), and a doublet from lactate (Lac) (Arnold and Matthews 1996). Excellent spectra also can be obtained using short echo time measurements, which allow the detection of a greater number of metabolites [including lipids and myo-inositol (mI)] (Arnold and Matthews 1996).

Changes in all of these metabolites can be seen within demyelinating lesions since the very early phase of the pathological process (de Stefano et al. 1995a) (Fig. 13.1a). Changes in the resonance intensity of Cho result mainly from increases in the steady state levels of phosphocholine and glycerolphosphocholine, both membrane phospholipids released during active myelin breakdown. Increases in Lac are likely to reflect the metabolism of inflammatory cells. In large, acute demyelinating lesions, decreases in Cr can also be seen (de Stefano et al. 1995a). Short echo time spectra give evidence for transient increases in mI (Koopmans et al. 1993) and lipids (Narayana et al. 1998), also released during myelin breakdown.

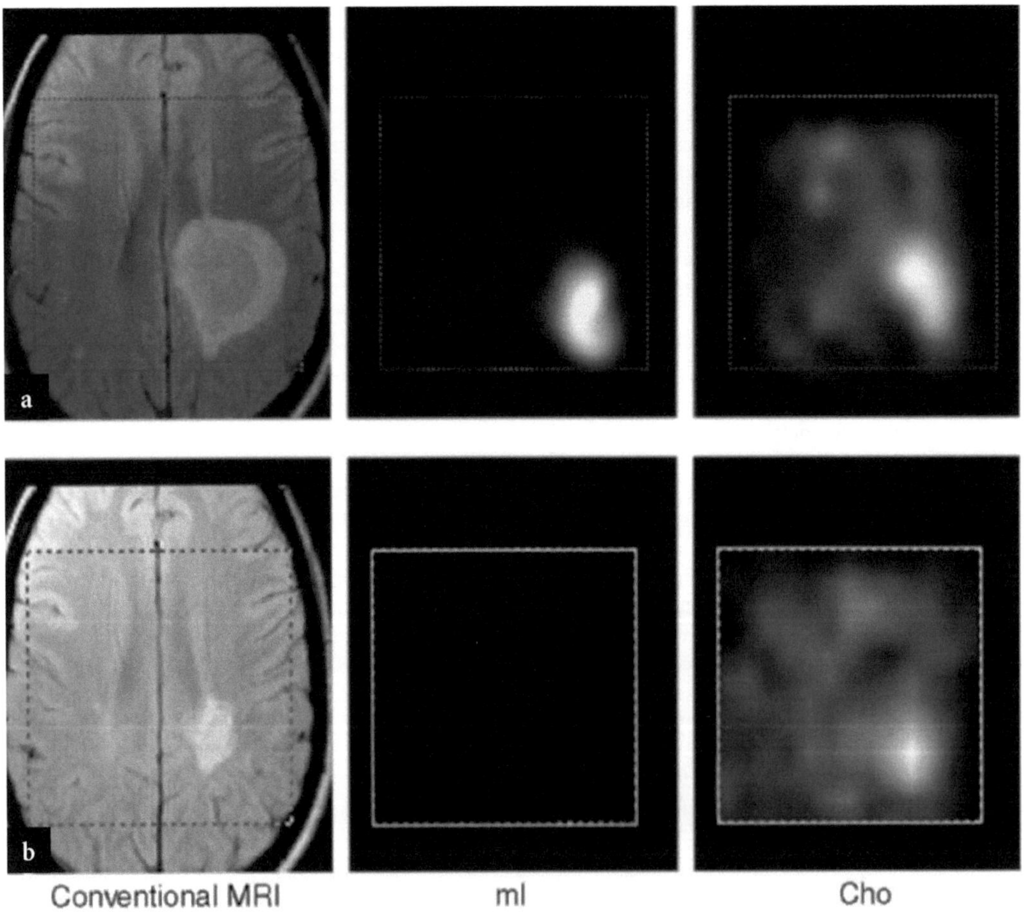

Fig. 13.1a,b. Conventional brain MRI in transversal orientation and spectroscopic images of myo-inositol (*mI*), choline (*Cho*), creatine (*Cr*), N-acetylaspartate (*NAA*) and lactate (*Lac*) of a patient with a single giant demyelinating lesion during acute (**a**) and chronic (**b**) stages. **a** During the acute stage, images of the different metabolites show focal increases in mI, Cho and Lac and

After the acute phase, metabolic modifications in the demyelinating lesion show a variable time course (DE STEFANO et al. 1995a) (Fig. 13.1b). Usually, resonance intensities of Cr and lipids return to normal within a few days. At this stage, small changes in Cr, due to changes in cellularity, can be found inside the demyelinating lesion (DAVIES et al. 1995). Resonance intensities of Lac show a progressive reduction over a period of weeks, whereas Cho and mI return to normal in months. The signal intensity of NAA remains decreased or may show a partial recovery (DE STEFANO et al. 1995b). Recovery of NAA may be related to resolution of edema, increases in the diameter of previously shrunken axons that are secondary to remyelination and clearance of inflammatory factors, and reversible metabolic changes in neurons (DE STEFANO et al. 1995b).

In slowly progressive disorders, such as many leukodystrophies, the loss of myelin can be very slow and released membrane phospholipids might not accumulate. Thus, MRS changes such as those detected in acute demyelination are not seen. In some cases, however, (i.e., adrenoleukodystrophy, Krabbe disease) the high membrane turnover may cause long-term increases in Cho (KRUSE et al. 1993; DE STEFANO et al. 2000a). In contrast, a decrease in Cho that is secondary to hypomyelination or vacuolar myelinopathy can be detected in spongiform leukoencephalopathies (VAN DER KNAAP et al. 1995, 1997; AUSTIN et al. 1991; GRODD et al. 1990) or mitochondrial disorders (MATTHEWS et al. 1993).

A number of brain MRS studies of patients with white matter disorders have also shown changes in the relative resonance intensity of mI. The function

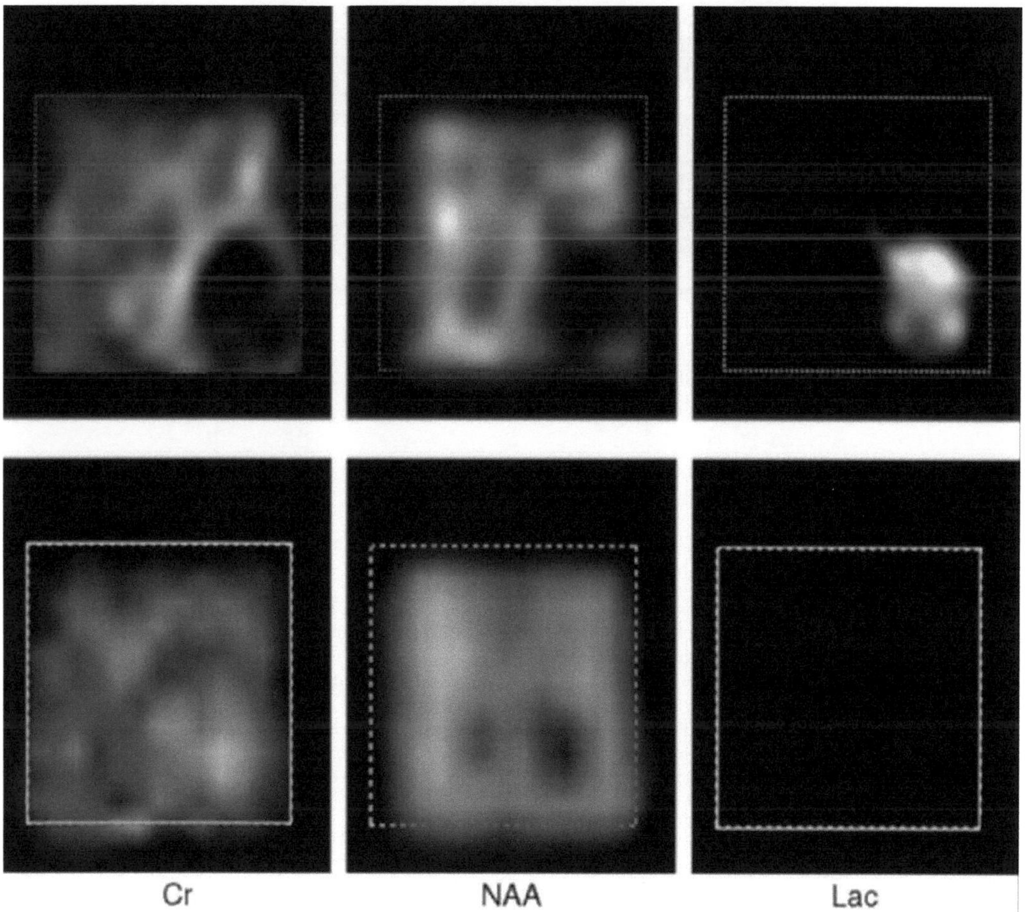

decreases in NAA and Cr that co-localize with the MRI lesion. **b** The examination performed 15 months later shows a reduction of the MRI lesion and normalization of mI, Cho, Cr and Lac metabolic images. NAA shows a partial recovery

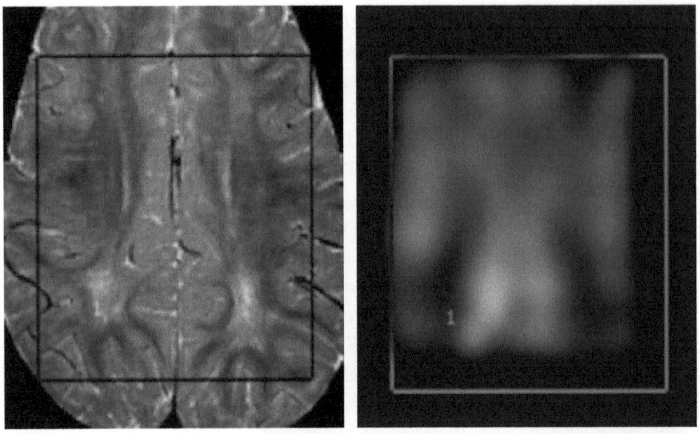

Fig. 13.2a,b. Conventional brain MRI in transversal orientation (**a**) and spectroscopic image of *N*-acetylaspartate (NAA) (**b**) of a patient with unknown leukoencephalopathy. The volume of interest of the multivoxel spectroscopic examination is shown in both images. In the metabolic image of NAA (**b**), note the decreases of the metabolite co-localized (1) with the white matter abnormalities on conventional MRI

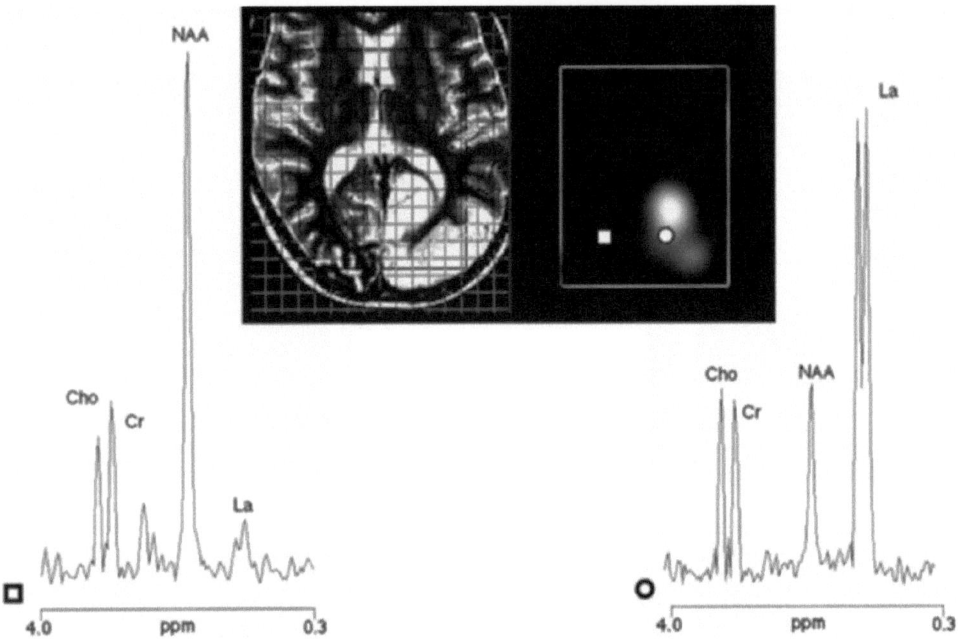

Fig. 13.3. Conventional brain MRI in transversal orientation (*central-left panel*) and spectroscopic image of lactate (*La*) relative to a patient with mitochondrial encephalopathy with lactic acidosis and stroke-like episodes during an acute attack of the disease (*central-right panel*). The grid of the spectroscopic volume of interest is shown in the transverse MRI. The conventional MR image shows the hyperintense signal in the right occipital region due to the recent stroke-like episode. Proton spectra from a voxel localized in the stroke-like region (*circle*) and in a homologous voxel of the contralateral hemisphere are also shown (*square*). The proton spectrum from a voxel localized to the stroke-like region shows a large decrease in *N*-acetylaspartate (*NAA*) and a striking increase in lactate. These changes are not found in the homologous voxel of the contralateral hemisphere

of mI in the human brain is not clear, but increases of this metabolite seem to be related to the presence of white matter gliosis and appear consistently in disorders associated with impaired myelination such as adrenoleukodystrophy, metachromatic leukodystrophies, phenylketonuria and Zellweger syndrome (Bruhn et al. 1992; Johannik et al. 1994; Kruse et al. 1993; Tzika et al. 1993).

Finally, a constant finding of all metabolic disorders affecting the brain white matter is the large decrease in cerebral NAA (de Stefano et al. 2000b) (Fig. 13.2). As NAA is found almost exclusively in neu-

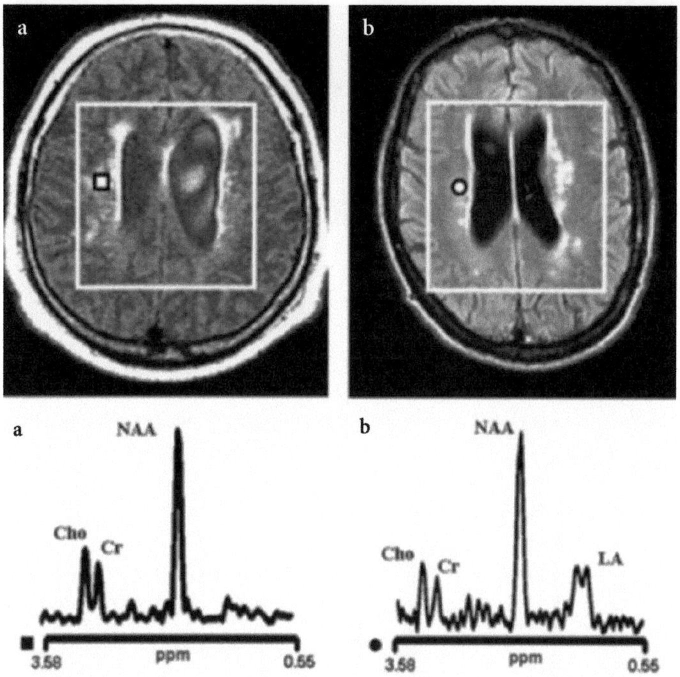

Fig. 13.4a,b. Conventional MRI of two elderly patients (over 70 year of age) with hypertension, loss of memory, previous cerebral transitory ischemic attacks (**a**, **b**) and their proton MR spectra coming from voxels localized to the deep periventricular white matter (*square* and *circle*, respectively). The volume of interest of the multi-voxel spectroscopic examination is shown in both images. In both patients, conventional MRI shows periventricular lesions suggestive of leukoaraiosis. In one patient (*right*), there is high resonance intensity of lactate (*LA*) in the proton spectrum. This patient was subsequently diagnosed as having MELAS (mitochondrial encephalopathy with lactic acidosis and stroke-like episodes), despite a stroke-like episode never being reported in the clinical history. The other patient (*left*) does not show changes in lactate resonance intensity and was subsequently diagnosed as having initial cerebrovascular dementia

rons and their processes in mature brains decreases in this metabolite are interpreted as an index of axonal damage (Matthews et al. 1998; Bjartmar et al. 2002). This is most likely due to a secondary axonal dysfunction and/or loss, suggestive of the relevance of neuro-axonal damage in both demyelinating and dysmyelinating disorders. Recent studies suggest that NAA may provide a surrogate measure that can be relevant to clinical disability in patients with several white matter disorders (de Stefano et al. 2000b).

13.3 Diagnostic-Specific MRS Changes in WM Disorders

As already mentioned, most of the metabolic changes detected in white matter disorders are not disease-specific. However, in some specific circumstances, proton MRS can offer information useful for the differential diagnosis beyond what is currently available in routine clinical use or can even provide typical brain metabolic patterns characteristic of a given disorder.

As proton MRS can provide a specific and accurate interpretation of the pathological processes underlying the white matter lesions, this can be used to differentiate brain lesions appearing similar on MRI. Different pathophysiology might be seen, for example, in hypoxic-ischemic white matter lesions with a complex pathogenesis existing in rare metabolic conditions such as mitochondrial encephalopathy with lactic acidosis and stroke-like episodes (MELAS) (Dubeau et al. 2000). Patients with MELAS can show very large increases in levels of brain parenchymal Lac in the area of the acute stroke (Fig. 13.3). Also, large increases in brain parenchymal Lac can be found in the brain tissue even in patients without history of acute ischemic attack (Fig. 13.4). Thus, proton MRS findings can allow for an accurate differentiation of this maternally inherited condition from any other acute and chronic cerebrovascular disorders.

In other very rare metabolic disorders such as ethylmalonic encephalopathy (Grosso et al. 2004) and cerebrotendinous xanthomatosis (de Stefano et al. 2001), the findings of diffuse brain mitochondrial impairment have strongly contributed to the interpretation of the complex pathogenetic mechanisms of these disorders. In the first case (Grosso et al. 2004), the diffuse MRS increase in brain Lac detected in a multi-voxel MRSI study (Fig. 13.5) was underlying a primary mitochondrial disorder, as later demonstrated by biochemical and genetic studies (Coburn

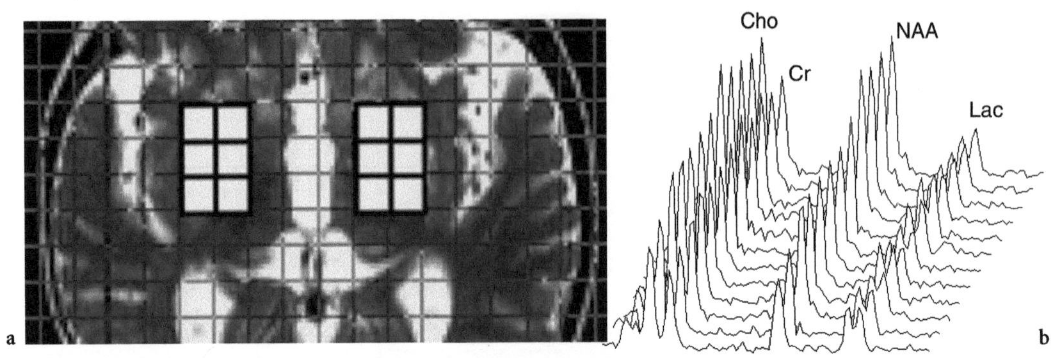

Fig. 13.5a,b. Conventional T2-weighted MRI with the superimposed grid of spectroscopy voxels (**a**) and proton MR spectra corresponding to brain voxels located in the basal ganglia of both cerebral hemispheres (**b**) in a patient with ethylmalonic encephalopathy. Each spectrum shows large pathological signals at 1.33 ppm coming from the methyl doublet of lactate (*Lac*)

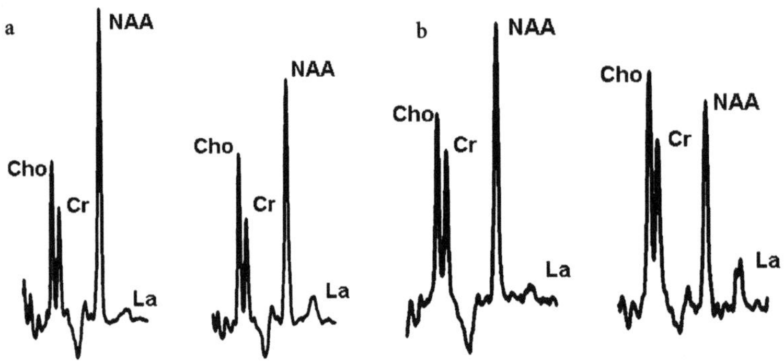

Fig. 13.6a,b. Single-voxel proton MR spectra relative to cerebral (**a**) and cerebellar (**b**) volume of interests of a normal control [*left panels* in (**a**) and (**b**)] and of a patient with cerebrotendinous xanthomatosis [*right panels* in (**a**) and (**b**)]. Note the cerebral and cerebellar increases in lactate in the patient's spectra with respect to normal control

2004). In the latter condition (DE STEFANO et al. 2001), single-voxel proton MRS data (Fig. 13.6) add to morphological and biochemical evidence of mitochondrial dysfunction (FEDERICO et al. 1991; DOTTI et al. 1995) (probably secondary to the toxic effect of high cholestanol and/or bile alcohol levels), suggesting the presence of a diffuse impairment of mitochondrial oxidative metabolism in patients with cerebrotendinous xanthomatosis.

There are also conditions in which proton MRS can provide typical brain metabolic patterns able to address the diagnosis. One example of a disease in which MRS provides a diagnostic pattern is a spongiform leukoencephalopathy known as Canavan disease. In this disorder, the deficiency of the enzyme aspartoacylase (which breaks down NAA) is responsible for abnormally high levels of NAA in the brain, which can be considered pathognomonic (AUSTIN et al. 1991; GRODD et al. 1990). Another characteristic metabolic MRS pattern has been shown recently in other spongiform leukoencephalopathies such as megalencephalic cystic leukoencephalopathy (MCL) (HANEFELD et al. 1993; VAN DER KNAAP et al. 1995) and childhood ataxia with diffuse CNS hypomyelination (CACH, also called vanishing white matter disease) (TEDESCHI et al. 1995; VAN DER KNAAP et al. 1997). In these disorders, conventional MRI findings of extensive white matter abnormalities with sparing of central brain structures are seen together with a peculiar MRS pattern. This is characterized by the almost complete disappearance of all normally detected metabolites in the white matter, presence of small increases in Lac and sparing of gray matter that is structurally and metabolically normal. In MCL, although MRS abnormalities tend to be more pronounced with increasing age, these are generally mild and the frontal white matter is significantly less involved than other white matter regions (Fig. 13.7). In patients with CACH disease, increases in glucose resonance intensities may also be present. This MRS metabolic profile is perhaps due to little brain white matter tissue left and the great increase in extracellular spaces. In both diseases, white matter increases in Lac resonance intensities are small and inconstant

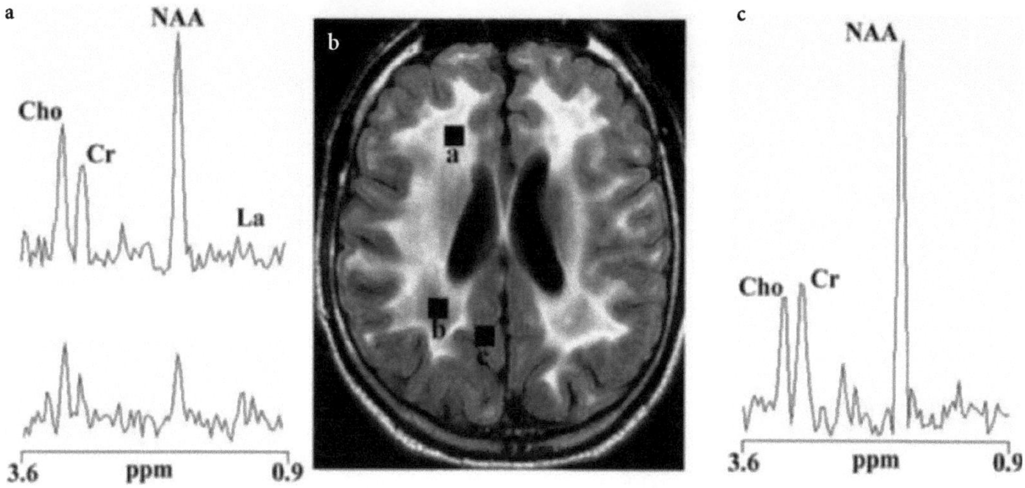

Fig. 13.7a–c. Conventional FLAIR image and proton MR spectra corresponding to brain voxels located in the frontal white matter (**a**), periventricular white matter (**b**) and grey matter (**c**) in the MRI/MRSI examination performed in a patient with megalencephalic cystic leukoencephalopathy at 25 years of age. Loss of signals in all the metabolites normally detected with the long echo time multi-voxel MRSI method are evident in white matter voxels. These abnormalities are relatively mild in the frontal white matter (**a**) and more pronounced in the periventricular white matter (**b**). Moderate increases in Lac resonance intensity can be seen in both white matter regions. No abnormalities are evident in grey matter voxels (**c**)

suggesting that they might be due to a disturbance in Lac removal after accumulation of foamy macrophages in pathologically active areas more than to a primary impairment of the oxidative metabolism. In any case, these MRS patterns appear to be sufficiently specific to differentiate these spongiform leukoencephalopathies from other white matter disorders with similar clinical and radiological appearance.

As mentioned before, distinctive white matter changes can also be seen in a number of mitochondrial encephalopathies (Bardosi et al. 1987; Burgeois et al. 1992; Leutner et al. 1994; Nakai et al. 1994). Significant decreases in Cho have been observed in some mitochondrial encephalopathies even in the absence of white matter abnormality on conventional MRI (Arnold and Matthews 1996; de Stefano et al. 1995c). These are likely related to be associated vacuolar myelinopathy which has been described pathologically in Kearns-Sayre syndrome and some of its variance (Matthews et al. 1993). Proton MRS studies also show decrease in NAA and increases in Lac relative resonance intensities in primitive mitochondrial encephalopathies (Matthews et al. 1993; Arnold and Matthews 1996). The latter, in particular, represents an important biochemical marker of these disorders. Lac levels are transiently increased in a number of acute pathological conditions associated with inflammatory cells (Arnold et al. 1992; Petroff et al. 1992; Arnold and Matthews 1996), but extensive pathological increases in Lac both within and outside of MRI lesions may be indicative of widespread energy failure associated with mitochondrial dysfunction (Matthews et al. 1993; de Stefano et al. 1995c). Accordingly, classical primitive mitochondrial such as pyruvate dehydrogenase deficiency, Leigh's and Kearns-Sayre syndromes show diffuse increases in brain parenchymal Lac (Fig. 13.8).

Other rare metabolic conditions also may provide diagnostic-specific proton MRS findings. In the phenylketonuria, patients show a specific peak due to the elevated phenylalanine and proton MRS can be used in patients with this metabolic disorder to follow the influx of phenylalanine from blood into brain tissue as well as to monitor the response of diet therapy (Kreis et al. 1995; Pietz et al. 2003). In the leukoencephalopathy associated with the disturbance of the metabolism of the polyols (van der Knaap et al. 1999), the diffuse decrease of all normally detected metabolites is associated with the increases of arabitol and sorbitol in both white and grey matter regions. In maple syrup disease, a relatively specific broad peak is detectable at 0.9 ppm. This region of the spectrum is usually attributed to lipids, but in maple syrup disease is believed to represent resonances of methyl protons from branched-chain amino-acids

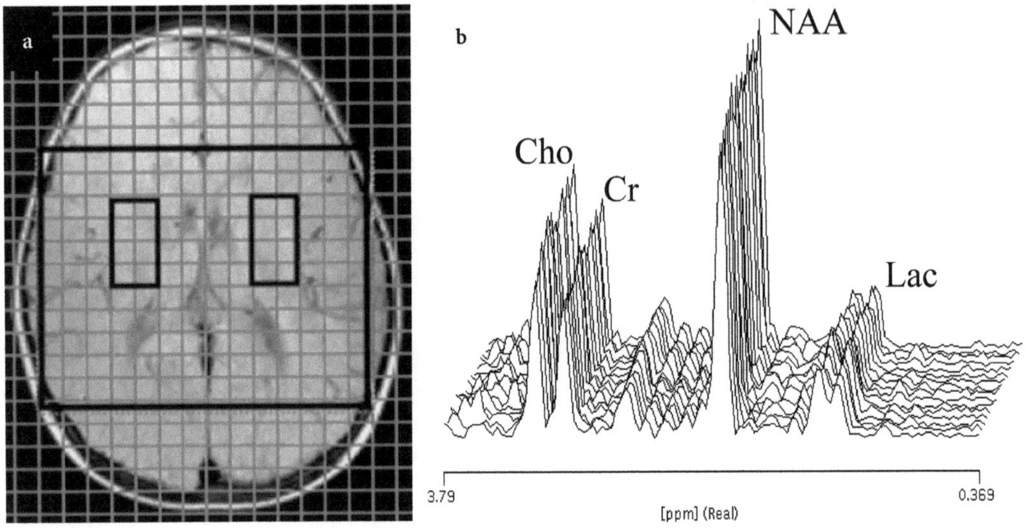

Fig. 13.8a,b. Conventional MRI with the superimposed grid of spectroscopy voxels (**a**) and proton MR spectra corresponding to brain voxels located in the basal ganglia of both cerebral hemispheres (**b**) in a patient with pyruvate dehydrogenase deficiency. Each spectrum shows large pathological signals at 1.33 ppm coming from the methyl doublet of lactate (*Lac*)

and branched-chain alpha-keto acids that accumulate as a result of defective oxidative decarboxylation of leucine, isoleucine and valine (Jan et al. 2003). Also proton MRS studies on patients with Niemann-Pick type C disease have shown increased resonance intensity of the lipid region of the spectrum (Fig. 13.9), probably due, in this case, to a defective metabolism of cholesterol with ceramide accumulation (Sylvain et al. 1994; Battisti et al. 2003). In both maple syrup and Niemann-Pick type C disease, the abnormal broad peak detectable at 0.9 ppm seem to decrease with appropriate therapy (Jan et al. 2003; Sylvain et al. 1994).

Finally, specific metabolic syndromes have recently been revealed by using proton MRS. This is the case of the creatine deficiency syndromes, which include defects in the guanidinoacetate methyltransferase and in the arginine-glycine amidinotransferase (Stockler et al. 1994; Schulze 2003), and the X-linked creatine deficiency syndrome (Bizzi et al. 2002). In the first two forms of the diseases, the Cr resonance intensity is undetectable in the brain on proton MRS, but cerebral levels of Cr do increase after creatine supplementation. In the X-linked form of creatine deficiency, as the metabolic defect is due to the transport of creatine into the central nervous system, patients are unresponsive to treatment and the Cr resonance intensity levels are unchanged after creatine supplementation (Fig. 13.10). Another condition with very specific proton MRS spectrum is the unique case of a child with minor developmental delay and absence of cerebral NAA, in whom the most prominent peak of proton MRS at 2.02 ppm was undetectable (Martin et al. 2001). Both creatine deficiency syndromes and the absence of NAA are characterized by mild or absent abnormalities on conventional MRI suggesting the unique potential of proton MRS in revealing metabolic abnormalities in MRI normal-appearing tissue.

13.4 Metabolic Changes Beyond MRI Lesions

As extensively reported in patients with multiple sclerosis (Fu et al. 1998), also in patients with both hereditary and acquired white matter disorders the detection of brain metabolic changes is not restricted to lesions (de Stefano et al. 2000b). Metabolic changes in normal-appearing white matter are usually less severe than those found inside the lesions and mostly consist in decreases in NAA and increases in Lac and Cho.

Because axons project through lesion volumes, any axonal dysfunction or loss should extend well beyond the borders of a lesion and into normal-appearing white matter, as an expression of anterograde and

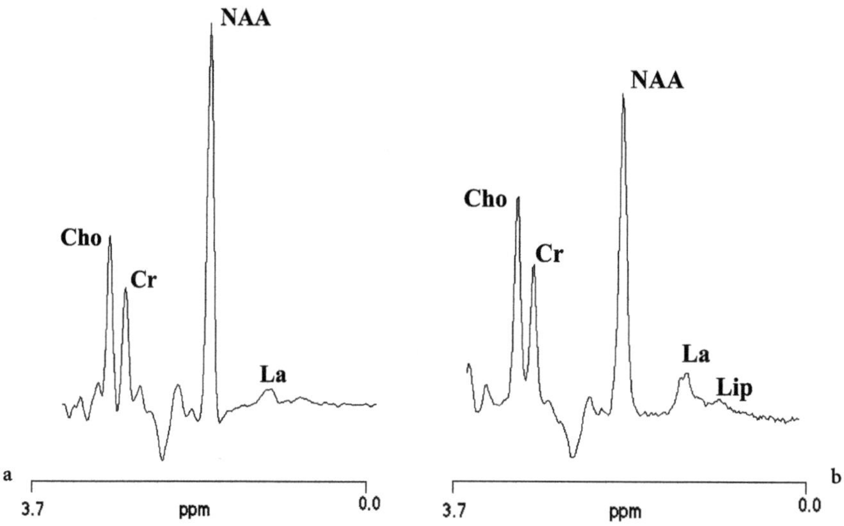

Fig. 13.9a,b. Single voxel proton MR spectra relative to a normal control (**a**) and a patient with Niemann-Pick type C disease (**b**). The spectra originate from homologous large volume of interest localized above the lateral ventricles and including grey and white matter of both cerebral hemispheres. Note the large decrease in *N*-acetyl aspartate and the increase in the lactate/lipids signals in the patient with Niemann-Pick type C disease respect to the normal control. Increases in lipids, rare in MR spectra at long echo times, are interpreted as due to ceramide accumulation

retrograde axonal degeneration. Thus, it should not be surprising that decreases in NAA can be observed beyond the borders of MS lesions as defined by T_2-weighted MRI. The analysis of serial multi-voxel proton MRSI studies from patients who present with large, solitary demyelinating lesions offers special opportunities in this respect. These studies showed that decreases in NAA can be seen well outside the demyelinating lesion (De Stefano et al. 1995a) and can be transiently evident even in homologous voxels of the hemisphere contralateral to the lesion (De Stefano et al. 1999).

Increases in Lac resonance intensities in the normal-appearing brain tissue represent a biochemical characteristic of mitochondrial encephalopathies. As mentioned before, Lac levels are transiently increased in a number of acute pathological conditions associated with inflammation (Arnold et al. 1992; Petroff et al. 1992), but pathological increases in Lac outside of MRI lesions may be indicative of widespread mitochondrial impairment (Matthews et al. 1993; De Stefano et al. 1995c).

Increases in Cho also could be detected in the normal-appearing WM in several WM conditions. This is the case, for example, in patients with rare, inherited diseases such as adrenoleukodystrophy (Kruse et al. 1994) and adult-onset Krabbe disease (De Stefano et al. 2000a) (Fig. 13.11). In all of these cases, the detec-

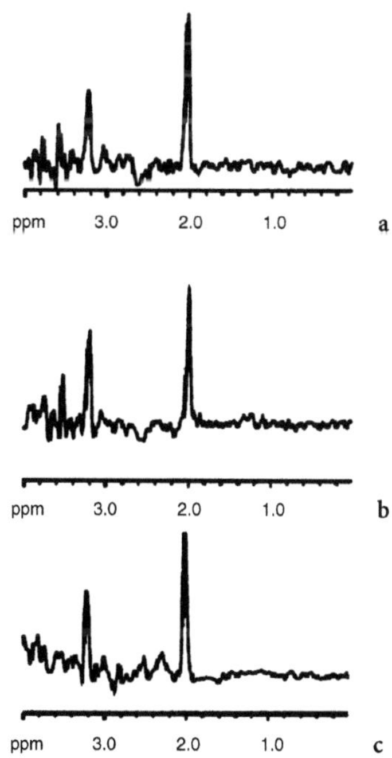

Fig. 13.10a–c. Proton brain MR spectra of a patient with X-linked creatine deficiency. The spectra show decreases in creatine resonance intensity (**a**), which remains unchanged after 3 months of oral creatine monohydrate supplementation at 400 mg/kg/day (**b**) and after 8 months of supplementation at 800 mg/kg/day (**c**). (Courtesy of Alberto Bizzi)

tion of metabolic changes in tissue appearing normal on MRI should be interpreted as the first sign of white matter pathology, not yet detectable by conventional MRI.

On the other hand, brain metabolic changes sometimes can be independent of the degree of abnormalities seen on conventional MRI. This can be found, for example, in CADASIL (cerebral autosomal dominant arteriopathy with subcortical infarcts and leukoencephalopathy) patients with mild and severe neurological impairment who can show similar white matter abnormalities on conventional MRI and, respectively, mild and severe brain metabolic abnormalities on multi-voxel proton MRSI (Fig. 13.12). Similarly, a single voxel study showed that this is also valid in other diseases such as in congenital muscular dystrophy where, in a patient with no central nervous system impairment, the MRS metabolic pattern was normal despite the diffuse white matter abnormalities on conventional MRI (Fig. 13.13). This confirms once again the lack of pathological specificity of the white matter lesions detected on conventional MRI and supports the hypothesis that brain lesions appearing similar on MRI may have a different pathophysiology and, as a consequence, different clinical relevance. In contrast, in both CADASIL and congenital muscular dystrophy as well as in other metabolic disorders cerebral levels of NAA correlated closely to patients' clinical status (De Stefano et al. 2000b) suggesting that the widespread cerebral neuro-axonal dysfunction and/or loss represents the most relevant mechanism of functional impairment in several metabolic disorders affecting the cerebral white matter.

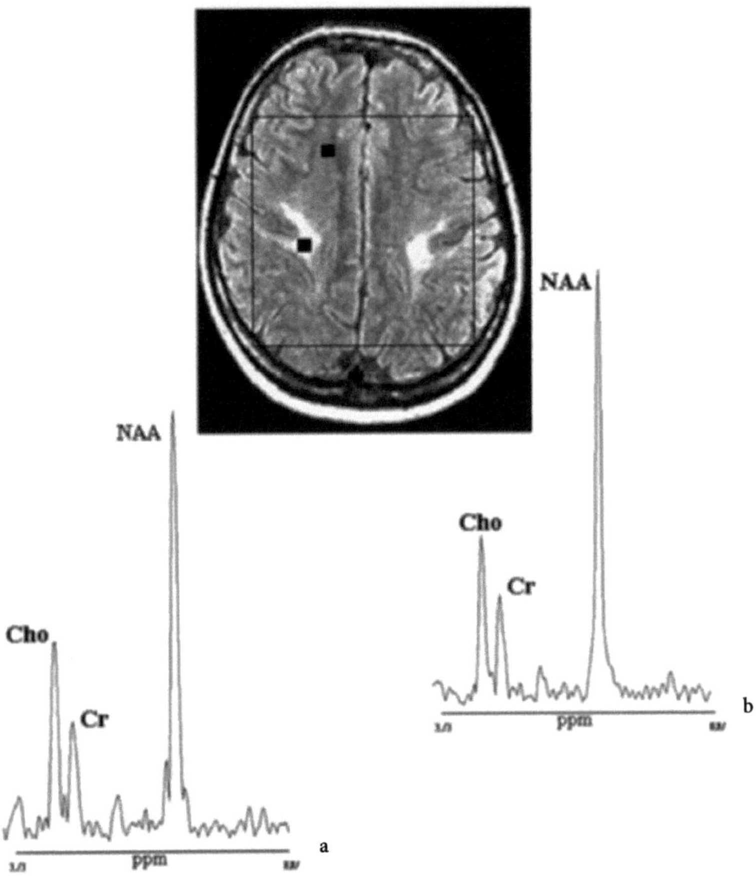

Fig. 13.11a,b. Proton brain MRI/MRSI examination of a patient with adult-onset Krabbe disease. Conventional MRI examination show abnormally high signal localized to the motor strips of both hemispheres. The volume of interest for spectroscopy is shown in the transverse MRI. Proton MRSI voxels were classified as inside the lesion if they were entirely filled with abnormal MRI signal (**a**) and as outside the lesion if there was no abnormal MRI signal within the voxel and in adjacent voxels (**b**). Proton MRSI spectra from voxels [*squares* in (**a**) and (**b**)] show abnormal increases in choline resonance intensities

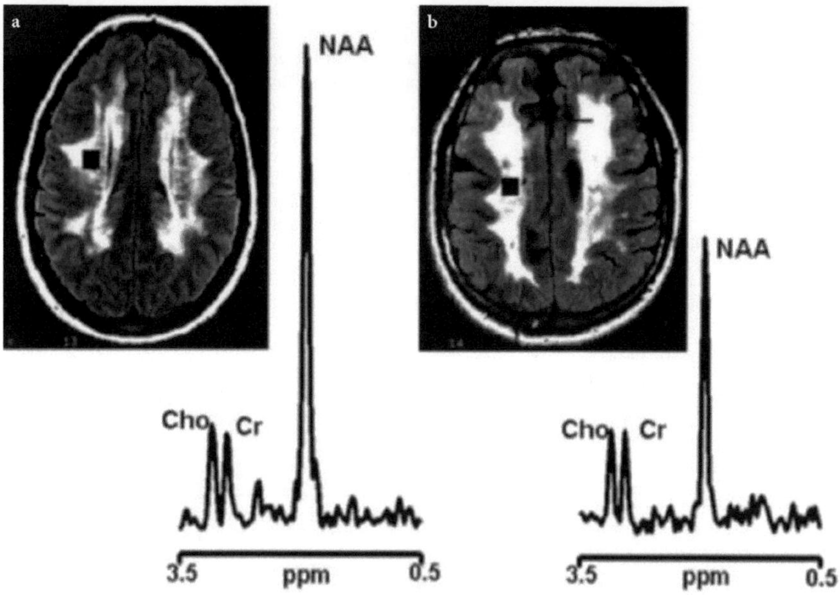

Fig. 13.12a,b. Proton brain MRI/MRSI examinations relative to two patients with cerebral autosomal dominant arteriopathy with subcortical infarcts and leukoencephalopathy (CADASIL) and mild (**a**) and severe (**b**) neurological impairment, respectively. Patients show similar white matter abnormalities on conventional MRI. In contrast, proton MRSI voxels localized in the deep white matter (*squares*) show metabolic changes which are independent of the degree of MRI white matter abnormalities and are very mild in the CADASIL patient with mild neurological impairment, and more pronounced in the CADASIL patient with severe clinical status

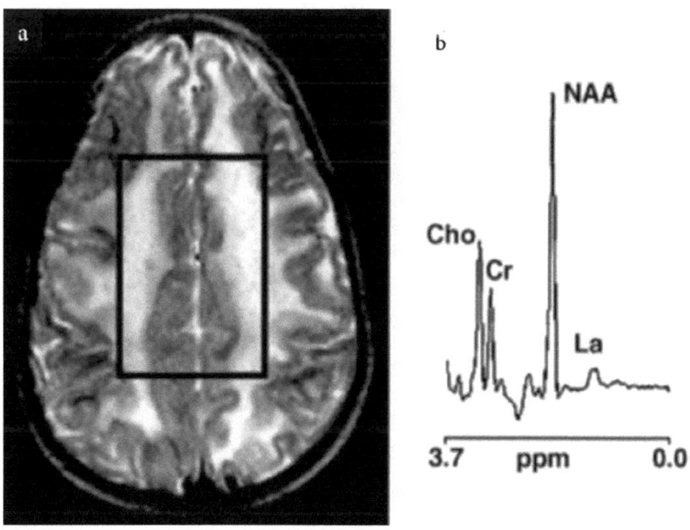

Fig. 13.13a,b. Conventional MRI in transversal orientation (**a**) and the single voxel proton MRS spectrum of a patient with congenital muscular dystrophy (**b**). The volume of interest for spectroscopy is shown in the transverse MRI. The conventional MR image shows diffuse white matter hyperintensity, but the MR spectrum is normal. The patient, despite the diffuse cerebral white matter abnormalities, did not have CNS impairment

13.5 Conclusions

Brain MRS provides chemical-pathological information that has the potential to improve both diagnostic classification and management of patients with metabolic disorders affecting the brain white matter. Metabolic indices provided by proton MRS and MRSI could be sensitive indicators of early neurological involvement, relevant to patients' clinical status. A more extensive use of a combination of MR modalities including volumetric MRI, MRS and other nonconventional MR techniques might yield a more complete description of the dynamics responsible for pathological changes in this heterogeneous group of disorders and allow a more accurate evaluation of disease progression and response to therapy. A wider use of proton MRS techniques should be encouraged in clinical studies of patients with metabolic disorders.

References

Arnold DL, Matthews PM (1996) Practical aspects of clinical applications of MRS in the brain. In: Young IR, Charles HC (eds) MR spectroscopy: clinical applications and techniques. Dunitz, London, pp 139-159

Arnold DL, Matthews PM, Francis GS, O'Connor J, Antel JP (1992) Proton magnetic resonance spectroscopic imaging for metabolic characterization of demyelinating plaques. Ann Neurol 31:235-241

Austin SJ, Connelly A, Gadian DG, Benton JS, Brett EM (1991) Localized 1H NMR spectroscopy in Canavan's disease: a report of two cases. Magn Reson Med 19:439-445

Bardosi A, Creutzfeldt W, DiMauro S, Felgenhauer K, Friede RL, Goebel HH et al (1987) Myo-, neuro-, gastrointestinal encephalopathy (MNGIE syndrome) due to partial deficiency of cytochrome-c-oxidase. A new mitochondrial multisystem disorder. Acta Neuropathol 74:248-258

Battisti C, Tarugi P, Dotti MT, De SN, Vattimo A, Chierichetti F et al (2003) Adult onset Niemann-Pick type C disease: a clinical, neuroimaging and molecular genetic study. Mov Disord 18:1405-1409

Bizzi A, Bugiani M, Salomons GS, Hunneman DH, Moroni I, Estienne M et al (2002) X-linked creatine deficiency syndrome: a novel mutation in creatine transporter gene SLC6A8. Ann Neurol 52:227-231

Bjartmar C, Battistuta J, Terada N, Dupree E, Trapp BD (2002) N-acetylaspartate is an axon-specific marker of mature white matter in vivo: a biochemical and immunohistochemical study on the rat optic nerve. Ann Neurol 51:51-58

Bruhn H, Kruse B, Korenke GC, Hanefeld F, Hanicke W, Merboldt KD et al (1992) Proton NMR spectroscopy of cerebral metabolic alterations in infantile peroxisomal disorders. J Comput Assist Tomogr 16:335-344

Burgeois M, Goutieres F, Chretien D, Rustin P, Munnich A, Aicardi J (1992) Deficiency in complex II of the respiratory chain, presenting as a leukodystrophy in two sisters with Leigh syndrome. Brain Dev 14:404-408

Coburn B (2004) A rare disorder, ethylmalonic encephalopathy, is caused by mutations in a mitochondrial protein. Clin Genet 65:460-462

Davies SE, Newcombe J, Williams SR, McDonald WI, Clark JB (1995) High resolution proton NMR spectroscopy of multiple sclerosis lesions. J Neurochem 64:742-748

De Stefano N, Matthews PM, Antel JP, Preul M, Francis G, Arnold DL (1995a) Chemical pathology of acute demyelinating lesions and its correlation with disability. Ann Neurol 38:901-909

De Stefano N, Matthews PM, Arnold DL (1995b) Reversible decreases in N-acetylaspartate after acute brain injury. Magn Reson Med 34:721-727

De Stefano N, Matthews PM, Ford B, Genge A, Karpati G, Arnold DL (1995c) Short-term dichloroacetate treatment improves indices of cerebral metabolism in patients with mitochondrial disorders. Neurology 45:1193-1198

De Stefano N, Narayanan S, Matthews PM, Francis GS, Antel JP, Arnold DL (1999) In vivo evidence for axonal dysfunction remote from focal cerebral demyelination of the type seen in multiple sclerosis. Brain 122:1933-1939

De Stefano N, Dotti MT, Mortilla M, Pappagallo E, Luzi P, Rafi MA et al (2000a) Evidence of diffuse brain pathology and unspecific genetic characterization in a patient with an atypical form of adult-onset Krabbe disease. J Neurol 247:226-228

De Stefano N, Narayanan S, Matthews PM, Mortilla M, Dotti MT, Federico A et al (2000b) Proton MR spectroscopy to assess axonal damage in multiple sclerosis and other white matter disorders. J Neurovirol 6 [Suppl 2]:121-129

De Stefano N, Dotti MT, Mortilla M, Federico A (2001) Magnetic resonance imaging and spectroscopic changes in brains of patients with cerebrotendinous xanthomatosis. Brain 124:121-131

Dotti MT, Manneschi L, Federico A (1995) Mitochondrial enzyme deficiency in cerebrotendinous xanthomatosis. J Neurol Sci 129:106-108

Dubeau F, De SN, Zifkin BG, Arnold DL, Shoubridge EA (2000) Oxidative phosphorylation defect in the brains of carriers of the tRNAleu(UUR) A3243G mutation in a MELAS pedigree. Ann Neurol 47:179-185

Federico A, Dotti MT, Volpi N (1991) Muscle mitochondrial changes in cerebrotendinous xanthomatosis (letter). Ann Neurol 30:734-735

Fu L, Matthews PM, De Stefano N, Worsley KJ, Narayanan S, Francis GS et al (1998) Imaging axonal damage of normal-appearing white matter in multiple sclerosis. Brain 121:103-113

Grodd W, Krageloh-Mann I, Petersen D, Trefz FK, Harzer K (1990) In vivo assessment of N-acetylaspartate in brain in spongy degeneration (Canavan's disease) by proton spectroscopy (letter). Lancet 336:437-438

Grosso S, Balestri P, Mostardini R, Federico A, De SN (2004) Brain mitochondrial impairment in ethylmalonic encephalopathy. J Neurol 251:755-756

Hanefeld F, Holzbach U, Kruse B, Wilichowski E, Christen HJ, Frahm J (1993) Diffuse white matter disease in three children: an encephalopathy with unique features on magnetic resonance imaging and proton magnetic resonance spectroscopy. Neuropediatrics 24:244-248

Jan W, Zimmerman RA, Wang ZJ, Berry GT, Kaplan PB, Kaye EM (2003) MR diffusion imaging and MR spectroscopy of maple syrup urine disease during acute metabolic decompensation. Neuroradiology 45:393-399
Johannik K, Van Hecke P, Francois B, Marchal G, Smet MH, Jaeken J et al (1994) Localized brain proton NMR spectroscopy in young adult phenylketonuria patients. Magn Reson Med 31:53-57
Kolodny EH (1993) Dysmyelinating and demyelinating conditions in infancy (review). Curr Opin Neurol Neurosurg 6:379-386
Koopmans RA, Li DK, Zhu G, Allen PS, Penn A, Paty DW (1993) Magnetic resonance spectroscopy of multiple sclerosis: in-vivo detection of myelin breakdown products (letter). Lancet 341:631-632
Kreis R, Pietz J, Penzien J, Herschkowitz N, Boesch C (1995) Identification and quantitation of phenylalanine in the brain of patients with phenylketonuria by means of localized in vivo 1H magnetic-resonance spectroscopy. J Magn Reson B 107:242-251
Kruse B, Barker PB, van Zijl PC, Duyn JH, Moonen CT, Moser HW (1994) Multislice proton magnetic resonance spectroscopic imaging in X-linked adrenoleukodystrophy. Ann Neurol 36:595-608
Kruse B, Hanefeld F, Christen HJ, Bruhn H, Michaelis T, Hanicke W et al (1993) Alterations of brain metabolites in metachromatic leukodystrophy as detected by localized proton magnetic resonance spectroscopy in vivo. J Neurol 241:68-74
Leutner C, Layer G, Zierz S, Solymosi L, Dewes W, Reiser M (1994) Cerebral MR in ophthalmoplegia plus. AJNR Am J Neuroradiol 15:681-687
Martin E, Capone A, Schneider J, Hennig J, Thiel T (2001) Absence of N-acetylaspartate in the human brain: impact on neurospectroscopy? Ann Neurol 49:518-521
Matthews PM, Andermann F, Silver K, Karpati G, Arnold DL (1993) Proton MR spectroscopic characterization of differences in regional brain metabolic abnormalities in mito chondrial encephalomyopathies. Neurology 43:2484-2490
Matthews PM, de Stefano N, Narayanan S, Francis GS, Wolinsky JS, Antel JP et al (1998) Putting magnetic resonance spectroscopy studies in context: axonal damage and disability in multiple sclerosis. Semin Neurol 18:327-336
Nakai A, Goto Y, Fujisawa K, Shigematsu Y, Kikawa Y, Konishi Y et al (1994) Diffuse leukodystrophy with a large-scale mitochondrial DNA deletion. Lancet 343:1397-1398
Narayana PA, Doyle TJ, Lai D, Wolinsky JS (1998) Serial proton magnetic resonance spectroscopic imaging, contrast-enhanced magnetic resonance imaging, and quantitative lesion volumetry in multiple sclerosis. Ann Neurol 43:56-71
Petroff OA, Graham GD, Blamire AM, al-Rayess M, Rothman DL, Fayad PB et al (1992) Spectroscopic imaging of stroke in humans: histopathology correlates of spectral changes. Neurology 42:1349-1354
Pietz J, Lutz T, Zwygart K, Hoffmann GF, Ebinger F, Boesch C et al (2003) Phenylalanine can be detected in brain tissue of healthy subjects by 1H magnetic resonance spectroscopy. J Inherit Metab Dis 26:683-692
Schiffmann R, van der Knaap MS (2004) The latest on leukodystrophies. Curr Opin Neurol 17:187-192
Schulze A (2003) Creatine deficiency syndromes. Mol Cell Biochem 244:143-150
Stockler S, Holzbach U, Hanefeld F, Marquardt I, Helms G, Requart M et al (1994) Creatine deficiency in the brain: a new, treatable inborn error of metabolism. Pediatr Res 36:409-413
Sylvain M, Arnold DL, Scriver CR, Schreiber R, Shevell MI (1994) Magnetic resonance spectroscopy in Neimann-Pick disease type C: correlation with diagnosis and clinical responce to cholestyramine and lovastatin. Pediatric Neurology 10:228-232
Tedeschi G, Schiffmann R, Barton NW, Shih HH, Gospe SMJ, Brady RO et al (1995) Proton magnetic resonance spectroscopic imaging in childhood ataxia with diffuse central nervous system hypomyelination. Neurology 45:1526-1532
Tzika AA, Ball WS Jr, Vigneron DB, Dunn RS, Nelson SJ, Kirks DR (1993) Childhood adrenoleukodystrophy: assessment with proton MR spectroscopy. Radiology 189:467-480
Van der Knaap MS (2001) Magnetic resonance in childhood white-matter disorders. Dev Med Child Neurol 43:705-712
Van der Knaap MS, Valk J, de Neeling N, Nauta JJ (1991) Pattern recognition in magnetic resonance imaging of white matter disorders in children and young adults. Neuroradiology 33:478-493
Van der Knaap MS, Barth PG, Stroink H, van Nieuwenhuizen O, Arts WF, Hoogenraad F et al (1995) Leukoencephalopathy with swelling and a discrepantly mild clinical course in eight children. Ann Neurol 37:324-334
Van der Knaap MS, Barth PG, Gabreels FJ, Franzoni E, Begeer JH, Stroink H et al (1997) A new leukoencephalopathy with vanishing white matter. Neurology 48:845-855
Van der Knaap MS, Wevers RA, Struys EA, Verhoeven NM, Pouwels PJ, Engelke UF et al (1999) Leukoencephalopathy associated with a disturbance in the metabolism of polyols. Ann Neurol 46:925-928

Demyelinating Diseases

14 Conventional MRI Techniques in Multiple Sclerosis

ANTHONY TRABOULSEE, DAVID K.B. LI, GUOJUN ZHAO, and DONALD W. PATY

CONTENTS

14.1 Introduction

The conventional MRI techniques used in MS in general are the sequences that are routinely used on a standard clinical MRI scanner. These typically include proton density (PD) and T2-weighted (T2W) spin-echo (SE) and fluid-attenuated inversion recovery (FLAIR) sequences for lesion identification, and gadolinium-enhanced T1-weighted imaging for identifying new lesion activity.

Despite the limitations of signal quality with the earliest MRI images (YOUNG et al. 1981) of MS patients it was quickly recognized that MRI provided a valuable tool for identifying lesions within the brain that were similar in shape and location to plaques seen pathologically. Since then, MRI, both conventional and non-conventional techniques, has transformed all aspects of MS research and clinical practice.

A. TRABOULSEE, MD, FRCPC
Instructor, Division of Neurology, Department of Medicine, The University of British Columbia, S195-2211 Wesbrook Mall, Vancouver, British Columbia, Canada, V6T 2B5
D.K.B. LI, MD, FRCPC
Professor, Department of Radiology, The University of British Columbia, Main Floor, 2211 Wesbrook Mall, Vancouver, British Columbia, Canada, V6T 2B5
G. ZHAO, MD
Research Associate, Division of Neurology, Department of Medicine, The University of British Columbia, Gerald McGavin Building, 2386 East Mall, Vancouver, British Columbia, Canada, V6T 1Z4
D.W. PATY, MD, FRCPC
Professor, Emeritus, Division of Neurology, Department of Medicine, The University of British Columbia, S195-2211 Wesbrook Mall, Vancouver, British Columbia, Canada, V6T 2B5

14.2 Technical Considerations

PD and T2W images are acquired simultaneously (double echo) with conventional SE techniques. Repetition times (TR) are long (2500–3000 ms), and lesion intensity increases with the longer echo time (TE) of the T2W (TE 80–120 ms) compared to PD (TE 15–40 ms) sequences (Fig. 14.1). Posterior fossa lesions are best seen on T2W images and periventricular lesions best seen with PD images. Faster acquisition sequences (fast or turbo spin echo) which allow additional signal averaging provide the ability to obtain thinner slices. This compensates for the occasional risk of missing smaller lesions due to the edge blurring associated with the shorter effective TE. Fast FLAIR is popular for periventricular and juxtacortical lesion identification because of the excellent suppression of cerebrospinal fluid (CSF) partial volume effects (RYDBERG et al. 1995). However, it may be less sensitive for some brainstem and spinal cord lesions (FILIPPI et al. 1996a; GAWNE-CAIN et al. 1997). Commonly used protocols range from 5 mm thick slices with 2.5 mm gaps to 3 mm contiguous slices. There is better reproducibility and slightly higher lesion volume detection using 3 mm rather than 5 mm slice thickness (FILIPPI et al. 1997; ROVARIS et al. 1998). The Consortium of MS Centers' MRI Working Group recommends contiguous 3 mm slice thickness with no gap for clinical MRI protocols.

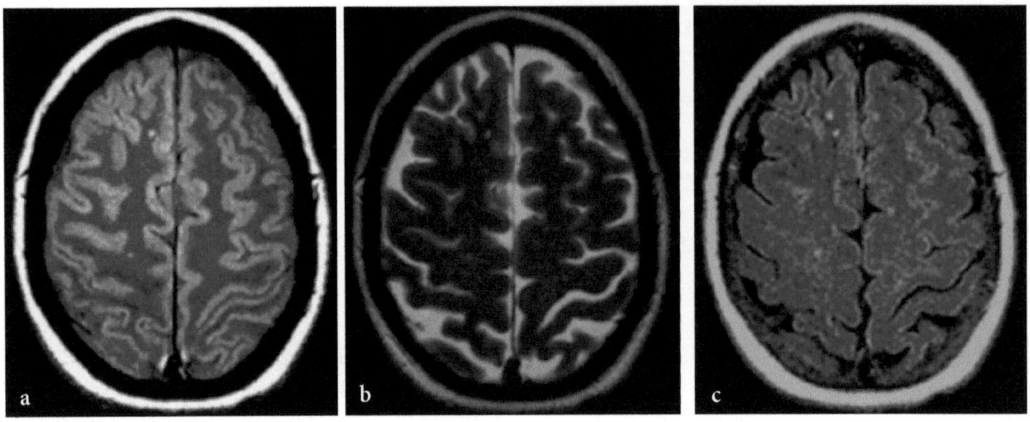

Fig. 14.1a–c. PD (**a**), T2W (**b**) and FLAIR (**c**) axial brain images with small MS lesions

14.3 Pathophysiology of MS

14.3.1 Lesion Morphology and Distribution

Post-mortem studies have validated that the T2 lesions seen on MRI correlate with the typical plaques of MS seen on gross pathology (Stewart et al. 1986). The classic MRI appearance is typically multiple white matter lesions with periventricular predominance (Fig. 14.2). MS plaques appear as bright T2 lesions because of the longer T2 relaxation times. However, the T2 lesions are not specific for plaque age, degree of myelin loss, amount of inflammation and edema, or the degree of axonal loss (Barnes et al. 1991). Most lesions have an expanded extracellular space, and it is possible that T2W lesions overestimate the extent of the pathology due to the edema, particularly with new inflammation (Newcombe et al. 1991). Lipids have a relatively short T2 relaxation time, making them effectively invisible on conventional MRI. Therefore, the lipid loss due to myelin sheath breakdown in demyelination probably does not directly contribute to the change seen on MRI. However, the loss of myelin lipid does create a more hydrophilic environment and the increased water content will lead to proton density increase and prolonged T1 and T2 relaxation times (increased intensity lesions on PD/T2W and decreased intensity lesions on T1W sequences). Thus, other pathologies, such as infarcts, infection, tumors and inflammation can produce similar MRI signal changes.

The most common location for MS lesions on MRI is periventricular and it would be unusual to have sparing of this region in MS. Lesions can occur in any CNS tissue where there is myelin, including the cortex. However, most of these lesions are missed with conventional MRI due to similarities in signal intensities of MS lesions and gray matter, and the partial volume effects of CSF within the adjacent sulci (Kidd et al. 1999). FLAIR sequences currently are preferred for the detection of cortical lesions (Boggild et al. 1996). Dawson fingers refer to the oval, elongated lesions in the corona radiata and the centrum semiovale. These lesions are oriented along subependymal veins that are perpendicular to the walls of the ventricles, representing perivenular inflammation that is a unique pathological feature of MS (Horowitz et al. 1989). These are best seen on sagittal PD/T2W or FLAIR images. The sagittal image is also useful for demonstrating lesions within the corpus callosum. Lesions are also often seen in the temporal lobes, at the gray-white matter junction (juxtacortical), brainstem and cerebellum. A fat-suppression technique improves the sensitivity to detect lesions within the optic nerves (Tien et al. 1991). Optic nerve involvement was detected on MRI in 76% of 25 patients investigated, only 4 of whom had a history of optic neuritis (Davies et al. 1998).

Spinal cord lesions are most common in the cervical cord (Fig. 14.3) (Bot et al. 2002) and they tend to involve the posterior and lateral regions and occupy less than half the area of the cord on axial images (Thielen and Miller 1996). These lesions rarely extend beyond two vertebral segments (Tartaglino et al. 1995). Spinal cord lesions can be found in 50–90%

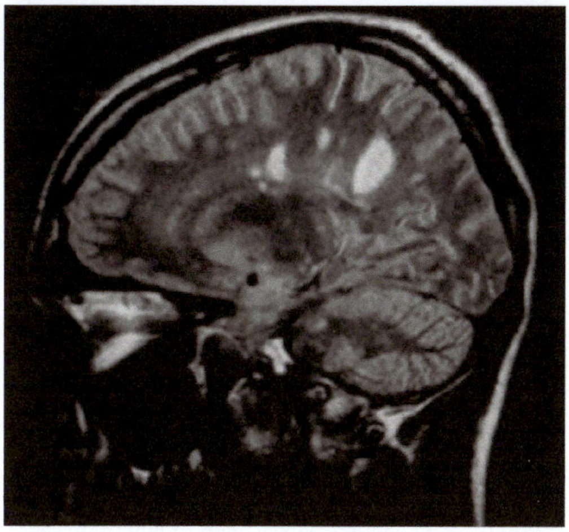

Fig. 14.2. Sagittal FLAIR brain image showing typical MS T2 lesions

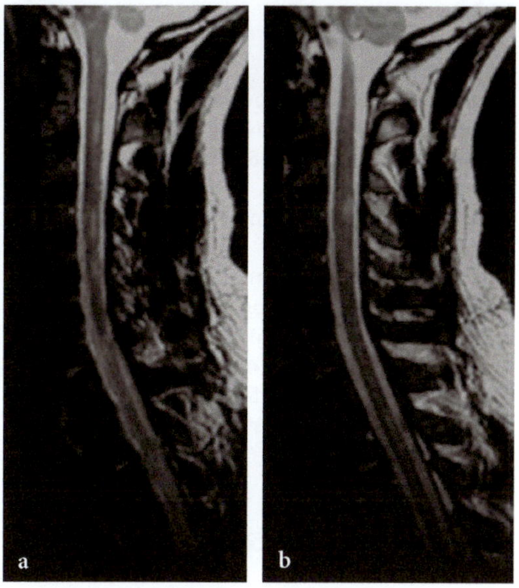

Fig. 14.3a,b. Consecutive sagittal T2W images of MS lesions in the cervical spinal cord

of MS patients, and in one study of 68 patients, 38 had multiple lesions (56%) (Tartaglino et al. 1995).

Not all lesions are discrete on MRI. There are diffuse changes throughout the normal-appearing brain tissues pathologically that can be investigated with non-conventional MRI techniques such as magnetization transfer imaging (Ostuni et al. 1999), diffusion-weighted imaging (Ciccarelli et al. 2001), MR spectroscopy (De Stefano et al. 2002), and myelin water imaging (Whittall et al. 2002). However, there can also be large, diffuse lesions visible on conventional MRI with poorly defined boundaries (Fig. 14.4). These areas of dirty-appearing white matter (DWM) are most common around the ventricles, especially adjacent to the occipital horn. DWM can extend over several contiguous slices and was present in 17% of relapsing-remitting MS (RRMS) patients in one study (Zhao et al. 2000). The degree of tissue abnormalities as determined with magnetization transfer imaging within DWM appears to be intermediate between normal-appearing brain tissue and lesions (Ge et al. 2003).

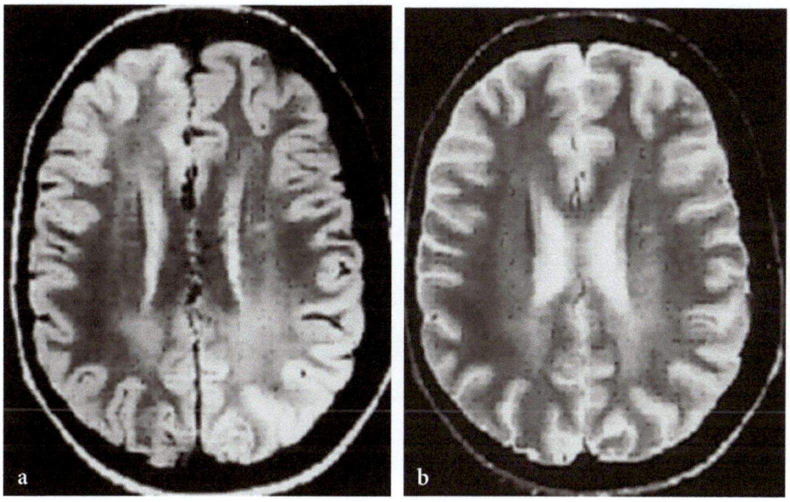

Fig. 14.4a,b. Dirty white matter (**a** PD image; **b** T2W image) refers to large diffuse areas of increased T2 hyperintensity. Unlike typical T2 lesions, DWM has poorly defined borders, and often extends through several slices. It is seen in fewer than 20% of RRMS patients

14.3.2 Lesion Development

Serial MRI studies have provided unique insights into the pathogenesis of new MS lesion formation (HARRIS et al. 1991; ISAAC et al. 1988; MCFARLAND et al. 1992; WILLOUGHBY et al. 1989). MRI is ideally suited for evaluating the cycle of dynamic changes in vivo, by providing full coverage of the CNS in a reasonable time frame, and without the safety concerns of radiation-based neuroimaging techniques. Perhaps the greatest impact of several MRI natural history studies is a better understanding of the degree of clinically silent MRI lesion activity that frequently occurs even during periods of clinical stability or remission.

14.3.3 Gadolinium-Enhancing Lesions

New disease activity (inflammation) can be detected by conventional MRI as gadolinium enhancement on the postcontrast T1W image, and as new and enlarging T2W lesions on serial studies (see below). Gadolinium enhancement (Fig. 14.5) can precede new T2W lesions by hours or days (MILLER et al. 1988) and represents breakdown of the blood–brain barrier as proinflammatory T cells infiltrate into the brain parenchyma (NESBIT et al. 1991). The enhancement is more often solid and homogeneous with fresh lesions, particularly when they are small and may appear ring-like with lesions that are larger and several weeks old. Enhancement usually lasts 4 weeks with a gradual decline during the next 2 to 4 weeks (KERMODE et al. 1990). It is extremely unusual for a MS lesion to have gadolinium enhancement beyond 3 months. This could help in distinguishing MS lesions from CNS tumors of the brain or spinal cord that can sometimes mimic early MS clinically. Gadolinium enhancement is sensitive to steroids and other antiinflammatory treatments. The majority of new T2W lesions will enhance with gadolinium. Preexisting T2W lesions can also enhance, indicating new activity, and in general newly enhancing lesions are seen twice as often as new T2 activity (new or enlarging T2W lesions). Higher ("double or triple") doses of gadolinium, longer delays between injecting the gadolinium and acquiring the postcontrast T1W images, thinner slices and incorporating a magnetization transfer sequence have been shown to increase the number of enhancing MS lesions as well as the intensity of some lesions (FILIPPI et al. 1996b; SILVER et al. 1997). For clinical MRI scans, the Consortium of MS Centers MRI Working Group recommends a standard dose of gadolinium of 0.1 mmol/kg with a minimum delay of 5 min.

Although the heaviest plaque burden in MS is usually found in the periventricular regions, we have observed that only 20% of enhancing lesions are immediately periventricular in distribution, 80% being nonperiventricular, 56% in the deep white matter and 24% at the gray–white matter junction. This difference in distribution between acute and chronic lesions raises questions about the genesis and ultimate fate of these new and dynamic lesions seen on MRI (LEE et al. 1999).

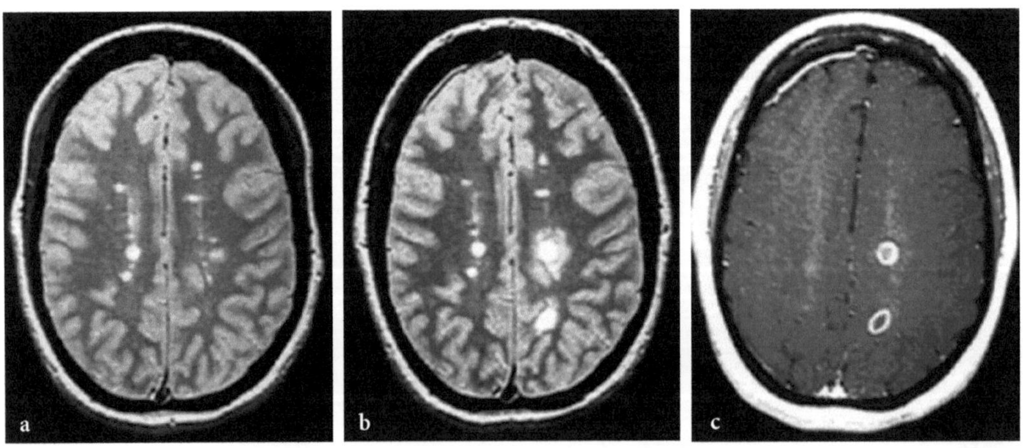

Fig. 14.5. a Baseline axial brain PDW image with multiple T2 lesions. **b** The registered image 1 month latter demonstrating several new T2 lesions that developed in the absence of any new clinical symptoms. **c** Corresponding axial postcontrast T1W image showing gadolinium enhancement of the new lesions

14.3.4
T2W Active Lesions

New T2W lesions represent new inflammation (Fig. 14.5). They increase in size during the acute phase mostly due to edema associated with inflammatory infiltrates, reaching their maximum size within 4 weeks (WILLOUGHBY et al. 1989). The process is self-limiting, and the lesions slowly decrease in size over the next 6 to 8 weeks as edema resolves and remyelination occurs. However, most lesions leave a smaller residual T2W lesion (KOOPMANS et al. 1989c).

14.3.5
Lesion Reactivation and Accumulation

On average, MS patients will develop four or five new MRI lesions per year with great variability amongst individuals (PATY 1988). Preexisting T2W lesions can reactivate with re-enhancement only, enlargement on T2W imaging, or both. The pathology within the chronic lesion is probably maturing to include gliosis and axonal loss in addition to demyelination. Eventually, after many reactivations, lesions will fuse with adjacent lesions. Thus, what may have started out as several small lesions may end up forming one large confluent lesion (KOOPMANS et al. 1989b).

Annually there is net accumulation of new and enlarging lesions that increases the total T2 volume or burden of disease (T2 BOD) of 5 to 10% per year (PATY et al. 1994). However, the variability between individuals is enormous, and this is not normally distributed. Thus, median values are the preferred descriptors when these are used as outcome measures in clinical trials. Monthly the T2 BOD can fluctuate due to the changes in disease activity especially if the baseline BOD is rather small (STONE et al. 1995). It is valuable if not essential to see an increase in T2 BOD in placebo groups for internal validation of any quantification methodology.

14.3.6
"Black Holes"

On the accompanying unenhanced T1W image, some T2 lesions may be isointense to surrounding white matter and therefore undetectable. However, some lesions will appear hypointense on the T1W (so-called T1 hypointensity or "black hole"; Fig. 14.6). A proportion of these black holes are acute lesions that enhance when gadolinium is given and almost half of these will resolve slowly over months (BAGNATO et al. 2003). Those that do not enhance represent (1) sub-acute or resolving lesions, and (2) chronic or stable lesions. We recommend that chronic black holes be defined as T2 lesions which are nonenhancing and hypointense T1W lesions, that persist for a minimum of 6 months after their first appearance, and have a signal intensity on T1W images less than or equal to that of gray matter. The chronic T1W hypointense black holes are associated with greater tissue destruction and axonal loss (VAN WALDERVEEN et al. 1999) compared to chronic, stable T2 lesions without a cor-

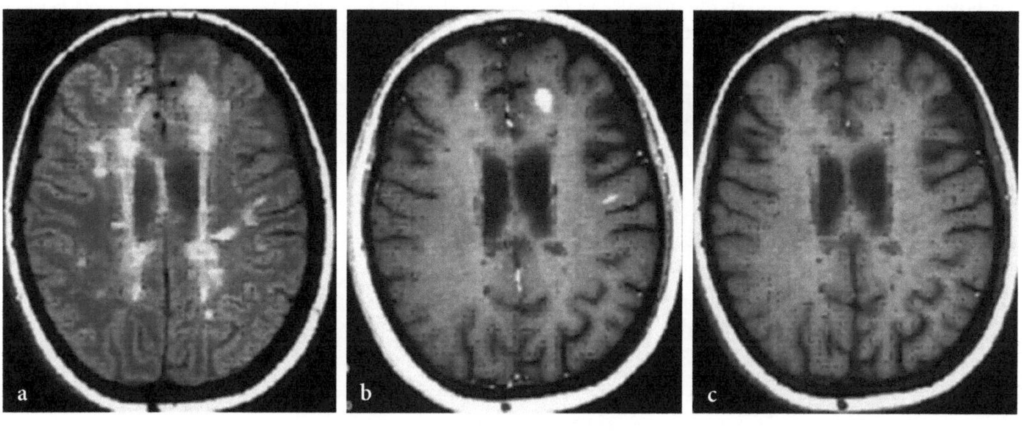

Fig. 14.6a–c. Chronic T1W hypointense lesions (black holes) are a subset of T2 lesions that do not enhance with gadolinium and have been present for at least 6 months. They are associated with greater tissue destruction and axonal loss than those T2 lesions that are isointense on T1W imaging. However, acute black holes can be commonly identified with new lesions, and many will resolve within 6–12 months

responding black hole. Furthermore, these lesions may have a better correlation with clinical disability because of their greater pathological specificity for severe axonal loss (Truyen et al. 1996) and have been suggested as a potential outcome measure in clinical trials for the degenerative processes of MS (Filippi et al. 2000).

14.3.7 Atrophy

Brain and spinal cord atrophy has been recognized in autopsy material from MS patients prior to the current widely available neuroimaging techniques. It is likely that axonal loss accounts for the irreversible and progressive clinical disability that occurs in MS (McDonald and Ron 1999) and atrophy is the result of axonal loss, in addition to myelin loss, and shrinkage due to gliosis. Thus, global brain atrophy is another important measure of the neurodegenerative component of MS (Miller et al. 2002).

An early CT study of 100 MS patients in 1978 demonstrated atrophy as a feature of MS brains and also demonstrated that it was progressive in a small subset of patients followed for up to 21 months (Cala et al. 1978). MRI studies have also shown that atrophy is common (Fig. 14.7), ranging from 47% to 100% of MS patients, depending on the population and technique (Filippi et al. 1998; Liu et al. 1999). It is more severe in patients with secondary progressive MS (SPMS) than RRMS (van Walderveen et al. 1998). It can be detected after a single attack of demyelination (clinically isolated syndrome, CIS) before the diagnosis of MS is made, and in the presence of only a small T2 lesion burden (Brex et al. 2000). Brain volume measurements are reliable and reproducible, with the majority of current techniques using MRI rather than CT data. Different methods have been used including: ventricular size (including linear measurements), corpus callosum area, measuring selected brain slices, segmentation of the entire brain to calculate a normalized brain parenchyma fraction or volume (BPF/BPV), and spinal cord cross-sectional area. Each method has unique strengths and limitations depending on the quality of the MRI data available, and the population being studied (Miller et al. 2002).

Atrophy is progressive during the course of MS. Patients with RRMS tend to lose 17.3 ml/year of BPV compared to 23.6 ml/year for SPMS (Ge et al. 2000). Ventricles increase in size by 1.6 ml/year in MS compared to 0.3 ml/year for control subjects, while the annual rate of cerebral atrophy in the same study was of 0.8% and 0.3%, respectively (Fox et al. 2000). Several other studies have shown similar annual rates of brain volume decrease in MS, ranging from 0.6% to 0.8% (Comi et al. 2001a; Rovaris et al. 2001; Rudick et al. 1999). Brain volume changes, however, are complex and may also be affected by inflammation, edema, and hydration. Furthermore, the use of high-dose intravenous steroids for an acute clinical relapse can temporarily decrease brain volumes (Hoogervorst et al. 2002), and it is possible that some of the disease-modifying therapies used in the treatment of MS could have a similar effect. There have been mixed reports of the relationships between the T2 BOD, T1 black hole BOD, gadolinium activity and the degree of brain atrophy (Losseff et al. 1996a; Paolillo et al. 2000; Zivadinov and Zorzon 2002). This suggests that any relationship between these measures is partial at best. Furthermore, this may indicate that the

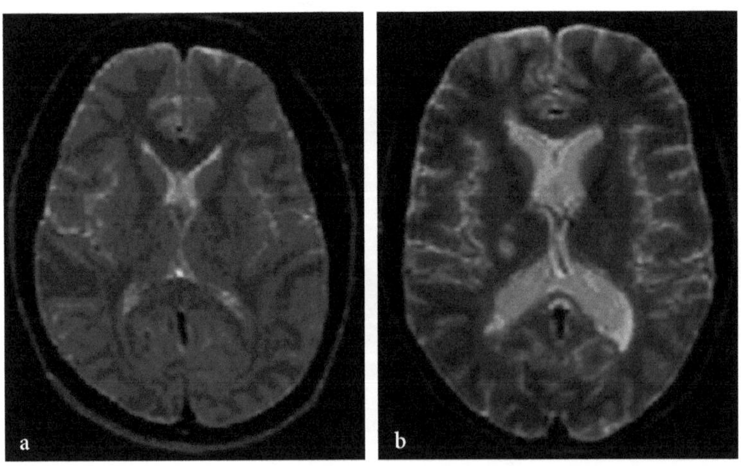

Fig. 14.7a,b. Compared to age-matched controls (**a**), MS patients (**b**) tend to have less brain parenchyma volume, increased size of the ventricles, and increased CSF spaces (i.e. atrophy)

pathological mechanisms underlying lesion formation are somewhat independent of the mechanisms leading to progressive tissue loss and atrophy.

14.4 Diagnosis

MS is a chronic disease, and most, if not all, MS patients will have T2 lesions on their brain and/or spinal cord images at some point in their disease course. The majority of MS patients have attacks of neurological dysfunction and a minority will have a slow progressive early course (Lublin and Reingold 1996). The clinical diagnosis requires two attacks or relapses consistent with demyelination of the central nervous system, and confirmed by a physician with adequate knowledge of the disease (McDonald et al. 2001; Poser et al. 1984). However, the interval between attacks is often years and this leads to a period of uncertainty for many patients who have suffered a single attack of demyelination (CIS). Although this group of patients are at risk for developing MS (recurrent attacks of demyelination), they are not necessarily destined to do so. The brain MRI findings at the time of a single clinical attack (CIS) are perhaps the best predictor of developing clinical MS (Brex et al. 2002; Cole et al. 2000).

The Optic Neuritis Treatment trial was one the earliest studies to systematically follow patients from multiple centers after a single event of demyelination. Approximately 50% of patients had a baseline brain MRI that had one or more T2 lesions. An abnormal MRI was the best predictor of converting to clinically definite MS (CDMS) at 10 years, with 56% of that group developed CDMS, whereas only 22% of those patients with a normal brain MRI at baseline subsequently developing CDMS (Beck et al. 2003). Similar results have been found by several groups investigating the natural history of developing MS after CIS including O'Riordan et al. (1998) after 10 years of follow-up. Subsequently Brex et al. (2002) followed the natural history cohort of O'Riordan et al. for up to 14 years since the first attack. This group included other typical forms of demyelination in addition to optic neuritis. In this population, approximately 88% of patients with an abnormal brain MRI at baseline converted to CDMS or laboratory-supported definite MS. However, only 19% of those with a normal initial brain MRI subsequently went on to MS. Although these studies differ in selection criteria and patients lost to follow-up, they support the prognostic value of early MRI abnormalities in MS.

The expanding knowledge of the predictive value of MRI in high-risk patients and that gained from the natural history of MRI changes in MS have led to a revision in the diagnostic criteria for MS proposed by an international panel of experts that met in London in 2000 (McDonald et al. 2001). In the appropriate clinical setting, MRI can support the diagnosis by providing additional evidence for disease dissemination that is separated in space and in time, especially in those patients who have only had the disease for a short period of time and lack sufficient clinical evidence to make the diagnosis. Table 14.1 summarizes how the MRI evidence required to support the diagnosis varies depending on the strength of the clinical findings. Table 14.2 illustrates the timing of serial MRI required to provide evidence for disease activity disseminated in time. The impact of using MRI in this manner is that patients can be diagnosed sooner with MS before they have new clinical symptoms. In a prospective natural history study of patients with a CIS, Dalton et al. found that only 20% of patients had had a second clinical attack at 2 years and met the Poser criteria, while 48% had a new clinically silent MRI activity and met the new international panel diagnostic criteria (Dalton et al. 2002). These patients included those with and without abnormalities on the baseline brain MRI. The specificity of the new criteria, compared to the traditional Poser criteria, was 95% (Dalton et al. 2003).

How valid these MRI criteria would be in atypical MS populations such as pediatric MS is not known. Furthermore, the evolution of MRI lesions in other white matter diseases such as neuroborreliosis, CNS angiitis, and CNS lupus have not been systematically studied to determine the specificity of these new diagnostic criteria. It is not uncommon to come across case series, such as with CNS involvement with Sjögren's disease (De Seze et al. 2001) where the MRI appearance and the clinical evolution resemble MS. Therefore, it must be emphasized that MRI plays a supportive role in the diagnosis, in the appropriate clinical situation, and always at the exclusion of alternative diagnoses (McDonald et al. 2001).

In diagnostically uncertain cases, the addition of spinal cord imaging can be extremely useful. Although the incidence of spinal cord lesions in MS is lower than that of brain lesions (present in 50–90% of patients with CDMS), the combination of spinal cord lesions with an abnormal brain MRI can improve the diagnostic confidence when other diseases are under consideration (Lycklama et al. 2003). An abnormal spinal cord MRI does not occur in normal controls, even in the elderly, and is much less com-

Table 14.1. International Diagnostic Criteria for MS (McDonald et al. 2001) (*RRMS* relapsing-remitting MS; *CIS* monosymptomatic, clinically isolated syndrome consistent with demyelination; *PPMS* primary progressive MS)

Clinical evidence		MRI evidence required to support diagnosis of MS	
Clinical attacks[a]	Physical signs[b]	Dissemination in space[c]	Dissemination in time[d]
Two or more (RRMS)	Two or more	Not needed (but recommended)	Not needed
Two or more (RRMS)	One	Required	Not needed
One (CIS)	Two or more	Not needed	Required
One (CIS)	One	Required	Required
None (PPMS)	One	Required[e] (and positive CSF)	Not needed (but helpful)

[a] Clinical attacks must be documented.
[b] Positive visual evoked potentials (delayed but well-preserved wave form) can substitute for one abnormal physical sign.
[c] MRI criteria for dissemination in space criteria in RRMS requires one of:
A. Two MRI lesions and positive CSF (oligoclonal IgG bands or elevated IgG index)
OR
B. Positive MRI by modified Barkhof criteria requires three of the following four criteria (one spinal cord lesion can substitute for one brain lesion, but a spinal cord lesion does not count as an infratentorial lesion):
One or more gadolinium-enhancing lesions OR nine or more T2 lesions
One or more infratentorial lesions
One or more juxtacortical lesions
Three or more periventricular lesions
[d] MRI criteria for dissemination in time (Table 2).
[e] Dissemination in space criteria for MRI in primary progressive MS (PPMS) requires positive CSF and one of:
Two or more spinal cord lesions
Three or more brain lesions and one spinal cord lesion and positive visual evoked potentials
Four or more brain lesions and one spinal cord lesion
Four or more brain lesions and positive VEPs
Nine or more T2 lesions (brain) only

Table 14.2. MRI evidence for dissemination in time

First scan (time since first attack, months)	Follow-up scan requirements for dissemination in time (not required if a second clinical attack occurs)	
Early (<3)	Second scan ≥3 months after attack but <3 months after first MRI	Gadolinium-enhancing lesion on second scan
Early (<3)	Second scan ≥3 months after first MRI	New T2 or gadolinium-enhancing lesion on second scan
Delayed– (≥3, and no gadolinium-enhancing lesions present)	Second scan ≥3 months after first MRI	New T2 or gadolinium-enhancing lesion on second scan
Delayed+ (≥3, and gadolinium-enhancing lesion present)	Follow-up scan not required	

mon with ischemia and other neurological diseases (6%) (Bot et al. 2002). Currently, the other recommended paraclinical tests used in the diagnosis of MS include cerebral spinal fluid analysis and visual evoked potentials. Although they lack the sensitivity of MRI, they can be helpful when the MRI abnormalities are indeterminate (McDonald et al. 2001).

MRI is not required for the diagnosis of MS. Nor are the individual lesions seen with conventional MRI techniques specific to MS. However, the pattern and evolution of MRI lesions, in the appropriate clinical setting, has made MRI abnormities important criteria for the early diagnosis of MS.

14.5 Clinical Correlations

14.5.1 Relapses

Most new MRI lesions are neurologically silent. The ability of conventional MRI to detect these lesions in the absence of clinical symptoms has contributed (ironically) to its generally poor correlation with overall clinical disability. The factors that determine neurological expression are probably a combination of location and the intensity and nature of pathology in the active lesion. Most clinical relapses are associated with new lesions on MRI (Smith et al. 1993; Thorpe et al. 1996) and RRMS patients can have new MRI lesions five to ten times more frequently than clinical relapses. Thus, only one of ten MRI active lesions hits an eloquent neurological tract and causes specific neurological symptoms to be identified as a clinical relapse. The severity of the pathological process in that lesion will affect the severity of the symptoms being expressed. Lesions that occur in relatively nonspecific areas of the brain such as the frontal lobes and the temporal lobes probably cause very subtle cognitive and emotional changes without necessarily producing specific neurological syndromes. Clinical relapses typically decrease in frequency with disease duration, and eventually most patients enter a phase of MS (SPMS) where progressive neurological deterioration occurs usually in the absence of clinical relapses. However, these patients continue to have a variable frequency of new lesion activity (Koopmans et al. 1989a).

14.5.2 Disability

Disability in MS can be transiently related to a clinical relapse or the result of incomplete recovery from a relapse, or be independent of relapses as a slow, relentless process. Disability has been traditionally measured on the ten-point Kurtzke expanded disability status scale (EDSS) (Kurtzke 1983). This scale can have significant inter- and intrarater variability, and tends to neglect cognitive dysfunction and fatigue. In most studies, there are significant but only modest correlations between EDSS and MRI active lesions and T2 BOD.

In contrast, cognitive abnormalities correlate well with the extent of involvement on the standard axial MRI image (Pozzilli et al. 1992). The location of the lesions may also be important as seen in a study of 39 MS patients where subcortical white matter disease was more strongly associated with cognitive dysfunction than total lesion load or cerebral atrophy (Damian et al. 1994). Modest associations can also be seen with regional atrophy measures, such as corpus callosum thinning (Edwards et al. 2001).

The poor correlation between MRI and clinical status is limited by the poor sensitivity of the clinical measures and by the inherent lack of tissue specificity of T2W images. Chronic black holes are associated with greater tissue destruction and have the potential for improved correlations with disability scales. In small studies, the correlations between the T1W black holes and EDSS have been modest but higher than those seen with T2 BOD for the same population (Truyen et al. 1996). However, a lack of a standardized approach to measuring and defining chronic black holes may limit future studies (Barkhof et al. 1998).

Brain and spinal cord atrophy are believed to be a common final pathway for the neurodegenerative aspects of MS that relate to irreversible disability. In general, correlations between global atrophy measures and disability have also only been modest (Miller et al. 2002). Regional atrophy of the spinal cord does tend to correlate better with disability. The cervical cord area measured using a technique with good reproducibility demonstrated a strong ($r=-0.7$) correlation between spinal cord area and disability measured by EDSS (Losseff et al. 1996b). At a mildly impaired EDSS of 3, the average cord area was reduced by 12% while at a severe level of disability (EDSS of 8) the average cord area was reduced by 35%. This may reflect the inherent bias of the EDSS for mobility that is reflected by spinal cord integrity.

Each MRI measure in isolation is only modestly correlated with clinical disability. This poor correlation between clinical and conventional MRI measures has, in part, fueled the need to develop additional MRI techniques such as magnetization transfer imaging and magnetic resonance spectroscopy. Efforts to combine multiple measures, including conventional and newer techniques, fail to fully explain the variance within a population's disability scores (Traboulsee et al. 2003). On the one hand, this reflects the limited nature of the EDSS scale which does not precisely quantify all aspects of clinical dysfunction. On the other hand, many T2 lesions are clinically silent and do not directly contribute to the disability, while functional reorganization may minimize the impact new lesions have on clinical disability. However, each of the conventional MRI measures reveals important and complimentary information that reflects the pathology of MS.

14.5.3 Prognosis

MRI measures are rarely used for prognosis because of this poor correlation with clinical outcome factors. One exception is for those patients presenting with a CIS who are at high risk of developing MS. The presence of MRI lesions in these patients is a strong predictor of MS and the baseline number, volume of lesions and rate of increase of total lesion volume over five years does have some prognostic value for future disability (Brex et al. 2002). A normal early scan also appears to predict a more benign course, although the numbers are quite small. However, for patients with established MS, the predictive value of new MRI lesions for short-term clinical outcomes such as relapses and disability remains poor (Kappos et al. 1999). A meta-analysis of 281 MS patients by Filippi (Filippi et al. 1995) found a significant but weak correlation between the development of new or enlarging T2 lesions over 2 to 3 years and worsening EDSS. It is possible that different mechanisms for disability dominate during different stages of the disease. There are several important long-term follow-up studies underway of patients with RRMS, originally enrolled in the pivotal interferon beta-1b and beta-1a clinical trials, that will include a comparison of their baseline MRI, with one obtained 7 to 10 years after starting treatment. It may be possible to use the baseline MRI characteristics to determine patterns of abnormalities that predict response to therapy and long-term prognosis.

14.6 Monitoring Treatment

Over the past decade there has been an increasing number of pivotal phase III clinical trials evaluating new therapies in MS. Conventional MRI measures of disease activity (new T2 and T1 gadolinium-enhancing lesions) and disease burden (T2 BOD and T1 hypointensities) have played an important role as a secondary outcome measures in the assessment and approval of these new treatments. The impact on new lesion activity varied from a suppression of less than 50% for new lesion formation or active scans compared to placebo for glatiramer acetate (Comi et al. 2001b) and interferon beta-1a 30 µg once weekly (Jacobs et al. 1996) to greater than 80% suppression for the higher dose interferons beta-1a (Li and Paty 1999) and beta-1b (Paty and Li 1993). The higher dose and higher frequency interferons beta-1a and beta-1b also had the greatest impact on reducing the accumulation of T2 BOD, with up to 4 years of follow-up (Prisms Study Group 2001). This pattern of response was consistent for drugs within the same class (interferon beta-1a and beta-1b) and with drugs that work by different mechanisms of action (glatiramer acetate).

The MRI measures were objectively quantified, blinded, and could be standardized for multicenter studies using clinical MRI scanners that varied in field strength, manufacturer, software and local expertise. Gadolinium-enhancing lesions, new T2 lesions and enlarging T2 lesions all represent new inflammation. It might be considered redundant information to detect all three types of lesions. However, it is useful to see a consistency in response across these measures, and in our experience, one measure may be more sensitive to a dose difference that would have been missed had only gadolinium-enhancing lesions been used (Li and Paty 1999). More recently, Wolinsky et al. have proposed a composite index of four MRI outcomes (contrast-enhancing lesion volume, T2 BOD, T1 hypointensity volume and CSF volume) as a potential outcome measure (Wolinsky et al. 2000) which would need to be evaluated and validated.

New lesion activity as detected by MRI has been favored as the primary outcome measure for phase I and phase II clinical trials of promising new therapies in MS. This is because it allows fairly rapid assessment using fewer patient because of the relatively higher frequency of MRI activity compared to clinical relapses. However, this could bias against the development of agents that have a potentially greater impact on the neurodegenerative aspects of the disease rather than inflammation.

Applying these results obtained from group or population outcomes from clinical trials to making treatment decisions for the individual patient remains unproven. The poor correlation between clinical status and MRI measures, and the yet-to-be proven long-term prognostic value of MRI limits its use for monitoring treatment response. There is also tremendous individual variation in the response to treatment, with almost a similar spread in response between those who are on placebo and those who have been treated. On the other hand, most would agree that MRI is an in vivo measure of the pathology of MS: new MRI activity reflects active inflammation and the accumulation of T2 burden, chronic black holes, and progressive brain and spinal cord atrophy likely reflect worsening disease irrespective of the clinical status. What is required before they can be used and applied in the management of the individual is the validation of what these changes mean for the long-term outcome of the individual patient and how they are modified and affected by treatment.

14.7 Summary

Conventional MRI techniques include measures of new inflammation (new and enlarging T2W lesions, gadolinium-enhancing T1W lesions), measures of acute and chronic disease (total T2 volume or BOD), and measures of degeneration (global brain and spinal cord atrophy, and chronic black holes on T1W images). Combined, they provide a unique insight into the dynamics of MS lesion development and the long-term pathological consequences on CNS tissues. The limited clinical correlation reflects, in part, the unique sensitivity of MRI to detect clinically silent disease. Although not required for the clinical diagnosis of MS, conventional MRI methods can be invaluable in establishing an earlier diagnosis. These techniques can also be standardized on routine clinical MRI scanners and used in multicenter therapeutic trials. Conventional MRI measures have become important outcome measures in clinical trials of new therapies for MS. It is likely that conventional MRI measures will be augmented, rather than replaced, by newer methods as the conventional methods reflect the basic pathological processes of MS. However, additional validation will be needed before they can be used to effectively monitor treatment response in the individual patient.

References

Bagnato F, Jeffries N, Richert ND, et al (2003) Evolution of T1 black holes in patients with multiple sclerosis imaged monthly for 4 years. Brain 126:1782–1789

Barkhof F, McGowan JC, van Waesberghe JH, et al (1998) Hypointense multiple sclerosis lesions on T1-weighted spin echo magnetic resonance images: their contribution in understanding multiple sclerosis evolution. J Neurol Neurosurg Psychiatry 64 [Suppl 1]:S77–S79

Barnes D, Munro PM, Youl BD, et al (1991) The longstanding MS lesion. A quantitative MRI and electron microscopic study. Brain 114:1271–1280

Beck RW, Trobe JD, Moke PS, et al (2003) High- and low-risk profiles for the development of multiple sclerosis within 10 years after optic neuritis: experience of the optic neuritis treatment trial. Arch Ophthalmol 121:944–949

Boggild MD, Williams R, Haq N, et al (1996) Cortical plaques visualised by fluid-attenuated inversion recovery imaging in relapsing multiple sclerosis. Neuroradiology 38 [Suppl 1]:S10–S13

Bot JC, Barkhof F, Lycklama A, et al (2002) Differentiation of multiple sclerosis from other inflammatory disorders and cerebrovascular disease: value of spinal MR imaging. Radiology 223:46–56

Brex PA, Jenkins R, Fox NC, et al (2000) Detection of ventricular enlargement in patients at the earliest clinical stage of MS. Neurology 54:1689–1691

Brex PA, Ciccarelli O, O'Riordan JI, et al (2002) A longitudinal study of abnormalities on MRI and disability from multiple sclerosis. N Engl J Med 346(3):158–164

Cala LA, Mastaglia FL, Black JL (1978) Computerized tomography of brain and optic nerve in multiple sclerosis. Observations in 100 patients, including serial studies in 16. J Neurol Sci 36:411–426

Ciccarelli O, Werring DJ, Wheeler-Kingshott CAM, et al (2001) Investigation of MS normal-appearing brain using diffusion tensor MRI with clinical correlations. Neurology 56:926–933

Cole SR, Beck RW, Moke PS, et al (2000) The National Eye Institute Visual Function Questionnaire: experience of the ONTT. Optic Neuritis Treatment Trial. Invest Ophthalmol Vis Sci 41:1017–1021

Comi G, Filippi M, Barkhof F, et al (2001a) Effect of early interferon treatment on conversion to definite multiple sclerosis: a randomised study. Lancet 357:1576–1582

Comi G, Filippi M, Wolinsky JS (2001b) European/Canadian multicenter, double-blind, randomized, placebo-controlled study of the effects of glatiramer acetate on magnetic resonance imaging-measured disease activity and burden in patients with relapsing multiple sclerosis. European/Canadian Glatiramer Acetate Study Group. Ann Neurol 49:290–297

Dalton CM, Brex PA, Miszkiel KA, et al (2002) Application of the new McDonald criteria to patients with clinically isolated syndromes suggestive of multiple sclerosis. Ann Neurol 52:47–53

Dalton CM, Brex PA, Miszkiel KA, et al (2003) New T2 lesions enable an earlier diagnosis of multiple sclerosis in clinically isolated syndromes. Ann Neurol 53:673–676

Damian MS, Schilling G, Bachmann G, et al (1994) White matter lesions and cognitive deficits: relevance of lesion pattern? Acta Neurol Scand 90:430–436

Davies MB, Williams R, Haq N, et al (1998) MRI of optic nerve and postchiasmal visual pathways and visual evoked potentials in secondary progressive multiple sclerosis. Neuroradiology 40:765–770

de Seze J, Devos D, Castelnovo G, et al (2001) The prevalence of Sjogren syndrome in patients with primary progressive multiple sclerosis. Neurology 57:1359–1363

De Stefano N, Narayanan S, Francis SJ, et al (2002) Diffuse axonal and tissue injury in patients with multiple sclerosis with low cerebral lesion load and no disability. Arch Neurol 59:1565–1571

Edwards SG, Liu C, Blumhardt LD (2001) Cognitive correlates of supratentorial atrophy on MRI in multiple sclerosis. Acta Neurol Scand 104:214–223
Filippi M, Paty DW, Kappos L, et al (1995) Correlations between changes in disability and T2-weighted brain MRI activity in multiple sclerosis: a follow-up study. Neurology 45:255–260
Filippi M, Yousry T, Baratti C, et al (1996a) Quantitative assessment of MRI lesion load in multiple sclerosis. A comparison of conventional spin-echo with fast fluid-attenuated inversion recovery. Brain 119:1349–1355
Filippi M, Yousry T, Campi A, et al (1996b) Comparison of triple dose versus standard dose gadolinium-DTPA for detection of MRI enhancing lesions in patients with MS. Neurology 46:379–384
Filippi M, Marciano N, Capra R, et al (1997) The effect of imprecise repositioning on lesion volume measurements in patients with multiple sclerosis. Neurology 49:274–276
Filippi M, Mastronardo G, Rocca MA, et al (1998) Quantitative volumetric analysis of brain magnetic resonance imaging from patients with multiple sclerosis. J Neurol Sci 158:148–153
Filippi M, Rovaris M, Rice GP, et al (2000) The effect of cladribine on T(1) 'black hole' changes in progressive MS. J Neurol Sci 176:42–44
Fox NC, Jenkins R, Leary SM, et al (2000) Progressive cerebral atrophy in MS: a serial study using registered, volumetric MRI. Neurology 54:807–812
Gawne-Cain ML, O'Riordan JI, Thompson AJ, et al (1997) Multiple sclerosis lesion detection in the brain: a comparison of fast fluid-attenuated inversion recovery and conventional T2-weighted dual spin echo. Neurology 49:364–370
Ge Y, Grossman RI, Udupa JK, et al (2000) Brain atrophy in relapsing-remitting multiple sclerosis and secondary progressive multiple sclerosis: longitudinal quantitative analysis. Radiology 214:665–670
Ge Y, Grossman RI, Babb JS, et al (2003) Dirty-appearing white matter in multiple sclerosis: volumetric MR imaging and magnetization transfer ratio histogram analysis. AJNR Am J Neuroradiol 24:1935–1940
Harris JO, Frank JA, Patronas N, et al (1991) Serial gadolinium-enhanced magnetic resonance imaging scans in patients with early, relapsing-remitting multiple sclerosis: implications for clinical trials and natural history. Ann Neurol 29:548–555
Hoogervorst EL, Polman CH, Barkhof F (2002) Cerebral volume changes in multiple sclerosis patients treated with high-dose intravenous methylprednisolone. Mult Scler 8:415–419
Horowitz AL, Kaplan RD, Grewe G, et al (1989) The ovoid lesion: a new MR observation in patients with multiple sclerosis. AJNR Am J Neuroradiol 10:303–305
Isaac C, Li DKB, Genton M, et al (1988) Multiple sclerosis: a serial study using MRI in relapsing patients. Neurology 38:1511–1515
Jacobs LD, Cookfair DL, Rudick RA, et al (1996) Intramuscular interferon beta-1a for disease progression in relapsing multiple sclerosis. The Multiple Sclerosis Collaborative Research Group (MSCRG). Ann Neurol 39:285–294
Kappos L, Moeri D, Radue EW, et al (1999) Predictive value of gadolinium-enhanced magnetic resonance imaging for relapse rate and changes in disability or impairment in multiple sclerosis: a meta-analysis. Gadolinium MRI Meta-analysis Group. Lancet 353:964–969
Kermode AG, Tofts PS, Thompson AJ, et al (1990) Heterogeneity of blood-brain barrier changes in multiple sclerosis: an MRI study with gadolinium-DTPA enhancement. Neurology 40:229–235
Kidd D, Barkhof F, McConnell R, et al (1999) Cortical lesions in multiple sclerosis. Brain 122:17–26
Koopmans RA, Li DK, Oger JJ, et al (1989a) Chronic progressive multiple sclerosis: serial magnetic resonance brain imaging over six months. Ann Neurol 26:248–256
Koopmans RA, Li DKB, Grochowski E, et al (1989b) Benign vesus chronic progressive multiple sclerosis: magnetic resonance imaging features. Ann Neurol 25:74–81
Koopmans RA, Li DKB, Oger JJF, et al (1989c) The lesion of multiple sclerosis: imaging of acute and chronic stages. Neurology 39:959–963
Kurtzke JF (1983) Rating neurologic impairment in multiple sclerosis: an expanded disability status scale (EDSS). Neurology 33:1444–1452
Lee MA, Smith S, Palace J, et al (1999) Spatial mapping of T2 and gadolinium-enhancing T1 lesion volume in multiple sclerosis: evidence for distinct mechanisms of lesion genesis? Brain 122:1261–1270
Li DK, Paty DW (1999) Magnetic resonance imaging results of the PRISMS trial: a randomized, double-blind, placebo-controlled study of interferon-beta1a in relapsing-remitting multiple sclerosis. Prevention of Relapses and Disability by Interferon-beta1a Subcutaneously in Multiple Sclerosis. Ann Neurol 46:197–206
Liu C, Edwards S, Gong Q, et al (1999) Three dimensional MRI estimates of brain and spinal cord atrophy in multiple sclerosis. J Neurol Neursurg Psychiatry 66:323–330
Losseff NA, Wang L, Lai HM, et al (1996a) Progressive cerebral atrophy in multiple sclerosis. A serial MRI study. Brain 119:2009–2019
Losseff NA, Webb SL, O'Riordan JI, et al (1996b) Spinal cord atrophy and disability in multiple sclerosis. A new reproducible and sensitive MRI method with potential to monitor disease progression. Brain 119:701–708
Lublin FD, Reingold SC (1996) Defining the clinical course of multiple sclerosis: results of an international survey. National Multiple Sclerosis Society (USA) Advisory Committee on Clinical Trials of New Agents in Multiple Sclerosis. Neurology 46:907–911
Lycklama G, Thompson A, Filippi M, et al (2003) Spinal-cord MRI in multiple sclerosis. Lancet Neurol 2:555–562
McDonald WI, Ron MA (1999) Multiple sclerosis: the disease and its manifestations (review). Philos Trans R Soc Lond B Biol Sci 354:1615–1622
McDonald WI, Compston A, Edan G, et al (2001) Recommended diagnostic criteria for multiple sclerosis: guidelines from the International Panel on the Diagnosis of Multiple Sclerosis. Ann Neurol 50:121–127
McFarland HF, Frank JA, Albert PS, et al (1992) Using gadolinium-enhanced magnetic resonance imaging lesions to monitor disease activity in multiple sclerosis. Ann Neurol 32:758–766
Miller DH, Rudge P, Johnson G, et al (1988) Serial gadolinium enhanced magnetic resonance imaging in multiple sclerosis. Brain 111:927–939
Miller DH, Barkhof F, Frank JA, et al (2002) Measurement of atrophy in multiple sclerosis: pathological basis, method-

ological aspects and clinical relevance. Brain 125:1676–1695
Nesbit GM, Forbes GS, Scheithauer BW, et al (1991) Multiple sclerosis: histopathologic and MR and/or CT correlation in 37 cases at biopsy and three cases at autopsy. Radiology 180:467–474
Newcombe J, Hawkins CP, Henderson CL, et al (1991) Histopathology of multiple sclerosis lesions detected by magnetic resonance imaging in unfixed postmortem central nervous system tissue. Brain 114:1013–1023
O'Riordan JI, Thompson AJ, Kingsley DP, et al (1998) The prognostic value of brain MRI in clinically isolated syndromes of the CNS. A 10-year follow-up. Brain 121:495–503
Ostuni JL, Richert ND, Lewis BK, et al (1999) Characterization of differences between multiple sclerosis and normal brain: a global magnetization transfer application. AJNR Am J Neuroradiol 20:501–507
Paolillo A, Pozzilli C, Gasperini C, et al (2000) Brain atrophy in relapsing-remitting multiple sclerosis: relationship with 'black holes', disease duration and clinical disability. J Neurol Sci 174:85–91
Paty DW (1988) Magnetic resonance imaging in the assessment of disease activity in multiple sclerosis. Can J Neurol Sci 15:266–272
Paty DW, Li DK (1993) Interferon beta-1b is effective in relapsing-remitting multiple sclerosis. II. MRI analysis results of a multicenter, randomized, double-blind, placebo-controlled trial. UBC MS/MRI Study Group and the IFNB Multiple Sclerosis Study Group. Neurology 43:662–667
Paty DW, Li DK, Oger JJ, et al (1994) Magnetic resonance imaging in the evaluation of clinical trials in multiple sclerosis. Ann Neurol [Suppl] 36:S95–S96
Poser CM, Paty DW, Scheinberg L, et al (1984) New diagnostic criteria for multiple sclerosis. Guidelines for research protocols. In: Poser CM, Paty DW, Scheinberg L, Ebers GC (eds) The diagnosis of multiple sclerosis. Thieme-Stratton, New York, pp 225–233
Pozzilli C, Fieschi C, Perani D, et al (1992) Relationship between corpus callosum atrophy and cerebral metabolic asymmetries in multiple sclerosis. J Neurol Sci 112:51–57
PRISMS Study Group (2001) PRISMS-4: long-term efficacy of interferon-beta-1a in relapsing MS. Neurology 56:1628–1636
Rovaris M, Rocca MA, Capra R, et al (1998) A comparison between the sensitivities of 3-mm and 5-mm thick serial brain MRI for detecting lesion volume changes in patients with multiple sclerosis. J Neuroimaging 8:144–147
Rovaris M, Comi G, Rocca MA, et al (2001) Short-term brain volume change in relapsing-remitting multiple sclerosis: effect of glatiramer acetate and implications. Brain 124:1803–1812
Rudick RA, Fisher E, Lee JC, et al (1999) Use of the brain parenchymal fraction to measure whole brain atrophy in relapsing-remitting MS. Multiple Sclerosis Collaborative Research Group. Neurology 53:1698–1704
Rydberg JN, Riederer SJ, Rydberg CH, et al (1995) Contrast optimization of fluid-attenuated inversion recovery (FLAIR) imaging. Magn Reson Med 34:868–877
Silver NC, Good CD, Barker GJ, et al (1997) Sensitivity of contrast enhanced MRI in multiple sclerosis. Effects of gadolinium dose, magnetization transfer contrast and delayed imaging. Brain 120:1149–1161
Smith ME, Stone LA, Albert PS, et al (1993) Clinical worsening in multiple sclerosis is associated with increased frequency and area of gadopentetate dimeglumine-enhancing magnetic resonance imaging lesions. Ann Neurol 33:480–489
Stewart WA, Hall LD, Berry K, et al (1986) Magnetic resonance imaging (MRI) in multiple sclerosis (MS): pathological correlation studies in eight cases. Neurology 36:320
Stone LA, Albert PS, Smith ME (1995) Changes in the amount of diseased white matter over time in patients with relapsing-remitting multiple sclerosis. Neurology 45:1808–1814
Tartaglino LM, Friedman DP, Flanders AE, et al (1995) Multiple sclerosis in the spinal cord: MR appearance and correlation with clinical parameters. Radiology 195:725–732
Thielen KR, Miller GM (1996) Multiple sclerosis of the spinal cord: magnetic resonance appearance. J Comput Assist Tomogr 20:434–438
Thorpe JW, Kidd D, Moseley IF, et al (1996) Serial gadolinium-enhanced MRI of the brain and spinal cord in early relapsing-remitting multiple sclerosis. Neurology 46:373–378
Tien RD, Hesselink JR, Szumowski J (1991) MR fat suppression combined with Gd-DTPA enhancement in optic neuritis and perineuritis. J Comput Assist Tomogr 15:223–227
Traboulsee A, Dehmeshki J, Peters KR, et al (2003) Disability in multiple sclerosis is related to normal appearing brain tissue MTR histogram abnormalities. Mult Scler 9:566–573
Truyen L, van Waesberghe JH, van Walderveen MA, et al (1996) Accumulation of hypointense lesions ("black holes") on T1 spin-echo MRI correlates with disease progression in multiple sclerosis. Neurology 47:1469–1476
van Walderveen MA, Barkhof F, Tas MW, et al (1998) Patterns of brain magnetic resonance abnormalities on T2-weighted spin echo images in clinical subgroups of multiple sclerosis: a large cross-sectional study. Eur Neurol 40:91–98
van Walderveen MA, Barkhof F, Pouwels PJ, et al (1999) Neuronal damage in T1-hypointense multiple sclerosis lesions demonstrated in vivo using proton magnetic resonance spectroscopy. Ann Neurol 46:79–87
Whittall KP, MacKay AL, Li DK, et al (2002) Normal-appearing white matter in multiple sclerosis has heterogeneous, diffusely prolonged T(2). Mag Reson Med 47:403–408
Willoughby EW, Grochowski E, Li DKB, et al (1989) Serial magnetic resonance scanning in multiple sclerosis: a second prospective study in relapsing patients. Ann Neurol 25:43–49
Wolinsky JS, Narayana PA, NoseworthyJH, et al (2000) Linomide in relapsing and secondary progressive MS: part II: MRI results. Neurology 54:1734–1741
Young IR, Hall AS, Pallis CA, et al (1981) Nuclear magnetic resonance imaging of the brain in multiple sclerosis. Lancet 2:1063–1066
Zhao GJ, Li DK, Wang XY, et al (2000) MRI of dirty-appearing white matter in MS. Neurology 54:A121
Zivadinov R, Zorzon M (2002) Is gadolinium enhancement predictive of the development of brain atrophy in multiple sclerosis? J Neuroimaging 12:302–309

15 Multiple Sclerosis: Other MR Techniques

MASSIMO FILIPPI and MARIA A. ROCCA

CONTENTS

15.1 Introduction

Multiple sclerosis (MS) is the commonest chronic inflammatory demyelinating disease affecting the central nervous system (CNS) of young adults in western countries, leading, in the majority of cases, to severe and irreversible clinical disability. Pathologically, the essential brain lesion in MS has always been considered the demyelinated plaques, which are widely distributed throughout the brain and spinal cord. The evolution of these lesions may be extremely variable in a given patient and between different patients.

M. FILIPPI, MD; M.A. ROCCA, MD
Neuroimaging Research Unit, Department of Neurology, Scientific Institute and University Ospedale San Raffaele, Milan, Italy.

The application of conventional magnetic resonance imaging (cMRI) to the study of MS has greatly improved our ability to diagnose MS and to monitor its evolution. The sensitivity of T2-weighted MRI in the detection of MS lesions and that of post-contrast T1-weighted images to detect lesions with an increased blood–brain barrier permeability associated with inflammatory activity make it possible to demonstrate the dissemination of MS lesions in space and time earlier than with clinical assessment and to detect disease activity with an increased sensitivity with respect to clinical evaluation of relapses (McDONALD et al. 2001). However, the magnitude of the relationship between cMRI measures of disease activity or burden and the clinical manifestations of the disease is weak (ROVARIS and FILIPPI 1999; MOLYNEUX et al. 2001). This clinical/MRI discrepancy is likely to be the result, at least partially, of the inability of cMRI to quantify the extent and to define the nature of MS-related tissue damage.

Pathological studies (LUMSDEN 1970; KIDD et al. 1999; PETERSON et al. 2001) have shown that MS is not exclusively a demyelinating disease and that demyelination alone is not sufficient to explain the neurological deficits of the disease. There are compelling pieces of evidence that axonal damage is one of the main contributors to the clinical manifestations of the disease and to its clinical worsening over time. Pathologically, marked axonal transection in inflamed MS lesions has been demonstrated by several authors (FERGUSON et al. 1997; TRAPP et al. 1998). The pathological heterogeneity of MS lesions, which can range from lesions which undergo a significant remyelination after their acute formation to lesions with permanent axonal loss, has to be considered among the factors responsible for the limited ability of cMRI to provide an accurate picture of MS-related tissue damage. In addition, lesions located in the gray matter (GM) have also been described in MS (LUMSDEN 1970; KIDD et al. 1999; PETERSON et al. 2001). Although MS cortical lesions are characterized by the paucity of inflammatory changes, they are associated with neuronal injury, including neuritic swelling, and dendritic and axonal transections (Peterson et al. 2001). These lesions are usually missed on conventional T2-weighted images because of their small size, their relaxation characteristics which result in poor contrast between them and the surrounding normal GM and because of partial volume effects with cerebrospinal fluid. Another reason for the clinical/MRI discrepancy in MS is the inability of cMRI to measure and quantify the presence and extent of normal-appearing tissue damage. Post-mortem studies have shown subtle changes in the normal-appearing brain tissue (NABT) from MS patients, which include diffuse astrocytic hyperplasia, patchy edema, and perivascular cellular infiltration, as well as axonal damage (Allen and McKeown 1979; Evangelou et al. 2000; Bjartmar et al. 2001).

Modern quantitative MR techniques have the potential to overcome some of the limitations of cMRI. Metrics derived from magnetization transfer (MT) (Filippi et al. 1999a) and diffusion-weighted (DW) (Filippi and Inglese 2001) MRI enable us to quantify the extent and severity of structural changes occurring within and outside cMRI-visible lesions of patients with MS. Proton MR spectroscopy (^{1}H-MRS) (Filippi et al. 2001a) can add information on the biochemical nature of such changes. Functional MRI (fMRI) (Filippi and Rocca 2003) can provide new insights into the role of cortical adaptive changes in limiting the clinical consequences of MS structural damage.

This chapter provides an update of the current "state-of-the-art" of the application of structural, metabolic and functional MR-based techniques to the study of MS pathophysiology.

15.2 MT MRI

The basic principles of MT MRI are described elsewhere in this book. An example of a magnetization transfer ratio (MTR) map is shown in Fig. 15.1. On MTR maps, the degree of signal loss depends on the density of macromolecules in a given tissue, and low MTR values indicate a reduced capacity of the macromolecules in the CNS to exchange magnetization with the surrounding water molecules, reflecting damage to myelin or to the axonal membrane. MT MRI has several advantages over cMRI in the assessment of MS. First of all, it provides quantitative information with a high specificity to demyelination and axonal loss, the more disabling substrates of MS pathology. Secondly, it enables us to assess the "invisible" disease burden in the brain tissue which does not show macroscopic abnormalities on cMRI. Thirdly, with the application of MTR histogram analysis, it provides, from a single procedure, multiple parameters influenced by both the macro- and microscopic lesion burden, that might also be used as paraclinical measures of MS evolution, either natural or modified by treatment.

A post-mortem study in MS (van Waesberghe et al. 1999) has provided the most compelling evidence that a marked reduction of MTR values in MS diseased tissues indicates severe structural damage, by showing strong correlations of MTR values from MS lesions and normal-appearing white matter (NAWM) with the percentage of residual axons and the degree of demyelination. More recently, a study performed on human specimens has confirmed the sensitivity

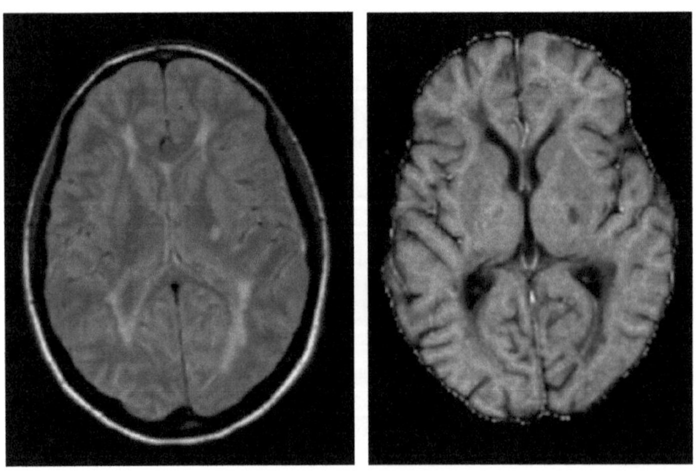

a b

Fig. 15.1a,b. Axial magnetic resonance images from a patient with multiple sclerosis. The proton-density weighted scan (**a**) shows multiple lesions. On the magnetization transfer (MT) map (**b**), lesions appear as hypointense areas. The degree of hypointensity is related to a decrease in the MT ratio and indicates damage to the myelin or to the axonal membranes of this technique towards the different pathological substrates of the disease, by showing that MTR values of remyelinated lesions are higher than those of demyelinated lesions and lower than those of the NAWM (Barkhof et al. 2003).

15.2.1 MT MRI Findings in Individual MS Lesions

The following are the main findings obtained by the application of MT MRI for the study of individual MS lesions:

1. New enhancing lesions are pathologically heterogeneous, as suggested by the demonstration that MTR values are higher: (a) in homogeneously enhancing lesions, which probably represent new lesions, than in ring-enhancing lesions, which may represent pre-existent, reactivated lesions (Silver et al. 1998); (b) in lesions enhancing on a single scan than in those enhancing on two or more serial scans (Filippi et al. 1998a); (c) in lesions enhancing after the injection of a triple dose of gadolinium than in those enhancing after the injection of a standard dose (Filippi et al. 1998b).
2. MTR changes can be detected in NAWM before lesion formation (Filippi et al. 1998c; Goodkin et al. 1998; Pike et al. 2000; Fazekas et al. 2002).
3. Longitudinal studies have shown that, in new enhancing lesions, MTR drops dramatically when the lesions start to enhance and can show a partial or complete recovery in the subsequent 1–6 months (Dousset et al. 1998; Filippi et al. 1998a,b; Goodkin et al. 1998; Silver et al. 1998; van Waesberghe et al. 1998).
4. Established MS lesions are also heterogeneous, as shown by the demonstration of lower MTR values in hypointense lesions than in lesions that are isointense to NAWM on T1-weighted scans (van Waesberghe et al. 1998).
5. Average lesion MTR has been found to be lower in patients with relapsing-remitting (RR) MS than in those with clinically isolated syndromes (CIS) suggestive of MS (Filippi et al. 1999), whereas no differences have been found in cross-sectional studies between patients with RRMS and those with secondary progressive (SP) MS (Filippi et al. 1999b) or between patients with SPMS and those with primary progressive (PP) MS (Rovaris et al. 2001). However, longitudinal studies have shown a more severe and faster decline of average lesion MTR values in SPMS patients than in patients with other disease phenotypes (Rocca et al. 1999; Filippi et al. 2000a), consistent with the unfavorable clinical evolution of these patients.

15.2.2 MT MRI Findings in NABT

The pathological abnormalities observed in the NAWM of MS patients (Allen and McKeown 1979; Evangelou et al. 2000; Bjartmar et al. 2001) have the potential to modify the relative proportions of mobile and bound protons in the affected tissue and, as a consequence, the corresponding MTR values. Therefore, MT MRI can show NABT microstructural abnormalities not detected when using conventional imaging. MT MRI analysis of the NABT can be performed using either a region of interest (ROI) approach, or, alternatively, a histogram analysis. More recently, with the development of new techniques capable of automatically segmenting the NAWM and the NAGM, it has become possible to study these two tissue compartments separately.

The following are the main results obtained by the application of MT MRI to the study of the NABT of MS patients:

1. Using ROI-analysis, a reduction of MTR values has been shown in the NAWM of MS patients with all the major MS phenotypes (Filippi et al. 1995; Loevner et al. 1995). More recently, MTR changes, of a lower magnitude than those observed in T2-visible lesions, have also been detected in the dirty-appearing white matter of MS patients (Ge et al. 2003).
2. The application of histogram analysis (Filippi et al. 1999b; Iannucci et al. 2000; Kalkers et al. 2001; Rovaris et al. 2001; Tortorella et al. 2000; Traboulsee et al. 2002) to the study of the NABT and of the NAWM confirmed and extended the previous findings obtained with ROI analysis, by showing that these abnormalities can be detected even in patients with CIS suggestive of MS (Iannucci et al. 2000; Traboulsee et al. 2002), are more pronounced in SPMS and PPMS patients than in patients with the other disease phenotypes (Tortorella et al. 2000), and are similar between patients with SPMS and those with PPMS (Rovaris et al. 2001) (Fig. 15.2).
3. NABT MTR values tend to decline over time in all MS phenotypes, even if these changes seem to be more pronounced in SPMS patients (Filippi et al. 2000a).
4. NABT MTR values are only partially correlated with the extent of macroscopic lesions and the

severity of intrinsic lesion damage (Tortorella et al. 2000), thus suggesting that NABT pathology does not only reflect Wallerian degeneration of axons traversing large focal abnormalities, but they may also represent small focal abnormalities beyond the resolution of conventional scanning and independent of larger lesions.

5. Using ROI (Cercignani et al. 2001) and histogram analysis (Cercignani et al. 2001; Ge et al. 2001, 2002; Dehmeshki et al. 2003), MT MRI abnormalities have also been shown in the NAGM of MS patients, including those with PPMS (Dehmeshki et al. 2003). As shown for the NABT, also NAGM changes are more pronounced in patients with SPMS than in those with RRMS (Ge et al. 2002).

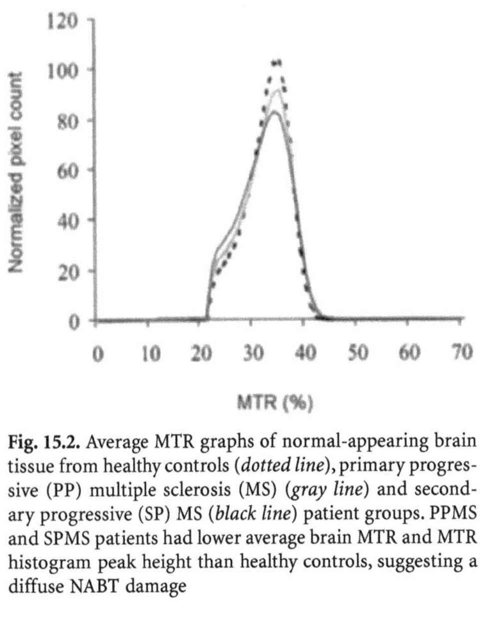

Fig. 15.2. Average MTR graphs of normal-appearing brain tissue from healthy controls (*dotted line*), primary progressive (PP) multiple sclerosis (MS) (*gray line*) and secondary progressive (SP) MS (*black line*) patient groups. PPMS and SPMS patients had lower average brain MTR and MTR histogram peak height than healthy controls, suggesting a diffuse NABT damage

15.2.3 Correlations with Clinical Manifestations and Disability

Due to its capability of quantifying the extent and the severity of tissue damage within T2-visible lesion and NABT, MT MRI is increasing the degree of correlation between MRI and clinical findings, as summarized below:

1. Moderate to strong correlations between various brain MTR histogram-derived metrics and the severity of physical disability have been shown by several studies (Iannucci et al. 1999; Dehmeshki et al. 2001; Kalkers et al. 2001; Traboulsee et al. 2003). These correlations have been found to be stronger in patients with RRMS and SPMS than in other disease phenotypes (Dehmeshki et al. 2001; Kalkers et al. 2001).
2. Subtle MTR changes in the NABT (Rovaris et al. 1998; van Buchem et al. 1998) and in the cortical/subcortical (Rovaris et al. 2000) brain tissue are well correlated with the presence of neuropsychological impairment in MS patients. In addition, a multivariate analysis of several MRI and MT MRI variables, has demonstrated that average NABT MTR is more strongly associated to cognitive impairment in MS patients than the extent of T2-visible lesions and their intrinsic tissue damage (Filippi et al. 2000b).
3. MTR histogram parameters from the cerebellum and brainstem of MS patients are significantly associated with impairment of these functional systems (Iannucci et al. 1999).
4. NAGM MTR metrics are correlated with the severity of clinical disability in patients with RR (Ge et al. 2001) and PP (Dehmeshki et al. 2003) MS.
5. Longitudinal studies (Iannucci et al. 2000; Santos et al. 2002; Rovaris et al. 2003) demonstrated that MT MRI metrics are useful markers to monitor disease evolution. In patients at presentation with CIS, the extent of NABT changes has been found to be an independent predictor of subsequent evolution to clinically definite MS (Iannucci et al. 2000); whereas in patients with established MS, NAWM MTR reduction has been shown to predict the accumulation of clinical disability over the subsequent 5 years (Santos et al. 2002; Rovaris et al. 2003).

15.2.4 MT MRI to Monitor Treatment Efficacy

MT MRI holds substantial promise to provide good surrogate markers for MS evolution (Filippi et al. 2002a). As a consequence, several recent MS clinical trials have already incorporated MT MRI, with a view to assessing the impact of treatment on demyelination and axonal loss. MT MRI has been used in phase II and phase III trials for RRMS (injectable and oral interferon beta-1a, interferon beta-1b, and oral glatiramer acetate) and SPMS (interferon beta-1b and immunoglobulins). In these phase III trials, MT MRI acquisition has been limited to highly-specialized MR centers and only subgroups of patients (about 50–100 per trial) have been studied using this technique. Two phase II studies have shown that treatment with interferon beta-1b (RICHERT et al. 2001) or interferon beta-1a (KITA et al. 2000) favorably modifies the recovery of MTR values which follows the cessation of gadolinium enhancement in newly-formed lesions from RRMS patients. On the contrary, RICHERT et al. (2001) did not find any significant difference in the MTR values of NAWM ROI before and during interferon beta-1b therapy, as well as in the parameters derived from whole brain MTR histograms (RICHERT et al. 1998) in RRMS patients. More recently, it has also been shown that treatment with interferon beta-1b does not affect the MTR loss seen in whole brain tissue and NAWM of patients with SPMS recruited in the European phase III trial (INGLESE et al. 2003a).

15.3 DW MRI

Diffusion is the microscopic random translational motion of molecules in a fluid system. In the CNS, diffusion is influenced by the microstructural components of tissue, including cell membranes and organelles. The diffusion coefficient of biological tissues (which can be measured in vivo by MRI) is, therefore, lower than the diffusion coefficient in free water and for this reason is named apparent diffusion coefficient (ADC) (LE BIHAN et al. 1986). Pathological processes which modify tissue integrity, thus resulting in a loss or increased permeability of "restricting" barriers, can determine an increase of the ADC. Since some cellular structures are aligned on the scale of an image pixel, the measurement of diffusion is also dependent on the direction in which diffusion is measured. As a consequence, diffusion measurements can give information about the size, shape, integrity, and orientation of tissues (LE BIHAN et al. 1991). A measure of diffusion which is independent of the orientation of structures is provided by the mean diffusivity (MD), the average of the ADCs measured in three orthogonal directions. A full characterization of diffusion can be obtained in terms of a tensor (BASSER et al. 1994), a 3×3 matrix which accounts for the correlation existing between molecular displacement along orthogonal directions. From the tensor, it is possible to derive MD, equal to the one third of its trace, and some other dimensionless indexes of anisotropy. One of the most used of these indices is named fractional anisotropy (FA) (PIERPAOLI et al. 1996). A more detailed description of technical aspects of DW MRI is provided in another chapter of this book.

The pathological elements of MS have the potential to alter the permeability or geometry of structural barriers to water molecular diffusion in the brain (Fig. 15.3). The application of DW MRI technology to MS is, therefore, appealing to provide quantitative estimates of the degree of tissue damage and, as a consequence, to improve the understanding of the mechanisms leading to irreversible disability.

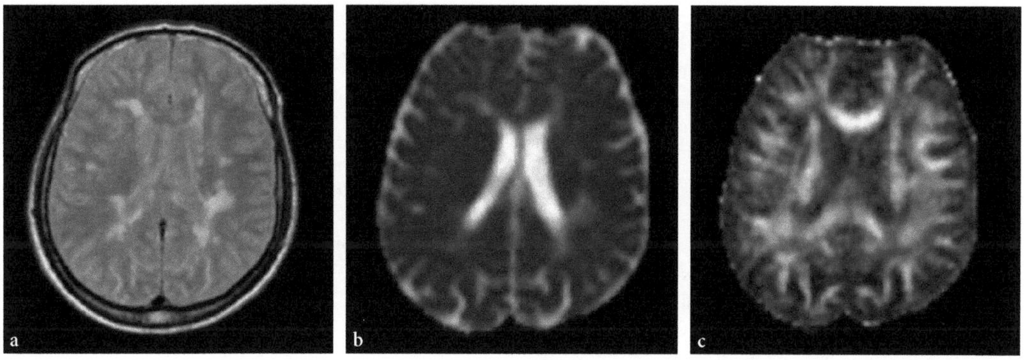

Fig. 15.3a–c. Axial magnetic resonance images from a patient with multiple sclerosis. The proton density-weighted scan (**a**) shows multiple lesions. On the mean diffusivity (MD) map (**b**), some of the lesions appear as hyperintense areas. The degree of hyperintensity is related to an increased MD and indicates a loss of structural barriers to water molecular motion. On the fractional anisotropy (FA) map (**c**), white matter pixels are bright because of the directionality of the white matter fiber tracts. Dark areas corresponding to some of the macroscopic lesions indicate a loss of FA and suggest the presence of structural disorganization

15.3.1 DW MRI Findings in Individual MS Lesions

The following are the main findings obtained by the application of DW MRI for the study of individual MS lesions:

1. Consistently with their pathological heterogeneity, T2-visible lesions are characterized by highly variable ADC, MD, and FA values (Horsfield et al. 1996; Droogan et al. 1999; Werring et al. 1999, 2000a; Filippi et al. 2000c, 2001b; Cercignani et al. 2000, 2001; Rocca et al. 2000). In particular, ADC and MD values have been shown to be higher in T1-hypointense than in T1-isointense lesions (Droogan et al. 1999; Werring et al. 1999; Filippi et al. 2000c, 2001b).
2. While FA values are consistently lower in enhancing than in non-enhancing lesions (Werring et al. 1999; Filippi et al. 2001b), conflicting results have been achieved when comparing ADC or MD between these two lesion populations. While some studies reported higher ADC or MD values in non-enhancing than in enhancing lesions (Droogan et al. 1999; Werring et al. 1999), others, based on larger samples of patients and lesions, did not report any significant difference between the two lesion populations (Filippi et al. 2000c, 2001b). The heterogeneity of enhancing lesions has also been underlined by the demonstration that water diffusivity is markedly increased in ring-enhancing lesions when compared to homogeneously-enhancing lesions (Roychowdhury et al. 2000), or in the non-enhancing portions of enhancing lesions when compared with enhancing portions (Roychowdhury et al. 2000).
3. As for MT MRI, DW MRI changes have been shown in regions that will develop new lesions (Rocca et al. 2000; Werring et al. 2000a).

15.3.2 DW MRI Findings in NABT

As for MT MRI, DW MRI analysis of regions that appear as "normal" on conventional imaging can be performed using either an ROI or histogram analysis. The major findings derived by the application of DW MRI to the assessment of NABT pathology of MS patients are the following:

1. ROIs of the NAWM of MS patients have increased ADC or MD and decreased FA values when compared to the corresponding white matter from controls. However, these abnormalities are milder than those measured in T2-visible lesions (Horsfield et al. 1996; Droogan et al. 1999; Werring et al. 1999, 2000a; Filippi et al. 2000c, 2001b; Cercignani et al. 2000, 2001; Rocca et al. 2000; Ciccarelli et al. 2001).
2. MD and FA changes in the whole brain and in the NABT have been shown also using histogram analysis in all the major MS clinical phenotypes (Cercignani et al. 2000, 2001; Nusbaum et al. 2000), including PPMS (Rocca et al. 2003a).
3. Using ROI (Cercignani et al. 2001) and histogram analysis (Cercignani et al. 2001; Bozzali et al. 2002; Rovaris et al. 2002a), MD changes have been shown to involve also the NAGM of MS patients (Fig. 15.4). Consistently with their worse clinical evolution, these changes tend to be more pronounced in patients with the progressive forms of the disease (Bozzali et al. 2002; Rovaris et al. 2002a), whereas no MD abnormalities have been detected in the NAGM and NAWM of patients with early RRMS (Griffin et al. 2001).
4. In a 1-year follow up study, Caramia et al. (2002) showed the development of MD abnormalities in the NAWM of CIS patients that evolved to definite MS. In an 18-month follow up study, Oreja-Guevara et al. (2003) showed that NAGM changes in patients with RRMS worsen over time.

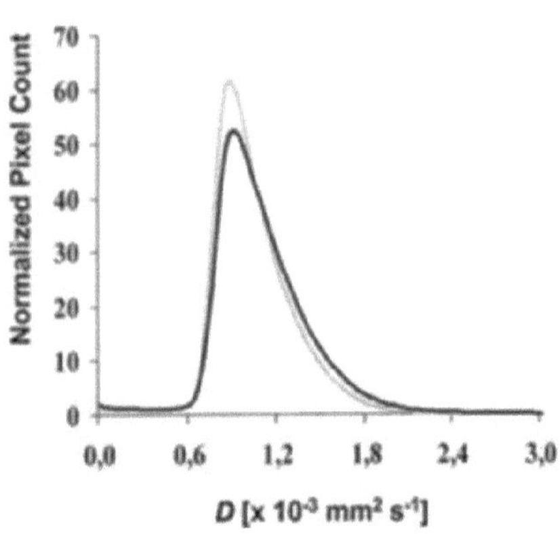

Fig. 15.4. Mean diffusivity (MD) histogram of the normal-appearing gray matter (NAGM) from a group of healthy controls (*gray line*) and a large sample of MS patients (*black line*). All MD histogram-derived metrics of the NAGM were significantly different between healthy controls and MS population, indicating the presence of structural damage of this tissue compartment

15.3.3 Correlations with Clinical Manifestations and Disability

The following are the major results obtained by the application of DW MRI to investigate the correlations between structural brain changes and the clinical manifestations of the disease:

1. While correlations between DW MRI findings and MS clinical manifestations or disability were not found in some of the earliest studies (Horsfield et al. 1996; Droogan et al. 1999; Cercignani et al. 2000; Filippi et al. 2000c), with improved DW MRI technology and increased numbers of patients studied, correlations between DW MRI findings and MS clinical manifestations or disability are now emerging (Castriota Scanderbeg et al. 2000; Nusbaum et al. 2000; Cercignani et al. 2001; Filippi et al. 2001b; Rovaris et al. 2002a).
2. In a large sample of MS patients, average lesion MD, but not average lesion FA, was found to be significantly correlated, albeit moderately, with clinical disability (Filippi et al. 2001b). Interestingly, in patients with SPMS a moderate and significant correlation was found between average lesion MD or FA and disability (Castriota Scanderbeg et al. 2000; Filippi et al. 2001b), whereas no significant correlation was found between disability and T2 lesion volume. On the contrary, a significant correlation between disability and T2 lesion volume was found in patients with RRMS, where, in turn, there was no correlation between average lesion MD or FA and disability (Filippi et al. 2001b). These findings suggest that mechanisms leading to disability are likely to be different in patients with RRMS and SPMS.
3. DW MRI metrics of specific brain structures, such as the pyramidal tracts (Wilson et al. 2003) or the cerebellar peduncles (Ciccarelli et al. 2001) are strongly correlated with the impairment of these functional systems.
4. In patients with RRMS, a moderate correlation between cognitive impairment and NAGM MD histogram metrics has been shown (Rovaris et al. 2002b).

15.4 ^{1}H-MRS

Water suppressed, proton MR spectra of normal human brain at long echo times reveal four major resonances: one at 3.2 ppm from tetramethylamines (mainly from choline-containing phospholipids [Cho]), one at 3.0 ppm from creatine and phosphocreatine (Cr), one at 2.0 ppm from N-acetyl groups (mainly NAA), and one 1.3 ppm from the methyl resonance of lactate (Lac). NAA is a marker of axonal integrity, while Cho and Lac are considered as chemical correlates of acute inflammatory/demyelinating changes (Filippi et al. 2001a). ^{1}H-MRS studies with shorter echo times can detect additional metabolites, such as lipids and myoinositol (mI), which are also regarded as markers of ongoing myelin damage. Additional technical information on ^{1}H-MRS are given elsewhere in this book.

^{1}H-MRS can complement cMRI in the assessment of MS patients, by defining simultaneously several chemical correlates of the pathological changes occurring within and outside T2-visible lesions. An immunopathologic study (Bitsch et al. 1999) has shown that a decrease in NAA levels is correlated with axonal loss, while an increase in Cho correlates with the presence of active demyelination and gliosis.

15.4.1 ^{1}H-MRS Findings in Individual MS Lesions

As shown by other non-conventional MRI techniques, ^{1}H-MRS can depict the heterogeneous pathological substrates of T2-visible MS lesions. The following are the major insights provided by the application of ^{1}H-MRS to the study of MS lesions:

1. ^{1}H-MRS of acute MS lesions at both short and long echo times reveals increases in Cho and Lac resonance intensities (Davie et al. 1994; De Stefano et al. 1995a), which reflect the releasing of membrane phospholipids and the metabolism of inflammatory cells, respectively. In large, acute demyelinating lesions, decreases of Cr can also be seen (De Stefano et al. 1995a). Short echo time spectra can detect transient increases in visible lipids, released during myelin breakdown, and mI (Narayana et al. 1998). All these changes are usually associated with a decrease in NAA. After the acute phase and over a period of days to weeks, there is a progressive reduction of raised Lac resonance intensities to normal levels. Resonance intensities of Cr also return to normal within a few days. Cho, lipid and mI resonance intensities return to normal over months. The signal intensity of NAA may remain decreased or show partial recovery, starting soon after the acute phase and lasting for several months (Arnold et al. 1992;

Davie et al. 1994; De Stefano et al. 1995a). Recovery of NAA may be related to resolution of edema, increases in the diameter of previously shrunk axons secondary to remyelination and clearance of inflammatory factors and reversible metabolic changes in neurons.

2. Chronic MS lesions are characterized by markedly reduced NAA/Cr peaks. These changes are more pronounced in severely hypointense MS lesions than in iso- or mildly hypointense lesions (van Walderveen et al. 1999) and in chronic lesions from patients with SPMS than in those from patients with benign MS (Falini et al. 1998).
3. Cho increase, probably reflecting an altered myelin chemistry or the presence of inflammation, and a decrease in NAA have been also shown in prelesional NAWM (Narayana et al. 1998; Sarchielli et al. 1999; Tartaglia et al. 2002).

15.4.2
^{1}H-MRS Findings in NABT

^{1}H-MRS also has the potential to provide information on MS pathological changes outside T2-visible lesions. The following are the main findings obtained from the study of the NABT in MS patients using ^{1}H-MRS:

1. Studies of limited and/or selected portions of the brain (Fu et al. 1998; Sarchielli et al. 1999; De Stefano et al. 2002) have shown that NAA reduction is not restricted to MS lesions, but also occurs in the NAWM. These changes are more severe in SPMS and PPMS patients than in those with RRMS (Fu et al. 1998; Suhy et al. 2000); however, they can be detected even in patients with no overt clinical disability (De Stefano et al. 2002) and in those in the early phase of the disease (De Stefano et al. 2001). Diffusely elevated Cho and Cr concentrations have also been described in the NAWM of RRMS (Inglese et al. 2003b) and PPMS (Suhy et al. 2000) patients.
2. The recent development of an unlocalized ^{1}H-MRS sequence for measuring NAA levels in the whole brain (WBNAA) (Gonen et al. 1998) has shown the presence of marked axonal pathology in clinically definite MS (Gonen et al. 2000; Bonneville et al. 2002) and in patients at the earliest clinical phases of MS (Filippi et al. 2003). Interestingly, no correlation has been found between WBNAA concentrations and T2-weighted lesion volumes in patients with RRMS (Bonneville et al. 2002) and in those at presentation with CIS (Filippi et al. 2003a). The lack of such a correlation is likely to be the result of the fact that T2-visible lesions represent just a small component of overall brain damage and calls for an accurate assessment of NABT pathology for a better understanding of MS pathophysiology.
3. Metabolite abnormalities, including decrease of NAA and Cho and increase of mI, have also been shown in the cortical GM of MS patients (Kapeller et al. 2001; Sarchielli et al. 2002; Sharma et al. 2001; Chard et al. 2002), since the early phases of the disease (Chard et al. 2002), but not in CIS patients (Kapeller et al. 2002). These changes are more pronounced in patients with SPMS than in those with RRMS (Adalsteinsson et al. 2003). More recently, NAA reduction has also been demonstrated in the thalamus of SPMS (Cifelli et al. 2002) and RRMS patients (Wylezinska et al. 2003).

15.4.3
Correlations with Clinical Manifestations and Disability

As already mentioned, axonal loss and/or dysfunction is likely to have a major role in the development of fixed clinical disability in MS. In agreement with this notion, a post-mortem study (Bjartmar et al. 2000) has shown a strong correlation between neurological impairment and both axonal density and NAA reduction in the spinal cord of patients with MS. The following are the main in vivo findings obtained from the application of ^{1}H-MRS to the understanding of MS-related disability:

1. Following an acute MS relapse, reversible decreases in NAA have been observed not only in macroscopic lesions responsible for the clinical symptomatology (De Stefano et al. 1995b; Reddy et al. 2000a), but also in the NAWM of the hemisphere contralateral to acute lesions (De Stefano et al. 1999) (Fig. 15.5) and have been correlated with reversal of functional impairment.
2. In patients with RRMS, a longitudinal decrease over time of NAA/Cr in the NAWM correlates strongly with EDSS worsening (De Stefano et al. 1998; Fu et al. 1998), suggesting that progressive axonal damage or loss may be responsible for functional impairment in MS. More recently, it has been demonstrated that brain axonal damage begins in the early stages of MS, develops more rapidly in the earlier clinical stages of the disease and correlates more strongly with disability in patients with mild than in those with more severe disease (De Stefano et al. 2001).

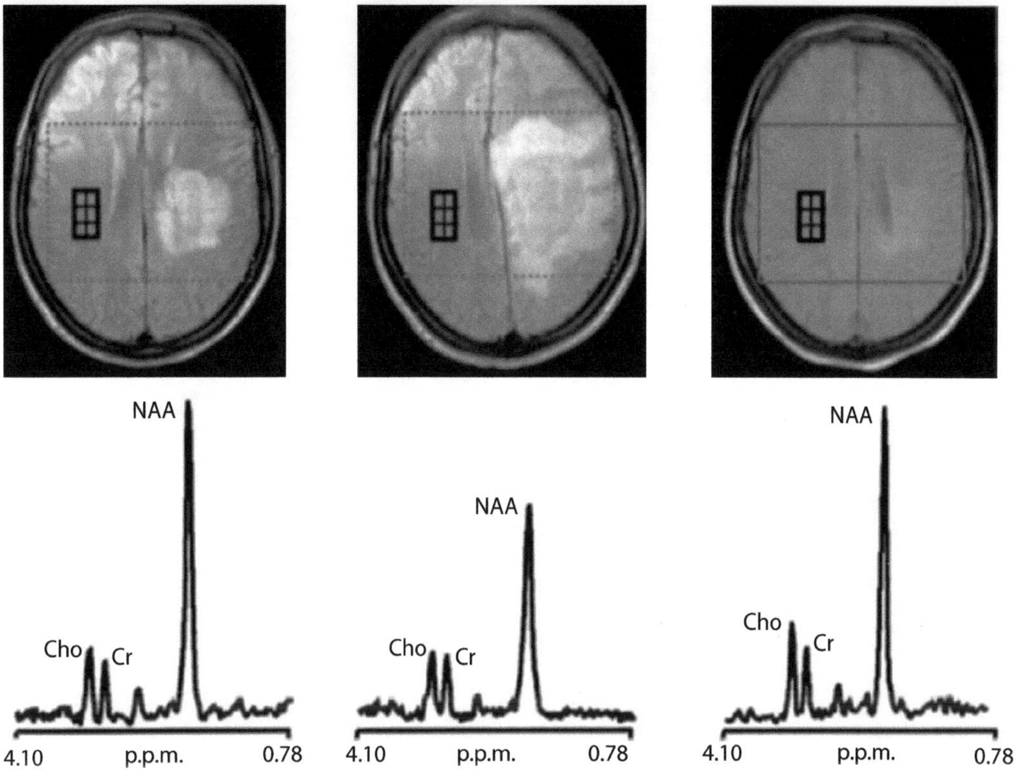

Fig. 15.5. Proton brain MRI/MRSI examinations of a multiple sclerosis patient performed during the acute phase of the disease (*left*), 1 month later (*center*) and 6 months later (*right*). Conventional proton MRI examinations show a solitary demyelinating lesion that enlarges to involve most of the hemisphere 1 month later (*top center*), and then decreases in size on the examination at 6 months (*top right*). Volumes of interest for spectroscopy are shown by the *dotted line* in each transverse MRI. Averaged spectra from voxels located in normal-appearing white matter contralateral and homologous to the demyelinating lesion (*small squares* in *top panels*) are shown in the *bottom panels*. Note the decrease in the NAA/Cr resonance intensity 1 month after the acute phase of the disease (*bottom center*). Complete recovery of NAA/Cr intensity ratios occurred at 6 months (*bottom right*)

3. NAA levels have also been quantified in specific brain regions, whose damage has been related to the impairment of the corresponding functional systems. Davie et al. (1995) showed a significant reduction of NAA concentration in the cerebellar WM of patients with MS and severe ataxia compared with those having little or no cerebellar deficits. Lee et al. (2000a) demonstrated an association between reduction of NAA in the internal capsule and selective motor impairment. Pan et al. (2001) found a relation between cognitive function and NAA levels in the periventricular WM. More recently, Gadea et al. (2004) found a relationship between attentional dysfunction in early RRMS patients and NAA/Cr values in the locus coeruleus nuclei of the pontine ascending reticular activation system.

15.4.4 ^{1}H-MRS to Monitor Treatment Efficacy

Only four studies have been conducted to evaluate the effect of disease-modifying MS treatments on ^{1}H-MRS-derived parameters (Sarchielli et al. 1998; Narayanan et al. 2001; Schubert et al. 2002; Khan et al. 2003). Using monthly ^{1}H-MRS scans, Sarchielli et al. (1998) found that treatment with interferon beta-1a is associated with increased Cho peaks in spectra of lesions from RRMS patients, suggesting an increase in lesion membrane turnover during the first period of treatment. Narayanan et al. (2001) found an increase of NAA/Cr in a small group of RRMS patients after 1 year of treatment with interferon beta-1b, suggesting a potential effect of treatment in preventing chronic, sublethal axonal injury. More recently, SCHUBERT et al. (2002) showed a stability of metabolite concentration over time in patients with RRMS treated with interferon beta-1b. Finally, KHAN et al. (2003) showed an increase of NAA/Cr levels in lesions and NAWM of RRMS patients after 2 years of treatment with glatiramer acetate.

15.5 Functional MRI

Although the resolution of acute inflammation, remyelination, redistribution of voltage-gated sodium-channels in persistently demyelinated axons, and recovery from sublethal axonal injury are all factors likely to limit the clinical impact of damaging MS pathology (WAXMAN and RITCHIE 1993; DE STEFANO et al. 1995b), other mechanisms have been recently recognized as potential contributors to the recovery or to the maintenance of function in the presence of irreversible MS-related axonal damage. Brain plasticity is a well known feature of the human brain which is likely to have several pathologic substrates, including an increased axonal expression of sodium channels (WAXMAN 1998), synaptic changes, increased recruitment of parallel existing pathways or "latent" connections, and reorganization of distant sites. All these changes might have a major adaptive role in limiting the functional consequences of axonal loss. The application of fMRI to the study of the motor, visual and cognitive systems in patients with MS has provided new insights into the mechanisms contributing to the progressive clinical worsening of these patients.

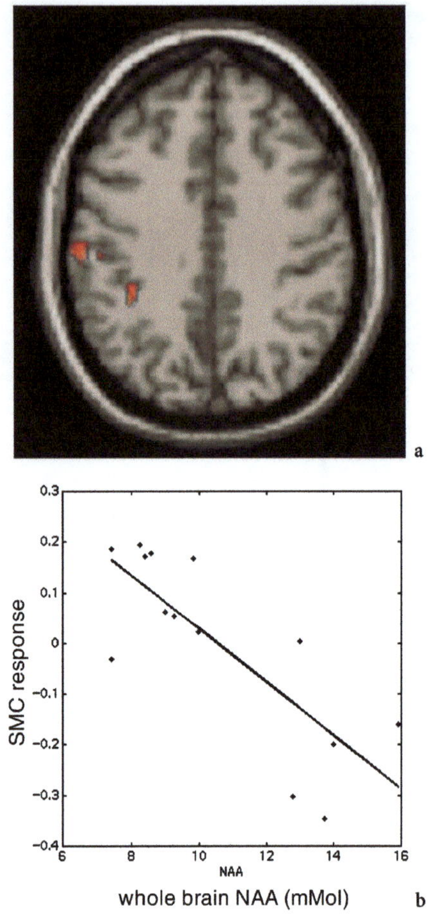

Fig. 15.6a,b. Relative contralateral primary sensory-motor cortex (SMC) activation in patients at presentation with clinically isolated syndromes suggestive of multiple sclerosis during the performance of a simple motor task with the right hand in comparison to healthy volunteers (**a**). The scatterplot of the correlation between the relative activation of the contralateral primary SMC and whole brain *N*-acetyl aspartate concentrations is shown in (**b**)

Functional cortical changes have been demonstrated in all MS phenotypes, using different fMRI paradigms. A study of the visual system (WERRING et al. 2000b), in patients who had recovered from a single episode of acute optic neuritis (ON), demonstrated that such patients had an extensive activation of the visual network compared to healthy volunteers. An altered brain pattern of movement-associated cortical activations, characterized by an increased recruitment of the contralateral primary sensorimotor cortex (SMC) during the performance of simple tasks (ROCCA et al. 2003b; FILIPPI et al. 2004a) (Fig. 15.6) and by the recruitment of additional "classical" and "higher-order" sensorimotor areas during the performance of more complex tasks (FILIPPI et al. 2004a) has been demonstrated in patients with CIS. An increased recruitment of several sensorimotor areas, mainly located in the cerebral hemisphere ipsilateral to the limb which performed the task has also been demonstrated in patients with early MS and a previous episode of hemiparesis (PANTANO et al. 2002a). Interestingly, in patients with similar characteristics, but who presented with an ON, this increased recruitment involved sensorimotor areas which were mainly located in the contralateral cerebral hemisphere (PANTANO et al. 2002b). In patients with established MS and a RR course, functional cortical changes have been shown during the performance of visual (ROMBOUTS et al. 1998), motor (LEE et al. 2000b; REDDY et al. 2000a, 2000b; FILIPPI et al. 2002b; ROCCA et al. 2002a), and cognitive (Staffen et al. 2002; Hillary et al. 2003; Parry et al. 2003) tasks. Movement-associated cortical changes, characterized by the activation of highly specialized cortical areas, have also been described in patients with SPMS (Rocca et al. 2003c) during the performance of a simple motor task. Two fMRI studies of the motor system (Filippi et al. 2002c; Rocca et al. 2002b) of patients with PPMS suggested a lack of "classical" adaptive mechanisms as a potential additional factor contributing to the accumulation of disability.

The results of all these studies suggest that there might be a "natural history" of the functional reorganization of the cerebral cortex in MS patients, which might be characterized, at the beginning of the disease, by an increased recruitment of those areas "normally" devoted to the performance of a given task, such as the primary SMC and the supplementary motor area (SMA) in case of a motor task. At a later stage, bilateral activation of these regions is first seen, followed by a widespread recruitment of additional areas, which are usually recruited in normal people to perform novel/complex tasks. This notion has been supported by the results of a recent study (Filippi et al. 2004b), which has provided a direct demonstration that MS patients, during the performance of a simple motor task, activate some regions, that are part of a fronto-parietal circuit, whose activation occurs typically in healthy subjects during object manipulation (Filippi et al. 2004b).

15.5.1 Correlations with Structural Tissue Damage

The following are the main findings supporting the adaptive role of functional cortical changes in MS:

a) An increased cortical recruitment with increasing T2 lesion load has been shown in patients with relapsing (Lee et al. 2000a; Pantano et al. 2002a; Rocca et al. 2002a), SP (Rocca et al. 2003c) and PP (Rocca et al. 2002b) MS.
b) The severity of intrinsic T2-visible lesion damage has been found to modulate the activity of some cortical areas. A strongly increased recruitment of the primary SMC has been shown to be correlated with the severity of lesion damage of the corticospinal tracts, measured using T1-weighted images (Pantano et al. 2002b) and with the whole brain average lesion MT ratio and mean diffusivity (Rocca et al. 2002a).
c) The severity of NABT damage, measured using ^{1}H-MRS (Reddy et al. 2000b; Rocca et al. 2003b), MT MRI or DW MRI (Filippi et al. 2002c; Rocca et al. 2002a; Rocca et al. 2003c) is another important factor modulating movement-associated cortical reorganization, as shown by studies of patients with various disease phenotypes and different levels of disability (Reddy et al. 2000b), patients at presentation with CIS suggestive of MS (Rocca et al. 2003b) (Fig. 15.6), patients with RRMS and no clinical disability (Rocca et al. 2002a), and PPMS and SPMS patients with different degrees of clinical involvement (Filippi et al. 2002c; Rocca et al. 2003c).
d) Subtle GM damage may play a role in modulating cortical excitability, as demonstrated in patients with SPMS (Rocca et al. 2003c) and in patients with clinically definite MS and non-specific (less than three lesions) cMRI findings (Rocca et al. 2003d).
e) Finally, the demonstration of strong correlations between cortical activations and cervical cord damage, quantified using MT MRI, in patients with PPMS (Filippi et al. 2002c), patients with a previous episode of acute myelitis of probable demyelinating origin (Rocca et al. 2003e), and patients with Devic's neuromyelitis optica (Rocca et al. 2004) suggests that not only brain, but also spinal cord pathology can induce cortical changes with the potential to limit the functional impact of the disease.

15.5.2 Correlations with Clinical Manifestations and Disability

Although the actual role of cortical reorganization on the clinical manifestations of MS remains unclear, the demonstration that MS patients may have a normal level of performance despite the presence of diffuse tissue damage suggests that cortical adaptive changes are likely to contribute in limiting the clinical consequences of MS-related structural damage (Filippi and Rocca 2003). The most compelling evidence that cortical reorganization may have a role in recovery from axonal damage derives from the study by Reddy et al. (2000a), who followed a patient after the onset of an acute hemiparesis and a new, large demyelinating lesion located in the corticospinal tract with serial 1H-MRS and fMRI exams. In this patient, clinical recovery preceded complete normalization of NAA and was accompanied by increased recruitment of ipsilateral primary SMC and SMA. In line with these findings, in a group of patients who complained of fatigue when compared to matched non-fatigued MS patients, there was a reduced activation of a complex movement-associated cortical/subcortical network, including the cerebellum, the rolandic operculum, the thalamus and the middle frontal gyrus (Filippi et al. 2002b). In these patients, a strong correlation between the reduction of thalamic activity and the clinical severity of fatigue was found, indicating that a less marked cortical recruitment might be associated to the appearance of clinical symptomatology in MS. Preliminary work has shown that the pattern of movement-associated cortical activations in MS is determined by both the extent of brain injury and disability and that these changes are distinct (Reddy et al. 2002).

15.6 Conclusions

The application of modern MRI techniques to the assessment of MS patients has considerably improved our understanding of MS pathophysiology and has provided new objective metrics that might be useful to monitor disease evolution, either in natural history studies or in treatment trials. However, none of the quantitative MR-based techniques considered, taken in isolation, is able to provide a complete picture of the complexity of the MS process and this should call for the definition of aggregates of MR quantities, thought to reflect different aspects of MS pathology, to improve our ability to monitor the disease. At present, longitudinal natural history data collected in large samples of MS patients using structural, metabolic and functional MR techniques are needed to gain additional insight into MS pathobiology and on the actual value of modern MR technologies in the management of MS.

References

Adalsteinsson E, Langer-Gould A, Homer RJ et al (2003) Gray matter N-acetyl aspartate deficits in secondary progressive but not relapsing-remitting multiple sclerosis. AJNR Am J Neuroradiol 24:1941–1945

Allen IV, McKeown SR (1979) A histological, histochemical and biochemical study of the macroscopically normal white matter in multiple sclerosis. J Neurol Sci 41:81–91

Arnold DL, Matthews PM, Francis GS et al (1992) Proton magnetic resonance spectroscopic imaging for metabolic characterization of demyelinating plaques. Ann Neurol 31:235–241

Barkhof F, Bruck W, De Groot CJ et al (2003) Remyelinated lesions in multiple sclerosis: magnetic resonance image appearance. Arch Neurol 60:1073–1081

Basser PJ, Mattiello J, Le Bihan D (1994) Estimation of the effective self-diffusion tensor from the NMR spin-echo. J Magn Reson B 103: 247–254

Bitsch A, Bruhn H, Vougioukas V et al (1999) Inflammatory CNS demyelination: histopathologic correlation with in vivo quantitative proton MR spectroscopy. AJNR Am J Neuroradiol 20:1619–1627

Bjartmar C, Kidd G, Mork S et al (2000) Neurological disability correlates with spinal cord axonal loss and reduced N-acetyl aspartate in chronic multiple sclerosis patients. Ann Neurol 48:893–901

Bjartmar C, Kinkel RP, Kidd G et al (2001) Axonal loss in normal-appearing white matter in a patient with acute MS. Neurology 57:1248–1252

Bonneville F, Moriarty DM, Li BS et al (2002) Whole-brain N-acetyl aspartate concentration: correlation with T2-weighted lesion volume and expanded disability status scale score in cases of relapsing-remitting multiple sclerosis. AJNR Am J Neuroradiol 23:371–375

Bozzali M, Cercignani M, Sormani MP et al (2002) Quantification of brain gray matter damage in different MS phenotypes by use of diffusion tensor MR imaging. AJNR Am J Neuroradiol 23:985–988

Caramia F, Pantano P, Di Legge S et al (2002) A longitudinal study of MR diffusion changes in normal appearing white matter of patients with early multiple sclerosis. Magn Reson Imaging 20:383–388

Castriota Scanderbeg A, Tomaiuolo F, Sabatini U et al (2000) Demyelinating plaques in relapsing-remitting and secondary-progressive multiple sclerosis: assessment with diffusion MR imaging. AJNR Am J Neuroradiol 21:862–868

Cercignani M, Iannucci G, Rocca MA et al (2000) Pathologic damage in MS assessed by diffusion-weighted and magnetization transfer MRI. Neurology 54:1139–1144

Cercignani M, Bozzali M, Iannucci G et al (2001) Magnetisation transfer ratio and mean diffusivity of normal-appearing white and gray matter from patients with multiple sclerosis. J Neurol Neurosurg Psychiatry 70:311–317

Chard DT, Griffin CM, McLean MA et al (2002) Brain metabolite changes in cortical grey and normal-appearing white matter in clinically early relapsing-remitting multiple sclerosis. Brain 125:2342–2352

Ciccarelli O, Werring DJ, Wheeler-Kingshott CA et al (2001) Investigation of MS normal-appearing brain using diffusion tensor MRI with clinical correlations. Neurology 56:926–933

Cifelli A, Arridge M, Jezzard P et al (2002) Thalamic neurodegeneration in multiple sclerosis. Ann Neurol 52:650–653

Davie CA, Hawkins CP, Barker GJ et al (1994) Serial proton magnetic resonance spectroscopy in acute multiple sclerosis lesions. Brain 117:49–58

Davie CA, Barker GJ, Webb S et al (1995) Persistent functional deficit in multiple sclerosis and autosomal dominant cerebellar ataxia is associated with axon loss. Brain 118:1583–1592

Dehmeshki J, Ruto AC, Arridge S et al (2001) Analysis of MTR histograms in multiple sclerosis using principal components and multiple discriminant analysis. Magn Reson Med 46:600–609

Dehmeshki J, Chard DT, Leary SM et al (2003) The normal appearing grey matter in primary progressive multiple sclerosis: a magnetisation transfer imaging study. J Neurol 250:67–74

De Stefano N, Matthews PM, Antel JP et al (1995a) Chemical pathology of acute demyelinating lesions and its correlation with disability. Ann Neurol 38:901–909

De Stefano N, Matthews PM, Arnold DL (1995b) Reversible decreases in N-acetyl aspartate after acute brain injury. Magn Reson Med 34:721–727

De Stefano N, Matthews PM, Fu L et al (1998) Axonal damage correlates with disability in patients with relapsing-remitting multiple sclerosis. Results of a longitudinal magnetic resonance spectroscopy study. Brain 121:1469–1477

De Stefano N, Narayanan S, Matthews PM et al (1999) In vivo evidence for axonal dysfunction remote from focal cerebral demyelination of the type seen in multiple sclerosis. Brain 122:1933–1939

De Stefano N, Narayanan S, Francis GS et al (2001) Evidence of axonal damage in the early stages of multiple sclerosis and its relevance to disability. Arch Neurol 58:65–70

De Stefano N, Narayanan S, Francis SJ et al (2002) Diffuse axonal and tissue injury in patients with multiple sclerosis with low cerebral lesion load and no disability. Arch Neurol 59:1565–1571

Dousset V, Gayou A, Brochet B et al (1998) Early structural changes in acute MS lesions assessed by serial magnetization transfer studies. Neurology 51:1150–1155

Droogan AG, Clark CA, Werring DJ et al (1999) Comparison of multiple sclerosis clinical subgroups using navigated spin echo diffusion-weighted imaging. Magn Reson Imaging 17: 653–661

Evangelou N, Esiri MM, Smith S et al (2000) Quantitative pathological evidence for axonal loss in normal appearing white matter in multiple sclerosis. Ann Neurol 47:391–395

Falini A, Calabrese G, Filippi M et al (1998) Benign versus secondary progressive multiple sclerosis: the potential role of ^{1}H MR spectroscopy in defining the nature of disability. AJNR Am J Neuroradiol 19:223–229

Fazekas F, Ropele S, Enzinger C et al (2002) Quantitative magnetization transfer imaging of pre-lesional white-matter changes in multiple sclerosis. Mult Scler 8:479–484

Ferguson B, Matyszak MK, Esiri MM et al (1997) Axonal damage in acute multiple sclerosis lesions. Brain 120:393–399

Filippi M, Inglese M (2001) Overview of diffusion-weighted magnetic resonance studies in multiple sclerosis. J Neurol Sci 186 [Suppl 1]:S37–S43

Filippi M, Rocca MA (2003) Disturbed function and plasticity in multiple sclerosis as gleaned from functional magnetic resonance imaging. Curr Opin Neurol 16:275–282 (review)

Filippi M, Campi A, Dousset V et al (1995) A magnetization transfer imaging study of normal-appearing white matter in multiple sclerosis. Neurology 45:478–482

Filippi M, Rocca MA, Comi G (1998a) Magnetization transfer ratios of multiple sclerosis lesions with variable durations of enhancement. J Neurol Sci 159:162–165

Filippi M, Rocca MA, Rizzo G et al (1998b) Magnetization transfer ratios in multiple sclerosis lesions enhancing after different doses of gadolinium. Neurology 50:1289–1293

Filippi M, Rocca MA, Martino G et al (1998c) Magnetization transfer changes in the normal appearing white matter precede the appearance of enhancing lesions in patients with multiple sclerosis. Ann Neurol 43:809–814

Filippi M, Grossman RI, Comi G (eds) (1999a) Magnetization transfer in multiple sclerosis. Neurology 53 [Suppl 3]

Filippi M, Iannucci G, Tortorella C et al (1999b) Comparison of MS clinical phenotypes using conventional and magnetization transfer MRI. Neurology 52:588–594

Filippi M, Inglese M, Rovaris M et al (2000a) Magnetization transfer imaging to monitor the evolution of MS: a 1-year follow-up study. Neurology 55:940–946

Filippi M, Tortorella C, Rovaris M et al (2000b) Changes in the normal appearing brain tissue and cognitive impairment in multiple sclerosis. J Neurol Neurosurg Psychiatry 68:157–161

Filippi M, Iannucci G, Cercignani M et al (2000c) A quantitative study of water diffusion in multiple sclerosis lesions and normal-appearing white matter using echo-planar imaging. Arch Neurol 57:1017–1021

Filippi M, Arnold DL, Comi G (eds) (2001a) Magnetic resonance spectroscopy in multiple sclerosis. Springer, Milan

Filippi M, Cercignani M, Inglese M et al (2001b) Diffusion tensor magnetic resonance imaging in multiple sclerosis. Neurology 56:304–311

Filippi M, Dousset V, McFarland HF et al (2002a) The role of MRI in the diagnosis and monitoring of multiple sclerosis. Consensus report of the "White Matter Study Group" of the International Society for Magnetic Resonance in Medicine. J Magn Reson Imag 15:499–504

Filippi M, Rocca MA, Colombo B et al (2002b) Functional magnetic resonance imaging correlates of fatigue in multiple sclerosis. NeuroImage 15:559–567

Filippi M, Rocca MA, Falini A et al (2002c) Correlations between structural CNS damage and functional MRI changes in primary progressive MS. NeuroImage 15:537–546

Filippi M, Bozzali M, Rovaris M et al (2003) Evidence for widespread axonal damage at the earliest clinical stage of multiple sclerosis. Brain 126:433–437

Filippi M, Rocca MA, Mezzapesa DM et al (2004a) Simple and complex movement-associated functional MRI changes in patients at presentation with clinically isolated syndromes suggestive of MS. Human Brain Mapping 21:108–117

Filippi M, Rocca MA, Mezzapesa DM et al (2004b) A functional MRI study of cortical activations associated with object manipulation in patients with MS. NeuroImage, in press

Fu L, Matthews PM, De Stefano N et al (1998) Imaging axonal damage of normal-appearing white matter in multiple sclerosis. Brain 121:103–113

Gadea M, Martinez-Bisbal MC, Marti-Bonmati L et al (2004) Spectroscopic axonal damage of the right locus coeruleus relates to selective attention impairment in early stage relapsing-remitting multiple sclerosis. Brain 127:89–98

Ge Y, Grossman RI, Udupa JK et al (2001) Magnetization transfer ratio histogram analysis of gray matter in relapsing-remitting multiple sclerosis. AJNR Am J Neuroradiol 22:470–475

Ge Y, Grossman RI, Udupa JK et al (2002) Magnetization transfer ratio histogram analysis of normal-appearing gray matter and normal-appearing white matter in multiple sclerosis. J Comput Assist Tomogr 26:62–68

Ge Y, Grossman RI, Babb JS et al (2003) Dirty-appearing white matter in multiple sclerosis: volumetric MR imaging and magnetization transfer ratio histogram analysis. AJNR Am J Neuroradiol 24:1935–1940

Gonen O, Viswanathan AK, Catalaa I et al (1998) Total brain N-acetyl aspartate concentration in normal, age-grouped females: quantitation with non-echo proton NMR spectroscopy. Magn Reson Med 40:684–689

Gonen O, Catalaa I, Babb JS et al (2000) Total brain N-acetyl

aspartate. A new measure of disease load in MS. Neurology 54:15–19
Goodkin DE, Rooney WD, Sloan R et al (1998) A serial study of new MS lesions and the white matter from which they arise. Neurology 51:1689–1697
Griffin CM, Chard DT, Ciccarelli O et al (2001) Diffusion tensor imaging in early relapsing-remitting multiple sclerosis. Mult Scler 7:290–297
Hillary FG, Chiaravalloti ND, Ricker JH et al (2003) An investigation of working memory rehearsal in multiple sclerosis using fMRI. J Clin Exp Neuropsychol 25:965–978
Horsfield MA, Lai M, Webb SL et al (1996) Apparent diffusion coefficients in benign and secondary progressive multiple sclerosis by nuclear magnetic resonance. Magn Reson Med 36:393–400
Iannucci G, Minicucci L, Rodegher M et al (1999) Correlations between clinical and MRI involvement in multiple sclerosis: assessment using T1, T2 and MT histograms. J Neurol Sci 171:121–129
Iannucci G, Tortorella C, Rovaris M et al (2000) Prognostic value of MR and magnetization transfer imaging findings in patients with clinically isolated syndromes suggestive of multiple sclerosis at presentation. AJNR Am J Neuroradiol 21:1034–1038
Inglese M, van Waesberghe JH, Rovaris M et al (2003a) The effect of interferon beta-1b on quantities derived from MT MRI in secondary progressive MS. Neurology 60:853–860
Inglese M, Li BS, Rusinek H et al (2003b) Diffusely elevated cerebral choline and creatine in relapsing-remitting multiple sclerosis. Magn Reson Med 50:190–195
Kalkers NF, Hintzen RQ, van Waesberghe JH et al (2001) Magnetization transfer histogram parameters reflect all dimensions of MS pathology, including atrophy. J Neurol Sci 184155–162
Kapeller P, McLean MA, Griffin CM et al (2001) Preliminary evidence for neuronal damage in cortical grey matter and normal appearing white matter in short duration relapsing-remitting multiple sclerosis: a quantitative MR spectroscopic imaging study. J Neurol 248:131–138
Kapeller P, Brex PA, Chard D et al (2002) Quantitative 1H MRS imaging 14 years after presenting with a clinically isolated syndrome suggestive of multiple sclerosis. Mult Scler 8:207–210
Khan O, Shen Y, Ching W et al (2003) Combining immunomodulation and neuroprotection: cerebral axonal recovery in relapsing-remitting multiple sclerosis patients treated with glatiramer acetate. Multiple Sclerosis 9:S63
Kidd D, Barkhof F, McConnell R et al (1999) Cortical lesions in multiple sclerosis. Brain 122:17–26
Kita M, Goodkin DE, Bacchetti P et al (2000) Magnetization transfer ratio in new MS lesions before and during therapy with IFNß-1a. Neurology 54:1741–1745
Le Bihan D, Breton E, Lallemand D et al (1986) MR imaging of intravoxel incoherent motions: application to diffusion and perfusion in neurologic disorders. Radiology 161:401–407
Le Bihan D, Turner R, Pekar J et al (1991) Diffusion and perfusion imaging by gradient sensitization: design, strategy and significance. J Magn Reson Imaging 1:7–8
Lee MA, Blamire AM, Pendlebury S et al (2000a) Axonal injury or loss in the internal capsule and motor impairment in multiple sclerosis. Arch Neurol 57:65–70
Lee M, Reddy H, Johansen-Berg H et al (2000b) The motor cortex shows adaptive functional changes to brain injury from multiple sclerosis. Ann Neurol 47:606–613
Loevner LA, Grossman RI, Cohen JA et al (1995) Microscopic disease in normal-appearing white matter on conventional MR images in patients with multiple sclerosis: assessment with magnetization-transfer measurements. Radiology 196:511–515
Lumsden CE (1970) The neuropathology of multiple sclerosis. In: Vinken PJ, Bruyn JW (eds) Handbook of clinical neurology. North-Holland, Amsterdam Vol 9, pp 217-309
McDonald WI, Compston A, Edan G et al (2001) Recommended diagnostic criteria for multiple sclerosis: guidelines from the International Panel on the diagnosis of multiple sclerosis. Ann Neurol 50:121–127
Molyneux PD, Barker GJ, Barkhof F et al (2001) Clinical-MRI correlations in a European trial of interferon beta-1b in secondary progressive MS. Neurology 57:2191–2197
Narayana PA, Doyle TJ, Lai D et al (1998) Serial proton magnetic resonance spectroscopic imaging, contrast-enhanced magnetic resonance imaging, and quantitative lesion volumetry in multiple sclerosis. Ann Neurol 43:56–71
Narayanan S, De Stefano N, Francis GS et al (2001) Axonal metabolic recovery in multiple sclerosis patients treated with interferon beta-1b. J Neurol 248:979–986
Nusbaum AO, Tang CY, Wei TC et al (2000) Whole-brain diffusion MR histograms differ between MS subtypes. Neurology 54:1421–1426
Oreja-Guevara C, Rovaris M, Caputo D et al (2003) Changes in cortical gray matter in untreated relapsing-remitting MS patients: a follow up study. Neurology 60 [Suppl 1]:A297
Pan JW, Krupp LB, Elkins LE et al (2001) Cognitive dysfunction lateralizes with NAA in multiple sclerosis. Appl Neuropsychol 8:155–160
Pantano P, Iannetti GD, Caramia F et al (2002a) Cortical motor reorganization after a single clinical attack of multiple sclerosis Brain 125:1607–1615
Pantano P, Mainero C, Iannetti GD et al (2002b) Contribution of corticospinal tract damage to cortical motor reorganization after a single clinical attack of multiple sclerosis. NeuroImage 17:1837–1843
Parry AM, Scott RB, Palace J et al (2003) Potentially adaptive functional changes in cognitive processing for patients with multiple sclerosis and their acute modulation by rivastigmine. Brain 126:2750–2760
Peterson JW, Bo L, Mork S et al (2001) Transected neurites, apoptotic neurons, and reduced inflammation in cortical multiple sclerosis lesions. Ann Neurol 50:389–400
Pierpaoli C, Jezzard P, Basser PJ et al (1996) Diffusion tensor MR imaging of the human brain. Radiology 201:637–648
Pike GB, De Stefano N, Narayanan S et al (2000) Multiple sclerosis: magnetization transfer MR imaging of white matter before lesion appearance on T2-weighted images. Radiology 215:824–830
Reddy H, Narayanan S, Matthews PM et al (2000a) Relating axonal injury to functional recovery in MS. Neurology 54:236–239
Reddy H, Narayanan S, Arnoutelis R et al (2000b) Evidence for adaptive functional changes in the cerebral cortex with axonal injury from multiple sclerosis. Brain 123:2314–2320
Reddy H, Narayanan S, Woolrich M et al (2002) Functional brain reorganization for hand movement in patients with multiple sclerosis: defining distinct effects of injury and disability. Brain 125:2646–2657

Richert ND, Ostuni JL, Bash CN et al (1998) Serial whole-brain magnetization transfer imaging in patients with relapsing-remitting multiple sclerosis at baseline and during treatment with interferon beta-1b. AJNR Am J Neuroradiol 19:1705–1713

Richert ND, Ostuni JL, Bash CN et al (2001) Interferon beta-1b and intravenous methylprednisolone promote lesion recovery in multiple sclerosis. Mult Scler 7:49–58

Rocca MA, Mastronardo G, Rodegher M et al (1999) Long-term changes of magnetization transfer-derived measures from patients with relapsing-remitting and secondary progressive multiple sclerosis. AJNR Am J Neuroradiol 20:821–827

Rocca MA, Cercignani M, Iannucci G et al (2000) Weekly diffusion-weighted imaging of normal-appearing white matter in MS. Neurology 55:882–884

Rocca MA, Falini A, Colombo B et al (2002a) Adaptive functional changes in the cerebral cortex of patients with non-disabling MS correlate with the extent of brain structural damage. Ann Neurol 51:330–339

Rocca MA, Matthews PM, Caputo D et al (2002b) Evidence for widespread movement-associated functional MRI changes in patients with PPMS. Neurology 58:866–872

Rocca MA, Iannucci G, Rovaris M et al (2003a) Occult tissue damage in patients with primary progressive multiple sclerosis is independent of T2-visible lesions-a diffusion tensor MR study. J Neurol 250:456–460

Rocca MA, Mezzapesa DM, Falini A et al (2003b) Evidence for axonal pathology and adaptive cortical reorganisation in patients at presentation with clinically isolated syndromes suggestive of MS. NeuroImage 18:847–855

Rocca MA, Gavazzi C, Mezzapesa DM et al (2003c) A functional magnetic resonance imaging study of patients with secondary progressive multiple sclerosis. NeuroImage 19:1770–1777

Rocca MA, Pagani E, Ghezzi A et al (2003d) Functional cortical changes in patients with MS and non-specific conventional MRI scans of the brain NeuroImage 19:826–836

Rocca MA, Mezzapesa DM, Ghezzi A et al (2003e) Cord damage elicits brain functional reorganization after a single episode of myelitis. Neurology 61:1078–1085

Rocca MA, Agosta F, Mezzapesa DM et al (2004) A functional MRI study of movement-associated cortical changes in patients with Devic's neuromyelitis optica. NeuroImage, in press

Rombouts SA, Lazeron RH, Scheltens P et al (1998) Visual activation patterns in patients with optic neuritis: an fMRI pilot study. Neurology 50:1896–1899

Rovaris M, Filippi M (1999) Magnetic resonance techniques to monitor disease evolution and treatment trial outcomes in multiple sclerosis. Curr Opin Neurol 12:337–344

Rovaris M, Filippi M, Falautano M et al (1998) Relation between MR abnormalities and patterns of cognitive impairment in multiple sclerosis. Neurology 50:1601–1608

Rovaris M, Filippi M, Minicucci L et al (2000) Cortical/subcortical disease burden and cognitive impairment in multiple sclerosis. AJNR Am J Neuroradiol 21:402–408

Rovaris M, Bozzali M, Santuccio G et al (2001) In vivo assessment of the brain and cervical cord pathology of patients with primary progressive multiple sclerosis. Brain 124:2540–2549

Rovaris M, Bozzali M, Iannucci G et al (2002a) Assessment of normal-appearing white and gray matter in patients with primary progressive multiple sclerosis. Arch Neurol 59:1406–1412

Rovaris M, Iannucci G, Falautano M et al (2002b) Cognitive dysfunction in patients with mildly disabling relapsing-remitting multiple sclerosis: an exploratory study with diffusion tensor MR imaging. J Neurol Sci 195:103–109

Rovaris M, Agosta F, Sormani MP et al (2003) Conventional and magnetization transfer MRI predictors of clinical multiple sclerosis evolution: a medium-term follow-up study. Brain 126:2323–2332

Roychowdhury S, Maldijan JA, Grossman RI (2000) Multiple sclerosis: comparison of trace apparent diffusion coefficients with MR enhancement pattern of lesions. AJNR Am J Neuroradiol 21:869–874

Santos AC, Narayanan S, De Stefano N et al (2002) Magnetization transfer can predict clinical evolution in patients with multiple sclerosis. J Neurol 249:662–668

Sarchielli P, Presciutti O, Tarducci R et al (1998) 1H-MRS in patients with multiple sclerosis undergoing treatment with interferon beta-1a: results of a preliminary study. J Neurol Neurosurg Psychiatry 64:204–212

Sarchielli P, Presciutti O, Pelliccioli GP et al (1999) Absolute quantification of brain metabolites by proton magnetic resonance spectroscopy in normal-appearing white matter of multiple sclerosis patients. Brain 122:513–521

Sarchielli P, Presciutti O, Tarducci R et al (2002) Localized (1) H magnetic resonance spectroscopy in mainly cortical gray matter of patients with multiple sclerosis. J Neurol 249:902–910

Schubert F, Seifert F, Elster C et al (2002) Serial 1H-MRS in relapsing-remitting multiple sclerosis: effects of interferon-beta therapy on absolute metabolite concentrations. MAGMA 14:213–222

Sharma R, Narayana PA, Wolinsky JS (2001) Grey matter abnormalities in multiple sclerosis: proton magnetic resonance spectroscopic imaging. Mult Scler 7:221–226

Silver NC, Lai M, Symms MR et al (1998) Serial magnetization transfer imaging to characterize the early evolution of new MS lesions. Neurology 51:758–764

Staffen W, Mair A, Zauner H et al (2002) Cognitive function and fMRI in patients with multiple sclerosis: evidence for compensatory cortical activation during an attention task. Brain 156:1275–1282

Suhy J, Rooney WD, Goodkin DE et al (2000) 1H MRSI comparison of white matter and lesions in primary progressive and relapsing-remitting MS. Mult Scler 6:148–155

Tartaglia MC, Narayanan S, De Stefano N et al (2002) Choline is increased in pre-lesional normal appearing white matter in multiple sclerosis. J Neurol 249:1382–1390

Tortorella C, Viti B, Bozzali M et al (2000) A magnetization transfer histogram study of normal-appearing brain tissue in MS. Neurology 54:186–193

Traboulsee A, Dehmeshki J, Brex PA et al (2002) Normal-appearing brain tissue MTR histograms in clinically isolated syndromes suggestive of MS. Neurology 59:126–128

Traboulsee A, Dehmeshki J, Peters KR et al (2003) Disability in multiple sclerosis is related to normal appearing brain tissue MTR histogram abnormalities. Mult Scler 9:566–573

Trapp BD, Peterson J, Ransohoff RM et al (1998) Axonal transection in the lesions of multiple sclerosis. N Engl J Med 338:278–285

van Buchem MA, Grossman RI, Armstrong C et al (1998)

Correlation of volumetric magnetization transfer imaging with clinical data in MS. Neurology 50:1609–1617

van Waesberghe JHTM, van Walderveen MA, Castelijns JA et al (1998) Patterns of lesion development in multiple sclerosis: longitudinal observations with T1-weighted spin-echo and magnetization MR. AJNR Am J Neuroradiol 19:675–683

van Waesberghe JH, Kamphorst W, De Groot CJ et al (1999) Axonal loss in multiple sclerosis lesions: magnetic resonance imaging insights into substrates of disability. Ann Neurol 46:747–754

van Walderveen MA, Barkhof F, Pouwels PJ et al (1999) Neuronal damage in T1-hypointense multiple sclerosis lesions demonstrated in vivo using proton magnetic resonance spectroscopy. Ann Neurol 46:79–87

Waxman SG (1998) Demyelinating diseases: new pathological insights, new therapeutic targets. New Engl J Med 338:323–326

Waxman SG, Ritchie JM (1993) Molecular dissection of the myelinated axon. Ann Neurol 33:121–136

Werring DJ, Clark CA, Barker GJ et al (1999) Diffusion tensor imaging of lesions and normal-appearing white matter in multiple sclerosis. Neurology 52:1626–1632

Werring DJ, Brassat D, Droogan AG et al (2000a) The pathogenesis of lesions and normal-appearing white matter changes in multiple sclerosis. A serial diffusion MRI study. Brain 123:1667–1676

Werring DJ, Bullmore ET, Toosy AT et al (2000b) Recovery from optic neuritis is associated with a change in the distribution of cerebral response to visual stimulation: a functional magnetic resonance imaging study. J Neurol Neurosurg Psychiatry 68:441–449

Wilson M, Tench CR, Morgan PS et al (2003) Pyramidal tract mapping by diffusion tensor magnetic resonance imaging in multiple sclerosis: improving correlations with disability. J Neurol Neurosurg Psychiatry 74:203–207

Wylezinska M, Cifelli A, Jezzard P et al (2003) Thalamic neurodegeneration in relapsing-remitting multiple sclerosis. Neurology 60:1949–1954

16 Variants of Multiple Sclerosis

Jack H. Simon and Bette K. Kleinschmidt-DeMasters

CONTENTS

16.1 Introduction

Around the turn of the last century, several unusual demyelinating conditions were described, including Devic's disease (1894, neuromyelitis optica), Marburg disease (1906, acute multiple sclerosis, "encephalitis periaxialis diffusa"), Schilder disease (1912, recognized as a childhood variant of Marburg encephalitis periaxialis diffusa by Schilder) and Balo disease (1928, "encephalitis periaxialis concentrica," concentric sclerosis, recognized by Balo to be similar to Marburg and Schilder diseases). All except Devic's disease were considered by the original authors to represent rare, acute, and/or severe variants of multiple sclerosis (MS).

Debate raged almost immediately as to whether these represented unique demyelinating disorders or MS variants as the original author had often contended. Since several of these original reports were only single cases it took some time before sufficient numbers of patients were accrued by other workers, with tissues reviewed by neuropathologists at autopsy, to put these cases in proper perspective. Adding to the confusion was the fact that Schilder himself subsequently reported two more children with acute demyelinating disorders which he thought represented acute childhood MS, but which subsequently proved to be adrenoleukodystrophy and subacute sclerosing panencephalitis (Prineas et al. 2002).

There are valid differences of opinion as to how rigidly these terms, especially "Devic" and "Balo", should be applied. Some workers use these eponymic designations when specific distribution patterns are predominantly, but not exclusively, present. An example of this would be the use of the term "Devic's disease" for MS patients in whom the initial presentation was severe optic nerve and/or spinal cord disease, but who later in the course of the disease develop pathologically proven demyelinative plaques in other central nervous system (CNS) sites. A second instance is the use of these terms when the key variant feature is only minimally or focally present. An example of this would be the use of "Balo disease" for cases of large acute demyelinating lesions that may contain one or more "rings" by neuroimaging studies only in a single lesion, as opposed to the original use of the term which required widespread multiple concentric ring formation throughout cerebral hemispheres, as documented pathologically at autopsy. A final difference is those experts who favor use of

J. H. Simon, MD, PhD
Departments of Radiology, Neurology, Neurosurgery, University of Colorado Health Sciences Center, 4200 E Ninth Ave, Denver, CO 80262, USA
B. K. Kleinschmidt-DeMasters, MD
Departments of Pathology, Neurology, Neurosurgery, University of Colorado Health Sciences Center, 4200 E Ninth Ave, Denver, CO 80262, USA

these terms to denote certain stereotypic sites of involvement irrespective of co-existent disorders. An example of this would be the use of "Devic's disease" for spinal cord and optic nerve lesions in autoimmune disorders or cancer.

Today, based on neuropathology and imaging, Marburg (acute MS), Schilder (large coalescent, usually childhood, MS with exclusive cerebral hemispheric involvement), and Balo (alternating concentric rings of myelin loss and preservation in MS) are accepted as variants of MS. Devic's disease (as defined by exclusive spinal cord and optic nerve involvement) on the other hand, from both an imaging and neuropathology perspective is less confidently categorized today as an MS variant, but if it is, it likely lies on the far-side of the spectrum of MS (Table 16.1).

All these variants result in diagnostic difficulty and errors disproportionate to their incidence. A few additional points are worth noting:

1) The initial clinical presentation of these MS variants is usually severe and rapidly progressive, making the differential diagnostic list broad.
2) Making the diagnosis at the very initial phases of any of these diseases (when the neuroradiologist is most likely to be confronted with the disorder by imaging studies) is virtually impossible. Only passage of time and evolution of clinical features of the disease, biopsy, or even autopsy provide the final and correct diagnosis.
3) All these MS variants are rare and heterogeneous within each category due to differing uses of the terms, as noted above. Although correct diagnosis is always desirable, in actuality, treatment decisions are more often guided by anecdote and desperation than by evidence-based studies.
4) Despite these difficulties, from a research perspective, these MS variants as "outliers" do provide important material with which to address questions related to variant host response, mechanisms of remyelination or barriers to remyelination, and issues surrounding new hypotheses of MS classification (Lucchinetti et al. 2000).

This chapter will attempt to outline the unique versus the overlapping clinical, pathological, and neuroimaging features of Marburg, Schilder, Balo, and Devic types of MS. Acute tumefactive demyelinating lesions will also be briefly discussed under the acute MS section.

16.2 Devic's Neuromyelitis Optica

16.2.1 General Features

Devic's neuromyelitis optica (DNO), originally described in 1894 (Devic 1894) is an inflammatory demyelinating disease with features that overlap with MS (Cree et al. 2002; de Seze et al. 2003; Weinshenker 2003). However, in contrast to the other MS variants discussed below, DNO has come to be understood as more distinct than similar to MS, based on clinical, pathological, immunological and imaging criteria.

The key clinical features of DNO include acute visual loss, often bilateral, and acute transverse myelitis, with the visual and spinal cord signs and symptoms often presenting nearly simultaneously (O'Riordan et al. 1996; de Seze et al. 2003; Wingerchuk et al. 1999). Despite striking and classic demyelination in the optic nerve and spinal cord, patients with "pure" DNO do not develop neurologic signs or symptoms or demyelination in other regions of the CNS; the brain remains normal or shows at most non-specific findings in the white matter on follow-up MRI (Filippi et al. 1999; Mandler et al. 1993; O'Riordan et al. 1996; Fazekas et al. 1994).

Many series of DNO patients suggest that visual symptoms usually precede spinal symptoms, but the reverse is not uncommon. Severe visual symptoms with blindness may become total and permanent within a few days and bilateral optic neuritis is most common. This contrasts with MS where bilateral optic neuritis is relatively uncommon and the initial visual compromise is usually limited and reversible (Weinshenker 2003). In patients who present with visual system difficulties, transverse myelitis characteristically develops within a few weeks, with severe paraplegia, sensory loss with a distinct level, and sphincter disturbances. Fixed weakness from onset, rather than improvement over time after the initial event, is the typical course. This contrasts with MS where weakness is frequently reversible in the early stages and the spinal cord presentation is that of only partial transverse myelitis. The interval separating the visual and spinal syndromes may be hours, days, or weeks, but in most cases is within 3 months. However, cases with a 2- or more year separation have been described. As no single criterion is specific for DNO, diagnostic criteria have been developed based on multiple factors, including MRI (Wingerchuk and Weinshenker 2003; Wingerchuk et al. 1999; de Seze et al. 2002).

Table 16.1. Classical features of the MS variants compared to relapsing MS

	Relapsing MS	Devic's NMO	Balo's concentric sclerosis	Schilder's disease	Acute (Marburg) MS
Age	Childhood to adult	Childhood to adult	Childhood to adult	Predominantly children	Childhood to adult; typically in young adult
Typical course	First events often subclinical Early deficits mostly reversible Relapsing early, then progressive in >50%	Acute onset Nearly synchronous myelopathy and optic neuropathy (either first) Fixed and severe deficits with each attack Monophasic or relapsing	Symptoms suggesting mass may occur Typical lesions (one or few) at presentation, may suggest mass Rarely can occur during course of typical relapsing MS By MRI more common and more benign Historically acute, severe but highly variable and MS-like	Headache, vomiting seizures, visual problems (cortical blindness or bilateral optic neuritis) No prodrome Variable	Acute onset, poorly responsive, death not uncommon within weeks or months Typically monophasic
MRI	Brain and cord with multifocal lesions, in brain periventricular >peripheral white Spinal cord short segments (<2 in height) Partial transverse involvement No T1-hypointensity, acute or chronic	Brain normal[a] Spinal cord swollen, diffuse, transverse, long vertical pathology Near full transverse involvement May show T1-hypointensity (acute and chronic)	Lamellar lesions in isolation or accompanying typical MS-like lesions Lamellar pattern at autopsy (not expected in vivo)	Large (3×2 cm), bihemispheric brain white matter lesions may show edge enhancement	Multifocal diffuse white matter lesions in brain or brainstem
CSF	OCB, in most	OCB uncommon >100 WBC; neutrophils common	Insufficient studies	Normal or not typical for MS	OCB may be absent in acute illness
Pathology	Demyelination with variable, but lesser, axonal injury; lesions of differing ages often detected at autopsy; most old lesions well demarcated from surrounding white matter; periventricular, subpial, gray-white junction plaques typical	Demyelination and necrosis with severe axonal injury and cavitation; damage predominantly or exclusively in optic nerve and spinal cord, often affected long segments of cord	Concentric zones of normal myelin alternating with demyelination, leading to a mosaic pattern of myelin damage in cerebral hemispheric white matter; histology may suggest aberrant remyelination	Severe myelin loss; large, well demarcated, bilateral white matter plaques involving cerebral hemispheric white matter, with fewer brainstem, cerebellar, and spinal cord lesions	Severe acute myelin loss with numerous LFB-positive macrophages; few if any old lesions; most lesions in cerebral hemispheres; lesions may be poorly demarcated due to acute nature

[a] Brain MRI may reveal non-specific white matter foci.
OCB, oligoclonal bands

The clinical course following presentation with DNO is variable. The disorder may be monophasic without recurrent attacks (but with fixed deficits) or the patient may experience multiple severe relapses with step-wise neurologic deterioration (Weinshenker 2003; Wingerchuk and Weinshenker 2003; Fardet et al. 2003). DNO may also follow an acute progressive and fatal course, with patients suffering respiratory failure and death related to cervical myelitis (Wingerchuk and Weinshenker 2003). Rarely there can be complete clinical recovery without relapse. Prognosis is poor compared to classic MS, with most patients demonstrating severe visual loss or inability to ambulate without assistance within 5 years of onset.

The early literature suggested that DNO was the predominant demyelinating disease in parts of Asia, where MS is relatively rare. There is now evidence from studies in Japan and elsewhere that many cases classified as DNO might better be classified as MS with disproportionate optic and spinal cord involvement. Nevertheless, DNO is still rare in these Asian countries compared to MS, and is even more rare in North America and Europe (Kuroiwa 1985a). An interesting co-association of DNO has been described with autoimmune and connective tissue disease, including systemic lupus erythematosus and Sjögren syndrome (de Seze et al. 2002; O'Riordan et al. 1996; Weinshenker 2003; Cree et al. 2002).

Early and correct diagnosis of DNO is important as current treatment recommendations vary from those for MS (Weinshenker 2003). Treatment of DNO with beta-interferon or glatiramer acetate has been described after an initial misdiagnosis of MS, but azathioprine may be the treatment of choice to suppress attacks (Mandler et al. 1998). DNO may respond to plasma exchange when steroid therapy fails (Keegan et al. 2002). DNO in the presence of anticardiolipin antibodies has been treated with antiplatelet and anticoagulant drugs (Karussis et al. 1998).

16.2.2 Neuropathology

DNO is characterized pathologically by considerably more tissue destruction and loss of axons than is seen in typical MS, with necrotizing demyelination in the spinal cord and optic nerves. The tissue involvement often extends over numerous spinal cord segments. In early cases the cord may be swollen, simulating a tumor, whereas in late stages there may be considerable shrinkage of the cord and cavitation due to the tissue destruction. DNO may show a greater B cell component, more prominent eosinophilic and neutrophilic infiltrates, complement activation, and vascular fibrosis, all rare in typical MS, along with the more MS-like features including T cell infiltrates and the presence of macrophages (Lucchinetti et al. 2002). Depending on how one defines the entity, the remainder of the CNS shows little or no demyelinative disease. The cerebrospinal fluid, in contrast to MS, reveals a pleocytosis of >50 leukocytes, is often neutrophilic, and in most cases there is absence of oligoclonal bands.

16.2.3 Imaging

The conventional MRI findings in the spinal cord in DNO differ from those in typical MS (Fig. 16.1). In DNO lesions of the spinal cord tend to be large, often exceeding three segments in height, across the full thickness of spinal cord on axial views. Both the gray and white matter and central cord may be abnormal, and the spinal cord may show striking swelling (O'Riordan et al. 1996; Filippi et al. 1999). This contrasts to the typical appearance of MS by MRI (Lycklama et al. 2003), where there is typically partial and asymmetric involvement observed on axial images, the vertical extent is usually two segments or less, and spinal cord swelling is relatively mild if present at all in the acute stages.

In acute MS the spinal cord is rarely if ever hypointense on T1-weighted images (Gass et al. 1998), while in DNO the cord may be diffusely hypointense. Chronic T1-hypointensity (T1-black holes) are notably absent in MS (Gass et al. 1998; Lycklama et al. 2003), but occur in DNO, probably related to tissue necrosis. In DNO, there may be longitudinally extensive and central enhancement of the spinal cord (Weinshenker 2003).

Cord atrophy does occur frequently in MS, but most often by visual criteria is localized and segmental (Simon 2000; Lycklama et al. 2003). In DNO, cord atrophy may be readily apparent, may be diffuse and prevalent (beyond the acute stages) when measurements are made (Filippi et al. 1999). These neuroimaging changes perfectly parallel the known neuropathological features described above. Imaging findings in the optic nerve or chiasm, including T2-hyperintensity, swelling or enhancement, do not distinguish DNO from typical MS.

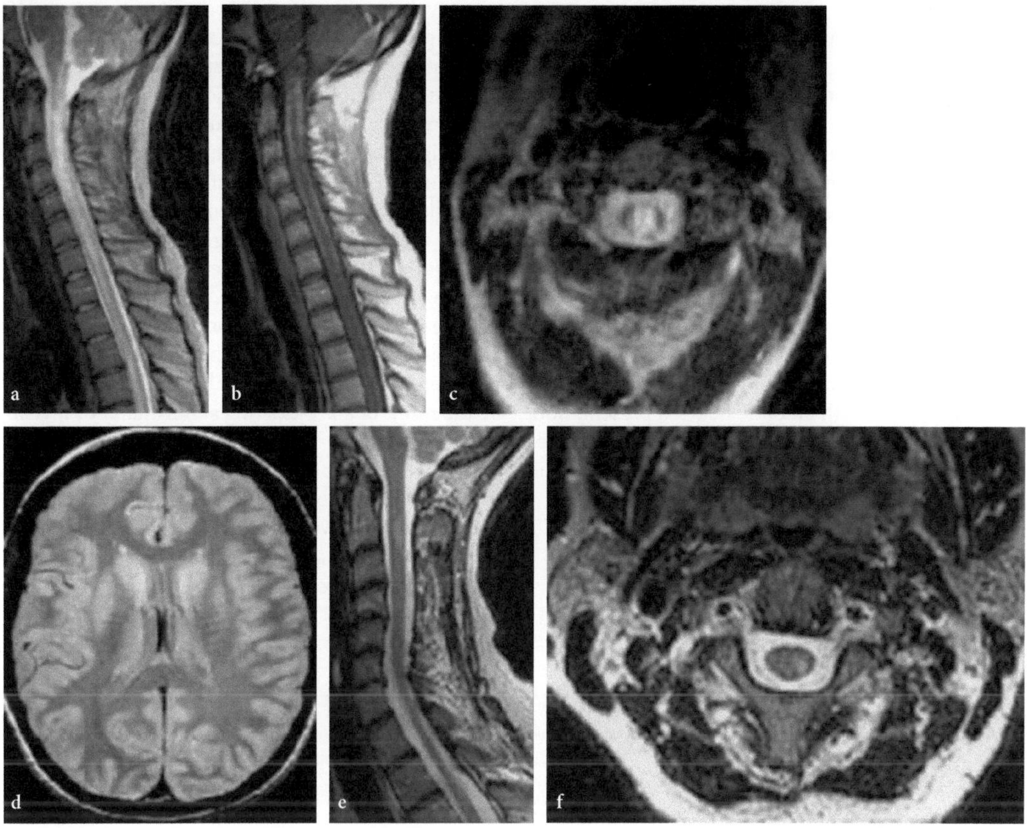

Fig. 16.1a-f. Devic's neuromyelitis optica. A relapsing spinal cord presentation included an episode with severe long segment, diffuse spinal cord involvement as seen on T2-weighted MRI (**a**), with corresponding T1-hypointensity (**b**), findings not associated with classic MS. On axial T2-weighted MRI (**c**), the cervical cord lesion is large, symmetric, and crosses the midline. The brain MRI in Devic's neuromyelitis optica is typically normal as shown here (**d**), but can include non-specific T2-hyperintensities. In MS, on T2-weighted sagittal images, the spinal cord lesion is often vertically oriented, but <2 segments in height. Involvement as seen on axial T2-weighted axial images (**f**) is classically asymmetric, corresponding to the clinical finding of partial transverse myelitis

While there is some variation depending on the criteria used to make the diagnosis of DNO, there is good evidence that the majority of cases will be characterized by a normal brain MRI at presentation (Wingerchuk et al. 1999; Wingerchuk and Weinshenker 2003; Mandler et al. 1993; de Seze et al. 2003; O'Riordan et al. 1996; Fazekas et al. 1994; Filippi et al. 1999). When T2-hyperintensities are seen in the brain, they tend to be non-specific, for example not abutting the ventricular surfaces, and without accompanying T1-hypointensity, either acute or chronic. On follow-up, cases of "pure" DNO do not tend to accumulate new T2-hyperintensities, in contrast to typical MS where new lesions are frequent and most often subclinical (Filippi et al. 1999).

Magnetization transfer imaging studies have provided further support for the concept of DNO as a more limited neuroanatomical disorder in contrast to typical MS. The magnetization transfer ratio (MTR) of focal non-specific brain lesions when they do occur in DNO is only mildly abnormal and considerably less abnormal than in MS. The MTR-based measures of normal-appearing white matter (NAWM) is normal in DNO, in contrast to the NAWM in MS which is consistently abnormal even in the relatively early stages of disease (Filippi et al. 1999). In keeping with a more severe spinal cord pathology, the MTR of spinal cord is significantly more abnormal in DNO than in typical MS (Filippi et al. 1999).

16.2.4 Differential Diagnosis

Depending on the initial presentation (spinal or optic), the differential diagnosis by imaging includes (for spinal presentations) transverse myelitis, acute disseminated encephalomyelitis (ADEM), including post-vaccination, viral and other infectious etiologies, and neoplasm. An abnormal brain MRI with typical demyelinating lesions in the cerebral hemispheres, cerebellum, and brainstem, and consistent laboratory findings makes MS more likely. Vascular insults and collagen vascular disease are not always separable from DNO without supporting laboratory or historical information. With an optic neuritis presentation, especially if unilateral, imaging findings are non-specific and the differential diagnosis will include optic neuritis from MS if the brain MRI is positive.

16.3 Acute MS (Marburg Type)

16.3.1 General Features

Rarely, an acute, idiopathic, inflammatory demyelinating disease may be relatively unresponsive to conventional therapy (corticosteroids), resulting in death or severe residual deficits, and may then be classified as acute MS of the Marburg type. Death may occur in weeks to months, either from severe widespread cerebral lesions or acute involvement of the lower brainstem or upper cervical cord (Mendez and Pogacar 1988). Patients who survive the acute presentation may be left with significant deficits or may develop severe exacerbations.

It must be acknowledged, however, that some patients who present with a large acute tumefactive demyelinative lesion that prompts biopsy, later go on to exhibit a classic chronic relapsing/remitting course of typical MS. These cases should perhaps not be considered "pure" Marburg type MS although at the time the patient presents the outcome may not be at all clear. For the individual patient, the difficulty is that at the time of clinical presentation there are no good predictors for whether he or she will follow a fulminant rapidly fatal course after biopsy, develop mild or severe MS, or even develop MS at all, despite several years follow-up (Kepes 1993). It has been suggested that some patients who present with acute tumefactive demyelinating lesions prompting biopsy might actually have disorders intermediate between MS and large coalescent ADEM (Kepes 1993). Hence, the appellation "Marburg" is best applied to severe, acute MS that meets both clinical and pathological criteria of a monophasic illness and may best be defined by its malignant course and acute, severe demyelination (Bitsch et al. 1999; Poser et al. 1992).

While poorly responsive to corticosteroids (the first line of therapy), there are suggestions that patients with Marburg-type MS may benefit from plasma exchange (Weinshenker 1999). Cases have also been described with response to combined corticosteroid and mannitol therapy (Giubilei et al. 1997).

Recently, Marburg MS has been hypothesized to be the result of a pre-existing abnormality of myelin basic protein in a developmentally immature (less cationic) form (Wood et al. 1994; Beniac et al. 1999). Alternatively, Marburg type of demyelination may simply lie at the severe, acute end of the clinical spectrum of MS (Coyle 2000), possibly reflecting factors related to a host response.

16.3.2 Neuropathology

In most patients who succumb, demyelinative lesions are usually all of the same acute age. The distribution of lesions is similar to typical MS, but there is a predilection for lesions to occur in the cerebral hemispheres, including near the gray-white matter junction. Virtually no older plaques can be identified at neuropathological examination, paralleling the patient's rapid clinical downhill course. This is in contradistinction to typical MS where the demyelinative lesions at autopsy are usually remote and/or show differing ages of myelin breakdown. The latter is assessed by several types of special stains, the most common of which is the histochemical stain for myelin (Luxol fast blue, LFB) with a periodic acid Schiff (PAS) counterstain. This stain allows distinction between very recently phagocytosed myelin within macrophages, which is as yet undigested and retains its LFB-positivity, versus myelin that has been broken down to neutral lipids in macrophages (PAS-positivity) as a result of a more advanced and subacute process. In Marburg type of acute MS, abundant LFB-positive macrophages are seen throughout the hypercellular demyelinative lesions. Acute MS shows less chronic gliosis, more edema, and even partial bands of preserved myelin (see description of Balo type in Sect. 16.4) than typical relapsing/remitting MS cases that come to autopsy. More abundant perivascular inflammation may also be present than is seen in typical MS.

16.3.3 Imaging

The classic MRI appearance is that of a first presentation with large, often confluent, lesions, sometimes involving the brainstem but more commonly affecting cerebral hemispheric white matter. Lesions may show enhancement and perilesional edema is often present. If a single lesion is the initial presentation of MS, the neuroimaging characteristic may be difficult to distinguish from a neoplasm.

16.3.4 Differential Diagnosis

The differential diagnosis at the time of presentation includes ADEM (Schwarz et al. 2001), which may be favored by an appropriate accompanying history of vaccination or recent viral or other infectious illness. If blood is present in the lesion at neuroimaging studies, the rare Hurst's disease (acute hemorrhagic leukoencephalitis) may also be a consideration, a disorder generally considered to represent a hyperacute form of perivenous encephalomyelitis (ADEM). Infectious and autoimmune diseases can usually be excluded by clinical and laboratory features or by neuropathology of the biopsy or at autopsy.

The difficulty with biopsies of tumefactive MS is that they may overlap with Marburg MS or be intermediate between ADEM and classic MS (Giang et al. 1992; Kepes 1993). While classic ADEM is distinguishable from classic MS by the presence of multifocal, small perivenous demyelinative lesions in ADEM, this feature is not generally present in acute demyelinative lesions that prompt biopsy. There are no morphological features in these biopsy specimens of single tumefactive demyelinative lesions that reliably predict whether the patient will go on to subsequently develop MS.

16.4 Balo's Concentric Sclerosis

16.4.1 General Features

Balo's concentric sclerosis (BCS) might be best characterized as a relatively rare expression of pathology that might be entirely within the classification of MS. The original case of Balo was that of acute disease, with death within 3 and a half months after onset in a 23-year-old male, prompting Balo himself to consider the disorder he described as a variant of acute MS; he named this process encephalitis periaxialis concentrica, paralleling the name given several years earlier by Marburg to acute MS (Balo 1928; Kuroiwa 1985a).

BCS by definition shows a peculiar pattern of pathology in cerebral hemispheric white matter consisting of a concentric, mosaic, or floral configuration of alternating bands of white matter whose basis is relatively preserved myelination alternating with regions of demyelination (Fig. 16.2).

The literature reflects two extremes of BCS – the earlier (pre-MRI) neuropathology literature is based primarily on autopsy material from cases after an acute, monophasic, fulminant disease process. In the autopsy BCS series, disease typically progresses over weeks to months, with severe disability or death as the typical outcome. Clinical symptoms typically include headache, aphasia, cognitive or behavioral dysfunction, and/or seizures.

In contrast, the MRI-era literature tends to reflect a far greater range of disease, from focal BCS lesions co-existing with typical MS-like lesions, but also acknowledging cases with a fulminant course ending in death. The more "benign" BCS has been described as monophasic with resolution of pathology and clinical findings over time, and as MS-like with a multiphasic but self-limited course, and responsive to therapy (Spiegel et al. 1989; Ng et al. 1999; Louboutin and Elie 1995; Sekijima et al. 1997; Karaarslan et al. 2001).

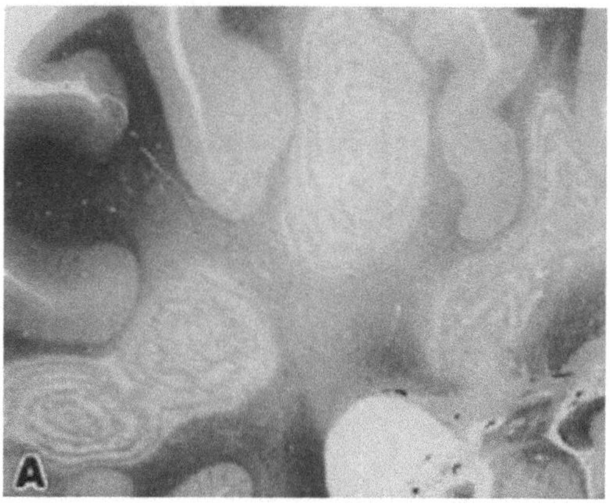

Fig. 16.2. Classic Balo's concentric sclerosis as a white matter lesion with partly myelinated and demyelinated bands arranged in concentric and mosaic patterns. Section stained with Luxol fast blue. [From Yao et al. (1994)]

The explanation for the pre-MRI and MRI era dichotomy is not known. One possibility may lie with a more detailed explanation of the pathological features of acute MS. Acute Marburg type MS often shows partial bands of preserved myelin at pathological examination, as explained above. Such cases with limited banding are classified as acute MS by neuropathologists, but might be considered as having "focal or limited Balo rings" based on imaging. Acute tumefactive demyelinative lesions with a few alternating bands of intact and damaged myelin may be the lesions that account for the diagnosis of "Balo rings" by MRI in some patients.

Co-existence of BCS lesions with typical MS-like (non-concentric) lesions has also been recognized in the neuropathology literature (Itoyama et al. 1985; Moore et al. 1985). BCS lesions have been found very rarely to develop after a typical relapsing-remitting course of typical MS (Moore et al. 2001), and Balo-like band pattern lesions have been described along the periphery of acute MS plaques (Moore et al. 2001).

While the early literature emphasized BCS within the cerebral hemispheric white matter of the brain, this process also occurs within the optic chiasm and spinal cord, and BCS lesions can occur in the brainstem and cerebellum (Itoyama et al. 1985; Moore et al. 1985).

16.4.2 Neuropathology

While much of the literature of BCS was interpreted as indicating that the abnormal bands (intermingled with normal bands) were the result of partial remyelination, more recent evidence suggests that the abnormal bands are more often areas of early demyelination alternating with preserved myelin (Yao et al. 1994). In some well documented cases there does appear to be remyelination of previously demyelinated fibers (Moore et al. 1985). BCS-like features, without the full blown BCS macroscopic pathology have also been described along the surface of chronic active MS plaques (Moore et al. 2001), suggesting that this pathology may not be characteristic of a separate disease, but reflects a variation in pathology or host response.

The mechanism(s) responsible for this peculiar pathology remain a mystery. Balo postulated a "lecithinolytic enzyme" centrifugally spreading from the center of a lesion (Kuroiwa 1985). A more recent hypothesis is based on downregulation of local demyelination by CD8 suppressor T-cells (Moore et al. 2001; Traugott et al. 1983), in both typical MS and BCS lesions, as might occur as well through cytokine action (Moore et al. 2001; Canella and Raine 1995). The suppression of demyelination along the surface of a lesion, surrounded by an external zone of activity and demyelination, and a sequential repeat of the process might then result in the repetitive alternating lamellae characteristic of BCS (Moore et al. 2001).

16.4.3 Imaging

With the introduction of MRI, the literature regarding BCS has evolved. BCS is currently described as consisting of a range appearances, from classic large BCS lesions in isolation associated with a fulminant clinical course, to cases in which the BCS pattern of focal lesions co-exists with typical MS-like lesions (Chen et al. 1996; Yao et al. 1994; Iannucci et al. 2000; Ng et al. 1999). There is also increasing recognition of borderline BCS-like lesions with only a few lamellae or rings. The co-existence and development of BCS lesions within typical MS lesions, though rare, is likely more common than development of only classic large BCS lesions throughout both cerebral hemispheres.

BCS lesions are readily identified on proton or T2-weighted images, but the concentric pattern may also be apparent on T1-weighted images (Fig. 16.3). There are reports of contrast enhancement in BCS, with alternating bands of enhancement and non-enhancement, the enhancing regions thought to correspond to zones of demyelination. Synchronously enhancing, sequentially enhancing, and transiently enhancing rings have been reported (Iannucci et al. 2000; Sekijima et al. 1997; Chen 2001;Chen et al. 1999; Ng et al. 1999; Bolay et al. 1996; Caracciolo et al. 2001; Kastrup et al. 2002) (Fig. 16.4).

By both imaging and neuropathology, most studies suggest a chronologic progression of rings, with the most recent pathology along the periphery. In some cases a more synchronous process has been suggested, possibly associated with a very rapid tempo of lesion progression, not unlike that of chronic active lesions in classic MS, where ongoing demyelination may occur along a lesion's perimeter (Moore et al. 2001; Sekijima et al. 1997; Ng et al. 1999).

In the few cases of BCS studied to date with MR spectroscopy, the principal metabolite ratios and other abnormal peaks (from lipid and lactate) are those observed from typical large MS lesions

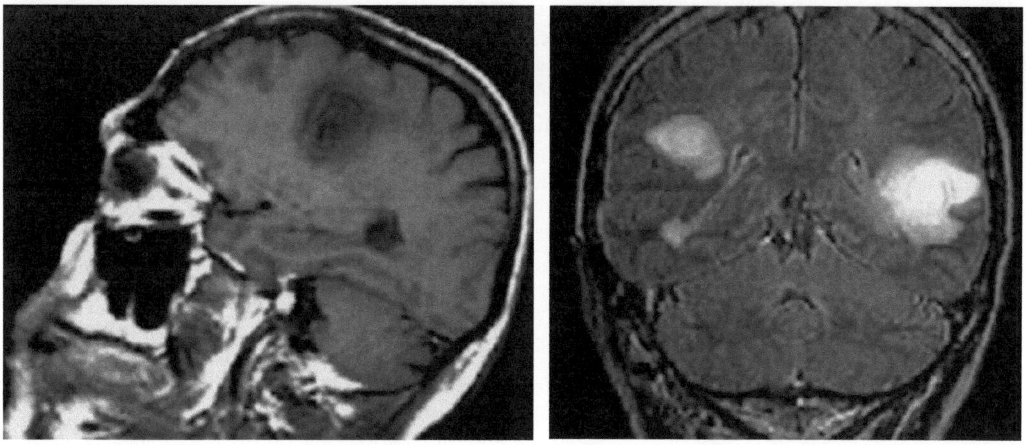

a b

Fig. 16.3a,b. Balo's concentric sclerosis. (**a**) A 52-year-old man presenting with acute left hemiparesis, ataxia and agitation. Sagittal T1-weighted image shows concentric rings, the lesion had peripheral enhancement (not shown). (**b**) A 48-year-old man developed acute sensorial aphasia 4 days before admission, the coronal fluid-attenuated inversion-recovery (FLAIR) series shows bilateral lesions, one with many rings in the left temporo-parietal lobe, and two right hemisphere lesions, one with few rings, one more classically MS-like along the ventricular surface. [From Karaarslan et al. (2001)]

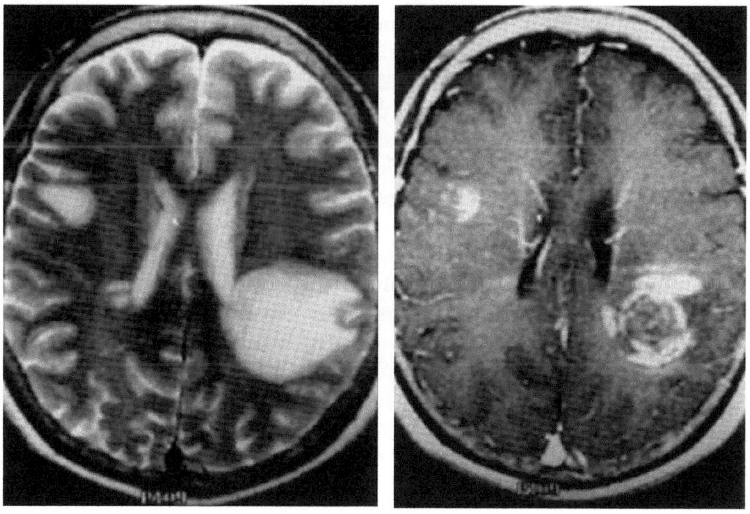

a b

Fig. 16.4a,b. Balo's concentric sclerosis. A 56-year-old woman with a 2-week history of progressive weakness, the axial T2-weighted MRI shows a left parietal and right frontal subcortical lesion, and small right periventricular lesions (**a**). The axial post-contrast T1-weighted image (**b**) shows concentric enhancement of the left lesion, arcuate enhancement of the right subcortical lesion, and enhancement at right angle to the ventricle surface in the smaller right periventricular lesion. Follow-up at 12 months showed regression but the laminated appearance remained on T2-weighted imaging (not shown). [From Ng et al. (1999)]

(Karaarslan et al. 2001; Kim et al. 1997; Chen et al. 2001). Based on a series of large concentric lesions in four patients in Taipei, Taiwan, with 2- to 23-month follow-up Chen et al. (2001) reported an increase in the choline-to-creatine ratio, a decrease in the N-acetyl aspartate-to-creatine ratio, and increased lactate. On follow-up, there was a return toward normal ratios and values. Lipid peaks were seen in early lesions, similar to those observed in MS by short echo time MR spectroscopy (Davie et al. 1994).

With increased sensitivity of MRI to Balo-like patterns in vivo, one of the difficult and intriguing questions is concerned with the definition of BCS. For example are lesions with only a few or one to two rings representative of BCS (Fig. 16.5), and its corresponding pathology, or are these better characterized as relatively rare presentations of the common demyelination characteristic of typical MS? Does identification of a minimal BCS pattern contain prognostic information, information relevant to discussions of subtypes of MS pathology or information relevant to optimal therapy?

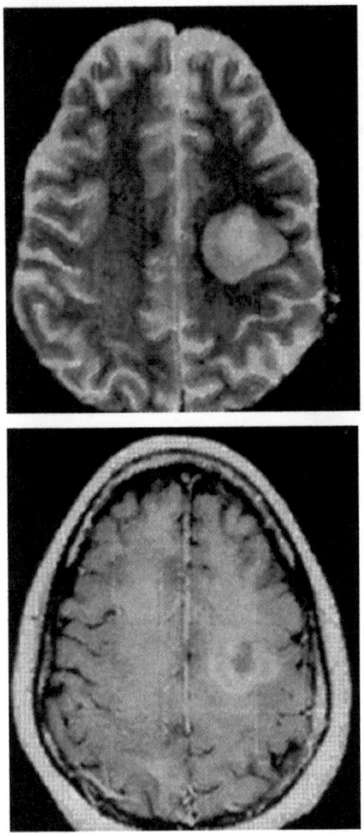

a b

Fig. 16.5a,b. Balo's concentric sclerosis pattern with few rings. Biopsy-proven inflammatory demyelinating process consistent with Balo's concentric sclerosis. T2-weighted image (**a**) shows two concentric zones of abnormal intensity. Post-contrast T1-weighted image (**b**) shows multiple concentric rings of enhancement. [From Caracciolo et al. (2001)]

16.4.4 Differential Diagnosis

Classic large and potentially mass-like BCS lesions may be confused with neoplasm or abscess, but when their appearance is equivocal, the course when followed by imaging should suggest a resolving (non-malignant) process. MR spectroscopy may also support the diagnosis of a demyelinating process (Chen et al. 2001).

16.5 Schilder's Disease

16.5.1 General Features

Schilder's disease, also known as diffuse myelinoclastic sclerosis, is a rare demyelinating disorder that is essentially a diagnosis of exclusion as its clinical and MRI appearance may overlap with inherited metabolic disorders of myelin, particularly adrenoleukodystrophy. Schilder's original three cases, under the umbrella of an entity known as encephalitis periaxialis diffusa, described in 1912, 1913, and 1924 were subsequently found to be three different disorders: myelinoclastic diffuse sclerosis (the 1912 case), adrenoleukodystrophy (the 1913 case), and subacute sclerosing panencephalitis (SSPE) (the 1924 case) (Poser 1985).

A practical definition proposed by Poser (1985) includes the following components: (1) a subacute or chronic myelinoclastic disorder with one or two roughly symmetrical plaques at least 2×3 cm in two of three dimensions; (2) involvement of the centrum semiovale; (3) these being the only lesions based on clinical, paraclinical or imaging findings; (4) adrenoleukodystrophy must be excluded.

Schilder's disease in its classic sense is acute MS that occurs in childhood. Analogous to other MS variants discussed above, both "pure" forms and "transitional" forms have been described. "Pure" forms predominate in childhood and have plaques confined to the cerebral white matter. "Transitional" forms affected a broader age range of adolescents and adults and show large cerebral plaques combined with more typical MS plaques elsewhere (Prineas et al. 2002).

Disease duration is highly variable. In the 70 cases collected by Poser (1957) the mean duration was 6.2 years, ranging from 3 days to 45 years, but duration was less than 1 year in 40%. The clinical course is diverse, but widespread white matter involvement usually produces subacute or chronic mental and neurological deterioration, spastic paresis, convulsion, and involvement of vision and hearing. Pure psychiatric forms have been described. Increased intracranial pressure, headache, and vomiting may suggest a mass lesion. The cerebrospinal fluid may be normal with only a slight elevation of protein or cell count. Treatment with corticosteroids and cyclophosphamide has been successful in some instances. Cases considered to be Schilder's disease at onset may follow a downhill progressive course or go on to develop relapsing/remitting disease. As noted above in the discussion of acute MS, it is not possible to determine prognosis. In general, however, early age onset often results in severe neurological deficits.

16.5.2 Neuropathology

The defining feature of Schilder's disease is sharply demarcated, giant coalescent plaques of demyelination, usually involving the majority of bilateral cerebral hemispheric white matter. Histologically, the features of Schilder's disease are nearly identical to MS. Using the eponymic designation more broadly to include cases of all ages that show massive bilateral cerebral white matter disease affecting the centrum semiovale, "Schilder's disease" is not distinguishable from severe MS. Indeed, in a study of 22 cases of MS compared to two of Schilder's disease, no differences could be found (GALLUCCI et al. 2001). The histological features, however, that linked Schilder's first MS case with his subsequent misdiagnosed two further cases (adrenoleukodystrophy and SSPE as noted above), however, was the prominent non-neoplastic lymphocytic cuffing in all three disorders. Even today, these three conditions may be included in the differential diagnosis by neuropathologists for large, inflammatory demyelinating diseases found at biopsy or autopsy. Normal ratios of very long chain fatty acids and absence of involvement of the peripheral nervous system exclude adrenoleukodystrophy.

16.5.3 Imaging

Imaging reveals large, bihemispheric lesions (EBLEN et al. 1991; MEHLER and RABINOWICH 1988) of white matter that may show enhancement at the perimeter (Fig. 16.6). Unfortunately these lesions can also be similar by neuroimaging studies to adrenoleukodystrophy or possibly acute disseminated encephalomyelitis (FERNANDEZ-JAEN et al. 2001;VALK and VAN DER KNAAP 1989). The lesions occurring in two hemispheres may be bridged by abnormal signal in the corpus callosum. Frank necrosis and cavitation may also occur.

16.5.4 Differential Diagnosis

Myelinoclastic diffuse sclerosis remains a rare disorder with few cases meeting rigorous diagnostic criteria (COYLE 2000). Cases coming to biopsy must be distinguished from tumor, abscess, or ADEM (HYNSON et al. 2001; NEJAT and EFTEKHAR 2002; KOTIL et al. 2002; KURUL et al. 2003) although as noted above, this is often only possible after histological assessment. As expected, the differential diagnosis for Schilder's disease is very similar to that for other acute forms of MS, such as Marburg type. The additional disorder in the differential diagnosis in children and adolescents is inherited metabolic disorders of demyelination.

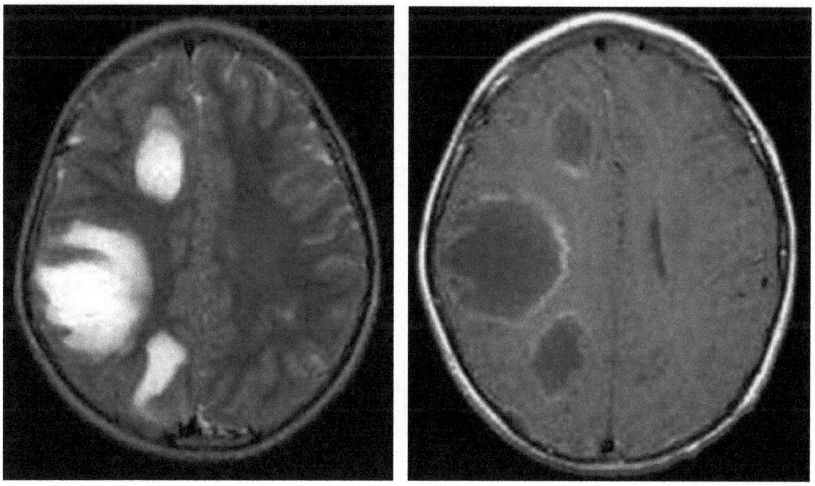

a b

Fig. 16.6a,b. Schilder's disease. A 10-year-old male presented with headache, vomiting, ataxia and foot drop. The MRI reveals multiple large hemispheric (predominantly T2-hyperintense) lesions (**a**) with ring enhancement (**b**). Adrenoleukodystrophy was excluded, and neuropathology findings were consistent with Schilder's disease. (Courtesy of John Strain MD, The Children's Hospital, Denver)

References

Balo J (1928) Encephalitis periaxialis concentrica. Arch Neurol Psychiatry 19:242-264

Beniac DR, Wood DD, Palaniyar N et al (1999) Marburg's variant of multiple sclerosis correlates with a less compact structure of myelin basic protein. Mol Cell Biol Res Commun 1:48-51

Bitsch A, Wegener C, da Costa C et al (1999) Lesion development in Marburg's type of acute multiple sclerosis: from inflammation to demyelination. Mult Scler 5:138-146

Bolay H, Karabudak R, Tacal T et al (1996) Balo's concentric sclerosis. Report of two patients with magnetic resonance imaging follow-up. J Neuroimaging 6:98-103

Cannella B, Raine CS (1995) The adhesion molecule and cytokine profile of multiple sclerosis lesions. Ann Neurol 37:424-435

Caracciolo JT, Murtagh RD, Rojiani AM et al (2001) Pathognomonic MR imaging findings in Balo concentric sclerosis. AJNR Am J Neuroradiol 22:292-293

Chen CJ (2001) Serial proton magnetic resonance spectroscopy in lesions of Balo concentric sclerosis. J Comput Assist Tomogr 25:713-718

Chen CJ, Chu NS, Lu CS et al (1999) Serial magnetic resonance imaging in patients with Balo's concentric sclerosis: natural history of lesion development. Ann Neurol 46:651-656

Chen CJ, Ro LS, Wang LJ et al (1996) Balo's concentric sclerosis: MRI. Neuroradiology 38:322-324

Chen CJ, Ro LS, Chang CN (1996) Serial MRI in pathologically verified Balo concentric sclerosis. J Comput Assist Tomogr 20:732-735

Coyle P (2000) Diagnosis and classification of inflammatory demyelinating disorders. In: Burks JS, Johnson KP (eds) Multiple sclerosis diagnosis, medical management, and rehabilitation. Demos, New York, pp 81-97

Cree BA, Goodin DS, Hauser SL (2002) Neuromyelitis optica. Semin Neurol 22:105-122

Davie CA, Hawkins CP, Barker GJ et al (1994) Serial proton magnetic resonance spectroscopy in acute multiple sclerosis lesions. Brain 117:49-58

de Seze J, Lebrun C, Stojkovic T et al (2003) Is Devic's neuromyelitis optica a separate disease? A comparative study with multiple sclerosis. Mult Scler 9:521-525

de Seze J, Stojkovic T, Ferriby D et al (2002) Devic's neuromyelitis optica: clinical, laboratory, MRI and outcome profile. J Neurol Sci 197:57-61

Devic E (1894) Myelite subaigue complique de nevrite optique. Bull Med 8:1033-1034

Eblen F, Poremba M, Grodd W et al (1991) Myelinoclastic diffuse sclerosis (Schilder's disease): cliniconeuroradiologic correlations. Neurology 41:589-591

Fardet L, Genereau T, Mikaeloff Y et al (2003) Devic's neuromyelitis optica: study of nine cases. Acta Neurol Scand 108:193-200

Fazekas F, Offenbacher H, Schmidt R et al (1994) MRI of neuromyelitis optica: evidence for a distinct entity. J Neurol Neurosurg Psychiatry 57:1140-1142

Filippi M, Rocca MA, Moiola L et al (1999) MRI and magnetization transfer imaging changes in the brain and cervical cord of patients with Devic's neuromyelitis optica. Neurology 53:1705-1710

Fernandez-Jaen A, Martinez-Bermejo A, Gutierrez-Molina M et al (2001) (Schilder's diffuse myelinoclastic sclerosis). Rev Neurol 33:16-21

Gallucci M, Caulo M, Cerone G et al (2001) Acquired inflammatory white matter disease. Child's Nerv Syst 17:202-210

Gass A, Filippi M, Rodegher ME et al (1998) Characteristics of chronic MS lesions in the cerebrum, brainstem, spinal cord, and optic nerve on T1-weighted MRI. Neurology 50:548-550

Giang DW, Poduri KR, Eskin TA et al (1992) Multiple sclerosis masquerading as a mass lesion. Neuroradiology 34:150-154

Giubilei F, Sarrantonio A, Tisei P et al (1997) Four-year follow-up of a case of acute multiple sclerosis of the Marburg type. Ital J Neurol Sci 18:163-166

Hynson JL, Kornberg AJ, Coleman LT et al (2001) Clinical and neuroradiologic features of acute disseminated encephalomyelitis in children. Neurology 56:1308-1312

Iannucci G, Mascalchi M, Salvi F et al (2000) Vanishing Balo-like lesions in multiple sclerosis. J Neurol Neurosurg Psychiatry 69:399-400

Itoyama Y, Tateishi J, Kuroiwa Y (1985) Atypical multiple sclerosis with concentric or lamellar demyelinated lesions: two Japanese patients studied post mortem. Ann Neurol 17:481-487

Karaarslan E, Altintas A, Senol U et al (2001) Balo's concentric sclerosis: clinical and radiologic features of five cases. AJNR Am J Neuroradiol 22:1362-1367

Karussis D, Leker RR, Ashkenazi A et al (1998) A subgroup of multiple sclerosis patients with anticardiolipin antibodies and unusual clinical manifestations: do they represent a new nosological entity? Ann Neurol 44:629-634

Kastrup O, Stude P, Limmroth V (2002) Balo's concentric sclerosis. Evolution of active demyelination demonstrated by serial contrast-enhanced MRI. J Neurol 249:811-814

Keegan M, Pineda AA, McClelland RL et al (2002) Plasma exchange for severe attacks of CNS demyelination: predictors of response. Neurology 58:143-146

Kepes JJ (1993) Large focal tumor-like demyelinating lesions of the brain: intermediate entity between multiple sclerosis and acute disseminated encephalomyelitis? A study of 31 patients. Ann Neurol 33:18-27

Kim MO, Lee SA, Choi CG et al (1997) Balo's concentric sclerosis: a clinical case study of brain MRI, biopsy, and pronton magnetic resonance spectroscopic findings. J Neurol Neurosurg Psychiatry 62:655-658

Kotil K, Kalayci M, Koseoglu T et al (2002) Myelinoclastic diffuse sclerosis (Schilder's disease): report of a case and review of the literature. Br J Neurosurg 16:516-519

Kurul S, Cakmakci H, Dirik E et al (2003) Schilder's disease: case study with serial neuroimaging. J Child Neurol 18:58-61

Kuroiwa Y (1985a) Concentric sclerosis. In: Koetsier JC (ed) Demyelinating diseases. Handbook of clinical neurology, vol 3, pp 409-417

Kuroiwa Y (1985b) Neuromyelitis optica (Devic's disease, Devic's syndrome). In: Koetsier JC (ed) Demyelinating diseases. Handbook of clinical neurology, vol 3, pp 397-408

Louboutin JP, Elie B (1995) Treatment of Balo's concentric sclerosis with immunosuppressive drugs followed by multimodality evoked potentials and MRI. Muscle Nerve 18:1478-1480

Lucchinetti C, Bruck W, Parisi J et al (2000) Heterogeneity of multiple sclerosis lesions: implications for the pathogenesis of demyelination. Ann Neurol 47:707-717

Lucchinetti CF, Mandler RN, McGavern D et al (2002) A role

for humoral mechanisms in the pathogenesis of Devic's neuromyelitis optica. Brain 125:1450-1461

Lycklama G, Thompson A, Filippi M et al(2003) Spinal-cord MRI in multiple sclerosis. Lancet Neurol 2:555-562

Mandler RN, Davis LE, Jeffery DR et al (1993) Devic's neuromyelitis optica: a clinicopathological study of 8 patients. Ann Neurol 34:162-168

Mandler RN, Ahmed W, Dencoff JE (1998) Devic's neuromyelitis optica: a prospective study of seven patients treated with prednisone and azathioprine. Neurology 51:1219-1220

Mendez MF, Pogacar S (1988) Malignant monophasic multiple sclerosis or "Marburg's disease". Neurology 38:1153-1155

Mehler MF, Rabinowich L (1988) Inflammatory myelinoclastic diffuse sclerosis. Ann Neurol 23:413-415

Moore GR, Neumann PE, Suzuki K et al (1985) Balo's concentric sclerosis: new observations on lesion development. Ann Neurol 17:604-611

Moore GR, Berry K, Oger JJ et al (2001) Balo's concentric sclerosis: surviving normal myelin in a patient with a relapsing-remitting clinical course. Mult Scler 7:375-382

Noseworthy JH, Lucchinetti C, Rodriguez M et al (2000) Multiple sclerosis. N Eng J Med 343:938-952

Nejat F, Eftekhar B (2002) Decompressive aspiration in myelinoclastic diffuse sclerosis or Schilder disease. Case report. J Neurosurg 97:1447-1449

Ng SH, Ko SF, Cheung YC et al (1999) MRI features of Balo's concentric sclerosis. Br J Radiol 72:400-403

O'Riordan JI, Gallagher HL, Thompson AJ et al (1996) Clinical, CSF, and MRI findings in Devic's neuromyelitis optica. J Neurol Neurosurg Psychiatry 60:382-387

Poser CM (1957) Diffuse disseminated sclerosis in the adult. J Neuropathol Exp Neurol 16:61-78

Poser CM (1985) Myelinoclastic diffuse sclerosis. In: Koetsier JC (ed) Demyelinating diseases. Handbook of clinical neurology, vol 3, pp 419-428

Poser S, Luer W, Bruhn H et al (1992) Acute demyelinating disease. Classification and non-invasive diagnosis. Acta Neurol Scand 86:579-585

Prineas JW, McDonald WI, Franklin RJM (2002) Demyelinating diseases. In: Adams JH, Corsellis JAN, Duchen LW (eds) Greenfield's neuropathology, 7th edn. John Wiley & Sons, New York

Schwarz S, Mohr A, Knauth M et al (2001) Acute disseminated encephalomyelitis: a follow-up study of 40 adult patients. Neurology 56:1313-1318

Sekijima Y, Tokuda T, Hashimoto T et al (1997) Serial magnetic resonance imaging (MRI) study of a patient with Balo's concentric sclerosis treated with immunoabsorption plasmapheresis. Mult Scler 2:291-294

Simon JH (2000) Brain and spinal cord atrophy in multiple sclerosis. Neuroimaging Clin N Am 10:753-770

Spiegel M, Kruger H, Hofmann E et al (1989) MRI study of Balo's concentric sclerosis before and after immunosuppressive therapy. J Neurol 236:487-488

Traugott U, Reinherz EL, Raine CS (1983) Multiple sclerosis. Distribution of T cells, T cell subsets and Ia-positive macrophages in lesions of different ages. J Neuroimmunol 4:201-221

Valk J, van der Knaap MS (1995) Multiple sclerosis, neuromyelitis optica, concentric sclerosis, and Schilder's diffuse sclerosis. In: Magnetic resonance of myelin, myelination, and myelin disorders. Springer-Verlag, Berlin-Heidelberg-New York, pp 179-205

Weinshenker BG (2003) Neuromyelitis optica: what it is and what it might be. Lancet 361:889-890

Weinshenker BG (1999) Therapeutic plasma exchange for acute inflammatory demyelinating syndromes of the central nervous system. J Clin Apheresis 14:144-148

Wingerchuk DM, Hogancamp WF, O'Brien PC et al (1999) The clinical course of neuromyelitis optica (Devic's syndrome). Neurology 53:1107-1114

Wingerchuk DM, Weinshenker BG (2003) Neuromyelitis optica: clinical predictors of a relapsing course and survival. Neurology 60:848-853

Wood DD, Bilbao JM, O'Connors P (1994) Acute multiple sclerosis (Marburg type) is associated with developmentally immature myelin basic protein. Ann Neurol 40:18-24

Yao DL, Webster HD, Hudson LD et al (1994) Concentric sclerosis (Balo): morphometric and in situ hybridization study of lesions in six patients. Ann Neurol 35:18-30

17 Acute Disseminated Encephalomyelitis

Stefan Schwarz and Michael Knauth

CONTENTS

17.1 Introduction

The first clinical descriptions of patients with "acute disseminated encephalomyelitis" (ADEM) originate from the begin of the 20th century. In a summary of these early case reports, McAlpine concluded in 1931 that ADEM typically occurs after an infection or immunization, but may also arise spontaneously. He further pointed out that the course of the disease is short, the mortality low, and, in contrast to the "disseminated sclerosis", the disease is monophasic (McAlpine 1931). Unfortunately, today, more than 70 years after McAlpine's landmark publication, a more detailed and precise definition of ADEM is still not available.

S. Schwarz, MD
Assistant Professor, Department of Neurology, Klinikum Mannheim, University of Heidelberg, Theodor Kutzer Ufer 1-3, 68167 Mannheim, Germany
M. Knauth, MD
Professor, Department of Neuroradiology, Zentrum Radiologie, Georg-August-University of Göttingen, Robert-Koch-Str. 40, 37075 Göttingen, Germany

Although the number of case reports and small case series has increased to date, generally accepted diagnostic criteria for the diagnosis ADEM have not been established. It remains debatable whether ADEM is a distinct disease entity or a subform of multiple sclerosis (MS). Because many neurologists, encouraged from the results of the CHAMPS (Jacobs et al. 2000) and ETOMS (Comi et al. 2001) trials, now tend to treat patients with a suspected MS already after the first clinical manifestation, it is of particular importance to identify those patients with a monophasic disease who would not need an improper, expensive and potentially hazardous preventive immunomodulatory medication. Applying the novel McDonald diagnostic criteria for MS (McDonald et al. 2001), in many of the patients previously diagnosed with ADEM, the diagnosis of MS could be made already during the first episode of symptoms using the clinical and MRI findings usually present in these patients. To complicate these diagnostic qualms even further, the discrimination of ADEM from other acute demyelinating syndromes such as "acute MS of the Marburg type", Schilder's diffuse sclerosis, Devic's neuromyelitis optica, or Hurst syndrome frequently is elusive. Because there have been no large systematic studies, the previous attempts for a classification of these syndromes depended on hypotheses and empirical clinical evidence only. Most authors agree that "Marburg disease" should be subsumed under ADEM, and the Hurst syndrome constitutes the most severe variant of ADEM.

The aim of this chapter is to give an overview of the neuroradiological features of ADEM. Because ADEM and its complex diagnostic problems cannot be understood on radiological grounds only, we also briefly review the clinical symptoms, pathological and laboratory findings. We will show that during the initial presentation of the patients there is a wide range of overlapping clinical symptoms and radiological findings with MS, and today, the diagnosis of ADEM can only be established with certainty after a long symptom-free follow-up.

17.2 Epidemiology

ADEM is an uncommon disease. Accurate epidemiological figures do not exist. MILLER et al. (1956) estimated the incidence of a parainfectious ADEM after acute measles infection to be 1:1000. However, these and other results from studies originating from the pre-MRI era must be interpreted with caution because, at this time, the diagnostic possibilities were hardly adequate. Before the introduction of MRI, an acute demyelinating disease could only be presumed from the patients' history and clinical findings; a definite diagnosis was only possible after a brain biopsy or autopsy. Because mild or transient symptoms rarely justify a brain biopsy, it can be presumed that severe or even lethal courses are overrepresented in the studies from the pre-MRI era. This is also the reason for the previously frequently held opinion that ADEM is a severe disease with a high mortality.

Supposedly, the incidence of ADEM is higher than previously assumed because the disease may be clinically completely asymptomatic or the symptoms are mild and transient, and further diagnostic procedures are not performed.

The incidence of ADEM is probably highest in children and declines with increasing age. In patients older than 40 years, ADEM is rare (WANG et al. 1996). However, few single patients with ADEM over 70 years have been described. As a rule of thumb, in patients over 40 years, the diagnosis of ADEM should be established only with great caution.

The occurrence of postinfectious and postvaccinal ADEM is not confined to populations with a high incidence of MS (MODI et al. 2001; MURTHY et al. 1999). Unfortunately, there are no systematic studies comparing the incidence of ADEM between countries with a high incidence of MS and countries where indigenous MS is virtually absent. However, the rate of "idiopathic" ADEM without preceding infection or vaccination seems to be higher in the European and North American countries than in Brazil (REIS et al. 1999) and India (MURTHY et al. 1999). The development of MS after the diagnosis of ADEM is also uncommon in these countries.

17.3 Etiology

In the majority of patients, an infection, or, rarely, a vaccination, precedes the onset of symptoms. This is particularly true for children: in 62 of 84 children an infection or vaccination preceded the onset of ADEM (TENEMBAUM et al. 2002). In contrast, in adults ADEM occurs more often spontaneously. The interval between infection and onset of symptoms is variable. Typically, the time interval is between 2 days and 4 weeks.

ADEM is associated with a large number of different, in particular viral, infections. The most common trigger is an unspecific upper respiratory tract infection. Many other viral infections have been reported: Coxsackie, HHV-6, EBV, HSV, CMV, HIV, HTLV-1, varicella, measles, mumps, and rubella. Arguably, the non-viral encephalomyelitis in HIV-infected patients with the "common variable immunodeficiency syndrome (CVID)" is a variant of ADEM (HAPPE and HUSSTEDT 2000).

Compared with the reports on viral infections and ADEM, associations with bacterial or parasitic infections are much more infrequent. Fairly often, an association with intracellular bacteria has been described, above all with *Mycoplasma*. Anecdotally, ADEM has been reported after infections with *Chlamydia*, *Leptospira*, *Legionella*, *Rickettsia*, *Streptococcus* and *Salmonella*.

Given the enormous number of vaccinations, ADEM should be considered as a very rare complication [for an overview, see STRATTON et al. (1994)]. Although the association between vaccination and ADEM may be purely coincidental in some patients, especially in children, in single patients, a causal association is obvious. A high rate of postvaccinal ADEM (0.83%) has been reported after vaccinations against rabies with Semple rabies vaccine produced on neural cell cultures. In developing countries, these sera are still in use due to lower production costs.

Apart from vaccinations and infections, ADEM has been associated with gold therapy, live lamb cell injection, parenteral therapy with herbal extracts (SCHWARZ et al. 2000), transplantation, bee sting and after accidental inoculation with guinea pig brain tissue.

17.4 Pathophysiological Hypotheses

The pathophysiology of ADEM has not yet been fully elucidated. There is only the general agreement that autoimmune mechanisms may play a key role in postvaccinal and parainfectious ADEM. In idiopathic ADEM, a genetic disposition (Idrissova et al. 2003) or other unidentified factors may also be present. Furthermore, it is unclear to which extent the pathophysiological mechanisms in ADEM are homogeneous or the same as those found in patients with MS. In recent years, convincing evidence has been accumulated that in MS there are several subgroups with differing pathophysiological mechanisms (Lucchinetti et al. 2000).

Autoreactive T-lymphocytes against myelin antigens (in particular, myelin basic protein and myelin oligodendrocytic glycoprotein) might contribute to the demyelinating process (Antel and Owens 1999). In patients with ADEM, autoreactive myelin basic protein T cells clones have been found (Pohl-Kappe et al. 1998). The mechanisms, by which these autoreactive T-cells are activated outside the CNS, are unknown. Under normal circumstances, the blood–brain barrier prevents contact between T-cells and myelin antigens. Therefore, an initial damage of the blood–brain barrier could be postulated. Structural homologies between microbial antigens and autoantigens of the myelin antigens may also switch on the autoimmune reaction in ADEM (Jorens et al. 2000).

Following the invasion of auto-reactive T-lymphocytes into the brain tissue, secondary inflammatory processes are initiated by the mass of pro-inflammatory cytokines, activation of macrophages, and interaction with B-lymphocytes secreting immunoglobulins into the CSF compartment (Martino et al. 2002). Compared with the cellular immunoreaction, humoral mechanisms probably are of minor importance for the progression of the pathological process. Antibodies against gangliosides (GM1, GD1a) can be found. However, it is still unknown which of the various inflammatory mechanisms found in MS and ADEM are epiphenomena or causative, and which ones have possible desirable or, alternatively, deleterious effects.

Relying on pathological findings of a predominantly perivascular localized demyelination ("disseminated vasculomyelinopathy"), Reik (1980) hypothesized that at the beginning of the pathological cascade, deposits of circulating antigen–antibody complexes in the vessel wall cause initial, local damage to the blood–brain barrier, expose myelin antigens, thus initiating the autoimmune reaction to myelin antigens. However, except for some single observations, this hypothesis could not be substantiated in patients with ADEM (Tachovsky et al. 1976).

17.5 Pathological Findings

Demyelinating lesions can be found in the white matter of the entire CNS. The gray matter, usually the deep cortical layers and the basal ganglia, may also be affected. The macroscopic examination may reveal small perivascular gray discolorations. The histological work-up shows multifocal, disseminated inflammatory infiltrates with predominant demyelination, typically located around small and medium-sized venous vessels ("perivenous encephalomyelitis"), occasionally accumulating to large lesions (Hart and Earle 1975). The inflammatory infiltrates primarily consist of lymphocytes, but may also exhibit a mixed picture with lymphocytes, neutrophils, and microglia/macrophages. Small perivascular hemorrhages may be present. A more or less pronounced reactive astrocytic proliferation is usually found. Frequently, there are additional subpial and subependymal small demyelinating areas. Patients with an acute hemorrhagic leukencephalitis ("Hurst syndrome"), in addition to the above-mentioned hallmarks of ADEM, show multiple hemorrhagic necrotizing foci, joining up to large lesions (Hurst 1941).

17.6 Clinical Symptoms

The neurological symptoms are unspecific and vary enormously, depending on the size and location of the demyelinating lesions. It is not possible to establish the diagnosis of ADEM on clinical grounds only. Fever is commonly recognized as a typical finding in patients with ADEM, but is present only in a minority of patients. Fever is more often found in children and in adults with a fulminant clinical course (Hynson et al. 2001). Meningism is another infrequent clinical sign, also associated with a severe clinical picture. In children, loss of consciousness of a variable degree until deep coma is more frequently observed (Anlar et al. 2003; Hynson et al. 2001; Tenembaum et al. 2002). In adults, loss of consciousness is uncommon. Patients with large space-occupying supratentorial or extensive lesions in the brainstem occasionally require intensive care therapy, intubation and artificial ventilation. In a few patients, aphasia or seizures, ranging from single focal fits to a status epilepticus, have been described. In MS patients, these clinical symptoms are not common, but not entirely exceptional. Remarkably, many patients present with behavioral abnormalities such as psychomotor slowing, slight to moderate personality changes and psychiatric symptoms occasionally imitating an acute psychosis (Nasr et al. 2000).

Spinal symptoms are present in a minority of patients. However, in general, even an isolated myelitis may be diagnosed as ADEM. There are no reasons for the assumption that different pathophysiological mechanisms are present in patients with an acute postinfectious myelitis. Poser (1989) suggested establishing the diagnosis of ADEM only if a complete transverse myelitis is present, but not in patients with partial spinal symptoms suggesting MS. However, there is no scientific evidence from radiological or clinical studies to support this empirical categorization.

A similar problem arises in patients with optic neuritis. Most authors agree that a unilateral optic neuritis should not be diagnosed as ADEM, even if it occurs after an infection. In contrast, bilateral optic neuritis is a characteristic finding in ADEM.

To complicate the attempts of a clinical classification even further, ADEM may occur in combination with demyelinating diseases of the peripheral nervous system. Anecdotally, an association with Guillain-Barré syndrome has also been reported (Nadkarni and Lisak 1993).

17.7 Cerebrospinal Fluid

CSF findings in patients with ADEM are variable. Therefore, the main reason for a lumbar puncture is to exclude other possible diagnoses. Apart from the conventional CSF parameters, a meticulous microbiological and serological examination of both CSF and blood for markers of infection with neurotropic viruses (HSV, EBV, CMV, VZV, HHV-6, HIV, JCV, measles, Coxsackie and enteroviruses, in endemic regions central European encephalitis), *Borrelia* spp. and lues is warranted.

In many patients, the lumbar puncture is completely unremarkable. However, in the majority of patients, the CSF is abnormal. The protein content is slightly to moderately raised. In particular in patients with severe clinical symptoms, the protein content may be markedly raised, indicating a disturbed blood–brain barrier.

In most patients, a slight lymphocytic pleocytosis is found. Leukocyte counts over 100 leukocytes per microliter are infrequent and usually associated with a severe clinical course. In these patients, a severe blood–brain barrier disruption is mostly present.

Although lymphocytes predominate, in some patients, a polymorphonuclear pleocytosis with a higher proportion of granulocytes is present. These patients require a meticulous search for other differential diagnoses, in particular infectious encephalitis.

CNS-specific oligoclonal IgG production is mostly absent. However, an oligoclonal IgG synthesis does not exclude the diagnosis of ADEM. Although it is frequently postulated that patients with a CNS-specific IgG production bear a greater risk for the progression to MS, there is not enough data to support this hypothesis.

The CSF content of myelin basic protein (MBP) may be raised in ADEM. It has been speculated that this finding may differentiate ADEM from MS (Nishikawa et al. 1999). Recently, Berger et al. (2003) reported that the presence of serum antibodies to myelin oligodendrocyte glycoprotein (MOG) and MBP in patients with a clinically isolated syndrome suggestive of MS predicts the interval to conversion to clinically definite MS. To date, the clinical significance of these antibodies in ADEM remains uncertain.

17.8 Therapeutic Options and Prognosis

There are no randomized, controlled studies in ADEM. The natural evolution of the disease is not known because after the diagnosis has been established, nearly all patients receive immunosuppressive therapy. However, spontaneous complete remission is possible. In patients with none or minor symptoms a wait-and-see strategy is justified. In analogy with the management of acute exacerbations in MS patients, iv methylprednisolone is generally considered as the standard first choice of therapy. Already 50 years ago, Miller (1953) reported a rapid improvement after infusion of adrenocorticotropic hormone. Now, there is an overwhelming body of evidence from prospective case series and numerous single reports that corticosteroids rapidly improve even severe symptoms in the majority of patients. After discontinuation of the corticosteroid therapy, a relapse is not uncommon (Anlar et al. 2003; Gupte et al. 2003). If corticoids fail, immunoglobulins are an option. Most authors recommend a dosage which has been shown to be effective in patients with idiopathic thrombotic purpura (0.4g/kgBW per day over 5 days). Alternatively, plasma separation in various protocols (e.g. five treatments every other day) can be employed.

In individual patients with a fulminant onset of severe clinical symptoms, favorable results have been published after high-dose therapy with cyclophosphamide even after the failure of standard methyl prednisolone therapy.

Therapeutic recommendations are summarized in Table 17.1. It has to be emphasized that these recommendations are based on "educated guesses" rather than "evidence-based" trials.

Table 17.1. Empirical therapy of ADEM

(1) In patients with minor or no symptoms, consider a "wait-and-see" strategy
(2) Initial standard therapy: 0.5 g methylprednisolone iv/day over 5 days
(3) If methylprednisolone iv is successful, but moderate to severe symptoms are still present after 5 days, continue methylprednisolone orally, starting with 100 mg/day and tapering over 4 weeks
(4) If (2) is unsuccessful or if contraindications for corticosteroids are present: immunoglobulins (0.4 g/kg BW per day over 5 days). Alternatively: plasma separation (second choice due to a higher rate of complications)
(5) If (4) is unsuccessful: cyclophosphamide (bolus 1 g iv, may be repeated at 4-week intervals depending on blood cell count and clinical symptoms)

Patients with large space-occupying lesions may develop a critical raise of the intracranial pressure. In single cases, decompressive surgery has also been performed. In addition to the craniectomy, Takata et al. (1999) employed therapeutic hypothermia, an option which might be theoretically sound, but which has not yet been used in a sufficient number of patients to draw any definite conclusion on its clinical efficacy.

In general, the prognosis of ADEM is favorable. Roughly 70% of all patients recover fully or nearly completely (Hynson et al. 2001; Schwarz et al. 2001; Tenembaum et al. 2002). This is true even for patients who present in a poor clinical state. However, fulminant clinical courses may lead to severe residual deficits or may even be lethal. Mild cognitive deficits escaping the standard neurological examination can persist even in patients in whom the MRI has normalized completely (Hahn et al. 2003).

17.9 The Problem of Relapsing or Multiphasic ADEM

The proportion of patients with "multiphasic" ADEM depends on the diagnostic criteria employed. Some authors differentiate even between "relapsing" and "multiphasic" ADEM which, in our opinion, is a quite elusive undertaking. The term "multiphasic ADEM", for which an acronym has already been coined (MDEM), is problematic, and its use should not be encouraged. These patients usually fulfill all criteria for MS, using either the Poser (Poser et al. 1983) or the McDonald criteria (McDonald et al. 2001). However, particularly in children after an infection-associated ADEM, a second episode after months to years which shows all characteristic signs of ADEM is not uncommon (Anlar et al. 2003; Hynson et al. 2001; Tenembaum et al. 2002). Most of these relapses occur within the first weeks up to a few months after the first episodes. Tenembaum et al. (2002) observed in their large study that 10% of all 84 patients with ADEM developed a second episode. These children seem not to be at risk to develop a typical MS in later life. However, Rust et al. (1997) published contradicting results: in their study, 17 of 121 children initially diagnosed with ADEM later developed various forms of MS. Tenembaum et al. (2002) argued that MS is unlikely in patients in whom the episodes are clearly associated with a preceding infection or immunization. Yet, this point remains unsatisfactory because also in MS patients, febrile infections frequently trigger a relapse. In contrast to pediatric studies, adults with the initial diagnosis of ADEM have a higher risk to develop MS. In our own series, 14 of 40 adult patients with the initial diagnosis of ADEM developed MS (Schwarz et al. 2001).

17.10 Differential Diagnosis

Because well-defined diagnostic criteria are absent, ADEM is a diagnosis which can only be made after the exclusion of several other diseases with similar symptoms and radiological findings. Table 17.2 gives

Table 17.2. Differential diagnosis of ADEM

- Multiple sclerosis (plus variants)
- Cerebral lymphoma
- Infectious encephalitis
  Viral: EBV, CMV, HSV1+2, JCV, HIV, HHV-6, FSME, HTLV, enteroviruses, measles, SSPE
  Bacterial: *Tropheryma whipplei*, *Mycoplasma*, *Listeria*, *Brucella* spp.
  Fungal (e.g., *Histoplasma* spp.)
- Other autoimmune diseases
  Vasculitis (e.g., Behçet's disease, panarteritis nodosa)
  Sarcoidosis
- Porphyrias
- Leukodystrophies
- Mitochondrial disorders (e.g., MELAS)
- Myelinolysis after electrolyte imbalances (e.g., central pontine myelinolysis)

an overview of the most important differential diagnoses.

In clinical practice, the differentiation between ADEM and viral encephalitis or CNS lymphoma can be challenging. The clinical symptoms as well as the CSF results may be identical. Moreover, in some forms of viral encephalitis (e.g. CMV, PML, enteroviruses, HIV, HHV-6), MRI shows focal lesions indistinguishable from those found in ADEM. Therefore, an extensive microbiological examination of the CSF with serological tests and PCR for antigens of neurotropic viruses is necessary. However, the microbiological work-up is limited, because only the most frequent and important viruses can be analyzed, and in addition, these analyses are usually expensive. Thus, routinely, only those infections were searched for which a specific therapy is available (Herpesviruses and HIV). In addition, many viral infections can only be diagnosed with certainty after approximately 2 weeks, when a second examination reveals a significant rise of the specific antibodies.

Some patients present with ambiguous CSF and MRI findings which make a clear differentiation between ADEM and a cerebral lymphoma impossible (Schwarz et al. 2002). Both diseases require different immediate emergency treatment. Unfortunately, in both diseases, corticosteroids usually lead to a rapid remission of the clinical and MRI abnormalities, and therefore, an improvement after steroid therapy does not clarify the diagnosis. Whenever a cerebral lymphoma is suspected, a brain biopsy should be performed. This is particularly important because after initiation of steroid treatment for suspected ADEM, the pathological diagnosis of a lymphoma can be difficult due to the regression of the lymphoma which can render the histopathological changes difficult to interpret. PCR-based analysis of immunoglobulins in the CSF is a highly sensitive means for identifying clonal B-cell responses, and provides additional criteria for the differentiation between acute demyelinating diseases of the CNS (monoclonal B-cell populations) and CNS lymphoma (polyclonal B-cell populations) (Wildemann et al. 2001).

17.11 Neuroradiology

17.11.1 Computed Tomography

MRI is the radiological gold standard for the diagnosis of ADEM. However, in many patients with unexplained neurological symptoms, a CT is first performed. In the CT, hypodense lesions, usually in the subcortical white matter, but occasionally also involving the cortex, the basal ganglia or brainstem, can be found, sometimes with enhancement after administration of contrast medium (Lukes and Norman 1983). Large lesions may have a space-occupying effect, imitating a brain tumor. Of course, the CT abnormalities are unspecific and offer a wide range of possible diagnoses. Moreover, in many patients with ADEM, CT findings may be completely normal.

17.11.2 Magnetic Resonance Imaging

Nowadays, without an MRI, the diagnosis of ADEM cannot be established. MRI serves not only to confirm the presence of demyelinating lesions, but also to exclude other diagnoses. Compared with CT, MRI enables a better differentiation from other diseases and has a high sensitivity which can be equal to 100% (Tenembaum et al. 2002). However, the lesions may develop over the course of several days after the onset of the clinical symptoms, and therefore, the initial MRI may be unremarkable. In a small case series, Honkaniemi et al. (2001) reported on three patients with ADEM in whom the initial MR scans showed no abnormalities until several weeks after the onset of the disease. Höllinger et al. (2002) found no MRI abnormalities at all in a few patients diagnosed with ADEM which led them to the unusual conclusion that MRI should not be considered mandatory in adult ADEM, and an EEG should be performed instead because of the higher rate of abnormal findings. However, these case reports are the exception. Generally, a completely normal MRI makes the diagnosis of ADEM improbable. In most patients, cranial MRI demonstrates multiple lesions of various size and shape, predominantly in the white matter of the hemispheres, the cerebellum and the brainstem (for an overview, see Table 17.3). In MRI theses lesions are hyperintense on T2-weighted images and hypo- to isointense on T1-weighted images (Figs. 17.1, 17.2) (Kesselring et al. 1990; O'Riordan et al. 1999; Singh et al. 1999). However, MRI findings in ADEM have a high variability. Although most patients have multiple, disseminated lesions, a solitary lesion is not uncommon (Figs. 17.3, 17.4). In principle, the lesions in ADEM cannot be differentiated with certainty from those in MS. A few radiological findings suggest – but are in no way definitive proof – ADEM. In contrast to MS, the basal ganglia and

Table 17.3. MRI findings in ADEM: results from five case series

	Dale et al. (2000)	Hynson et al. (2001)	Tenembaum et al. (2002)	Murthy et al. (2002)	Schwarz et al. (2001)
Number with MRI (%)	32 (91)	31 (100)	70 (94)	15 (83)	26 (100) Only confirmed ADEM
Population	Pediatric	Pediatric	Pediatric	Pediatric	Adult
Lesion site (%)					
White matter	91	90	Not stated	93	100
Periventricular	44	29	Not stated	60	54
Corpus callosum	Not stated	29	Not stated	7w	23
Subcortical/deep	91	80	Not stated	93	38
Cortical gray matter	12	Not stated	Not stated	80	8
Brainstem	56	42	Not stated	47	57
Cerebellum	31	Not stated	Not stated	13	31
Thalamus	41	32	13 (bilateral)	27	15 (includes basal ganglia)
Basal ganglia	28	39	Not stated	20	15 (includes thalamus)
Spinal cord	Not stated	67	Not stated	71	Not stated
Number with gadolinium enhancement (%)	Not stated	8 (29)	10 (37)	7 (47)	20 (95)
Number with follow-up MRI (%)	19 (59)	8 (26)	Not stated	14 (93)	20 (77)
MRI follow-up in years (range)	0.2–9	Not stated	Not stated	0.2–2	0.04–1.5
Original brain lesion change (%)					
Complete resolution	37	?	Not stated	7	30
Partial resolution	53	6	Not stated	57	55
Unchanged	10	?	Not stated	21	0
New lesions	0	3 (all clinical relapses)	0	14 (all within 8 weeks)	15 (no clinical relapses)

the thalami are more often affected, and the lesions of ADEM are typically located in the subcortical white matter, and sometimes involve the cortex. A further criteria which has been claimed to be helpful for the radiological differentiation between MS and ADEM is the predominant infratentorial location of the lesions, which are frequently found within the brainstem and cerebellar peduncles. Although this sign is habitually emphasized, it is probably of no particular diagnostic value since infratentorial lesions are also characteristic for MS. Moreover, the total lesion load does not differentiate between ADEM and MS, although it has sometimes been suggested, that a very high lesion load would be indicative for ADEM.

There is only a weak association between the initial MRI, clinical findings, and the long-term prognosis. Even patients with a high lesion load may recover completely. Tenembaum et al. (2002) tried to establish an MRI classification into four MRI groups (small lesions, large lesions, additional bithalamic involvement, acute hemorrhagic encephalomyelitis). However, there was no association found between these MRI subgroups and long-term disability.

Some patients have confluent demyelinating lesions, often with a striking space-occupying effect,

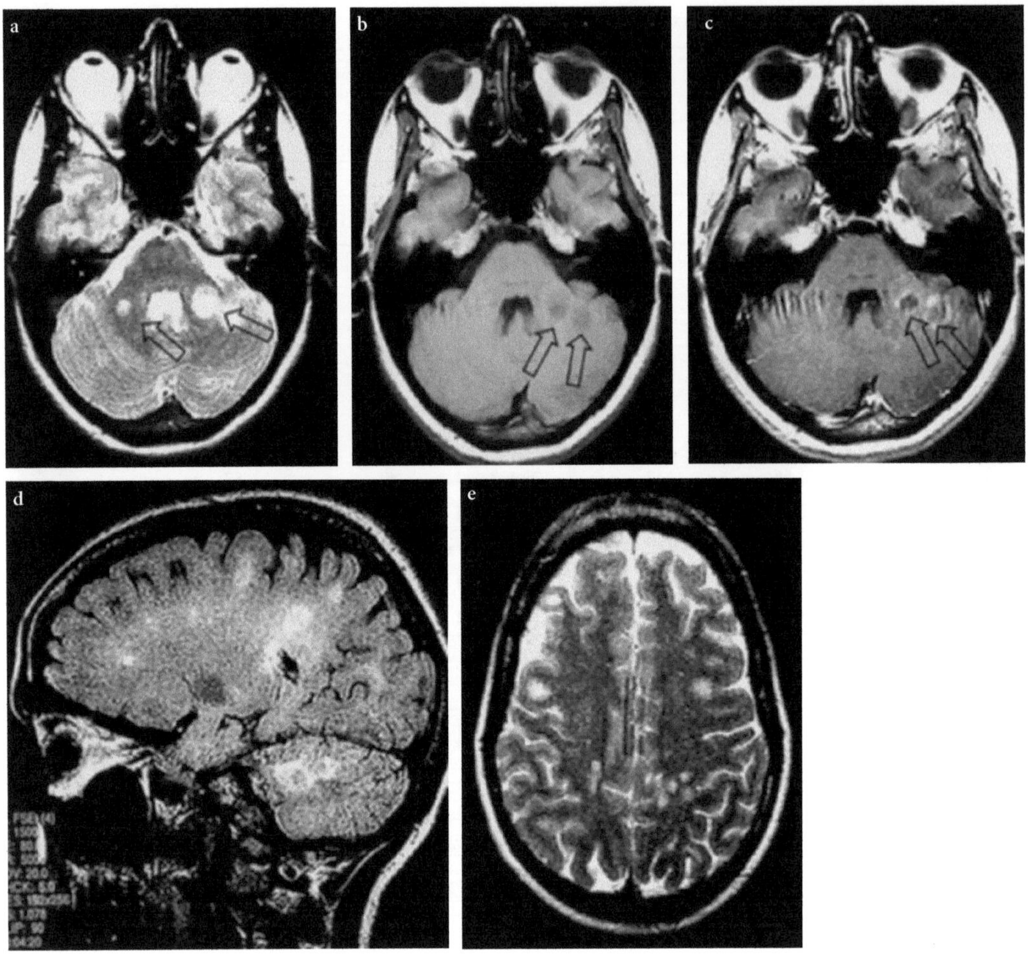

Fig. 17.1a–e. A few days after unspecific signs of a systemic viral infection, this 32-year-old woman developed dysarthria, gait ataxia, and double vision. The lumbar puncture revealed 16 lymphocytes/µl. The MRI showed several lesions in the cerebellum and cerebellar peduncles (*arrows*), which are hyperintense in the T2-weighted images (**a**) and hypointense in the native T1-weighted images (**b**). After administration of gadolinium, there was a ring-shaped enhancement (**c**). The FLAIR images (**d**) and T2-weighted images (**e**) showed the diffuse supratentorial involvement

resembling a brain tumor (Fig. 17.5). It remains disputable whether these findings indicate a distinct disease or merely a subgroup of ADEM (Kepes 1993).

Patients with a fulminant clinical course (Hurst syndrome) have lesions with a pronounced perifocal brain edema and a central area of necrosis, typically with a hemorrhagic transformation. In these patients, the most important clinical as well as radiological differential diagnoses are brain abscess or glioblastoma.

The incidence of spinal lesions in ADEM has not yet been systematically evaluated. In most patients, spinal lesions occur together with cerebral lesions. However, there are patients with isolated spinal lesions diagnosed as having ADEM (Baum et al. 1994; Kesselring et al. 1990). The lesions seen on the spinal MRI are not specific and do not allow a clear differentiation from other causes of myelitis such as MS or infections (Simon 2000; Singh et al. 1999). Some authors proposed that, compared with MS, the spinal lesions in ADEM extend over more segments of the cord and their diameter exceeds the half of the cord. This speculation is still unproven.

The previously held opinion that all lesions in ADEM appear simultaneously and, therefore, show a uniform contrast enhancement, has not yet been con-

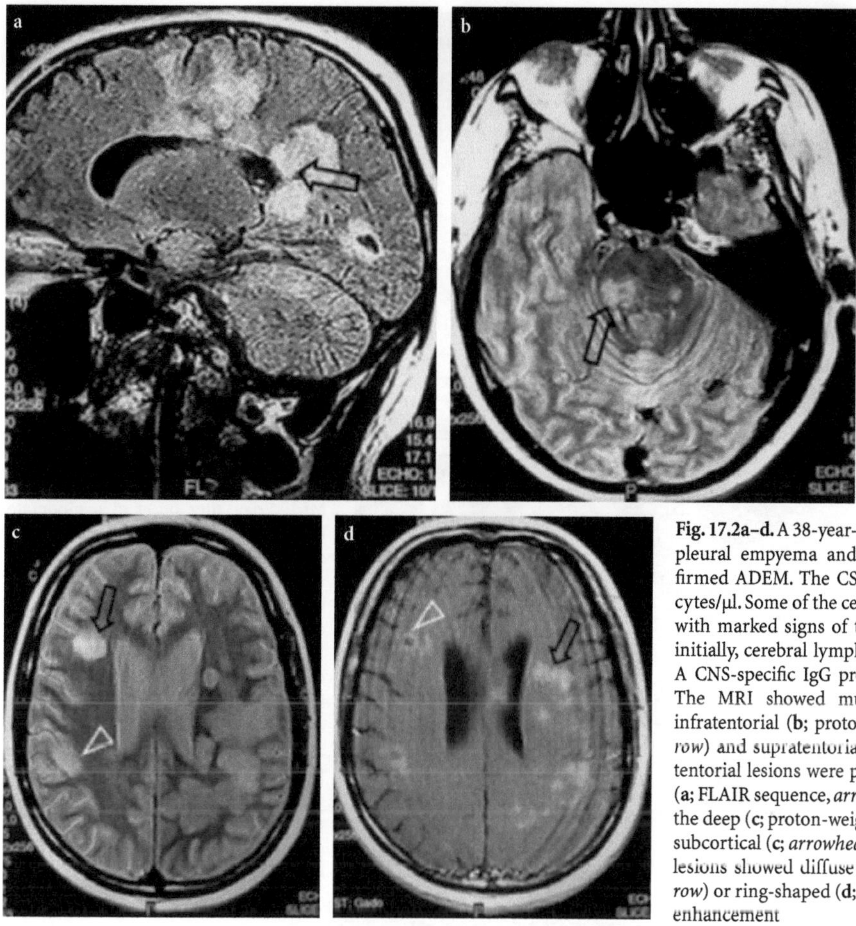

Fig. 17.2a–d. A 38-year-old man with chronic pleural empyema and pathologically confirmed ADEM. The CSF revealed 23 leukocytes/µl. Some of the cells were lymphocytes with marked signs of transformation, thus, initially, cerebral lymphoma was suspected. A CNS-specific IgG production was found. The MRI showed multiple disseminated infratentorial (**b**; proton-weighted MRI, *arrow*) and supratentorial lesions. The supratentorial lesions were partly periventricular (**a**; FLAIR sequence, *arrow*), partly located in the deep (**c**; proton-weighted MRI, *arrow*) or subcortical (**c**; *arrowhead*) white matter. The lesions showed diffuse (**d**; T1-weighted, *arrow*) or ring-shaped (**d**; *arrowhead*) contrast enhancement

firmed in CT studies (Atlas et al. 1986). In the majority of patients with multiple lesions, at one single point of time, non-enhancing as well as enhancing lesions are present (Singh et al. 2000). The ratio between enhancing and non-enhancing lesions could be a useful criteria for the diagnosis of ADEM; however, this has not been evaluated yet. The pattern of contrast enhancement is not specific. Nodular, diffuse nodular, amorphous, gyral, spotty, and ring-like patterns of contrast enhancement have all been described. Recently, the ring-like pattern of contrast enhancement has been suggested as an important criteria for the differentiation between lymphoma (complete ring enhancement) and demyelinating lesions ("open ring sign") (Masdeu et al. 2000). However, in patients with MS and ADEM, the contrast enhancement can also have the appearance of a complete ring (Lim et al. 2003). Therefore, the diagnostic value of the "open ring sign" is questionable.

Systematic short-time interval follow-up examinations have only been undertaken in a few selected patients (Honkaniemi et al. 2001). In most patients under therapy, at least a partial, rapid remission of size and number of the lesions can be seen. In ADEM, the lesions can disappear completely (O'Riordan et al. 1999). However, in some patients, new lesions may appear even after clinical recovery (Honkaniemi et al. 2001). There are also patients with new lesions at follow-up examinations without new clinical symptoms. It is not known whether these patients have a greater risk for the development of a clinically definite MS. Because of the lack of larger prospective, systematic MRI follow-up studies, a statement on the point of time of the appearance of these new lesions cannot be made. It has been repeatedly noted that new lesions predominantly appear within the first 4 weeks after the onset of symptoms.

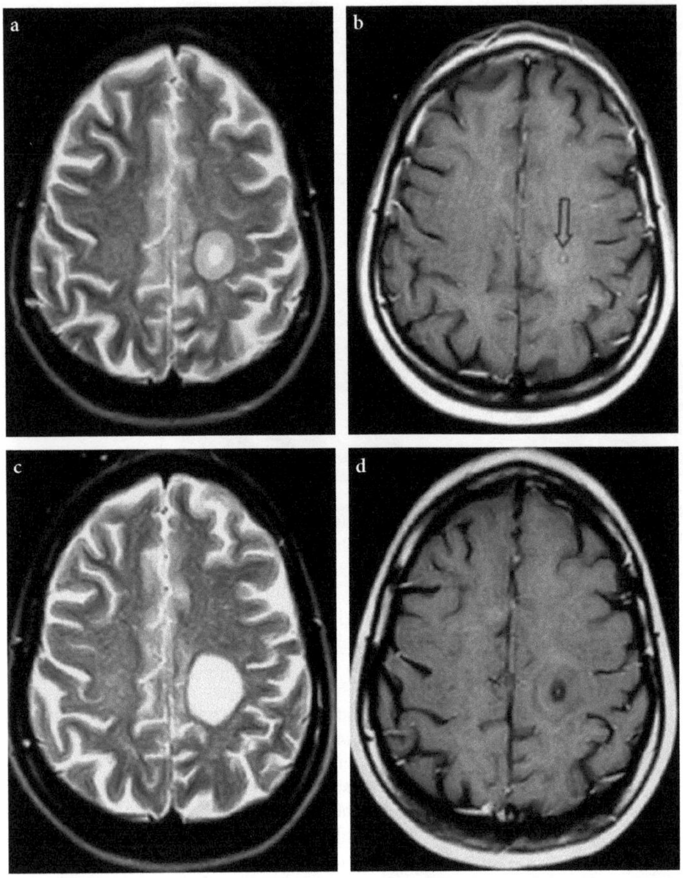

Fig. 17.3a-d. Images from a 47-year-old woman with spontaneous ADEM. Her mother suffers from MS. The initial MRI, 1 day after onset of a moderate hemiparesis, demonstrated a single lesion, which was hyperintense on T2-weighted images (**a**) with a ring-shaped halo, showing contrast enhancement in the center (**b**; T1-weighted, *arrow*). After 10 days of treatment with high-dose corticoid therapy, the size of the lesion increased (**c**), but contrast enhancement disappeared (**d**). The CSF was normal, as well as an extensive search for differential diagnosis. In the subsequent course, the clinical symptoms disappeared completely. Two years later, the clinical as well as the MRI findings remain normal

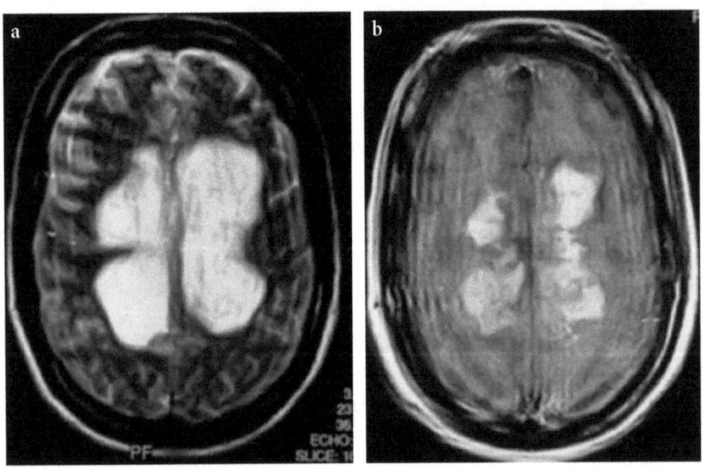

Fig. 17.4a,b. This 40-year-old woman was suffering from a subacute progressive weakness in the right hand. The CSF was normal. The T2-weighted images showed a single lesion with a hypointense margin in the left precentral gyrus (**a**; *arrow*) with massive enhancement, slightly off the center of the lesion (**b**; T1-weighted images, after gadolinium). Initially, a brain abscess or metastasis were suspected. However, systemic signs of infection were absent, and a meticulous search for a tumor was negative. The patient refused a brain biopsy. The symptoms resolved spontaneously. Two years later, the patient is asymptomatic; the MRI reveals a very small residual lesion

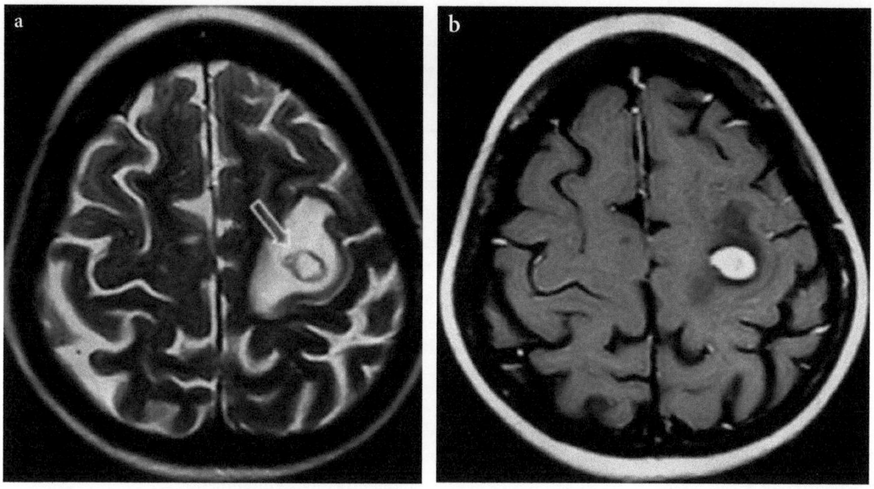

Fig. 17.5a,b. Within a few days of disease onset, this 30-year-old woman developed Broca aphasia, moderate sensorimotor hemiparesis, and slight personality changes. A history of infection or vaccination was absent. The MRI revealed peri- and supraventricular large hypointense lesions on the T2-weighted images (**a**) with diffuse contrast enhancement (**b**; T1-weighted). Initial treatment with methylprednisolone was ineffective. After interval therapy with cyclophosphamide, a remission of the symptoms was achieved. After 2 years, only slight neuropsychological deficits are still present

17.11.3 New MRI Techniques

Because of the above outlined shortcomings of conventional MRI to achieve a definite diagnosis of ADEM, more specific methods that can potentially separate ADEM and other white matter diseases from MS are warranted. Currently, none exists. Hopefully, new MRI methods and the use of novel contrast agents such as small iron oxide particles might improve the diagnostic specificity of MRI in the future.

Using magnetization transfer and diffusion tensor MRI, Inglese et al. (2002) demonstrated in a small, heavily selected sample of patients after ADEM that, in contrast to a control group of patients with MS, the normal appearing brain tissue and spinal cord are spared from the pathological changes. All MR studies were performed after the acute phase of the disease. These results are in agreement with those of a recent MR follow-up study in which diffuse brain atrophy was detectable already within a 3-month period in untreated patients with an active relapsing remitting MS (Hardmeier et al. 2003). These studies offer the perspective that short-term MRI follow-up studies could separate the patients with MS from those with monophasic ADEM in whom an immunomodulatory long-term treatment would be improper.

There are only sparse reports on MR spectroscopy in ADEM. Bizzi et al. (2001) presented a patient with ADEM who showed transient low levels of NAA on the initial MR spectroscopic imaging during the acute phase which normalized after clinical recovery. Unlike other demyelinating diseases, choline levels remained normal in all stages of the disease. Harada et al. (2000) compared the differences in water diffusion and lactate production in two patients with ADEM and acute necrotizing encephalopathy. In these two patients, the diffusion of brain water indicated the reversibility of neuronal impairment whereas the extent of lactate production did not correlate with the prognosis.

17.12 Variant of MS or Distinct Disease Entity?

The differentiation between ADEM and MS remains an unsolved issue. Possibly, in the future, new MRI techniques and innovative serological markers such as the presence of antimyelin antibodies may help to identify those patients with a monophasic disease who do not require preventive treatment already after the first episode of symptoms due to a demyelinating CNS syndrome and who could reliably be assured that they do not need to live with a possibly devastating disease.

Since the time of the first review on ADEM in 1931 (McAlpine 1931), it has, so far unsuccessfully, been repeatedly tried to identify reliable criteria for the differentiation between ADEM and MS. The larger follow-up examinations generally show a varying rate up to one third of all patients initially diagnosed with ADEM who later develop MS (Hynson et al. 2001; Rust et al. 1997; Schwarz et al. 2001). Moreover, terms such as Marburg disease, acute MS, multiphasic ADEM, which were often used as synonyms to ADEM, add to the confusion. Table 17.4 summarizes frequently assumed criteria to distinguish the two diseases. However, it has to be emphasized that none of these unspecific criteria are evidence-based. Thus, these criteria may only provide hints toward the correct diagnosis. During or immediately after the first episode of a demyelinating CNS disease, a definite diagnosis of ADEM is probably not possible. So far, the differentiation between ADEM or the first symptom of an MS can only be ascertained after a longer follow-up.

Table 17.4. Empiric criteria for the differentiation between ADEM and MS. These points should be acknowledged as relative criteria only. Exceptions are common. There are no well-established criteria for the diagnosis of ADEM vs. MS. Specificity and sensitivity of none of these points have been evaluated in a prospective study

	ADEM	MS
Age	Highest incidence in children	Onset in childhood possible, but uncommon
Symptoms	Various neurological symptoms May be oligo- or asymptomatic Rapid onset Bilateral optic neuritis Transverse myelitis In children: fever, meningism, stupor	Frequently oligosymptomatic Unilateral optic neuritis Partial transverse myelitis
History	Preceding infection or immunization	Preceding infection possible, but infrequent
CSF	May be normal; often slight to moderate lymphocytic pleocytosis Oligoclonal IgG synthesis usually absent	Slight to moderate lymphocytic pleocytosis Oligoclonal IgG synthesis mostly detectable
Course	Acute onset Monophasic Favorable long-term prognosis	Relapsing or progressive Long-term prognosis dubious
MRI	Multiple, diffuse, symmetrically distributed lesions in the supra- and infratentorial white matter Typically subcortical Involvement of the basal ganglia possible No new lesions or atrophy during the long-term follow-up	Often unilateral, asymmetric lesions Typically periventricular Involvement of the basal ganglia rare New lesions and atrophy during the long-term follow-up

References

Anlar B, Basaran C, Kose G et al (2003) Acute disseminated encephalomyelitis in children: outcome and prognosis. Neuropediatrics 34:194-199

Antel JP, Owens T (1999) Immune regulation and CNS autoimmune disease. J Neuroimmunol 100:181-189

Atlas SW, Grossman RI, Goldberg HI et al (1986) MR diagnosis of acute disseminated encephalomyelitis. J Comput Assist Tomogr 10:798-801

Baum PA, Barkovich AJ, Koch TK et al (1994) Deep gray matter involvement in children with acute disseminated encephalomyelitis. AJNR Am J Neuroradiol 15:1275-1283

Berger T, Rubner P, Schautzer F et al (2003) Antimyelin antibodies as a predictor of clinically definite multiple sclerosis after a first demyelinating event. N Engl J Med 349:139-145

Bizzi A, Ulug AM, Crawford TO et al (2001) Quantitative proton MR spectroscopic imaging in acute disseminated encephalomyelitis. AJNR Am J Neuroradiol 22:1125-1130

Comi G, Filippi M, Barkhof F et al (2001) Effect of early interferon treatment on conversion to definite multiple sclerosis: a randomised study. Lancet 357:1576-1582

Dale RC, de Sousa C, Chong WK et al (2000) Acute disseminated encephalomyelitis, multiphasic disseminated encephalomyelitis and multiple sclerosis in children. Brain 123:2407-2422

Gupte G, Stonehouse M, Wassmer E et al (2003) Acute disseminated encephalomyelitis: a review of 18 cases in childhood. J Paediatr Child Health 39:336-342

Hahn CD, Miles BS, MacGregor DL et al (2003) Neurocognitive outcome after acute disseminated encephalomyelitis. Pediatr Neurol 29:117-123

Happe S, Husstedt IW (2000) Successful treatment of acute encephalomyelitis associated with common variable immunodeficiency syndrome (CVID): case report and review of the literature. J Neurol 247:562-565

Harada M, Hisaoka S, Mori K et al (2000) Differences in water diffusion and lactate production in two different types of postinfectious encephalopathy. J Magn Reson Imaging 11:559-563

Hardmeier M, Wagenpfeil S, Freitag P et al (2003) Atrophy is detectable within a 3-month period in untreated patients with active relapsing remitting multiple sclerosis. Arch Neurol 60:1736-1739
Hart MN, Earle KM (1975) Haemorrhagic and perivenous encephalitis: a clinical-pathological review of 38 cases. J Neurol Neurosurg Psychiatry 38:585-591
Höllinger P, Sturzenegger M, Mathis J et al (2002) Acute disseminated encephalomyelitis in adults: a reappraisal of clinical, CSF, EEG, and MRI findings. J Neurol 249:320-329
Honkaniemi J, Dastidar P, Kahara V, Haapasalo H (2001) Delayed MR imaging changes in acute disseminated encephalomyelitis. AJNR Am J Neuroradiol 22:1117-1124
Hurst AE (1941) Acute haemorhagic leucoencephalitis: a previously undefined entitiy. Med J Aust 1:1-6
Hynson JL, Kornberg AJ, Coleman LT et al (2001) Clinical and neuroradiologic features of acute disseminated encephalomyelitis in children. Neurology 56:1308-1312.
Idrissova Zh R, Boldyreva MN, Dekonenko EP et al (2003) Acute disseminated encephalomyelitis in children: clinical features and HLA-DR linkage. Eur J Neurol 10:537-546
Inglese M, Salvi F, Iannucci G et al (2002) Magnetization transfer and diffusion tensor MR imaging of acute disseminated encephalomyelitis. AJNR Am J Neuroradiol 23:267-272
Jacobs LD, Beck RW, Simon JH et al (2000) Intramuscular interferon beta-1a therapy initiated during a first demyelinating event in multiple sclerosis. CHAMPS Study Group. N Engl J Med 343:898-904
Jorens PG, VanderBorght A, Ceulemans B et al (2000) Encephalomyelitis-associated antimyelin autoreactivity induced by streptococcal exotoxins. Neurology 54:1433-1441
Kepes JJ (1993) Large focal tumor-like demyelinating lesions of the brain: intermediate entity between multiple sclerosis and acute disseminated encephalomyelitis? A study of 31 patients. Ann Neurol 33:18-27
Kesselring J, Miller DH, Robb SA et al (1990) Acute disseminated encephalomyelitis. MRI findings and the distinction from multiple sclerosis. Brain 113:291-302
Lim KE, Hsu YY, Hsu WC et al (2003) Multiple complete ring-shaped enhanced MRI lesions in acute disseminated encephalomyelitis. Clin Imaging 27:281-284
Lucchinetti C, Bruck W, Parisi J et al (2000) Heterogeneity of multiple sclerosis lesions: implications for the pathogenesis of demyelination. Ann Neurol 47:707-717
Lukes SA, Norman D (1983) Computed tomography in acute disseminated encephalomyelitis. Ann Neurol 13:567-572
Martino G, Adorini L, Rieckmann P et al (2002) Inflammation in multiple sclerosis: the good, the bad, and the complex. Lancet Neurol 1:499-509
Masdeu JC, Quinto C, Tenner M et al (2000) Open-ring imaging sign. Neurology 54:1427-1433
McAlpine D (1931) Acute disseminated encephalomyelitis. Lancet 1:846-852
McDonald WI, Compston A, Edan G et al (2001) Recommended diagnostic criteria for multiple sclerosis: guidelines from the International Panel on the diagnosis of multiple sclerosis. Ann Neurol 50:121-127
Miller HG (1953) Acute disseminated encephalomyelitis treated with A.C.T.H. Brit Med J:177-183
Miller HG, Stanton JB, Gibbons JL (1956) Para-infectious encephalomyelitis and related symptoms. J Med 25:427-505
Modi G, Mochan A, Modi M et al (2001) Demyelinating disorder of the central nervous system occurring in black South Africans. J Neurol Neurosurg Psychiatry 70:500-505
Murthy JM, Yangala R, Meena AK et al (1999) Clinical, electrophysiological and magnetic resonance imaging study of acute disseminated encephalomyelitis. J Assoc Physicians India 47:280-283
Murthy SN, Faden HS, Cohen ME et al (2002) Acute disseminated encephalomyelitis in children. Pediatrics 110:e21
Nadkarni N, Lisak RP (1993) Guillain-Barré syndrome (GBS) with bilateral optic neuritis and central white matter disease. Neurology 43:842-843
Nasr JT, Andriola MR, Coyle PK (2000) ADEM: literature review and case report of acute psychosis presentation. Pediatr Neurol 22:8-18
Nishikawa M, Ichiyama T, Hayashi T et al (1999) Intravenous immunoglobulin therapy in acute disseminated encephalomyelitis. Pediatr Neurol 21:583-586
O'Riordan JI, Gomez-Anson B, Moseley IF et al (1999) Long term MRI follow-up of patients with post infectious encephalomyelitis: evidence for a monophasic disease. J Neurol Sci 167:132-136
Pohl-Koppe A, Burchett SK, Thiele EA et al (1998) Myelin basic protein reactive Th2 T cells are found in acute disseminated encephalomyelitis. J Neuroimmunol 91:19-27
Poser CM (1989) Magnetic resonance imaging in asymptomatic disseminated vasculomyelinopathy. J Neurol Sci 94:69-77
Poser CM, Paty DW, Scheinberg L et al (1983) New diagnostic criteria for multiple sclerosis: guidelines for research protocols. Ann Neurol 13:227-231
Reik L (1980) Disseminated vasculomyelinopathy: An immune complex disease. Ann Neurol 7:291-296
Reis F, Kobayashi E, Maciel EP et al (1999) Ressonancia magnética e características clínicas em adultos com doencas desmielinizantes monofásicas. Encefalomielite aguda disseminada ou uma variante da esclerose múltipla? Arq Neuropsiquiatr 57:853-859
Rivers TM, Sprunt DH, Berry GP (1933) Observations on attempts to produce acute disseminated encephalomyelitis in monkeys. J Exp Med 58:39-53
Rust RS, Dodson W, Prensky A et al (1997) Classification and outcome of acute disseminated encephalomyelitis. Ann Neurol 42:491
Schwarz S, Knauth M, Schwab S et al (2000) Acute disseminated encephalomyelitis after parenteral therapy with herbal extracts: a report of two cases. J Neurol Neurosurg Psychiatry 69:516-518
Schwarz S, Mohr A, Knauth M et al (2001) Acute disseminated encephalomyelitis: a follow-up study of 40 adult patients. Neurology 56:1313-1318
Schwarz S, Zoubaa S, Knauth M et al (2002) Intravascular lymphomatosis presenting with a conus medullaris syndrome mimicking disseminated encephalomyelitis. Neuro-Oncology 4:187-191
Simon JH (2000) The contribution of spinal cord MRI to the diagnosis and differential diagnosis of multiple sclerosis. J Neurol Sci 172:S32-S35
Singh S, Alexander M, Korah IP (1999) Acute disseminated encephalomyelitis: MR imaging features. AJR 173:1101-1107
Storch MK, Stefferl A, Brehm U et al (1998) Autoimmunity to myelin oligodendrocyte glycoprotein in rats mimics the spectrum of multiple sclerosis pathology. Brain Pathol 8:681-694

Stratton KR, Howe CJ, Johnston RB (1994) Adverse events associated with childhood vaccines. Washington, National Academy Press

Tachovsky TG, Lisak RP, Koprowski H (1976) Circulating immune complexes in multiple sclerosis and other neurological diseases. Lancet 2:997-999

Takata T, Hirakawa M, Sakurai M et al (1999) Fulminant form of acute disseminated encephalomyelitis: successful treatment with hypothermia. J Neurol Sci 165:94-97

Tenembaum S, Chamoles N, Fejerman N (2002) Acute disseminated encephalomyelitis: a long-term follow-up study of 84 pediatric patients. Neurology 59:1224-1231

Wang PN, Fuh JL, Liu HC et al (1996) Acute disseminated encephalomyelitis in middle-aged or elderly patients. Eur Neurol 36:219-223

Wildemann B, Jansen O, Haas J et al (2001) Rapid distinction of acute demyelinating disorders and central nervous system lymphoma by molecular analysis of cerebrospinal fluid cells. J Neurol 248:127-130

18 Demyelinating Diseases of the Spinal Cord

Roland Bammer, Franz Fazekas, and Siegrid Strasser-Fuchs

CONTENTS

18.1 Introduction

Magnetic resonance imaging (MRI) has opened a new window on the visualization of abnormalities associated with white matter diseases in the brain. The contribution of MRI with regard to delineating such disorders in the spinal cord is even more impressive considering the fact that MRI has been the first technique to allow for a direct and detailed in vivo evaluation of morphological abnormalities of the spinal cord at all. Of course, MRI of the spinal cord still poses technical difficulties and may thus be more variable in quality than MRI of the brain. Not all pulse sequences which contribute to our understanding of cerebral disorders can easily and equally be applied to this region of the body. The small size of the cord, its position within the dural sac surrounded by pulsating cerebrospinal fluid (CSF), and the motion of the body and its organs during the examination are all factors that may degrade image quality and have to be considered in the examination protocol. Also signal intensities and resulting contrasts between tissue classes generated by conventional sequences are somewhat different from the brain due to the specific texture of the cord. This is also relevant for the detection of lesions within the cord and necessitates the choice of appropriate sequences. A recent review addressed these technical aspects of spinal cord imaging especially with regard to multiple sclerosis (MS) as the most frequent demyelinating disease of the spinal cord (Lycklama et al. 2003).

Applying these techniques, characteristic MRI findings can be elicited for a distinction between the various demyelinating disorders of the cord and their separation from other diseases which may also affect the spinal cord (Fazekas and Kapeller 1999; Bot et al. 2002). Herein we concentrate especially on the patterns which are typically seen with the different so-called idiopathic inflammatory demyelinating disorders (Weinshenker and Miller 1998). Despite obvious specifics, it needs to be emphasized that the interpretation of MRI abnormalities must always take place in the context of clinical findings and, where necessary, together with other biological (e.g. CSF) and electrophysiologic investigations (Transverse Myelitis Consortium Working Group 1999). In addition to primarily diagnosis-related issues, we also review current possibilities for a quantitation of spinal cord damage from demyelinating diseases especially in relation to function, and we speculate on future prospects for the evaluation of this important part of the central nervous system by MRI.

18.2 Multiple Sclerosis

Multiple sclerosis most commonly causes distinct lesions within the spinal cord (Fazekas et al. 1999; Bot et al. 2004). These lesions typically occupy less than half of the cross-sectional area of the cord and affect both white and grey matter (Tartaglino et al.1995; Thielen and Miller 1996).

R. Bammer, PhD
Lucas MRS/I Center, Department of Radiology, Stanford, California, USA
F. Fazekas, MD
Department of Neuroradiology, Medical University Graz, Auenbruggerplatz 22, 8036 Graz, Austria
S. Strasser-Fuchs, MD
Department of Neurology, Medical University Graz, Auenbruggerplatz 22, 8036 Graz, Austria

With advancing disease focal MS lesions may merge to larger areas of high signal intensity (Fig. 18.4). A small proportion of MS patients also show only diffuse abnormalities of the spinal cord (Lycklama et al. 1997; Bot et al. 2004). These abnormalities consist mostly of a subtle increase of signal intensity on proton-density-weighted images and have been observed especially in patients with high disability and a primary progressive course of the disease (Lycklama et al. 1998). MRI–histopathological correlations have shown that both diffuse and focal signal hyperintensities in the spinal cord correspond primarily to demyelination (Nijeholt et al. 2001). Axonal damage, however, appears to occur largely independent of intramedullary T2-hyperintensities (Bergers et al. 2002a). This may also explain why a large proportion of spinal cord lesions obviously remain asymptomatic and can at least partly account for reportedly disappointing correlations between clinical symptoms and imaging findings on conventional MRI of the spinal cord (Kidd et al. 1993; Lycklama et al. 1998; O'Riordan et al. 1998; Brex et al. 1999).

Some investigators have found a prevalence of up to 30-40% of spinal cord lesions in patients with a clinically isolated syndrome suggestive of MS, i.e. at the first clinical presentation of the disease, and even in those presenting with optic neuritis (O'Riordan et al. 1998; Brex et al. 1999). In patients with established MS, the prevalence of intramedullary lesions increases to 80% and higher (Bot et al. 2004). Including diffuse cord changes, probably more than 90% of MS patients have some form of spinal involvement at some point in their disease (Lycklama et al. 1998).

In later stages of MS and with advanced disability spinal cord atrophy becomes readily apparent as well. Volume changes of the spinal cord, although occurring much earlier, can otherwise be reliably established only by the use of exact measurement techniques as described below. Distinct focal areas of cord atrophy are rarely seen except following recovery from very large MS lesions. Different from the brain, spinal cord lesions also do not evolve into so-called black holes, i.e. cystic lesions within the cord are not seen in typical MS. It is also common for the signal hyperintensity of spinal cord MS lesions to decrease over time, and together with the shrinkage of the lesion, causes them to disappear, or at least to

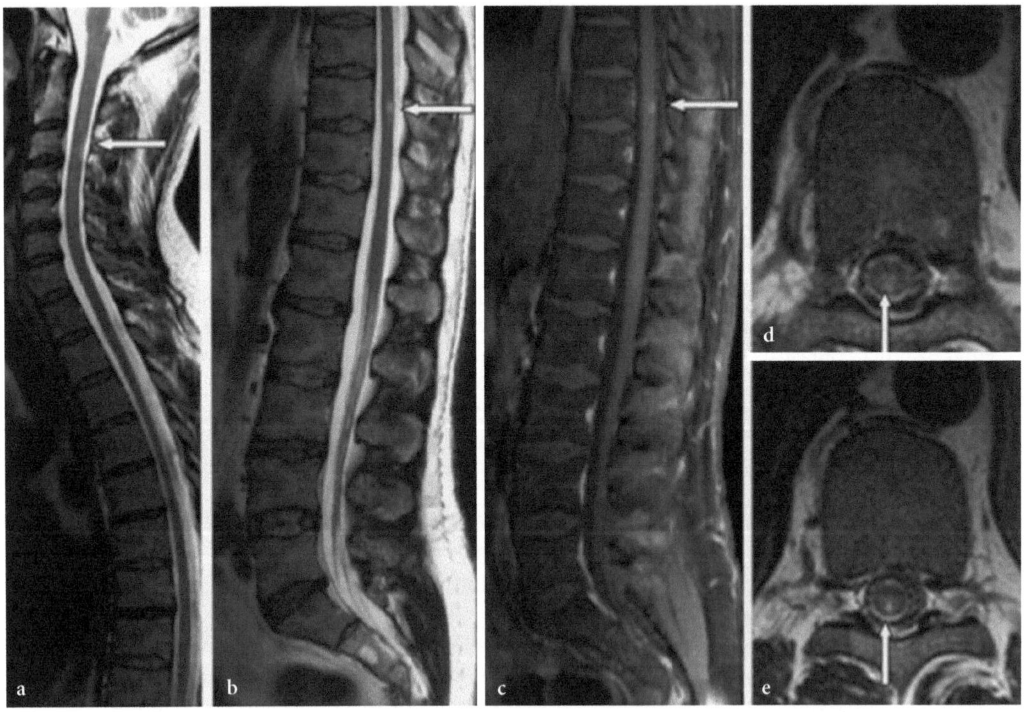

Fig. 18.1a–e. Patient with a second episode of spinal cord symptoms. A sensory level and gait ataxia correspond to an acute lesion at T10 which shows minimal swelling on T2 (**b**) and faint contrast enhancement (**c**). The lesion affects primarily the centre of the cord and the posterior tracts in a wedge-shaped manner (**d,e**). An old lesion at C3/C4 is barely seen (**a**)

Fig. 18.2a–c. Patient with relapsing–remitting multiple sclerosis (MS). Multiple hyperintense intramedullary lesions without mass effect on T2-weighted fast-spin-echo images (**a,b**). One of the lesions shows contrast enhancement (**c**)

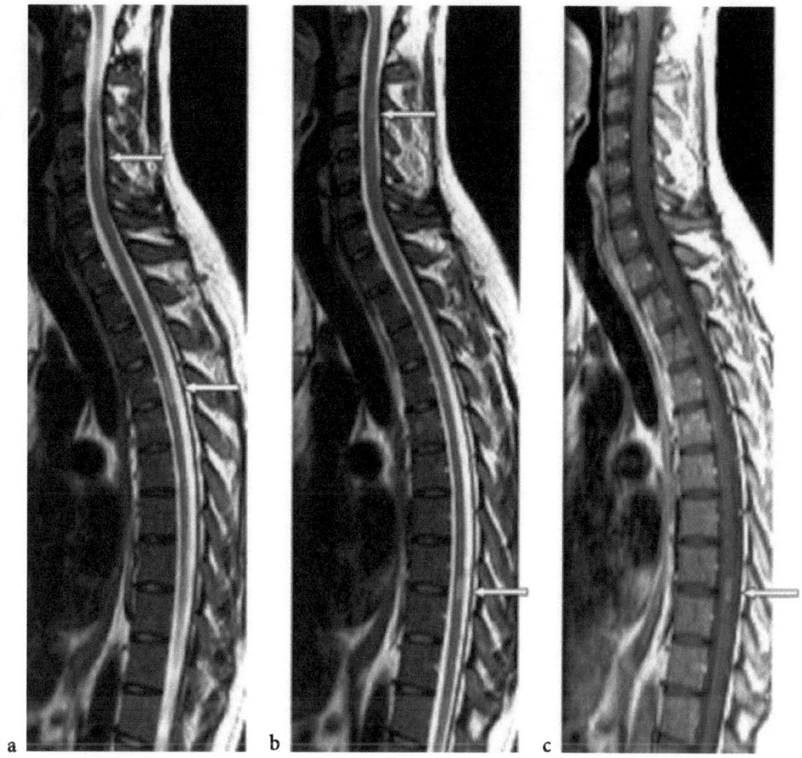

Fig. 18.3a–d. Unusually large intramedullary lesion with marked oedema (**a**) and contrast enhancement (**c,d**) in a patient who subsequently developed clinically definite MS

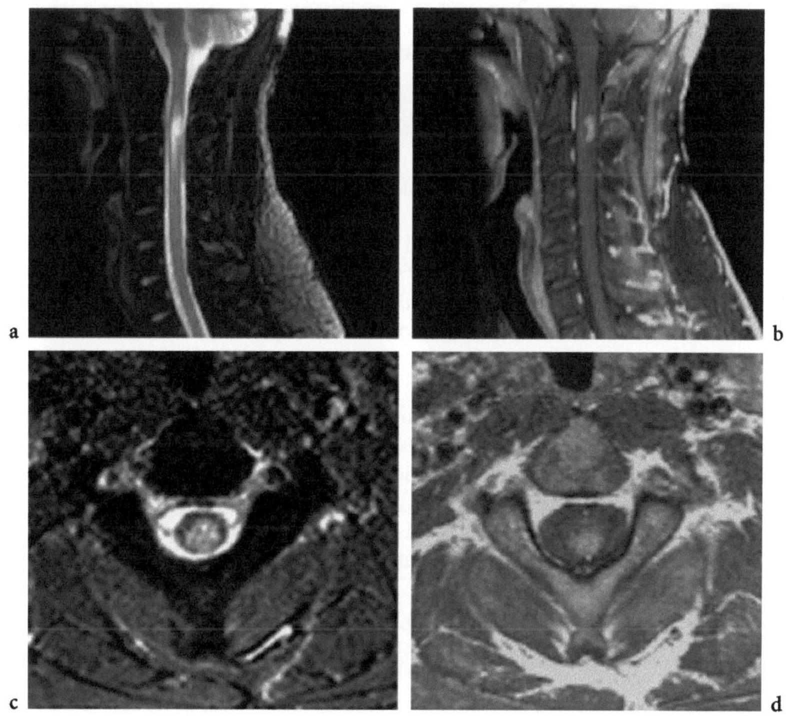

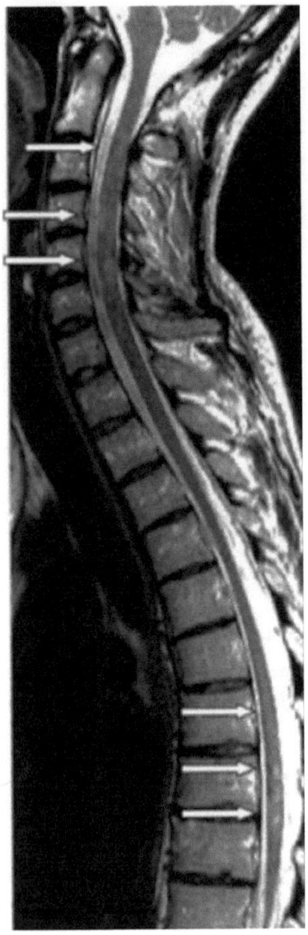

Fig. 18.4 Confluence of intramedullary lesions in a patient with secondary progressive MS

become very difficult to detect on routine follow-up scanning (Fig. 18.2).

Formal integration of spinal cord MRI findings in MS into current diagnostic criteria may still be viewed as suboptimal (McDonald et al. 2001; Bot et al. 2004; Miller et al. 2004). Earlier limitations regarding MRI examinations of the spinal cord at a high resolution with reproducibly good quality and a paucity of data regarding the diagnostic and prognostic value of the demonstration of MS lesions in the cord made the International Panel simply state that "one spinal cord lesion can be substituted for one brain lesion" (McDonald et al. 2001). Whether this substitution simply is additive to the number of total brain lesions or could also serve to fulfil the requirement of an infratentorial lesion, as defined by Barkhof's criteria, remains unclear. Similarly, the proposed diagnostic criteria for primary progressive MS have remained somewhat vague (Thompson et al. 2000; McDonald et al. 2001) but recognise the higher specificity of spinal cord lesions compared with brain lesions, as they do not occur with ageing per se (Thorpe et al. 1993). In addition to previous recommendations on the role of spinal cord MRI in the algorithm for MS diagnosis, which focussed primarily on the need to rule out other disorders (Fazekas et al. 1999), recent data also confirm a higher probability to prove disease dissemination in space by such examination. In a cohort of 104 patients with newly diagnosed MS, Bot et al. (2004) found that substitution of one spinal cord lesion for one brain lesion increased the sensitivity of the McDonald's dissemination in space criteria from 66 to 85%, and it reached 94% when allowing for an unlimited substitution of brain lesions by spinal cord lesions. In a more selective manner such contribution has already been reported previously for patients with suspected MS, but no or only very few cerebral lesions (Thorpe et al. 1996b). Whether evidence for spinal cord lesions also conveys some prognostic information is still a matter of debate (Lycklama et al. 2003).

18.2.1 Acute Disseminated Encephalomyelitis

By definition, acute disseminated encephalomyelitis (ADEM) is a monophasic demyelinating disorder which usually follows a viral infection (Wingerchuk 2003) or vaccination. Children are more frequently affected than adults. The MRI findings in the brain consist of multiple, frequently large lesions with perifocal oedema and contrast enhancement as evidence of their acute nature. Lesions can involve the cerebral white matter as well as the basal ganglia, the brain-stem and cerebellum and, according to their appearance and distribution, have been categorized into different patterns including a haemorrhagic variant (acute haemorrhagic encephalomyelitis; Tenenbaum et al. 2002). As part of the central nervous system, the spinal cord can also be involved. In comparison with MS, ADEM lesions of the spinal cord are typically larger and more oedematous (Fig. 18.5).The clinical presentation following a potentially triggering event and the absence of oligoclonal bands should point towards such a diagnosis. A corresponding MRI of the brain with multiple, exclusively acute-appearing lesions is also very suggestive of ADEM (Fig. 18.5).The notion that normal-appearing brain white matter of ADEM patients is truly unaffected (Inglese et al. 2002), while in contrast more severe damage is found in the basal gan-

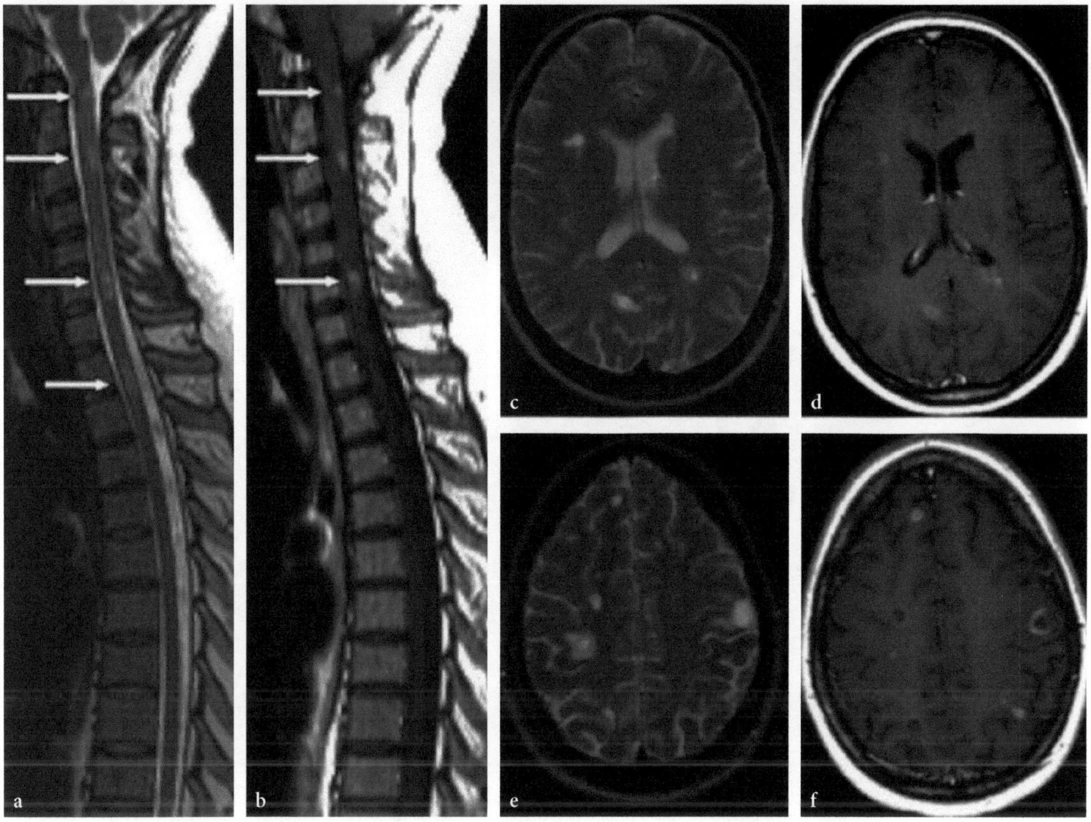

Fig. 18.5a–f. Patient presenting with rapidly progressing multifocal neurological symptoms shortly after an upper respiratory tract infection. Multiple hyperintense intramedullary lesions were seen on T2-weighted scans of the spinal cord (**a**) and tended to markedly enhance following the application of Gd-DTPA (**b**). A similar but more diverse lesion pattern was also seen on MRI of the brain (**c,d** T2-weighted scans; **e,f** corresponding contrast-enhanced scans). The patient fully recovered and for the next years experienced no further bouts of disease, supporting the diagnosis of acute disseminated encephalomyelitis

glia (Holtmannspötter et al. 2003), may also help to differentiate ADEM from MS. In individual cases, however, this may still be difficult, at least in the early stages (Dale et al. 2000; Tenenbaum et al. 2002). Contrast enhancement needs not to occur absolutely simultaneously in all lesions caused by ADEM. At the same time, contrast enhancement of both lesions in the brain and spinal cord is not uncommon for MS, as mentioned previously (Thorpe et al. 1996a). With more advanced MS, however, there is almost always a larger proportion of non-enhancing lesions, with some appearing as T1 hypointensities or so-called black holes, that strongly argue against ADEM. Nevertheless, in many instances clinical and imaging follow-up is necessary to make a final diagnosis from the absence of further disease activity, although it is known that a second bout of ADEM may also occur (Tenenbaum et al. 2002).

18.2.2 Neuromyelitis Optica

Neuromyelitis optica (NMO), or Devic's syndrome, is a severe form of idiopathic inflammatory demyelinating disease and is increasingly considered as a separate entity (Weinshenker 2003). The specific features include its topographic restriction to the optic nerve and spinal cord, and a greater attack severity than MS (Wingerchuk et al. 1999). This is also reflected by much more extensive spinal cord lesions on MRI than those seen in MS (Fig. 18.6). These lesions usually involve large segments of the cord with diffuse swelling and extensive contrast enhancement. The necrotising character of this type of demyelination is also evidenced in the post-acute phase by the frequent occurrence of cystic areas within the cord together with severe focal or diffuse atrophy as

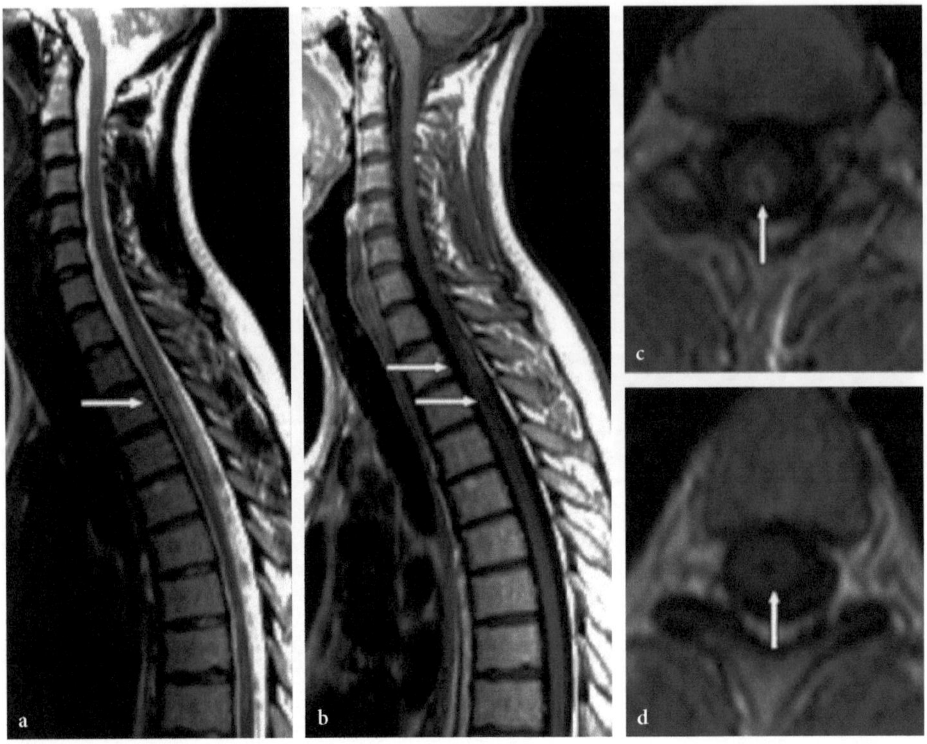

Fig. 18.6a–d. A 25-year-old patient with recurrent spastic paraparesis and complete visual loss of the left eye. The mid-thoracic spinal cord is diffusely swollen and hyperintense (**a**). Slight enhancement after application of contrast material surrounding and above intramedullary areas with signal isointense to cerebrospinal fluid consistent with necrotising inflammation (**b–d**). Magnetic resonance imaging of the brain was normal and there was no evidence of oligoclonal bands

indicators of extensive tissue destruction (Figs. 18.6, 18.7).

In terms of disease evolution, it is important to note that NMO can have both a monophasic and a relapsing course. In a review of 70 patients with NMO at the Mayo Clinic, patients with a monophasic course usually presented with rapidly sequential index events with moderate recovery. Two thirds of patients, however, presented with an extended interval between index events followed within 3 years by clusters of severe relapses isolated to the optic nerves and spinal cord. In these patients severe disability developed in a stepwise manner; thus, a prolonged interval between damage to the spinal cord and optic nerves does not rule against a diagnosis of NMO (Wingerchuk et al. 1999).

Absence of brain MRI changes is a hallmark finding of NMO and part of the diagnostic criteria for this disorder [30]. Unaffected brain white matter has also been shown in one study using magnetisation transfer (Filippi et al. 1999). Non-specific abnormalities, however, do not preclude a diagnosis of NMO.

18.3 Transverse Myelitis

Acute transverse myelitis can be caused by a number of bacterial, viral, fungal or parasitic infections, by connective tissue diseases, such as sarcoidosis, Behçet's disease, Sjögren's syndrome, systemic lupus erythematosus, antiphospholipid syndrome, and mixed connective tissue disease, and can be the presenting feature of NMO and less likely also of MS (Transverse Myelitis Consortium Working Group 2002). In rare cases no aetiology can be defined, and it may therefore be suggested to group such disorders under the umbrella of the idiopathic inflammatory demyelinating disorders as well. Some

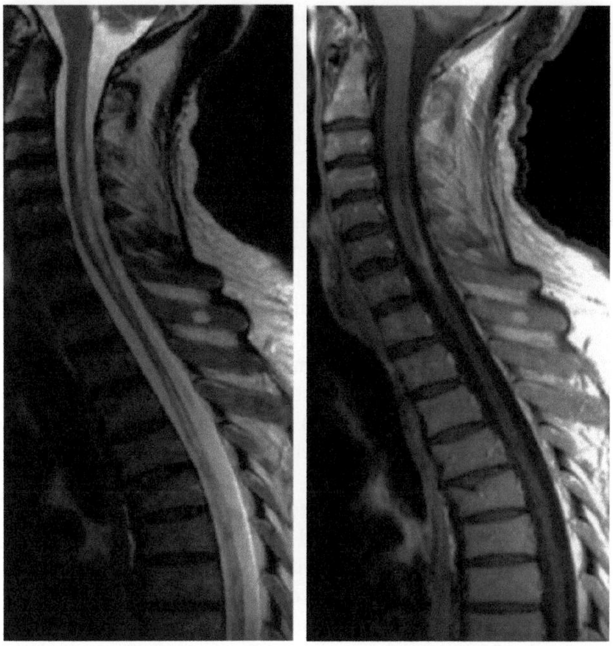

Fig. 18.7 Patient with recurrent transverse myelitis. Note the swelling and enhancement of the cervical portion of the spinal cord as evidence of acute inflammation in comparison with the atrophic thoracic portion with diffuse signal abnormality from previous inflammation

reports and our own experience suggest a similarity of spinal cord abnormalities with those observed in NMO. This has been especially true for patients with relapsing acute transverse myelitis (Fig. 7; T. Seifert et al., submitted). Support for this hypothesis comes from the fact that some of the patients with relapsing transverse myelitis subsequently also developed optic neuritis but otherwise showed a normal or at least non-specific MRI of the brain (Katz and Ropper 2000). Marked inflammatory CSF changes and the absence of oligoclonal bands are also more commonly found in this type of spinal cord disorder than with MS (Transverse Myelitis Consortium Working Group 2002).

18.3.1 MRI Evaluation of Spinal Cord Damage in Relation to Function

Spinal cord lesions do correlate with spinal cord symptoms as shown in cross-sectional and follow-up studies (Thorpe et al. 1996a; Lycklama et al. 1998); however, the relationship between a patient's symptoms and spinal cord findings frequently remains limited. The reasons for this are manifold. As in the brain, conventional MRI cannot serve to grade the severity of axonal destruction within lesions or display other factors which may impact on functioning also at non-morphological levels (Caramia et al. 2004). In addition, it is even more difficult to quantify the total extent of damage in the spinal cord than in the brain. This has also been seen in histopathological comparisons where the actual spinal cord damage was frequently much more pronounced than would have been expected from imaging alone (Bergers et al. 2002b). Finally, quantification of tissue loss, i.e. of spinal cord atrophy, is also not satisfactory by visual analysis. For this reason it has been attempted to use various MRI metrics for the global description of spinal cord damage from demyelinating diseases, especially in MS.

Much work has been done on the measurement and longitudinal follow-up of spinal cord atrophy (Zivadinov and Bakshi 2004). Measuring the cross-sectional size of the spinal cord, however, always has to be performed at the exactly same cervical level, and various technical problems may cause significant variance in the measurements. With the appropriate techniques, however, longitudinal follow-up can show small but statistically significant decreases in spinal cord area (Stevenson et al. 1998) and a relatively strong relationship between degree of spinal cord atrophy and EDSS values has been reported (Losseff et al. 1996). Especially in primary progressive MS, atrophy measurements may be more important in relation to function than those of lesion volumes (Ukkonenen et al. 2003).

In the brain, magnetisation transfer imaging (MTI) has shown the capability of detecting white matter abnormalities not accessible with conventional MRI (Filippi 2003). It was therefore speculated that this technique should also allow delineation of diffuse changes of the spinal cord from and independent of focal abnormalities. First studies in relatively small cohorts of patients confirmed that the cervical cord of MS patients had lower MTR values than those of controls (Inglese et al. 2002). Histogram analyses, however, showed that compared with control subjects patients with relapsing, -remitting MS had similar cervical cord MTR histogram-derived measures, whereas those with primary progressive and secondary progressive MS had abnormal MTR histograms (Filippi et al. 2000). More importantly, the cervical cord MTR histogram parameters were independent predictors of loco-motor disability. A further study confirmed that MTR metrics do not differ between primary and secondary progressive MS, and they also appear to be independent of the cerebral lesion load (Rovaris et al. 2000, 2001).

With technical advances it has also become possible to apply diffusion-weighted MRI (DWI) to the spinal cord (Bammer et al. 2002; Clark and Werring 2002). A preliminary study assessed water diffusion in seven cord lesions of three MS patients with loco-motor disability and found increased diffusivity compared with healthy volunteers (Weeler-Kingshott et al. 2002); however, for the individual patient no useful contribution can yet be expected from DWI, and especially in the early phase of MS only very subtle changes appear detectable (Mezzapesa et al. 2004). The development of techniques which allow to incorporate tractography into spinal cord MRI may be an important next step. Currently, DWI of the spinal cord still faces significant technical challenges that can limit the reproducibility of quantitative measurements. Specifically, motion of the patient and the cord itself, and the inhomogeneous magnetic environment within and around the spinal column, can cause deleterious artefacts.

Magnetization transfer imaging and DWI promise to provide complementary biophysical information about microstructural changes of the spinal cord. While MT is more targeted to the chemical–structural environment of the myelin sheath, DWI probes for potential changes in the micro-environment that may impair or facilitate the mobility of protons. In combination or individually these two biophysical mechanisms can help to provide insight and improve contrast beyond conventional MRI methods.

Recent technological developments in MR hardware, especially improved radio-frequency (RF) coils and higher field strengths, have furthered MRI's capability to image the spinal cord at highest spatial resolution. At numerous centres, neuroimaging is currently migrating from 1.5 to 3 T or even higher, trying to capitalize on the increased signal strength afforded by the stronger magnetic field. Here, especially for the spinal cord, the excessive signal-to-noise ratio can be invested in greatly improved spatial resolution. In combination with dedicated spine arrays, this strategy allows imaging of the entire spinal cord at once and at a higher spatial resolution, which should definitely impact diagnostic sensitivity and also specificity.

One issue associated with higher field strength that has to be kept in mind is the increased energy deposition in the patient's body, especially when transmitting with the large-body-volume coil. This can have major implications for pulse sequences with relatively high RF duty cycles, such as MT sequences. Fortunately, if only the spine needs to be imaged, its unique location in the body allows for the use of transmit/receive coils which demonstrate much fewer problems with energy deposition. Thus far, only little has been reported on the overall benefits of using higher magnetic fields in demyelinating diseases, especially when focused on the spinal cord. One should also be aware that the T1 relaxation times of semi-solid tissues changes with field strength, while CSF remains almost unchanged; therefore, certain adaptations in pulse sequence are mandatory to maintain contrast properties, and the altered relaxation properties should be kept in mind when interpreting/comparing studies performed at different field strengths.

18.4 Conclusion

Magnetic resonance imaging of the spinal cord provides characteristic patterns of abnormalities in different demyelinating diseases. It has to be recognised, however, that other aetiologies may mimic these abnormalities and have to be considered in the differential diagnosis as described elsewhere (Fazekas and Kapeller 1999; Bot et al. 2002). On the other hand, the recognition of spinal cord abnormalities as a consequence of demyelinating diseases makes an important contribution to their diagnosis. Future developments also promise to generate insights beyond these diagnostic contributions in terms of information relevant for function and repair.

References

Bammer R, Augustin M, Prokesch RW et al (2002) Diffusion-weighted imaging of the spinal cord: interleaved echo-planar imaging is superior to fast spin-echo. J Magn Reson Imaging 15:364–373

Bergers E, Bot JC, de Groot CJ et al (2002a) Axonal damage in the spinal cord of MS patients occurs largely independent of T2 MRI lesions. Neurology 59:1766–1771

Bergers E, Bot JC, van der Valk P et al (2002b) Diffuse signal abnormalities in the spinal cord in multiple sclerosis: direct postmortem in situ magnetic resonance imaging correlated with in vitro high-resolution magnetic resonance imaging and histopathology. Ann Neurol 51:652–656

Bot J, Barkhof F, Lycklama a Nijeholt G et al (2002) Differentiation of multiple sclerosis from other inflammatory disorders and cerebrovascular disease: value of spinal MR imaging. Radiology 223:46–56

Bot J, Barkhof F, Polman CH et al (2004) Spinal cord abnormalities in recently diagnosed MS patients. Added value of spinal MRI examination. Neurology 62:226–233

Brex P, O'Riordan JI, Miszkiel KA et al (1999) Multisequence MRI in clinically isolated syndromes and the early development of MS. Neurology 53:1184–1190

Caramia M, Palmieri MG, Desiato MT et al (2004) Brain excitability changes in the relapsing and remitting phase of multiple sclerosis: a study with transcranial magnetic stimulation. Clin Neurophysiol 115:956–965

Clark C, Werring D (2002) Diffusion tensor imaging in spinal cord: methods and applications – a review. NMR Biomed 15:578–586

Dale RC, de Sousa C, Chong WK et al (2000) Acute disseminated encephalomyelitis, multiphasic disseminated encephalomyelitis and multiple sclerosis in children. Brain 123:2407–2422

Fazekas F, Kapeller P (1999) Diseases of the spinal cord. In: Greenberg J (ed) Neuroimaging: a companion to Adam and Victor's principles of neurology. McGraw-Hill, New York, pp 521–542

Fazekas F, Barkhof F, Filippi M et al (1999) The contribution of magnetic resonance imaging to the diagnosis of multiple sclerosis. Neurology 53:448–456

Filippi M (2003) Magnetization transfer MRI in multiple sclerosis and other central nervous system disorders. Eur J Neurol 10:3–10

Filippi M, Rocca MA, Moiola L et al (1999) MRI and magnetization transfer imaging changes in the brain and cervical cord of patients with Devic's neuromyelitis optica. Neurology 53:1705–1710

Filippi M, Bozzali M, Horsfield MA et al (2000) A conventional and magnetization transfer MRI study of the cervical cord in patients with MS. Neurology 54:207–213

Holtmannspötter M, Inglese M, ROvaris M et al (2003) A diffusion tensor MRI study of basal ganglia from patients with ADEM. J Neurol Sci 15:27–30

Inglese M, Salvi F, Iannucci G et al (2002) Magnetization transfer and diffusion tensor MR imaging of acute disseminated encephalomyelitis. Am J Neuroradiol 23:267–272

Katz J, Ropper A (2000) Progressive necrotic myelopathy: clinical course in 9 patients. Arch Neurol 57:355–361

Kidd D, Thorpe JW, Thompson AJ et al (1993) Spinal cord MRI using multi-array coils and fast spin echo. II. Findings in multiple sclerosis. Neurology 43:2632–2637

Losseff N, Webb SL, O'Riordan J et al (1996) Spinal cord atrophy and disability in multiple sclerosis. A new reproducible and sensitive MRI method with potential to monitor disease progression. Brain 119:701–708

Lycklama à Nijeholt G, Barkhof F, Scheltens P et al (1997) MR of the spinal cord in multiple sclerosis: relation to clinical subtype and disability. Am J Neuroradiol 18:1041–1048

Lycklama à Nijeholt G, van Walderveen MAA, Castelijns JA et al (1998) Brain and spinal cord abnormalities in multiple sclerosis. Correlation between MRI parameters, clinical subtypes and symptoms. Brain 121:687–697

Lycklama G, Thompson AJ, Filippi M et al (2003) Spinal-cord MRI in multiple sclerosis. Lancet Neurol 2:555–562

McDonald W, Compston A, Edan G et al (2001) Recommended diagnostic criteria for multiple sclerosis: guidelines from the International Panel on the Diagnosis of Multiple Sclerosis. Ann Neurol 50:121–127

Mezzapesa D, Rocca MA, Falini A et al (2004) A preliminary diffusion tensor and magnetization transfer magnetic resonance imaging study of early-onset multiple sclerosis. Arch Neurol 61:366–368

Miller DH, Filippi M, Fazekas F et al (2004) The role of MRI within diagnostic criteria for multiple sclerosis: a critique. Ann Neurol (in press)

Nijeholt G, Bergers E, Kamphorst W et al (2001) Post-mortem high-resolution MRI of the spinal cord in multiple sclerosis: a correlative study with conventional MRI, histopathology and clinical phenotype. Brain 124:154–166

O'Riordan J, Losseff NA, Phatouros C et al (1998) Asymptomatic spinal cord lesions in clinically isolated optic nerve, brain stem, and spinal cord syndromes suggestive of demyelination. J Neurol Neurosurg Psychiatry 64:353–357

Rovaris M, Bozzali M, Santuccio G et al (2000) Relative contributions of brain and cervical cord pathology to multiple sclerosis disability: a study with magnetisation transfer ratio histogram analysis. J Neurol Neurosurg Psychiatry 69:723–727

Rovaris M, Bozzali M, Santuccio G et al (2001) In vivo assessment of the brain and cervical cord pathology of patients with primary progressive multiple sclerosis. Brain 124:2540–2549

Silver N, Good CD, Sormani MP et al (2001) A modified protocol to improve the detection of enhancing brain and spinal cord lesions in multiple sclerosis. J Neurol 248:215–224

Stevenson V, Leary SM, Losseff NA et al (1998) Spinal cord atrophy and disability in MS: a longitudinal study. Neurology 51:234–238

Tartaglino LM, Friedman DP, Flanders AE et al (1995) Multiple sclerosis in the spinal cord: MR appearance and correlation with clinical parameters. Radiology 195:725–732

Tenembaum S, Chamoles N, Fejerman N (2002) Acute disseminated encephalomyelitis. A long-term follow-up study of 84 pediatric patients. Neurology 59:1224–1231

Thielen K, Miller G (1996) Multiple sclerosis of the spinal cord: magnetic resonance appearance. J Comput Assist Tomogr 20:434–438

Thompson AJ, Montalban X, Barkhof F et al (2000) Diagnostic criteria for primary progressive multiple sclerosis: a position paper. Ann Neurol 47:831–835

Thorpe J, Kidd D, Kendall BE et al (1993) Spinal cord MRI using multi-array coils and fast spin echo. I. Technical aspects and findings in healthy adults. Neurology 43:2625–2631

Thorpe J, Kidd D, Moseley IF et al (1996a) Spinal MRI in patients with suspected multiple sclerosis and negative brain MRI. Brain 119:709–714

Thorpe JW, Kidd D, Moseley IF et al (1996b) Serial gadolinium-enhanced MRI of the brain and spinal cord in early relapsing-remitting multiple sclerosis. Neurology 46:373–378

Transverse Myelitis Consortium Working Group (2002) Proposed diagnostic criteria and nosology of acute transverse myelitis. Neurology 59:499–505

Ukkonen M, Dastidar P, Heinonen T et al (2003) Volumetric quantitation by MRI in primary progressive multiple sclerosis: volumes of plaques and atrophy correlated with neurological disability. Eur J Neurol 10:663–669

Weinshenker B (2003) Neuromyelitis optica: what it is and what it might be. Lancet 361:889–890

Weinshenker B, Miller DH (1998) MS: One disease or many? In: Siva A, Kesselring J, Thompson AJ (eds) Frontiers in multiple sclerosis. Dunitz, London

Wheeler-Kingshott C, Hickman SJ, Parker GJ et al (2002) Investigating cervical spinal cord structure using axial diffusion tensor imaging. Neuroimage 16:93–102

Wingerchuk DM (2003) Postinfectious encephalomyelitis. Curr Neurol Neurosci Rep 3:256–264

Wingerchuk D, Hogancamp WF, O'Brien PC et al (1999) The clinical course of neuromyelitis optica (Devic's syndrome). Neurology 53:1107–1114

Zivadinov R, Bakshi R (2004) Role of MRI in multiple sclerosis II: brain and spinal cord atrophy. Front Biosci 9:647–664

19 Demyelinating Diseases of the Optic Nerve

Simon J. Hickman and David H. Miller

CONTENTS

19.1 Introduction

The principal disease that will be discussed here will be optic neuritis, which is the prototypical demyelinating disease of the optic nerve and has been studied in most detail. Other conditions such as neuromyelitis optica and sarcoidosis will be considered principally in terms of the optic nerve imaging features that help in diagnosis. Magnetic resonance imaging (MRI) of the optic nerves presents many technical difficulties which will be discussed.

S. J. Hickman, MB, MRCP
D. H. Miller, MD, FRCP
NMR Research Unit, Department of Neuroinflammation, Institute of Neurology, University College London, Queen Square, London, WC1N 3BG, UK

19.2 Technical Aspects of Optic Nerve Imaging

Magnetic resonance imaging of the optic nerve presents many challenges (Barker 2000), principally due to:

1) Its small size and tortuosity
2) Its mobility
3) The surrounding cerebrospinal fluid (CSF) sheath
4) Orbital fat
5) The bones of the orbital canal and air–fluid interfaces from the adjacent sphenoid and ethmoid sinuses

The optic nerves are approximately 40–50 mm long and 3–5 mm in diameter (Sadun 1998; Tamraz 1994; Williams et al. 1989). Resolution of the small structures or lesions contained within the nerves is dependent upon the voxel size. If the voxel size is too large then resolution will be impaired due to partial volume effects (i.e. mixing of signal from neighbouring structures). The voxel size can be reduced by increasing the matrix size; however, if the voxel size is too small then there may not be enough signal resolved to produce an image because the signal-to-noise ratio (SNR) is reduced. Resolution and SNR can be increased by increasing the acquisition time or by increasing the magnetic field strength. Increasing the magnetic field strength, however, will increase the longitudinal relaxation time of the tissue being imaged, also potentially leading to increased acquisition time. There is also the possibility of more susceptibility artefacts (see later) from surrounding tissues at higher field strengths leading to worsening of the SNR (Horsfield 2000). Signal averaging can also improve the SNR and thereby improve the resolution, again at the expense of increased acquisition time (Barker 2000). Increasing acquisition time will lead to more movement artefact, particularly in the mobile optic nerve. Fast imaging techniques are therefore required to give high SNR with an acceptable acquisition time (Gass et al. 1995).

The optic nerves are surrounded by a CSF-filled nerve sheath and, in the orbit, by lipid (Sadun 1998;

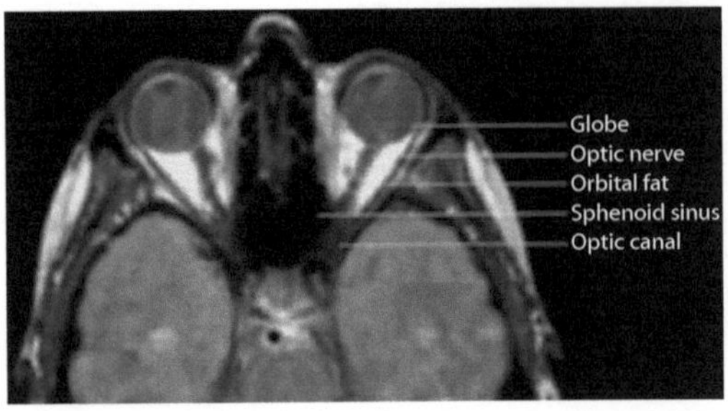

Fig. 19.1. Axial PD-weighted fast spin echo image demonstrating optic nerve anatomy

Williams et al. 1989). Due to its high proton density (PD) lipid typically gives high signal intensity on both T1- and PD/T2-weighted imaging (Fig. 19.1). CSF gives high signal intensity on PD- and T2-weighted imaging. This may cause problems due to obscuring the edge of the optic nerves and hence CSF suppression may be desirable. In certain circumstances, however, the bright CSF may assist in identification of the nerve (Barker 2000).

19.2.1 Artefacts

There is also a considerable potential for artefact in optic nerve imaging, more so than in the brain. The most important sources of artefact with possible solutions are discussed below.

19.2.1.1 Chemical Shift Artefacts

As has been discussed, the optic nerves are surrounded by lipid in the orbits. Chemical shift artefacts can occur at lipid-water boundaries. Due to their differing chemical environments protons in lipid have a lower precession frequency than protons in water. The lipid protons are therefore misregistered relative to the water protons in the frequency encoding direction (Soila et al. 1984). This can lead to decreased signal where the lipid is displaced away from water and high signal where lipid and water overlap. This chemical shift artefact is more prominent at higher field strengths (Barker 2000). High signal and chemical shift artefacts from orbital fat can be suppressed using short *tau* inversion recovery (STIR) imaging (Johnson et al. 1987) or a frequency-selective fat saturation excitation pulse prior to imaging time (Gass et al. 1995).

19.2.1.2 Motion Artefacts

Motion in a structure causes image blurring in the direction of movement and "ghost" artefacts in the phase-encoding direction due to the signal being reconstructed over and over. The major motion problem in optic nerve imaging is random motion due to eye movements. On ocular movement the intra-orbital portion of the optic nerve shifts against the direction of gaze with an increasing extent from the relatively fixed posterior part at the orbital apex anteriorly (Liu et al. 1992). Motion artefacts can be reduced by using fast imaging techniques with multiple signal acquisitions and signal averaging or by using gradient echo (GE) rather than spin echo techniques because a 180° refocusing pulse is not required in GE imaging (mobile protons may have moved before the 180° pulse has been applied) (Barker 2000; Taber et al. 1998). Subjects undergoing optic nerve imaging can also be encouraged to relax, close their eyes and avoid deliberate eye movements.

19.2.1.3 Susceptibility Artefacts

Susceptibility artefacts occur at interfaces between different tissues, due to the different magnetic properties of the tissues. It is more apparent at higher field strengths and can cause rapid dephasing of spins with signal loss and mismapping artefacts (Hashemi and Bradley Jr 1997). It is a particular problem in the canalicular portion of the optic nerves due to the bony cavity of the optic canal and air from the adjacent sphenoid and ethmoid sinuses. Metals, particularly iron, can cause a lot of image distortion and subjects should be carefully screened for metal in clothing before imaging commences. Susceptibility artefacts can be reduced by using spin echo rather than GE or echo-planar imaging (EPI) because the spin echo sequence includes a refocusing pulse (Barker 2000).

Imaging of the optic nerves is therefore a trade-off between imaging time, resolution, SNR and the amount of artefact induced.

19.3 MRI in the Diagnosis of Demyelinating Diseases

Optic neuritis can usually be diagnosed on its clinical features (Hickman et al. 2002b). The principal use of MRI is in assessing the brain for asymptomatic lesions which gives an indication of the risk of subsequent development of multiple sclerosis (MS) (Optic Neuritis Study Group 1997). If there is doubt about the diagnosis, in particular if a compressive lesion is suspected then optic nerve, MRI is very useful. In optic neuritis, it will usually demonstrate the lesion, either with conventional or gadolinium-enhanced imaging (Fig. 19.2). It will also demonstrate, in most cases, any compressive lesions (Fig. 19.3).

In neuromyelitis optica (Devic's disease) high signal and enhancement may be seen in both optic nerves (Eggenberger 2001), usually in combination with a long confluent spinal cord lesion extending over a number of vertebral segments (Fardet et al. 2003; Filippi et al. 1999). Optic nerve sheath enhancement may be seen in cases of sarcoidosis, optic perineuritis, or optic nerve sheath meningioma (Fig. 19.4) (Atlas and Galetta 1996; Carmody et al. 1994; Purvin et al. 2001). This feature has also been reported in demyelinating optic neuritis (Atlas and Galetta 1996) and we have witnessed it occurring in several of our own cases.

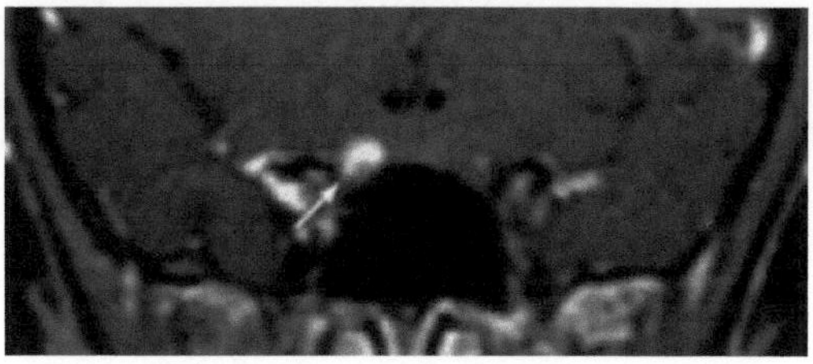

Fig. 19.4. Optic nerve sheath enhancement (*arrow*)

19.4 Conventional MRI Studies in Optic Neuritis

MRI provides a valuable opportunity for in vivo study of the pathological evolution of optic neuritis and, by inference, other central nervous system inflammatory/demyelinating lesions with clinical and electrophysiological correlation. There follows a summary of the studies and pulse sequences used in optic neuritis.

19.4.1 STIR Imaging

The first imaging technique used to investigate optic neuritis was the STIR sequence. In a study of 37 patients following an episode of optic neuritis using STIR imaging, lesions were detected in 84% of symptomatic nerves and 20% of asymptomatic

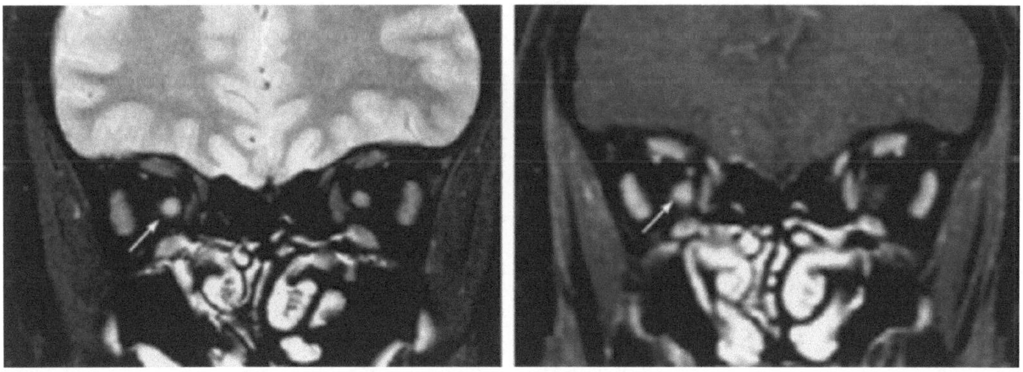

a b

Fig. 19.2a,b. Fat-saturated proton-density fast spin echo image of acute right-sided optic neuritis (**a**). Gadolinium-enhanced fat-saturated T1-weighted image from the same patient (**b**). The diseased optic nerve is indicated by an *arrow* in both images

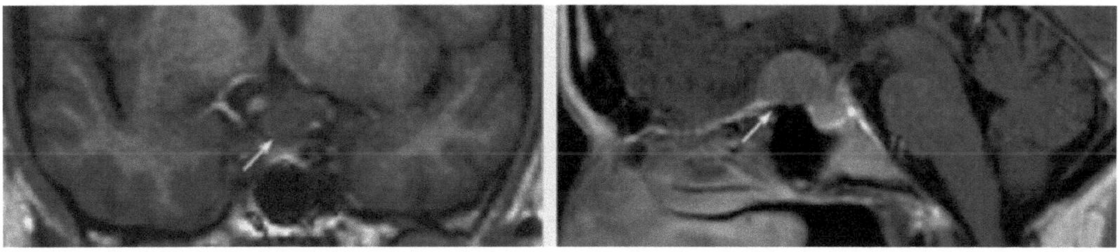

a b

Fig. 19.3a,b. Coronal (**a**) and sagittal (**b**) gadolinium-enhanced T1-weighted image from a patient with a left-sided sphenoid-wing meningioma (*arrow* in both images) causing a left optic neuropathy, initially diagnosed clinically as optic neuritis nerves (Miller et al. 1988). Slow (>4 weeks for vision to improve to 6/9) or poor (<6/9 at 6 months) visual recovery was associated with longer lesions (mean number of abnormal 5-mm coronal slices 3.50 versus 1.84, $p<0.01$), although there was no correlation between lesion length and latency or amplitude of the P100 response of the visual evoked potential (VEP). Of 15 patients with lesions involving the optic canal, 11 (73%) also had a poor recovery which was thought to be due to compression of the swollen optic nerve within the tight confines of the bony canal. These findings were confirmed by Dunker and Wiegand (1996). They examined 22 patients acutely and again after a mean of 4.7 years (range 2.5–8 years) with STIR MRI of the optic nerves. Lesions less than 17.5 mm long either acutely or chronically were correlated with complete visual recovery (visual acuity >20/25, no visual field, colour vision or contrast sensitivity defect). Intracanalicular lesions correlated with incomplete visual recovery (visual acuity >20/25 but other deficits present).

Kakisu et al. (1991) demonstrated that, although the lesion length on STIR was not correlated with pattern-reversal VEP findings in the acute phase, there was a significant correlation in the chronic phase ($r=0.68, p<0.005$). There was, however, no correlation between lesion length and visual acuity.

High signal in the optic nerves following optic neuritis usually persists despite improvements in vision and VEP findings (Youl et al. 1996) and may be seen in MS in the absence of acute attacks of optic neuritis (Davies et al. 1998).

19.4.2 Fat Saturated Fast Spin Echo Imaging

For optic nerve imaging with fat saturation the fast spin echo (FSE) sequence allows for increased resolution and image quality with an acceptable acquisition time. In a study comparing STIR with fat-saturated FSE, lesions were detected in 18 out of 21 symptomatic optic nerves with acute optic neuritis using STIR compared with 20/21 using FSE (Gass et al. 1996). Mean lesion length was 15.4 mm on STIR images and 17.3 mm on FSE images. Using fat-saturated FSE dual echo imaging is possible giving both PD- and T2-weighted images from the same acquisition if appropriate TE_{efs} are chosen (Barker 2000).

19.4.3 Combined Fat and Water Suppression Imaging

On FSE and, particularly the lower resolution STIR, CSF gives high signal which may obscure the signal from the optic nerves (Gass et al. 1996). It is possible to suppress the signal from CSF using fluid-attenuated inversion recovery (FLAIR) techniques. The FLAIR sequence uses an inversion pulse with a long inversion time for CSF suppression which increases the acquisition time. For optic nerve imaging fat saturation and fast acquisitions are required, hence a combined selective partial inversion recovery pre-pulse with a FLAIR sequence and FSE acquisition (SPIR-FLAIR) has been developed to try to achieve these aims (Jackson et al. 1998). SPIR-FLAIR was compared with both SPIR and STIR imaging in the assessment of optic neuritis. Both SPIR-FLAIR and SPIR detected lesions in all 21 symptomatic optic nerves imaged whereas STIR imaging detected only 20/21. Lesion lengths were also longest on the SPIR-FLAIR images (17.2 mm on SPIR-FLAIR, 15.8 mm on SPIR and 13.8 mm on STIR, $p<0.01$) even though the in-plane resolution was less than with SPIR imaging.

19.5 New Pulse Sequences and Methods of Analysis in Optic Neuritis

Although the above conventional MRI techniques are sensitive in detecting the lesions of optic neuritis there is a lack of pathological specificity to allow prediction of the chronological age of these lesions. This is because oedema, demyelination, axonal loss and gliosis all cause high signal on T2-weighted images (Miller et al. 1998). As has been discussed, imaging of the optic nerves is particularly limited by issues of poor resolution. Increasing the SNR requires very large increases in acquisition time. Using conventional imaging techniques at present is therefore limited by the technology available (Horsfield 2000). The only pointers to age the lesion have been a subjective impression of optic nerve swelling in the acute phase and atrophy in the chronic phase (Gass et al. 1996; Jackson et al. 1998; Kapoor et al. 1998; Miller et al. 1988). Other techniques have been developed which are able to study the optic nerves in order to understand better the pathophysiology of optic neuritis. These have principally been applied in brain imaging in MS but, with recent technological advances, optic nerve imaging using these techniques has also been possible.

19.5.1 Gadolinium "Enhancement"

Dimeglumine gadopentetate (gadolinium-DTPA) is the most common contrast agent used in MRI as gadolinium is a paramagnetic substance. In areas of acute inflammation where there is blood vessel wall leakage gadolinium will accumulate and show up as high signal on T1-weighted imaging due to shortening of T1. Optic nerve imaging imposes some constraints due to the need for fat suppression. If STIR imaging is used then the signal from gadolinium is also suppressed hence a drop in signal is indicative of acute inflammation and gadolinium "leakage" rather than gadolinium enhancement (Brown and Semelka 1999). In a study of 18 patients with acute optic neuritis (2 with bilateral simultaneous disease) STIR imaging was performed before and after injection of 0.02mmol/kg gadolinium (Youl et al. 1991). Ten of the patients (one with bilateral simultaneous optic neuritis) had MRI twice, once a mean 6.4 days (range: 2–13 days) after onset of symptoms and again a mean 27.8 days (range: 20–32 days later). Clinical and electrophysiological examination was also performed at each occasion. Of the 31 examinations in total, gadolinium leakage was seen in 6/6 lesions where the time since onset of optic neuritis was less than 7 days, in 7/8 lesions where time since onset was 7–13 days but in only 5/17 lesions where the age of the lesion was at least 14 days. Gadolinium leakage in the hyper-acute phase was associated with decreased visual acuity, pain on eye movement, a relative afferent pupillary defect, swelling of the optic disc (p=0.001 for each clinical feature compared with the asymptomatic optic nerves) and decreased amplitude of the P100 component of VEP (p<0.001). There was a trend for patients with longer lesions to have worse visual acuity (acuity <6/9 in 4/5 patients with gadolinium leakage on ≥3 slices, compared with 4/8 studies with leakage on 1–2 slices, p=0.1). In those patients who had a follow-up MRI, gadolinium leakage had ceased in 9/11 symptomatic optic nerves. This was associated with an improvement in all the above clinical features and increased P100 amplitude (p=0.02) compared with the first examination. It was concluded that acute inflammation is associated with conduction block in the optic nerve and that resolution of inflammation plays an important role in the recovery process.

A recent report confirmed that gadolinium enhancement is a consistent feature of acute optic neuritis and that the lesion length had clinical significance at presentation (Kupersmith et al. 2002). In this retrospective series 101/107 (94%) symptomatic optic nerves demonstrated enhancement following gadolinium on fat saturated T1-weighted imaging. Optic nerves with ≥17 mm enhancing segment on axial images had poorer baseline Snellen visual acuity (p=0.02), Humphrey 24-2 threshold perimetry (p=0.009) and colour vision on Ishihara plates (p=0.01). Canalicular involvement was associated with poorer colour vision (p=0.04). The location and length of the initial lesion, however, was not predictive of the degree of visual recovery in the 93 patients (68 treated with corticosteroids) with clinical follow-up after 6 months.

Triple-dose (0.3 mmol/kg dimeglumine gadopentetate) gadolinium increases the sensitivity for detecting enhancing lesions in MS by 66%–75% compared with the use of single-dose gadolinium (Filippi et al. 1996, 1998; Silver et al. 1997). In a serial study of patients with acute optic neuritis imaged with a triple dose gadolinium-enhanced fat-saturated T1-weighted spin echo sequence the symptomatic lesion was identified in 27 out of 28 cases (Hickman et al. 2002c). The lesion length correlated significantly with both baseline logarithm of the minimal angle of resolution (logMAR) visual acuity (r=0.38, p=0.044) and 30-2 Humphrey mean deviation (r=0.57, p=0.002) at baseline in agreement with the previous studies and suggesting that acute inflammation causes conduction block in the optic nerve. The median duration of enhancement was 63 days (range 0–113 days). After 1 year 30-2 Humphrey mean deviation was related to the initial lesion length (parameter estimate -0.09dB, 95% confidence intervals: 0.01, 0.20, p<0.05), but not duration of enhancement (Hickman et al. 2003b). Use of triple-dose gadolinium may therefore improve the ability to predict prognosis for recovery although the correlation was only modest.

19.5.2 Optic Nerve Size

Optic nerve size can be judged on MRI both subjectively and objectively.

19.5.2.1 Optic Nerve Swelling

Optic nerve swelling, suggesting the presence of acute inflammation and oedema, on STIR MRI was reported in three out of 37 cases (8%) of acute optic neuritis (Miller et al. 1988). It had been thought to be a rare occurrence in optic neuritis and if swelling was present then a glioma or meningioma should be suspected (Cornblath and Quint 1997). However, in a further study of acute optic neuritis using STIR imaging, swelling was reported in 12 out of 40 cases (40%) with, and in four out of 26 cases (15%) without canalicular involvement (Kapoor et al. 1998). Also, using formal measurement of optic nerve size with callipers from the intraorbital optic nerve on hard copy STIR images from ten patients, Youl et al. (1996) reported that the mean area of symptomatic optic nerves with acute optic neuritis (mean disease duration 6 days) was 20.0 mm^2 compared with 14.4 mm^2 for asymptomatic contralateral optic nerves ($p=0.001$). After a mean follow-up period of 28 days the mean area of the symptomatic optic nerves had decreased to 15.5 mm^2 ($p=0.01$) whereas the asymptomatic optic nerves had a mean area of 14.1 mm^2 (p=not significant [n.s.]). Both visual acuity and VEP amplitudes improved on follow-up, although VEP latencies showed no significant improvement. This suggested that resolution of acute inflammation was associated with resolution of optic nerve swelling.

19.5.2.2
Optic nerve atrophy

An expected end result of demyelination and axonal loss is atrophy of tissue. Measurement of atrophy may help in the quantification of the amount of tissue destruction and help in studies investigating disability in MS. There have been many studies of brain atrophy in MS using MRI (Losseff et al. 1996; Simon et al. 1999). Being able to quantify the degree of optic nerve atrophy following optic neuritis would be useful since optic neuritis is a model for the effects of lesions in MS. This is technologically very demanding for the reasons outlined above.

Youl et al. (1996) also studied 22 patients with a mean disease duration of 60 days. Optic nerve mean area in both symptomatic and asymptomatic nerves was 16.8 mm^2. After a mean of 405 days the patients were re-imaged. The mean area of symptomatic nerves decreased to 12.8 mm^2 ($p<0.001$) and the asymptomatic nerves to 16.3 mm^2 (p=n.s.). This was despite improvement in visual acuity, VEP amplitude ($p=0.03$) and VEP latency (p=n.s.) in the affected eyes. The STIR sequence Youl et al. (1996) used had the disadvantages of low resolution (pixel size 1.2×0.6 mm), the presence of high signal from CSF obscuring the edge of the optic nerve and the inclusion of optic nerve sheath leading to an overestimation of optic nerve area.

The combined CSF and fat suppression of SPIR-FLAIR imaging has allowed optic nerve atrophy to be detected qualitatively following optic neuritis. Inter-observer assessment of optic nerve size was 1.0 using a weighted Cohen κ test for SPIR-FLAIR compared with 0.85 for SPIR and 0.61 for STIR (sequences which were not CSF suppressed) (Jackson et al. 1998).

Inglese et al. (2002) imaged 30 patients with relapsing-remitting and secondary progressive MS who had had a previous episode of optic neuritis. A T1-weighted spin echo sequence was used. The mean volume of the optic nerves was calculated from the mean areas from 11 slices using a local thresholding segmentation technique. The mean volume was 93.3 ml in 18 age-matched controls, 89.2 ml for clinically healthy nerves from patients ($n=18$), 89.4 ml for diseased optic nerves with visual recovery to at least 20/25 ($n=20$), 79.0 ml for diseased optic nerves with vision worse than 20/25 ($n=22$) ($p=0.002$, versus optic nerves with good recovery) and 82.0 ml for optic nerves from patients with Leber's hereditary optic neuropathy (LHON) ($n=20$). Optic nerve volume from MS patients was correlated with both visual acuity ($r_S=0.39, p=0.01$) and VEP P100 latency ($r_S=-0.31$, $p=0.05$). The functional significance of optic nerve atrophy was therefore apparent although the correlations were modest. The volumes of optic nerves from MS patients with poor recovery were similar to those from patients with LHON, a condition where axonal loss has been demonstrated histologically (Saadati et al. 1998).

In a study of 17 patients who had had a previous single episode of unilateral optic neuritis Hickman et al. (2001) evaluated a coronal-oblique fat saturated short echo fast fluid attenuated inversion recovery (sTE fFLAIR) sequence for the measurement of optic nerve area. This sequence has potential advantages as it is CSF and lipid suppressed with low T2-weighting. The mean cross-sectional area of the intra-orbital portion of both optic nerves was 11.2 mm^2 in diseased eyes, 12.9 mm^2 in the contralateral eyes ($p=0.006$ compared with the diseased eye) and 12.8 mm^2 in controls ($p=0.03$ compared with the patients' diseased eyes) (Fig. 19.5). There was a significant negative correlation between disease duration and the size of the diseased optic nerve ($r=-0.59, p=0.012$).

At 1 year follow-up in a subgroup of patients, some years following the acute event in many, it was demonstrated that the mean area of diseased optic nerves decreased from 11.1 mm^2 to 10.2 mm^2 ($p=0.01$). Baseline visual acuity ($p=0.02$), decreased VEP amplitudes ($r_S=0.65$, $p=0.02$) and increased VEP latencies ($r_S=-0.61, p=0.04$) were associated with optic nerve

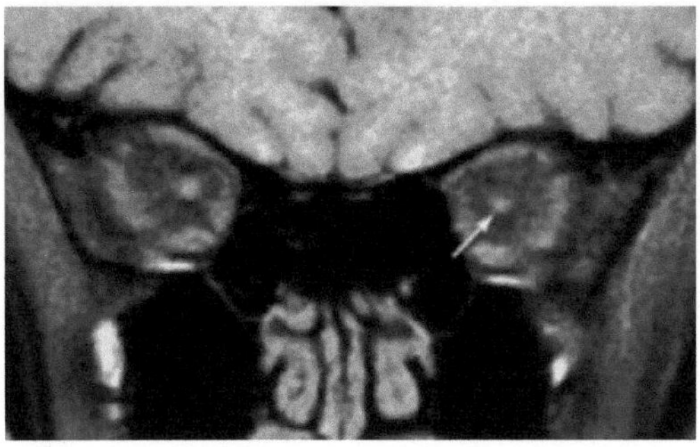

Fig. 19.5. sTE fFLAIR image demonstrating left optic nerve atrophy (*arrow*) following optic neuritis

mean area (Hickman et al. 2002a). The findings of these studies suggest that atrophy develops in a focal demyelinating lesion, it may evolve over several years, and may have functional significance. The continuing atrophy may be due to ongoing axonal loss in a persistently demyelinated lesion, or Wallerian degeneration following axonal damage during the acute inflammatory phase of the disease.

19.5.3 Magnetization Transfer Imaging

Magnetization transfer (MT) imaging provides a means by which tissues can be examined in more detail, going beyond the T1 and T2 characteristics. Use of MT allows the hitherto invisible bound water such as is held in myelin sheaths to be examined and provides a means of increasing contrast. It also provides a means of producing quantitative images by calculating the degree of exchange between bound and free protons. If images are produced of the same slice both with and without an MT pre-pulse the MT ratio (MTR) can be calculated which is an indication of the amount of signal reduction that has occurred due to the MT pulse. The higher the MTR, the greater the reduction in signal and hence the greater the bound water pool is.

From studies in MS (Filippi 1999) it is thought that low MTR results from a decreased capacity for exchange due to oedema, demyelination and gliosis. Axonal loss combined with demyelination results in even greater falls in MTR. Remyelination can result in restoration of MTR. It is not an absolute measure but is dependent on the amplitude and frequency offset of the MT pulse as well as the time delay between the MT pulse and the excitation pulse. It also varies between imagers and in the same imager due to coil non-uniformity, thus requiring accurate repositioning of patients in serial studies. Analysis of the images to give the MTR can be done in two ways. The conventional approach is to examine a region-of-interest (ROI) placed manually or using semi-automated techniques. This is useful when examining a particular tissue or a lesion. An alternative approach is to generate histograms containing information from all the pixels in the tissue to be examined. This can give an indication of the global burden of disease and can detect subtle changes in what appears to be normal tissue. The optic nerve is small and therefore imaging does not produce enough voxels for meaningful histogram analysis. An ROI-based approach is therefore required.

In a study of 39 patients with acute optic neuritis and 50 controls (selected from patients having brain imaging for other indications) Boorstein et al. (1997) placed eight pixel ROIs in the intraorbital portions of optic nerves on MT images. The MTR was 41.1 percent units (pu) in control optic nerves, 30.6 pu in 22 optic nerves in which either a high signal lesion was present on T2-weighted images or contrast-enhancement was seen and 36.3 pu in 12 of the remaining 18 patients who had no high signal lesion but who demonstrated a reduction in MTR. MTR was therefore more sensitive than conventional imaging at detecting abnormalities in affected optic nerves although no clinical or electrophysiological correlations were presented.

Thorpe et al. (1995) imaged six controls and 20 patients between 3 months and 16 years following optic neuritis (five of whom had MS, three with both eyes affected). One slice was acquired in the intraorbital portion of each optic nerve incorporating a lesion where possible. The MTR was recorded from a four pixel ROI placed in the centre of the nerve. The mean MTR was 49 pu in controls, 48 pu in clinically unaffected nerves and 42 pu in affected nerves ($p<0.005$ versus unaffected nerves and control nerves). The MTR was correlated with VEP whole field latency ($r_S=-0.554$, $p<0.01$) but not Snellen visual acuity. Lesion length on T2-weighted FSE images was correlated with visual acuity ($p<0.02$). The negative correlation between MTR and VEP latency supports the idea that some of the MTR reduction may be due to demyelination. The lack of correlation of MTR with clinical measures was concordant with the complex relationship between demyelination and vision that had previously been shown in VEP studies of optic neuritis (Halliday et al. 1973).

In addition to the optic nerve atrophy measurements in MS described above, Inglese et al. (2002)

also measured MTR in the optic nerves using a four pixel ROI from the whole length of the optic nerve from a two-dimensional GE sequence. The mean MTR was 35.3 pu in 18 age-matched controls, 35.1 pu for clinically healthy nerves (n=18), 34.6 pu for diseased optic nerves with visual recovery to at least 20/25 (n=20), 29.6 pu for diseased optic nerves with vision worse than 20/25 (n=22) ($p<0.001$, versus optic nerves with good recovery) and 30.2 pu for optic nerves from patients with LHON (n=20). When MTR was correlated with clinical and electrophysiological tests opposite results to Thorpe et al. were obtained. MTR correlated with visual acuity (r_S=0.49, p=0.01) but not VEP P100 latency (r_S=–0.10). A possible explanation for the latter finding was that this cohort was biased towards those with a limited visual recovery, over 50% having a visual acuity worse than 20/25. Axonal loss in the optic nerve may have been more pronounced in this group.

In a study of 29 patients with acute optic neuritis with 21 followed serially up to 1 year using a three-dimensional GE sequence, the mean MTR, defined using threshold-based segmentation, at baseline was 47.3 pu compared with 47.9 pu (from healthy contralateral optic nerves (p= n.s.) (Hickman et al. 2004). The diseased optic nerve MTR declined over time with a nadir at about 240 days at a mean MTR value of 44.2 pu, consistent with demyelination and axonal damage. The late nadir compared with studies of MS lesions may have been due to slow clearance of myelin debris. Subsequently, diseased optic nerve MTR appeared to rise, possibly due to remyelination: after 1 year the diseased optic nerve mean MTR was 45.1 pu, although the difference was not significant compared with the nadir value. Time-averaged VEP central field latency was shorter by 6.1 ms (95% confidence intervals 1.5, 10.7, p=0.012) per 1-pu rise in time-averaged diseased optic nerve MTR, supporting the idea that MTR can give an indication of the degree of demyelination/remyelination in a lesion.

19.5.4 Diffusion-Weighted Imaging

Diffusion of water molecules in vivo is affected by the structure of the tissue. In white matter tracts, of which the optic nerve is an example, the structure is in the form of tightly packed axons. Diffusion occurs preferentially along the orientation of the axons. In the direction orthogonal to the axons, cellular membranes act as barriers to the water molecule, hindering and restricting the process of water diffusion. Because of the complexity of the diffusion mechanism in tissue in vivo the measurements are dependent on the observation time, hence the term "apparent diffusion coefficient" (ADC) was introduced to indicate this dependency and its difference from the free diffusion coefficient of water. The directional dependence of the ADC in vivo is called anisotropy and is one of several parameters which can be derived from the diffusion tensor (Basser et al. 1994). If the white matter tracts are disrupted or the permeability of axonal membranes is increased then the ADC will increase and the fractional anisotropy (FA), a measure of the alignment of tissues, will decrease.

Studies in MS have revealed increased ADC values and decreased FA values in both lesions and normal appearing white matter (Ciccarelli et al. 2001; Filippi et al. 2001; Filippi and Inglese 2001). DWI of the optic nerves presents many challenges due to the reasons outlined above. The following issues need to be principally addressed: the need for high resolution whilst minimising susceptibility distortions; the need to reduce CSF and lipid contamination; and the need to minimise misregistration problems.

To sample the full diffusion tensor it is necessary to acquire a minimum of seven images: one without any diffusion weighting and six with diffusion weighting applied along six non-collinear directions (Basser and Pierpaoli 1998). This makes it very sensitive to motion occurring between each acquisition. Ideally, one would wish to implement a registration algorithm capable of correcting the possible variable spatial position of the ON. An alternative is to acquire several images with the same diffusion weighting and average them after reconstruction to determine the central position of the optic nerve, with the drawback of longer acquisition times. Hence, most DWI studies of optic nerve have concentrated on measuring the ADC along fewer directions (rather than the full diffusion tensor) as fewer acquisitions are required (Freeman et al. 1998; Iwasawa et al. 1997; Wheeler-Kingshott et al. 2002).

Iwasawa et al. (1997) studied the optic nerves with a spin-echo sequence and cardiac gating for a single slice through the orbital optic nerve. Three acquisitions were performed with the diffusion gradients in the x, y and z directions, respectively. Due to motion artefacts the ADC could only be measured in the y and z directions, and not always reliably then. The ADC was measured from a 1-mm diameter circular ROI placed in the centre of the nerve. In seven controls the mean ADC was $982\times10^{-6}\text{mm}^2/\text{s}$ in the y direction and $1559\times10^{-6}\text{mm}^2/\text{s}$ in the z direction. In four nerves with acute optic neuritis the mean ADC was

$843 \times 10^{-6} mm^2/s$ in the y direction and $941 \times 10^{-6} mm^2/s$ in the z direction. In nine nerves with previous optic neuritis the mean ADC was $1560 \times 10^{-6} mm^2/s$ in the y direction and $4180 \times 10^{-6} mm^2/s$ in the z direction ($p<0.001$ versus controls and acute optic neuritis).

EPI is a fast multi-echo imaging technique similar to FSE which uses no spin echoes during data acquisition but acquires gradient echoes (Warach et al. 1998). It allows for high resolution with high SNR but at the expense of susceptibility and chemical shift artefacts. For optic nerve DWI a fat- and CSF-suppressed zonal oblique multi-slice EPI (ZOOM-EPI) has been recently developed (Wheeler-Kingshott et al. 2002). This sequence uses a limited field-of-view along the phase-encoding direction, shortening the echo train length, which reduces susceptibility artefacts and therefore image distortions. In a pilot study, ZOOM-EPI DWI was carried out on three controls. After off-line post-processing with magnitude signal averaging and noise correction the mean ADC from the optic nerves as a combination of the x, y and z gradients could be calculated over the length of the optic nerves and was found to be 1058 (SD 101)$\times 10^{-6} mm^2/s$ in the three subjects measured.

Recently, Chabert et al. (2002) developed an axial fast spin-echo acquisition which could measure the ADC and FA in individual eyes. In four volunteers the mean diffusivity was 1670 (SD 450)$\times 10^{-6} mm^2/s$ with a mean FA of 0.59 (SD 0.08), reflecting strong anisotropy in the nerve. The fibre directions followed the expected nerve fibre directions on anisotropy maps. The sequence was free of susceptibility artefacts; however, it was neither fat- nor CSF-suppressed.

DWI offers the potential to offer more pathologically specific imaging with measures that are thought to be sensitive to changes in nerve structure, particularly axonal disruption. Further application of DWI in both patients acutely affected by, and recovering from, optic neuritis would be of interest. The functional significance of any changes measured would need to be elucidated with reference to clinical and electrophysiological tests.

19.6 Optic Nerve MRI in Treatment Monitoring

There has been only one study of the use of optic nerve imaging in treatment monitoring. Based on the observation that long and canalicular lesions on STIR were associated with a poorer prognosis (Miller et al. 1988), a prospective study was designed to assess whether stratification of patients may assist in targeting corticosteroids to those patients who might be predicted to have a worse outcome (Kapoor et al. 1998). A total of 66 patients with acute unilateral optic neuritis had their optic nerves imaged with the STIR sequence. They were then randomized to receive either 1 g/day intravenous methylprednisolone (IVMP) for 3 days or placebo. Patients were stratified into those with short or long (≥3 involved coronal slices) lesions. The presence of canalicular involvement was also noted. Patients with longer lesions tended to present earlier (mean 8.4 versus 12.1 days, $p<0.05$); however, there was no correlation between initial visual acuity and initial lesion length. Treatment with IVMP was not associated with improved visual outcome at 6 months in those patients with long or canalicular lesions and treatment did not affect 6-month lesion length on repeat imaging. An association between initial canalicular involvement and poor recovery was not seen; however, after 6 months canalicular involvement was seen in all 16 patients with a poor visual recovery compared with only 31 out of 45 patients with a good recovery ($p<0.01$).

A subsequent reanalysis of the data was performed to measure orbital optic nerve mean area (Hickman et al. 2003a). At 6 months following randomization optic nerve area was 17.4 mm^2 in healthy optic nerves and 16.4 mm^2 in all diseased optic nerves ($p=0.02$). The mean area of diseased optic nerves at 6 months in the IVMP group was 15.9 mm^2 compared with 16.9 mm^2 in the placebo group ($p=0.19$ for a test of no difference between the two groups in the ratio 6-month diseased/6-month healthy optic nerve area and $p=0.92$ for the ratio 6-month diseased nerve area/baseline diseased nerve area). It was concluded that acute treatment with a course of IVMP did not prevent the subsequent short-term development of optic nerve atrophy following acute optic neuritis.

19.7 Conclusion

While optic nerve MRI presents many challenges, it can be a useful tool in diagnosing optic neuritis, or in ruling out other conditions that might mimic optic neuritis, particularly compressive lesions (Hickman et al. 2002b). Conventional and enhanced imaging studies suggest that longer lesions and canalicular involvement may be associated with a poorer outcome; however, these observations have not been universally seen.

Optic nerve swelling occurs in acute optic neuritis followed by the development of optic nerve atrophy that was not prevented by acute treatment with IVMP in the one study to investigate this. In patients imaged some years from an attack of optic neuritis worsening optic nerve atrophy was associated with poorer vision. Optic nerve MT imaging and DWI offer the potential for more pathologically specific imaging. With current technology spectroscopy in the optic nerves has not been possible due to their small size and the surrounding CSF and orbital fat. There has been only one trial to date in optic neuritis incorporating optic nerve imaging. In future treatment trials of novel agents including remyelination therapy, optic nerve imaging, incorporating the newer sequences, would be useful in assessing the response to treatment in conjunction with clinical and electrophysiological measures.

References

Atlas SW, Galetta SL (1996) The orbit and visual system. In: Atlas SW (ed) Magnetic resonance imaging of the brain and spine. Lippincott-Raven Publishers, Philadelphia, pp 1007-1092

Barker GJ (2000) Technical issues for the study of the optic nerve with MRI. J Neurol Sci 172[Suppl.1]:S13–S16

Basser PJ, Pierpaoli C (1998) A simplified method to measure the diffusion tensor from seven MR images. Magn Reson Med 39:928–934

Basser PJ, Mattiello J, LeBihan D (1994) MR diffusion tensor spectroscopy and imaging. Biophys J 66:259–267

Boorstein JM, Moonis G, Boorstein SM et al (1997) Optic neuritis: imaging with magnetization transfer. AJR Am J Roentgenol 169:1709–1712

Brown MA, Semelka RC (1999) MR imaging abbreviations, definitions, and descriptions: a review. Radiology 213:647–662

Carmody RF, Mafee MF, Goodwin JA et al (1994) Orbital and optic pathway sarcoidosis: MR findings. AJNR Am J Neuroradiol 15:775–783

Chabert S, Molko N, Cointepas Y et al (2002) "Functional" diffusion tensor imaging of the optic nerve using a non CPMG fast spin echo sequence. Proc Intl Soc Magn Reson Med 10:1115

Ciccarelli O, Werring DJ, Wheeler-Kingshott CA et al (2001) Investigation of MS normal-appearing brain using diffusion tensor MRI with clinical correlations. Neurology 56:926–933

Cornblath WT, Quint DJ (1997) MRI of optic nerve enlargement in optic neuritis. Neurology 48:821–825

Davies MB, Williams R, Haq N et al (1998) MRI of optic nerve and postchiasmal visual pathways and visual evoked potentials in secondary progressive multiple sclerosis. Neuroradiology 40:765–770

Dunker S, Wiegand W (1996) Prognostic value of magnetic resonance imaging in monosymptomatic optic neuritis. Ophthalmology 103:1768–1773

Eggenberger ER (2001) Inflammatory optic neuropathies. Ophthalmol Clin North Am 14:73–82

Fardet L, Genereau T, Mikaeloff Y et al (2003) Devic's neuromyelitis optica: study of nine cases. Acta Neurol Scand 108:193–200

Filippi M (1999) Magnetization transfer imaging to monitor the evolution of individual multiple sclerosis lesions. Neurology 53[Suppl.3]:S18–S22

Filippi M, Inglese M (2001) Overview of diffusion-weighted magnetic resonance studies in multiple sclerosis. J Neurol Sci 186[Suppl.1]:S37–S43

Filippi M, Yousry T, Campi A et al (1996) Comparison of triple dose versus standard dose gadolinium-DTPA for detection of MRI enhancing lesions in patients with MS. Neurology 46:379–384

Filippi M, Rovaris M, Capra R et al (1998) A multi-centre longitudinal study comparing the sensitivity of monthly MRI after standard and triple dose gadolinium-DTPA for monitoring disease activity in multiple sclerosis. Implications for phase II clinical trials. Brain 121:2011–2020

Filippi M, Rocca MA, Moiola L et al (1999) MRI and magnetization transfer imaging changes in the brain and cervical cord of patients with Devic's neuromyelitis optica. Neurology 53:1705–1710

Filippi M, Cercignani M, Inglese M et al (2001) Diffusion tensor magnetic resonance imaging in multiple sclerosis. Neurology 56:304–311

Freeman AJ, Ballinger R, Werner M et al (1998) Diffusion weighted EPI of the human optic nerve at 3T. Proc Intl Soc Magn Reson Med 6:1265

Gass A, Barker GJ, MacManus D et al (1995) High resolution magnetic resonance imaging of the anterior visual pathway in patients with optic neuropathies using fast spin echo and phased array local coils. J Neurol Neurosurg Psychiatry 58:562–569

Gass A, Moseley IF, Barker GJ et al (1996) Lesion discrimination in optic neuritis using high-resolution fat- suppressed fast spin-echo MRI. Neuroradiology 38:317–321

Halliday AM, McDonald WI, Mushin J (1973) Delayed pattern-evoked responses in optic neuritis in relation to visual acuity. Trans Ophthalmol Soc UK 93:315–324

Hashemi RH, Bradley Jr WG (1997) MRI the basics. Lippincott Williams and Wilkins, Baltimore

Hickman SJ, Brex PA, Brierley CM et al (2001) Detection of optic nerve atrophy following a single episode of unilateral optic neuritis by MRI using a fat-saturated short-echo fast FLAIR sequence. Neuroradiology 43:123–128

Hickman SJ, Brierley CM, Brex PA et al (2002a) Continuing optic nerve atrophy following optic neuritis: a serial MRI study. Mult Scler 8:339–342

Hickman SJ, Dalton CM, Miller DH et al (2002b) Management of acute optic neuritis. Lancet 360:1953–1962

Hickman SJ, Toosy AT, Miszkiel KA et al (2002c) Serial magnetic resonance imaging in optic neuritis using triple dose gadolinium. Neuro-ophthalmology 27:223–224

Hickman SJ, Kapoor R, Jones SJ et al (2003a) Corticosteroids do not prevent optic nerve atrophy following optic neuritis. J Neurol Neurosurg Psychiatry 74:1139–1141

Hickman SJ, Toosy AT, Miszkiel KA et al (2003b) Predicting visual recovery following acute optic neuritis: a clinical,

electrophysiological and magnetic resonance imaging study. Mult Scler 9[Suppl1]:S95
Hickman SJ, Toosy AT, Jones SJ et al (2004) Serial magnetization transfer imaging in acute optic neuritis. Brain 127:692–700
Horsfield MA (2000) Imaging the cerebral hemispheres: technical issues. J Neurol Sci 172[Suppl 1]:S54–S56
Inglese M, Ghezzi A, Bianchi S et al (2002) Irreversible disability and tissue loss in multiple sclerosis: a conventional and magnetization transfer magnetic resonance imaging study of the optic nerves. Arch Neurol 59:250–255
Iwasawa T, Matoba H, Ogi A et al (1997) Diffusion-weighted imaging of the human optic nerve: a new approach to evaluate optic neuritis in multiple sclerosis. Magn Reson Med 38:484–491
Jackson A, Sheppard S, Laitt RD et al (1998) Optic neuritis: MR imaging with combined fat- and water-suppression techniques. Radiology 206:57–63
Johnson G, Miller DH, MacManus D et al (1987) STIR sequences in NMR imaging of the optic nerve. Neuroradiology 29:238–245
Kakisu Y, Adachi-Usami E, Fujimoto N (1991) Pattern visually evoked cortical potential and magnetic resonance imaging in optic neuritis. J Clin Neuroophthalmol 11:205–212
Kapoor R, Miller DH, Jones SJ et al (1998) Effects of intravenous methylprednisolone on outcome in MRI-based prognostic subgroups in acute optic neuritis. Neurology 50:230–237
Kupersmith MJ, Alban T, Zeiffer B et al (2002) Contrast-enhanced MRI in acute optic neuritis: relationship to visual performance. Brain 125:812–822
Liu C, Youl B, Moseley I (1992) Magnetic resonance imaging of the optic nerve in extremes of gaze. Implications for the positioning of the globe for retrobulbar anaesthesia. Br J Ophthalmol 76:728–733
Losseff NA, Wang L, Lai HM et al (1996) Progressive cerebral atrophy in multiple sclerosis. A serial MRI study. Brain 119:2009–2019
Miller DH, Grossman RI, Reingold SC et al (1998) The role of magnetic resonance techniques in understanding and managing multiple sclerosis. Brain 121:3–24
Miller DH, Newton MR, van der Poel JC et al (1988) Magnetic resonance imaging of the optic nerve in optic neuritis. Neurology 38:175–179
Optic Neuritis Study Group (1997) The 5-year risk of MS after optic neuritis. Experience of the optic neuritis treatment trial. Neurology 49:1404–1413
Purvin V, Kawasaki A, Jacobson DM (2001) Optic perineuritis: clinical and radiographic features. Arch Ophthalmol 119:1299–1306
Saadati HG, Husu HY, Heller KB et al (1998) A histopathologic and morphometric differentiation of nerves in optic nerve hypoplasia and Leber hereditary optic neuropathy. Arch Ophthalmol 116:911–916
Sadun AA (1998) Anatomy and physiology of the optic nerve. In: Miller NR, Newman NJ (eds) Walsh and Hoyt's clinical neuro-ophthalmology. Williams and Wilkins, Baltimore, pp 57–83
Silver NC, Good CD, Barker GJ et al (1997) Sensitivity of contrast enhanced MRI in multiple sclerosis. Effects of gadolinium dose, magnetization transfer contrast and delayed imaging. Brain 120:1149–1161
Simon JH, Jacobs LD, Campion MK et al (1999) A longitudinal study of brain atrophy in relapsing multiple sclerosis. Neurology 53:139–148
Soila KP, Viamonte M Jr, Starewicz PM (1984) Chemical shift misregistration effect in magnetic resonance imaging. Radiology 153:819–820
Taber KH, Herrick RC, Weathers SWet al (1998) Pitfalls and artifacts encountered in clinical MR imaging of the spine. Radiographics 18:1499–1521
Tamraz J (1994) Neuroradiologic investigation of the visual system using magnetic resonance imaging. J Clin Neurophysiol 11:500–518
Thorpe JW, Barker GJ, Jones SJ et al (1995) Magnetisation transfer ratios and transverse magnetisation decay curves in optic neuritis: correlation with clinical findings and electrophysiology. J Neurol Neurosurg Psychiatry 59:487–492
Warach S, Hajnal JV, Rovaris M et al (1998) The role of techniques characterised by faster acquisition times in the evaluation of multiple sclerosis. J Neurol Neurosurg Psychiatry 64[Suppl 1]:S59–S65
Wheeler-Kingshott CA, Parker GJ, Symms MR et al (2002) ADC mapping of the human optic nerve: increased resolution, coverage, and reliability with CSF-suppressed ZOOM-EPI. Magn Reson Med 47:24–31
Williams PL, Warwick R, Dyson M et al (1989) Gray's anatomy 37th edn. Churchill Livingstone, Edinburgh
Youl BD, Turano G, Miller DH et al (1991) The pathophysiology of acute optic neuritis. An association of gadolinium leakage with clinical and electrophysiological deficits. Brain 114:2437–2450
Youl BD, Turano G, Towell AD et al (1996) Optic neuritis: swelling and atrophy. Electroencephalogr Clin Neurophysiol 46[Suppl]:173–179

Immune-Mediated Disorders

20 Primary Angiitis of the Central Nervous System

Darin T. Okuda and Timothy L. Vollmer

CONTENTS

20.1 Introduction

Vasculitis is defined as an inflammation of the vessel wall with or without the presence of vessel wall necrosis. This condition may involve the central nervous system (CNS), peripheral nervous system (PNS), or both. The term "primary nervous system angiitis" is reserved for a vasculitic process restricted only to the CNS. In addition, systemic symptoms, such as fever, malaise, rash, myalgias, arthritis, arthralgias, and single or multi-organ involvement, usually are not present. Secondary nervous system vasculitides may involve both the CNS as well as the PNS (Table 20.1). They are associated with systemic involvement and occur in the setting of an identifiable cause such as an infectious or inflammatory process, connective tissue disorder, malignancy, drug, or toxin.

D. T. Okuda, MD; T. L. Vollmer, MD
St. Joseph's Hospital & Medical Center, Barrow Neurological Institute, Division of Neurology, 350 W. Thomas Road, Phoenix, Arizona 85013, USA

20.2 Primary Angiitis of the Central Nervous System

Primary angiitis of the central nervous system (PACNS) is a unique clinicopathological condition characterized by inflammation of blood vessels with or without vessel wall necrosis restricted to the CNS. In this disorder, both cerebral and meningeal vessels may be affected. This disease entity is more commonly seen involving the brain; however, a number of cases involving the spinal cord have been reported (Campi et al. 2001b; Cupps et al. 1983; Giovanini et al. 1994). Although the etiology is unclear, it is not known to be secondary to a systemic process. A hypothesis relating to a viral cause has been suggested by some investigators (Reyes et al. 1976).

Our knowledge of this disease process is greatly limited due to its rarity. The lack of multi-center, randomized, controlled therapeutic trials further hinders our understanding of the treatment modalities for this condition. In addition, our current understanding of the disease process is derived from a collection of small case series and individual case reports. Further confounding the data, neurodiagnostic studies rather than histological confirmation from brain and/or meningeal tissue were used to make the diagnosis of PACNS in these previous case series.

Primary angiitis of the CNS is most often observed in the fourth to sixth decade; however, a number of pediatric cases have also been reported (Gallagher et al. 2001; Giovanini et al. 1994; Lanthier et al. 2001; Katsicas et al. 2000; Matsell et al. 1990; Moore and Richardson 1998; Nishikawa et al. 1998; Stone et al. 1994). Men and women are thought to be equally affected (Moore and Richardson 1998); however, a

Table 20.1. Primary and secondary angiitis of the nervous system.

Primary
- Primary angiitis of the central nervous system (isolated angiitis of the CNS, granulomatous angiitis of the CNS).

Secondary

Drug induced
- Amphetamines
- Cocaine
- Ephedrine
- Heroin

Systemic diseases
- Systemic lupus erythematosis
- Churg-Strauss syndrome
- Polyarteritis nodosa
- Wegener's granulomatosis
- Behset's disease
- Sarcoidosis

Malignancy related
- Hodgkin's lymphoma
- Non-Hodgkin's lymphoma
- Leukemia
- Metastatic disease

Infectious causes
- *Mycobacterium tuberculosis*
- *Treponema pallidum*
- *Cocciodes immitis*
- *Borrelia burgdoferi*
- *Toxoplasma gondii*
- HIV
- CMV
- VZV
- Herpes simplex virus
- Hepatitis B, C

female:male ratio of 4:3 has been reported (Hajj-Ali et al. 2000). This condition is rarely diagnosed given the non-specific symptoms frequently reported.

The earliest report of PACNS dates back to 1922 when Harbitz (1992) reported two patients presenting with complaints of worsening headaches, hallucinations, confusion, and ataxia. A previously unreported cerebral vasculitis was identified in these patients on post-mortem examination of the brain and meninges. Newman and Wolf (1952) first identified a granulomatous angiitis based on histopathological findings observed; however, it was Cravioto and Feigin (1959) who delineated the clinicopathological syndrome of granulomatous angiitis after evaluating two cases involving a non-infectious granulomatous angiitis with a predilection for both leptomeningeal and intraparenchymal arteries. This disease entity has also been referred to as an isolated angiitis of the CNS (IAC; Moore 1994). It is important to emphasize that PACNS is synonymous with IAC and granulomatous angiitis of the nervous system (GANS); however, the term PACNS and IAC are preferred as the presence of granulomata composed of multinucleated giant cells and epithelioid cells are not consistent findings histologically (Younger et al. 1997). The terms PACNS and IAC also emphasize the restriction of involvement rather than its histopathology. There have been instances in which limited involvement outside of the CNS has occurred; however, these are rare and the term PACNS is preferred.

Regardless of the nomenclature, this condition is associated with a high degree of morbidity and mortality, if left untreated. In the past, PACNS was viewed as uniformly fatal; however, with aggressive immunosuppressive therapy the overall prognosis has improved. Yet, there is still much to be learned regarding this condition given the limited number of cases, heterogeneity of the disease process, and lack of specific physical exam findings or serological tests. In addition, data comparing treatment efficacy as well as long-term follow-up information providing insight into the natural history of the disease process are lacking.

20.3 Histopathology

The etiology and pathogenesis of PACNS remains unknown; however, the histopathological features have been well described (S. Coons 2003, personal communication; Kolodny et al. 1968; Koo and Massey 1988; Langford 2003; Lie 1992; Moore and Cupps 1983; Reik et al. 1983; Siva 2001; Vanderzant et al. 1988). Variability exists with respect to the pattern of histological change and presence of inflammatory cell types seen, suggesting that multiple etiologies may be responsible for the development of PACNS. The pathological mechanism, by which some histopathological features are present in some cases but not in others, has not been elucidated.

In PACNS, both small- and medium-size leptomeningeal, cortical, and subcortical arteries may be involved, in addition to veins and venules; however, arteries are more frequently involved than veins (Siva 2001; Vanderzant et al. 1988). Systemic vasculitides also can involve all vessel sizes but with a different histopathological picture observed (Langford 2003). Transmural involvement of the vessel wall is commonly seen with dense infiltration of inflammatory cells, primarily lymphocytes and larger mononuclear cells (Vanderzant et al. 1988). In addition, involvement of the ventricular vessels has been reported in the past (Reik et al. 1983). Segmental inflammation and necrosis involving the small leptomeningeal and parenchymal blood vessels is more commonly seen; however larger vessels may at times be involved (Moore and Cupps 1983).

Fibrin thrombosis has also been reported (Vanderzant et al. 1988). Kolodny et al. (1968) reported a higher predilection for leptomeningeal involvement compared with parenchymal vessels. The experience of Barrow Neurological Institute supports this observation. The surrounding brain parenchyma may also demonstrate areas of both gross and microscopic ischemic and hemorrhagic infarction in evolving stages in addition to reactive astrocytosis (Kolodny et al. 1968). The presence of reactive changes in the surrounding brain parenchyma is not a consistent feature. In addition, loss of myelin with or without axonal degeneration may also be present (S. Coons, pers. commun.). The inflammatory infiltrate is comprised of macrophages, lymphocytes, multinucleated giant cells, and plasma cells, with or without the presence of granulomata (Moore and Cupps 1983). The focal, segmental, and heterogeneous nature of the disease process may lead to patchy granulomata formation as well as areas free of granuloma. A necrotizing vasculitis may be seen along side a non-granulomatous PACNS (Lie 1992). Necrotic changes within granulomata and presence of eosinophils are usually not observed (Koo and Massey 1988). Focal and segmental involvement is not limited solely to brain parenchyma and meninges, but can also be present in the spinal cord.

Aside from the standard pathological techniques utilizing a variety of stains, other techniques are also available to determine the presence of PACNS. The role of electron microscopy is yet to be determined in the diagnosis of PACNS; however, it is useful for assessing the presence of viral inclusion particles. Immunofluorescence is useful in detecting the presence of infectious agents but is of little value in the diagnosis of PACNS.

20.4 Immunological Mechanisms

The primary events that initiate this disease process remain unknown at present. In addition, the immunological mechanisms that result in the histopathological changes seen in PACNS are not completely understood. In some cases an immune complex-mediated process is responsible for damage to the intimal surface of blood vessels and cell-mediated immune mechanisms, as is suggested by the presence of granulomata. This is also supported by the presence of a lymphomononuclear cell infiltrate seen in addition to endothelial cell proliferation (Moore 1995).

20.5 Clinical Presentation

Nearly every neurological symptom has been reported at least once in cases of PACNS (Calabrese et al. 1997). Headache and confusion are the most common presenting symptoms. Hemiparesis, language difficulties (expressive and receptive aphasia), hemisensory loss, cranial nerve abnormalities, and seizures may also be observed during the disease process. Myelopathic symptoms may also be seen as a result of spinal cord involvement (Giovanini et al. 1994). In addition, patients may also present with symptoms correlating with diffuse white matter disease (Finelli et al. 1997). Visual disturbances and hallucinations have also been reported (Cravioto and Feigin 1959; Nurick et al. 1972). Focal and multi-focal abnormalities occur in more than 80% of cases (Moore and Cupps 1983) with focal seizures reported in approximately 5% of cases (Moore and Richardson 1998). Some cases presenting with intracranial hemorrhage have also occurred (Kumar et al. 1997; Yasuda et al. 1993). In the case series by Duna et al. (1995), CNS hemorrhage was documented in 11% (18 of 168) of patients studied.

Diffuse neurological dysfunction is seen in aggressive cases with resultant coma and death. In PACNS, systemic symptoms, such as fever, rash, arthralgias, myalgias, or arthritis, are usually not observed. When systemic symptoms are present, the focus must be directed towards a systemic disease process with secondary CNS involvement. The progression of symptoms may vary greatly in cases of PACNS owing to the heterogeneity of the natural history of the disease. There are no specific symptoms pathognomonic for PACNS.

20.6 Benign Angiopathy of the Central Nervous System

Reports of a benign angiopathy of the CNS (BACNS) have been proposed as a subset of PACNS in previously published studies (Bettoni et al. 1994;

Calabrese et al. 1993; Hajj-Ali et al. 2002; Snyder and McClelland 1978). These patients differ with respect to their clinical presentation, requirements for long-term immunosuppression, and prognosis.

Calabrese et al. (1993) first proposed the existence of patients with PACNS who had a more "benign" course compared to individuals with pathologically documented granulomatous angiitis of the CNS. Their course was described as monophasic rather than progressive. It was observed that they were primarily females (female:male ratio 4.3:1) who presented most commonly with complaints of headache with or without the presence of a focal neurological deficit. In addition, cerebrospinal fluid (CSF) studies were normal to mildly abnormal along with findings on cerebral angiogram consistent with vasculitis. Moreover, these individuals required less immunosuppressive treatment than traditionally used. Although the underlying pathogenesis was not clearly understood, reversible vasoconstriction or vasospasm was proposed as the most likely cause of BACNS as compared with an inflammatory process in PACNS.

An evaluation of 16 cases of presumed BACNS without histological confirmation was reported by Hajj-Ali et al. (2002). Angiographic follow-up data on 10 of 16 cases were analyzed, in addition to clinical outcomes as assessed by phone interview utilizing the Barthel index and a specifically designed cognitive index (Hajj-Ali et al. 2002). Results showed improvement in all repeat cerebral angiograms obtained after treatment had consisted of varying courses of glucocorticoids, calcium channel blockers, and cytotoxic medications. Clinical recovery was seen in 94% of cases. No deaths were reported; however, there was a 6% relapse rate observed. In those patients evaluated by the Barthel index, there was no lasting disability in 71% of cases. A different outcome was reported by Woolfenden et al. (1998) who published retrospective data on 10 patients with angiographically defined PACNS. They concluded that these patients neither had a benign outcome nor monophasic course.

Further data are needed to determine if such a distinct group of patients exist. The presumed pathological mechanisms underlying this proposed subtype is still lacking. It is noteworthy that the cases included in the study by both Calabrese et al. (1993) and Hajj-Ali et al. (2002) lacked histopathological confirmation. In previously published studies, a fair amount of patients who underwent brain biopsy for presumptive PACNS were found to have other diagnoses (Alrawi et al. 1999; Chu et al. 1998).

At our institution, we feel that a form of "benign" angiopathy or angiitis is a misnomer as there usually is nothing benign about the patient's clinical presentation or course. More studies are needed to determine whether in fact there is a separate subgroup and, if so, its natural history and pathogenesis.

20.7 Diagnostic Studies

20.7.1 Serological Tests

No specific serological diagnostic test(s) exist for PACNS. Instead, a comprehensive serological workup is performed to exclude other disorders. Recommended tests include a complete blood count, comprehensive metabolic panel including liver function tests, and C-reactive protein. Erythrocyte sedimentation rate (ESR), a common serological marker assessed in the PACNS, is usually negative. The ESR was found to be positive in 8–35% in two studies (Calabrese and Mallek 1988; Lie 1992). Patients should also be evaluated for connective tissue disorders (e.g., anti-nuclear antibody, anti-neutrophil cytoplasmic antibody). Depending on the clinical context, human immunodeficiency virus (HIV), hepatitis, syphilis, Lyme disease, and sarcoidosis also need to be considered in the differential diagnosis.

20.7.2 Cerebrospinal Fluid Analysis

In general, CSF studies are important in the diagnosis of PACNS. Abnormal CSF profiles are seen in 80–90% of pathologically documented cases of PACNS (Calabrese et al. 1997). Characteristically, a mononuclear pleocytosis with or without increased protein levels are seen (Oliveira et al. 1994; Vollmer et al. 1993). A previous report of 40 cases of pathologically proven PACNS demonstrated moderately to markedly elevated protein levels, and normal or mild decreased glucose levels (Vollmer et al. 1993). Oligoclonal bands and increased IgG synthesis may also be present. Oliveira et al. (1994) suggested that following the plasmatic albumin transudation and intrathecal IgG synthesis profiles may be a reliable marker for monitoring the disease process and therapeutic response. The appropriate stains, cultures, and studies [herpes simplex virus–polymerase chain reaction (HSV–PCR), *Cocciodes immitis*, syphilis, etc.] should be performed to evaluate for the presence of infectious etiologies.

20.7.3 Brain Computed Tomography

Computed tomography (CT) of the brain is abnormal in up 67% of cases (Siva 2001). This imaging modality, however, is not sensitive in the diagnosis of PACNS. Findings may include areas of low signal intensity suggestive of an ischemic event. Intraparenchymal or subarachnoid hemorrhage are uncommonly seen but have been reported. CT is also valuable during instances when magnetic resonance imaging (MRI) cannot be performed or is unavailable.

Stone et al. (1994) compared the diagnostic sensitivities of CT, lumbar puncture and magnetic resonance imaging in 20 patients with angiographically proven PACNS (ages ranging from 7-72 years). Of the 17 patients who underwent brain CT, 11 were found to be abnormal with 35% of cases failing to demonstrate any significant abnormality. They concluded that CT is a useful diagnostic tool when used as an adjunct with CSF studies.

20.7.4 Magnetic Resonance Imaging

Magnetic resonance imaging of the brain and spinal cord has been proven to be valuable in the evaluation of PACNS (Fig. 20.1). Although abnormalities seen are not pathognomonic for PACNS, this non-invasive and reproducible technique is sensitive to parenchymal changes regardless of the size of vessels involved by a vasculitic process (Harris et al. 1994). Patients who fail to demonstrate abnormalities on MRI are unlikely to manifest changes on angiography or brain biopsy suggestive for PACNS. Cases have been reported, however, in which patients with angiographically proven PACNS have had negative brain CT and MRI scans (Greenan et al. 1992; Stone et al. 1994).

In their review of six patients (two biopsy proven) with PACNS, Campi et al. (2001) reported discrete or diffuse supra- and infratentorial lesions involving the deep and subcortical white matter (Campi et al. 2001a). This is consistent with other reported cases of PACNS (Ehsan et al. 1995; Greenan et al. 1992; Scully 1989). The lesions in PACNS are usually enhancing in up to 90% of cases. In addition to the brain, enhancement has been noted in the Virchow-Robin spaces and spinal cord (cervical and thoracic segments). Other authors have reported a predominance of white matter involvement on T2-weighted images suggestive of demyelinating disease (Alhalabi and Moore 1994). Non-specific scattered focal and linear areas of high-signal abnormality involving the brainstem, cerebellum, and cere-

a
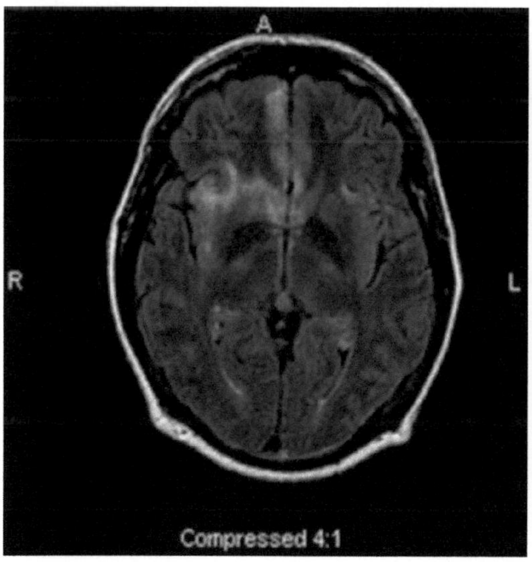

b
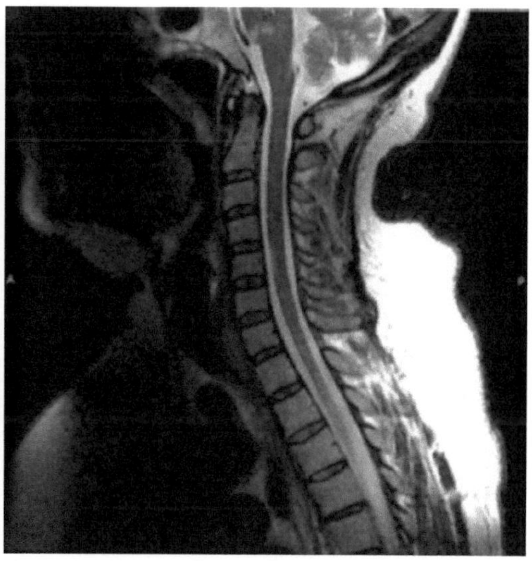

Fig. 20.1 a Axial brain fluid-attenuated inversion recovery (FLAIR) FSEIR magnetic resonance imaging (MRI) scan of a patient with primary angiitis of the central nervous system (PACNS) demonstrates high-signal abnormality involving the cortex and subcortical white matter of the right frontal lobe, anterior temporal lobe, and right insular region. **b** Sagittal T2-weighted MRI scan of the cervical cord demonstrates a region of high-signal abnormality involving the anterior cervical cord at C5 in a patient with PACNS

bral white matter has also been seen in addition to areas of recent infarction (Koo and Massey 1988; Shoemaker et al. 1994). Leptomeningeal enhancement with modest parenchymal involvement has also been reported (Negeshi and Sze 1993). Johnson et al. (1989) reported a case of granulomatous angiitis masquerading as a mass lesion with MRI findings revealing bilateral high signal intensity parieto-occipital lesions extending across the splenium of the corpus callosum. Idiopathic granulomatous angiitis of the CNS was also reported as manifesting as diffuse white matter disease in a patient presenting with progressive spastic paraparesis (Finelli et al. 1997).

Harris et al. (1994) studied the utility of MRI as a screening tool in 92 patients who underwent angiography for "exclude vasculitis" as the indication. The MRI data from 70 of the 92 patients were evaluated. Of the 92 patients studied, 11 patients were found of have intracranial vasculitis, 8 of which displayed abnormalities on angiography. The MRI data was available on 9 of the 11 cases, with all 9 demonstrating significant abnormalities. The authors advocated that brain MRI be performed in patients with suspected intracranial vasculitis. They concluded that a negative MRI was more valuable than a negative angiogram when trying to exclude the possibility of an intracranial vasculitis.

Currently, there are no MRI findings that are pathognomonic for PACNS; however, this modality is excellent in monitoring the natural history of the disease in addition to utilizing it as a tool for assessing for the presence of a treatment response (Ehsan et al. 1995).

20.7.5 Cerebral Angiography

Angiography is reportedly the most sensitive diagnostic modality available for the diagnosis of PACNS, although it is variable with respect to abnormalities seen (Alhalabi and Moore 1994; Ferris and Levine 1973; Leeds and Goldberg 1971; Moore 1995). Sensitivities do vary based on the study reviewed. A retrospective review of 30 consecutive patients who underwent brain biopsy and/or cerebral angiography for the evaluation of PACNS revealed that cerebral angiography had a sensitivity and positive predictive value (PPV) of <30% (Duna and Calabrese 1995). Vollmer et al. (1993) reported 56% of 41 angiograms were abnormal in biopsy-proved cases of idiopathic granulomatous angiitis of the CNS; however, only 27% (11 of 41) of these cases demonstrated findings thought to be diagnostic of vasculitis. On the other hand, a sensitivity of 89% was achieved with angiography by Alhalabi and Moore (1994) when retrospectively evaluating angiograms in 19 patients.

Angiography identifies large and medium-sized vessel abnormalities suggestive of vasculitis, but findings cannot unequivocally establish the diagnosis for PACNS, and a distinction between primary and secondary causes of vasculitis cannot be made based on the data. The angiographic abnormalities of PACNS cannot be differentiated from secondary causes of angiitis of the CNS; these include, among others, infectious causes (Engelter et al. 2002; Lehrer 1966; Mackenzie et al. 1981; Rabinov 1963; Ramos and Mandybur 1975; Rosenblum and Hatfield 1972; Walker et al. 1973), neoplasms (Giang 1994; Greco et al. 1976), collagen vascular diseases (Liem et al. 1996; Trevor et al. 1972), illicit drugs (Gertner and Hamlar 2002; Giang 1994; Glick et al. 1994; Margolis and Newton 1971), and other causes that may mimic a CNS vasculitis (Behcet's disease; Siva et al. 2001), Moya-moya disease (Coakham et al. 1979), fibromuscular dysplasia (Houser and Baker 1968), vasospasm, atherosclerosis (Ferris and Levine 1973), radiation injury, hypertensive vasculopathy, sickle cell anemia (Merkel et al. 1978), atrial myxoma embolism (Marazuela et al. 1989), refractory dermatomyositis (Regan et al. 2001), and medication toxicity (Berlit 1994; Giang 1994; Regan et al. 2001; Rumbaugh et al. 1971; Siva 2001).

Unlike magnetic resonance angiography (MRA), conventional angiography is an invasive procedure with associated risks. Previously published complication rates vary depending on the institution at which the procedure is performed. The complication rate at our institution following the evaluation of 1000 prospectively studied consecutive cases performed on 688 patients revealed a 1% overall incidence for a neurological deficit and a 0.5% incidence of a persistent deficit (Heiserman et al. 1994). The complications observed were seen in patients with a history of a cerebrovascular accident, transient ischemic attack, or carotid bruit (Heiserman et al. 1994).

Focal and/or multifocal segmental involvement of both small and medium-sized leptomeningeal and parenchymal blood vessels are angiographic findings seen in PACNS (Fig. 20.2). More commonly, single areas of focal abnormality are observed in a number of vessels rather than extensive areas of involvement on a single vessel (Alhalabi and Moore 1994). Also seen are vascular occlusions, collateral vessel formation, and prolonged circulation time (Alhalabi and

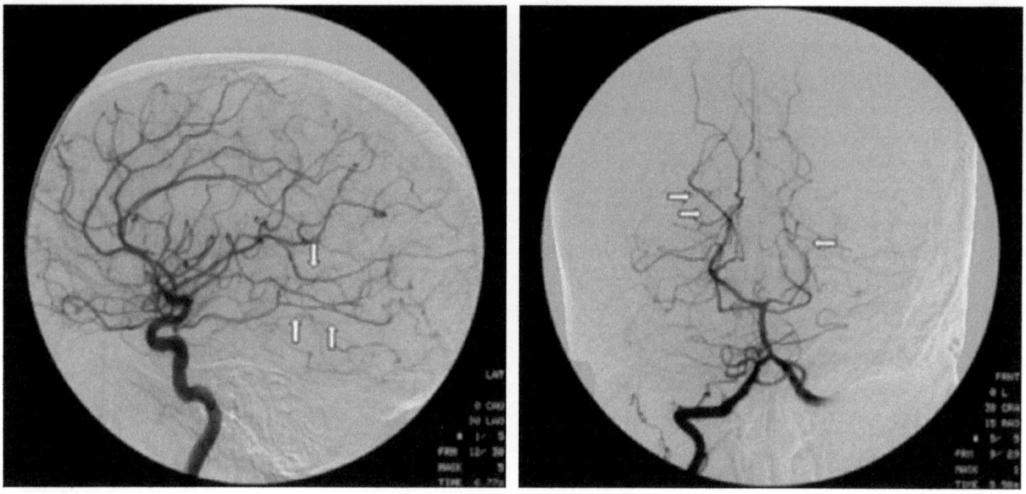

a b

Fig. 20.2 **a** Angiogram of the left common carotid artery (lateral view) demonstrates diffuse irregularity involving the distal branches of the middle cerebral and posterior cerebral artery (arrows). No branch occlusions are observed. **b** Angiogram of the posterior circulation reveals diffuse irregularity involving the distal posterior cerebral artery branches bilaterally

Moore 1994; Lie 1992). Aneurysms have also been identified (Nishikawa et al. 1998). Abnormalities observed on angiography do not always correlate with significant findings observed on MRI of the brain, likely owing to the extent of involvement of smaller vessels.

Alhalabi and Moore (1994) compared retrospective angiograms in 19 patients with PACNS along with prospective angiograms during the course of the disease. They noted areas of segmental narrowing were reversible if treatment was instituted early in the course of the disease. The initial areas of segmental narrowing were hypothesized to be secondary to inflammation and vasospasm. They also observed that areas of narrowing increased over time and that later in the course of the disease they were less likely to resolve. They suggested that serial angiography may be used to guide immunosuppressive therapy.

Although the sensitivity is highly variable, angiography provides another modality to help diagnose PACNS; however, brain and meningeal biopsies remain the gold standard for diagnosis.

20.7.6 Brain Biopsy

Histopathological confirmation by leptomeningeal and brain parenchymal biopsy remains the gold standard for the diagnosis of PACNS. Brain biopsy is the most specific diagnostic modality in PACNS. The optimal technique is wedge cortical biopsy with leptomeningeal tissue which permits better histological definition and a reduction in artifact (Moore 1989). Considerable debate exists as to whether stereotactic biopsy is as effective as open-wedge biopsy in the diagnosis of PACNS, although the experience of Alrawi et al. (1999) demonstrated no significant difference between these two approaches.

There are several retrospective studies which have calculated the specificity to be between 60 and 97% (Alrawi et al. 1999; Chu et al. 1998; Duna and Calabrese 1995). A false-negative rate of approximately 10% has been previously reported in premortem biopsies (Calabrese et al. 1993). False-positive results are rare and may occur in the setting of lymphoproliferative disease. Histological confirmation is necessary for a definitive diagnosis; however, the data must be correlated with the clinical history and information obtained from other diagnostic tests. Cases of PACNS with the presence of concomitant cerebral amyloid angiopathy have been reported in the past which may complicate the pathological diagnosis in some patients (Fountain and Eberhard 1996; Riemer et al. 1999; Schwab et al. 2003).

In addition to verifying the presence of a vasculitic process, the biopsy is also necessary to exclude other conditions that may affect the intracranial vasculature and mimic vasculitis. These include demyelinating conditions [acute disseminated encephalomyelitis (ADEM), multiple sclerosis]; infections (HIV [Nogueras et al. 2002], cytomegolovirus [CMV], herpes zoster, progressive multifocal leukoencephalopathy, Creutzfeldt-Jakob disease, Coxsackie A9, brain abscess, *Cocciodes immitis*); reaction to various toxic substances (heroin, cocaine, amphetamine use); neoplasia (lymphoma, malignant histiocytosis, metastatic small cell carcinoma); sterile infarction; and sarcoidosis.

Biopsy material should be examined with routine and special stains in addition to tissue cultures to exclude other diagnoses. It is of benefit to examine tissue by electron microscopy to identify the presence of viral inclusions or ultrastructural abnormalities that may be present.

Brain biopsy often is deferred due to concern for potential complications surrounding the procedure as well as the possibility of a false-negative result. The morbidity of the procedure has been reported to be 3.3% by Chu et al. (1998) and a similar morbidity rate of 4.9% was observed by Alrawi et al. (1999) in their analysis of 61 consecutive biopsy patients.

The site of the biopsy should be determined by location of active lesions observed on MRI. Biopsy of a radiographically abnormal region increases the sensitivity of the procedure and diagnostic accuracy is enhanced by sampling both the leptomeninges and cortical and subcortical tissues (Calabrese et al. 1992; Chu et al. 1998; Parisi and Moore 1994). Data from Alrawi et al. (1999) contradict this data as all identified cases of PACNS contained brain parenchyma involvement and only 77% demonstrated involvement of the leptomeninges. It is important to note, however, that sampling of the leptomeninges allows for the diagnosis of processes other than PACNS. The optimal location for biopsy would be a site of active disease on MRI, providing it is in a non-sensitive area of the brain; otherwise, sampling the anterior lip of the non-dominant temporal lobe is preferred and least harmful to the patient. Due to the focal and segmental nature of PACNS, biopsy results may vary with only 66–75% of biopsies being diagnostic (Siva 2001).

Duna and Calabrese (1995) reported results of 15 brain biopsies (7 stereotactic and 8 via craniotomy) in the diagnosis of PACNS. The sensitivity was 53%, specificity 87%, PPV 80%, and negative predictive value (NPV) 70%. One false-positive result was observed in a patient who was subsequently diagnosed with CNS lymphoma. Of the four true-positive biopsies, one demonstrated vasculitic changes in the cortex alone, one in the leptomeninges alone, and the other two with both parenchymal and leptomeningeal involvement (Duna and Calabrese 1995). A low sensitivity of 36% was observed in the report published by Alrawi et al. (1999). A specific diagnosis, however, was observed in 75% of the cases. This highlights the value of brain biopsy in not only identifying cases of PACNS but also those processes that it may mimic (Alrawi et al. 1999). The low sensitivities observed in both of these studies suggest that a negative biopsy result does not rule out the possibility of PACNS.

A retrospective analysis of 25 patients, 10 treated with immunosuppressive medications and 15 untreated, with PACNS were studied to assess the prognosis of those patients who had a negative brain biopsy (Alreshaid and Powers 2003). The addition of immunosuppressive therapy did not significantly enhance the outcome of these patients compared with the untreated group. Patients were stratified into two groups; "good", if the patient was residing at home; and "poor" if the patient resided in an extended-care facility or died. However, one should be cautioned that treatment regimens were not disclosed in this report and no specific treatment criteria were noted for those who received therapy. Additionally, it was not clear if other medical or social factors influenced their results.

20.7 Other Diagnostic Modalities

The role of positron emission tomography (PET), single-photon-emission computed tomography (SPECT), magnetic resonance spectroscopy (MRS), and transcranial doppler (TCD) is still undetermined (Ritter et al. 2002). These diagnostic modalities are neither sensitive nor specific in the diagnosis of PACNS.

Table 20.2 contains modified diagnostic criteria recommended by Moore (1989) for the diagnosis of PACNS.

Table 20.2. Antemortem diagnostic criteria for primary angiitis of the central nervous system modified from Moore (1989, 1998).

1. Clinical features consistent with recurrent, multifocal, or diffuse disease
2. Exclusion of an underlying systemic inflammatory process or infection
3. Neuroradiographic studies - cerebral angiography demonstrating findings supporting the diagnosis of a vasculopathy
4. Brain biopsy to establish the presence of vascular inflammation and exclude infection, neoplasia or alternate causes of vasculopathy
5. A CSF study consistent with CNS inflammation (pleocytosis, increased protein) and excluding infection and neoplasia

20.8 Treatment

Currently, the optimal treatment regimen for PACNS is not clearly delineated. To date, there have been no multicenter, randomized, or placebo-controlled studies investigating the efficacy of varying treatment regimens. This is most likely due to the paucity of documented cases. Our understanding and clinical approach therefore is based primarily on anecdotal experience and data from previously published individual case reports and modest case series. In general, there is agreement that the underlying pathogenesis of this condition is neuro-immunological, and thus treatment is directed towards modulating the immune system. Because of the clinical, radiological, and histopathological heterogeneity, it can be argued that the optimal treatment for one patient may not be as efficacious for another.

PACNS in previous years was viewed as uniformly fatal. There are now newer methods of modulating the patient's immune system, and with this availability the prognosis has become more favorable. At present, standard treatment recommendations include the use of high-dose corticosteroids and immunosuppressive agents. Azathioprine, methotrexate, and antiplatelet treatment for maintenance therapy have also been used in the past (Craven and French 1985; Griffin et al. 1973; Oliveira et al. 1994; Siva 2001; Zivkovic and Moore 2000). The role of IVIg, plasmapheresis, the interferons, and monoclonal antibody therapy in PACNS remains unclear.

Currently, it is generally agreed upon that aggressive immunotherapy should be instituted in cases where progressive neurological decline is present. This is with the understanding that an attempt to confirm the diagnosis of PACNS by histopathology, as well as conventional diagnostic modalities, has been made, and that other causes for the presenting symptoms have been investigated and ruled out. This approach is also advocated by other investigators (Calabrese et al. 1997). The optimal duration of treatment is not clearly established. Recommendations for a treatment period of 6–12 months after the clinical symptoms have stabilized have been made, although there is no conclusive evidence to support this (Calabrese 1995; Moore 1994). Treatment duration should be guided by patient response to therapy and current clinical status.

Most commonly, the treatment regimen used in PACNS includes high-dose methylprednisolone at a dose of 1000 mg/day for 3–7 days followed by oral prednisone at 60 mg/day with slow taper. The experience with cyclophosphamide in the treatment of PACNS has been extensively reported (Barron et al. 1993; Fountain and Lopes 1999; Mandybur and Balko 1992; Moore 1989; Riemer et al. 1999; Siva 2001; Woolfenden et al. 1998). Cyclophosphamide, oral or intravenous, is administered concomitantly with steroids at a dose of 2.0–2.5 mg/kg day^{-1}. If intravenous therapy is selected, pulsed intravenous cyclophosphamide (500–1000 mg/m^2) can be administered every second week for the first 6 weeks followed by monthly intervals.

Reviewing five patients with biopsy-proven PACNS, Moore (1989) recommended for the initial 6 weeks of therapy a regimen of prednisone at 40–60 mg/day combined with cyclophosphamide, dose of 100 mg/day (Moore 1989). Oral prednisone alone at a dose of 40–100 mg/day has also been advocated in a report by Crane et al. (1991) in their review of 11 patients with angiographically proven IACNS. Of the 11 patients studied, 10 achieved clinical remission following this regimen of steroid therapy alone. Cupps et al. (1983) reported four cases of biopsy proven (1) and unproven (3) PACNS. The single biopsy-proven case involved isolated spinal cord involvement as no brain abnormalities were identified. Sustained clinical remission was achieved with a combination of cyclophosphamide and alternate-day prednisone therapy in all patients (Cupps et al. 1983). The successful use of the prednisone and cyclophosphamide combination has also been seen in pediatric patients (Lanthier et al. 2001; Barron et al. 1993). Lanthier et al. (2001) reported on two pathologically proven cases of IACNS. One case was successfully treated with a regimen of prednisone 2 mg/kg day^{-1} and cyclophosphamide 2 mg/kg day^{-1}, the other with prednisone alone. The patient who received cyclophosphamide in addition to steroids remained symptom free for 6 years after discontinuation of therapy. A successful response was achieved in a 12-year-old patient with cerebral angiogram presumed IACNS with monthly pulse cyclophosphamide (750 mg/m^2) for 6 months followed by treatment every 3 months for 1 year (Barron et al. 1993).

The most sensitive as well as specific modality for monitoring the response to treatment in PACNS continues to be investigated. At present, serial brain MRI scans is the most sensitive means of monitoring disease progression. This imaging modality has been utilized in the past by other investigators to monitor both disease progression and response to treatment (Ehsan et al. 1995). Serial cerebral angiograms have also been used to assess the efficacy of the treatment regimen utilized (Alhalabi and Moore 1994; Stein et al. 1987). Some authors have proposed the use of subsequent serial CSF profiles as a guideline for monitoring disease activity and response to therapy (Oliveira et al. 1994). There have been, however, no reports of repeat histopathological analysis to assess therapeutic success. Since PACNS is such a heterogeneous disorder, it is unclear if repeat analysis of the leptomeninges or brain parenchyma would provide conclusive evidence of therapeutic success, since a lack of non-inflammatory findings may represent disease suppression rather than cure.

Further investigations are necessary to not only determine the optimal therapeutic regimen for PACNS, but also to prevent treatment complications. The sequelae of short- and long-term steroid use are well known. Cyclophosphamide has several well-known side effects primarily related to bone marrow suppression (Bradley et al. 1989). Riemer et al. (1999) reported on a single case of PACNS that was treated for 5 years with cyclophosphamide (cumulative dose 100 g). The patient ultimately died of cyclophosphamide-induced myelodysplastic syndrome. Post-mortem evaluation revealed vascular scarring and amyloid angiopathy; however, evaluation of the brain parenchyma revealed the absence of inflammation (Riemer et al. 1999).

Ideally, a national database encompassing patients with biopsy-proven and unproven PACNS, and their response to treatment, may help to define the optimal treatment regimen for this disorder.

20.9 Prognosis

The prognosis for patients with PACNS is variable due to the heterogeneity of the disease process with respect to progression and response to treatment. In addition, the natural history of the disease and long-term outcomes, for the most part, are unknown. Clearly important in improving the overall outcome is the rapid definitive diagnosis of PACNS with institution of appropriate treatment.

20.10 Case Discussion

The following case seen at this institution exemplifies the heterogeneity of PACNS, both clinically and pathologically, and the inherent difficulties in diagnosis and treatment. Some of the histopathological findings described here are unique and have not yet been reported in cases of PACNS.

A previously healthy right-handed 31-year-old man with no significant medical history initially presented with complaints of headache and transient right arm and leg weakness which began 7 days prior. His headache was described as being constant and unremitting with sharp pain located bi-frontally.

His general medical examination was unremarkable. No focal findings were observed on neurological examination. A complete blood count (CBC), comprehensive metabolic panel (CMP), including liver function tests, erythrocyte sedimentation rate (ESR), C-reactive protein (CRP), urine toxicology screen (U-TOX), serum protein electrophoresis (SPEP), extended anti-nuclear antibody panel (ANA), complement level, serum amino acids, and lactate level, were ordered and found to be within normal limits. On CSF analysis his opening pressure was 17 cm H_20, RBC 1/mm^3, nucleated cells 11/mm^3 (88% lymphocytes, 4% polymorphonuclear cells), glucose 74 mg/dl, and protein 35 mg/dl. The CSF cultures were negative for growth. The CSF cytology was negative for malignant cells and herpes simplex virus–polymerase chain reaction (HSV–PCR) test was negative.

An electroencephalogram (EEG) demonstrated focal slowing of the background rhythm over the left hemisphere. No electrographic seizure events or epileptiform activity were observed. An MRI of the brain demonstrated non-contrast enhancing, diffusion-negative T2 signal hyperintensities involving the left frontal and temporal lobe regions (Fig. 20.3a,b).

The patient was treated with high-dose methylprednisolone (1 g/day) for 3 days and was discharged to home where he completed a 15-day course of acyclovir. Improvement of his symptoms was reported at the time of discharge.

One month later, the patient returned to the hospital with complaints of language difficulty. He reported "mixing up" his words during conversation. He also had complaints of increased headache, confusion, muscle aches, fatigue, and left thumb twitching lasting seconds to minutes. Neurological examination was again found to be non-focal. A CBC, CMP, ESR, and CRP were again ordered and found to be within normal limits. Coagulation studies and rheumatoid factor were also found to be within normal limits. Repeat CSF analysis revealed nine nucleated cells per cubic millimeter (74% polymorphonuclear cells, 17% lymphocytes), RBC 0/mm^3, glucose 74 mg/dl, and protein 58 mg/dl. The CSF cultures and HSV–PCR were negative. The CSF lactate was within normal limits.

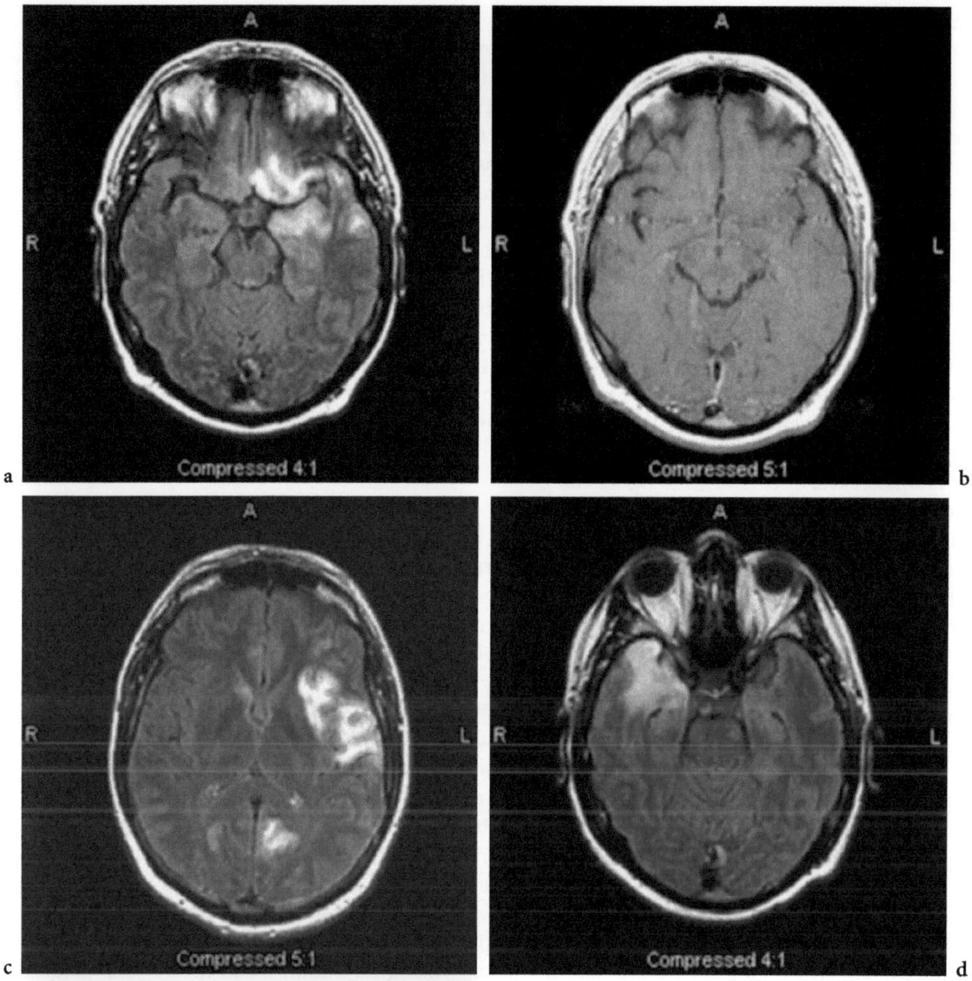

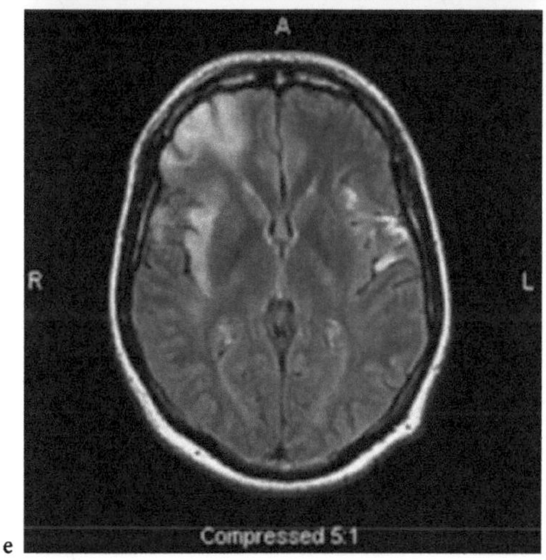

Fig. 20.3 **a** Axial brain FLAIR MRI image demonstrates cortical and subcortical high-signal abnormalities involving the left inferior frontal lobe, left posterior frontal lobe, and left temporal lobe. **b** Axial brain MRI T1-weighted image with gadolinium. No contrast enhancement is observed. **c** Axial brain FLAIR MRI image demonstrates left frontal lobe, medial parietal lobe, and left occipital lobe high-signal abnormalities. **d** Right temporal lobe high-signal abnormality on axial FLAIR MRI imaging. **e** Axial brain FLAIR MRI scan demonstrates new region of confluent high-signal abnormality involving the cortex and subcortical white matter of the right frontal lobe, right anterior temporal lobe, and right insular region

The patient underwent a repeat EEG with focal background slowing observed over the left fronto-temporal region. No discrete electrographic seizure events were captured and no epileptiform activity was observed. A repeat MRI of the brain with gadolinium demonstrated non-contrast-enhancing and diffusion-negative T2-hyperintensities involving the left frontal, temporal, and occipital lobes (Fig. 20.3c). The patient underwent the same treatment course as his previous hospitalization with modest improvement of his symptoms and was discharged.

Two months following his second discharge from the hospital, the patient presented after a generalized tonic–clonic seizure preceded by reports of automatisms and abdominal discomfort. He also had complaints of right ear numbness and fullness, left forearm numbness, chest discomfort, and right hemispheric headaches. Neurological examination again was non-focal. An HIV test was ordered which was negative. Serological tests were ordered once again (p-antineutrophil cytoplasmic antibody, c-antineutrophil cytoplasmic antibody, extended ANA panel, serum lactate, Lyme disease serologies, CRP) and found to be normal. He underwent a muscle biopsy to exclude the possibility of a mitochondrial disorder. Histological evaluation of the muscle architecture revealed normal findings. A four-vessel cerebral angiogram was normal with no signs of vasculitis observed. Magnetic resonance imaging revealed abnormalities now involving the right hemisphere with marked improvement of T2-hyperintensities observed previously involving the left hemisphere (Fig. 20.3d,e).

A stereotactic biopsy of the right frontal region was performed. Histopathology revealed lymphocytic invasion of both the meninges and vasculature (Fig. 20.4a–d). The surrounding parenchyma was significant for areas of infarction. There were no signs of hemorrhage observed. Staining of the cortex with von Kossa was positive, demonstrating spiculated calcium deposits throughout infarcted brain tissue (Fig. 20.4e). This was further confirmed by electron microscopy studies which had been performed initially to determine the presence of fungal and viral inclusion particles. Electron microscopy of brain tissue was negative for any infectious process. The sampled tissue was, however, significant for areas of dystrophic calcification in addition to abnormal calcium deposits adjacent to dendrites (Figs. 20.5, 20.6). Dystrophic calcification was also observed involving the mitochondria (Fig. 20.5c,d). Although the role of calcium in cell injury has been greatly studied, this finding has not been described or previously reported in cases of vasculitis involving the CNS (Trump et al. 1980).

The patient was treated with daily oral prednisone (60 mg/day with slow taper over 1 year) and cyclophosphamide (2 g IV every month for 6 months followed by infusions once every 2 months) with good result. Azathioprine was also added to his treatment regimen. He continued on phenytoin and lamotrigine for his seizures. Since completing the treatment regimen, the patient has remained symptom free for 18 months. Serial MRI scans of the brain have demonstrated signs of encephalomalacia but no progression of disease or areas of increased T2-signal abnormality.

20.11 Conclusion

Physicians are faced daily with the challenges of accurately diagnosing patients by employing the current diagnostic criteria, recommended structural neuroimaging techniques, and/or guidelines put forth by ad hoc committees, consensus groups, and data from large, multicenter, placebo-controlled studies. A comprehensive understanding of the approach to PACNS from the etiology to optimal treatment is currently not clearly defined. This is a rare disorder that represents a unique diagnostic challenge for the neurologist given the lack of uniformity with respect to the clinical presentation, radiological and histopathological findings, and the varying natural history of the disease. This condition is restricted to the CNS with no signs of systemic involvement and biopsy of the brain parenchyma and leptomeninges is paramount in the diagnosis. A delay in the diagnosis and proper treatment of the disorder may cause increased morbidity and death. Current treatment strategies should be initiated aggressively, but only after confirmation of the diagnosis has been made. The diagnosis should not be made based on any single study. Instead, historical, clinical, serological, radiological, and histopathological correlation is needed for an accurate diagnosis. It is only by this approach that appropriate treatment interventions can be instituted in a timely manner to increase the likelihood of a better outcome. Future studies may focus on the genetic predilection for this condition which may provide insight into its pathogenesis and varied clinical course as well as treatment response.

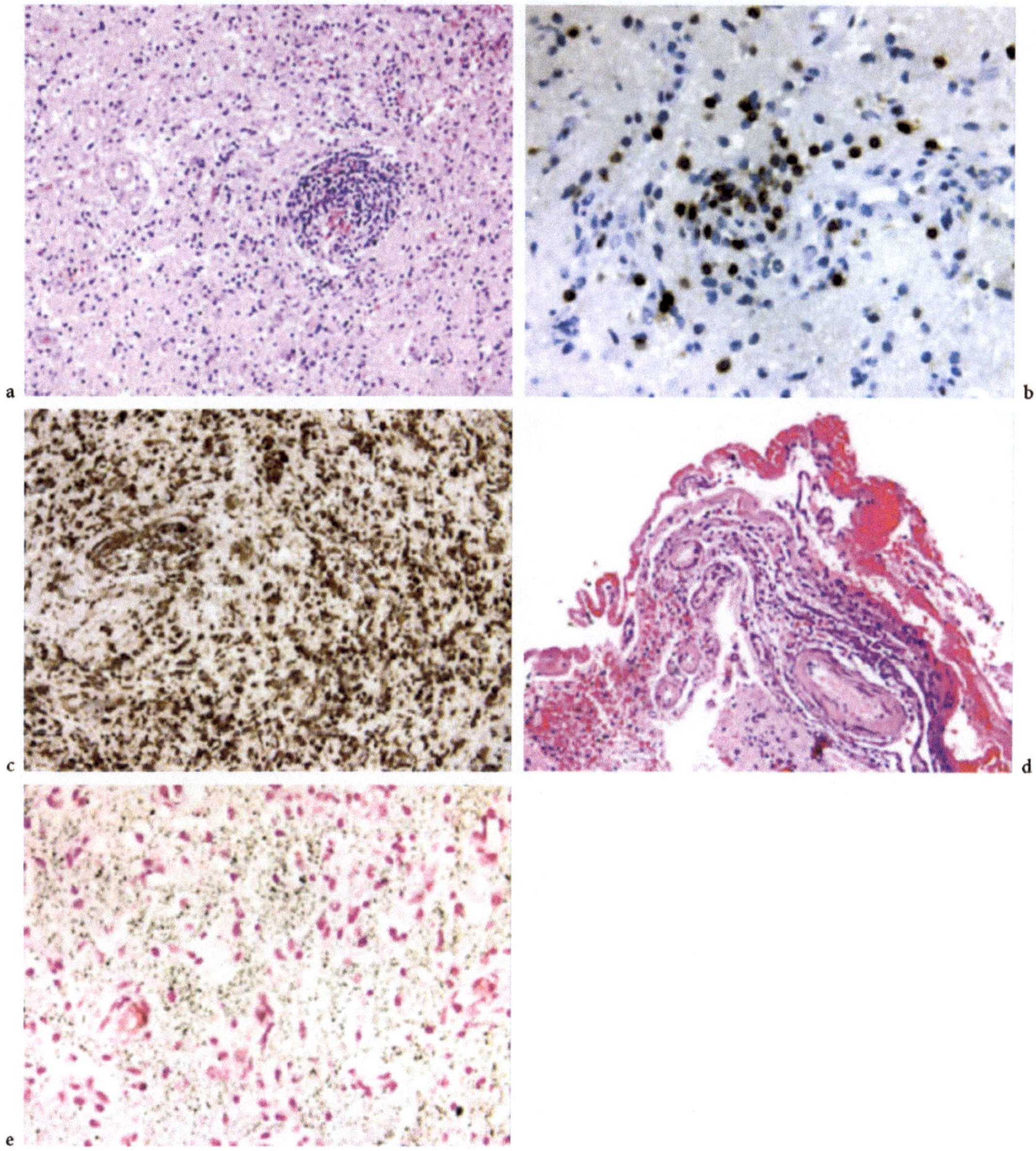

Fig. 20.4 a The cerebral cortex is edematous with numerous parenchymal mononuclear cells. Focal marked perivascular mononuclear cuffing is also present (hematoxylin–eosin stain, original magnification ×200). **b** Histopathological slide of brain tissue demonstrating numerous perivascular mononuclear cells. Abundant small lymphocytes reactive for the T-cell marker CD-3 are seen. Diaminobenzidine and hematoxylin–eosin stain (original magnification, ×400). **c** Many of the perivascular cells are reactive for CD-68, a marker for monocytes, macrophages, and microglia. In addition, numerous CD-68 reactive cells are seen throughout the brain parenchyma. Diaminobenzidine and hematoxylin–eosin stain (original magnification ×200). **d** Histopathological slide of meninges demonstrating scattered small lymphoid cells (hematoxylin–eosin stain, original magnification ×200). **e** Numerous coarse black granules of calcium are scattered throughout the parenchyma (von Kossa, original magnification ×400)

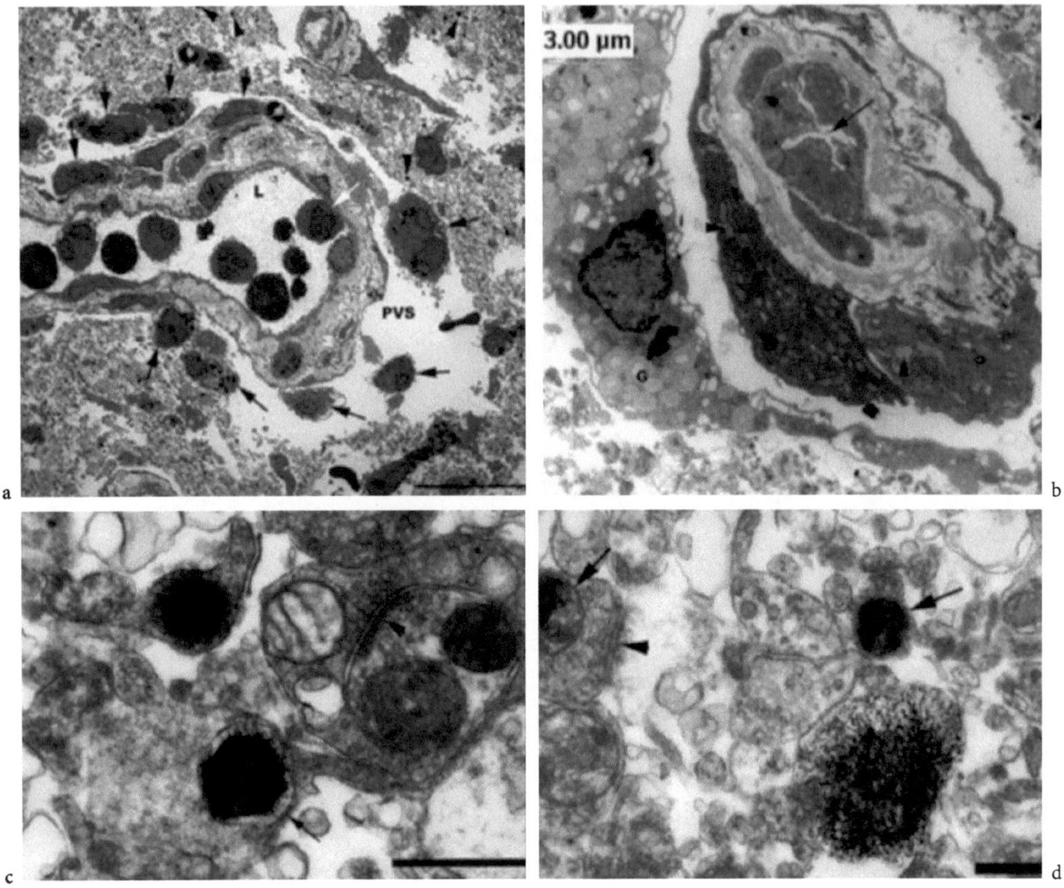

Fig. 20.5 a Low magnification (Bar=20µm) electron micrograph. Lumen *(L)* of this gray matter venule contains numerous leucocytes, one of which *(white arrow)* is attached to the endothelium in the process of emigration. The perivascular space *(PVS)* exhibits numerous inflammatory cells *(black arrows)*. The PVS as well as the extracellular spaces are significantly widened consistent with vasogenic edema. The highly disorganized neuropil contains numerous calcium deposits; a few are shown with black arrowheads. **b** The lumen (arrow) of this microvessel is compromised due to endothelial hypertrophy. Perivascular inflammatory cells with long processes encircle the vessel. Extensive arrays of dilated rough endoplasmic cisternae (arrowheads) are filled with a fine granular material. Ultrastructurally these cells appear as plasma cells. Gitter (foam) cells *(G)* also occupy the perivascular space. **c** Neuropil debris consists of neural processes, two of which contain calcium deposits. One deposit is localized within the matrix of a mitochondrion; arrow identifies the outer mitochondrial membrane. Among the cellular debris an intact axon-dendritic synaptic contact is seen; arrowhead identifies the post-synaptic specialization of the dendrite. In the axon terminal, a cluster of clear round synaptic vesicles are near the presynaptic membrane. Bar = 0.5 µm. **d** A mitochondrion with a calcium deposit can be seen *(arrow)*. The post-synaptic membrane *(arrowhead)* is the only remains of this disintegrated dendrite. A neural element below the right arrow contains calcium deposits in the form of thin spicules (see Fig. 20.6c) that appear free (non-membrane bound) within the cytoplasm. Bar = 0.5 µm

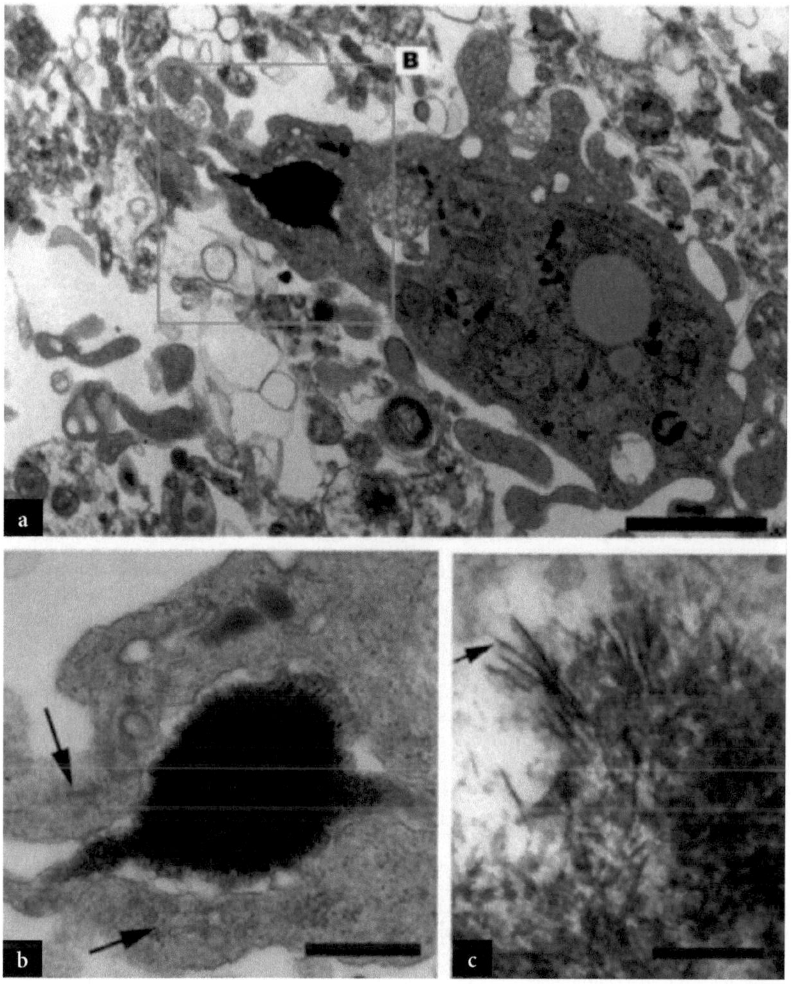

Fig.20.6 a A macrophage is in the process of phagocytizing a neural process containing a calcium deposit. Bar= 1.5 µm. A higher magnification of the boxed area is shown in inset **b** which demonstrates macrophage pseudopods *(arrows)* engulfing the calcium deposit. Bar = 0.5 µm. These deposits appear to be composed of thin spicules (~6nm in diameter) which radiate outwardly at the periphery of the deposit. *(inset C)* Bar = 100 nm

References

Alhalabi M, Moore PM (1994) Serial angiography in isolated angiitis of the central nervous system. Neurology 44:1221–1226

Alreshaid AA, Powers WJ (2003) Prognosis of patients with suspected primary CNS angiitis and negative brain biopsy. Neurology 61:831–833

Alrawi A, Trobe JD, Blaivas M et al (1999) Brain biopsy in primary angiitis of the central nervous system. Neurology 11/53:858–860

Alreshaid AA, Powers WJ (2003) Prognosis of patients with suspected primary CNS angiitis and negative brain biopsy. Neurology 61:831–833

Ay H, Sahin G, Saatci I et al (2002) Primary angiitis of the central nervous system and silent cortical hemorrhages. Am J Neuroradiol 23:1561–1563

Barron TF, Ostrov BE, Zimmerman RA et al (1993) Isolated angiitis of CNS: treatment with pulse cyclophosphamide. Pediatr Neurol 9:73–75

Berlit P (1994) The spectrum of vasculopathies in the differential diagnosis of vasculitis. Semin Neurol 14:370–379

Bettoni L, Bortjuvatta G, Lecki A (1984) Isolated benign cerebral vasculitis. Arch Neurol 84:161–163

Bradley JD, Brandt KD, Katz BP (1989) Infectious complications of cyclophosphamide treatment of vasculitis. Arthritis Rheum 32:45–53

Calabrese LH (1995) Vasculitis of the central nervous system. Rheum Dis Clin North Am 21:1059–1076
Calabrese LH, Mallek JA (1988) Primary angiitis of the central nervous system: report of eight new cases, review of literature and proposal for diagnostic criteria. Medicine 67:20–39
Calabrese LH, Furlan AJ, Gragg LA (1992) Primary angiitis of the central nervous system: diagnostic criteria and clinical approach. Cleve Clin J Med 59:293–306
Calabrese LH, Gragg LA, Furlan AJ (1993) Benign angiopathy: a distinct subset of angiographically defined primary angiitis of the central nervous system. J Rheumatol 20:2046–2050
Calabrese LH, Duna GF, Lie JT (1997) Vasculitis in the central nervous system. Arthritis Rheum 40:1189–1201
Campi A, Benndorf G, Filippi M et al (2001a) Primary angiitis of the central nervous system: serial MRI of brain and spinal cord. Neuroradiology 43:599–607
Campi A, Benndorf G, Martinelli V et al (2001b) Spinal cord involvement in primary angiitis of the central nervous system: a report of two cases. Am J Neuroradiol 22:577–582
Chu TC, Gray L, Goldstein B et al (1998) Diagnosis of intracranial vasculitis: a multidisciplinary approach. J Neuropathol Exp Neurol 57:30–38
Coakham HM, Duchen LW, Scaravilli F (1979) Moya-moya disease: clinical and pathological report of a case with associated myopathy. J Neurol Neurosurg Psychiatry 42:289–297
Crane R, Kerr LD, Spiera H (1991) Clinical analysis of isolated angiitis of the central nervous system: a report of 11 cases. Arch Intern Med 151:2290–2294
Craven RS, French JK (1985) Isolated angiitis of the central nervous system. Ann Neurol 18:263–265
Cravioto H, Feigin I (1959) Noninfectious granulomatous angiitis with a predilection for the nervous system. Neurology 9:599–609
Cupps TR, Moore PM, Fauci AS (1983) Isolated angiitis of the central nervous system: prospective diagnostic and therapeutic experience. Am J Med 74:97–105
Duna GF, Calabrese LH (1995) Limitations of invasive modalities in the diagnosis of primary angiitis of the central nervous system. J Rheumatol 22:662–667
Duna GF, George T, Rybicki L (1995) Primary angiitis of the central nervous system: an analysis of unusual presentations (abstract). Arthritis Rheum 38 (Suppl 9):S340
Ehsan T, Hasan S, Powers JM et al (1995) Serial magnetic resonance imaging in isolated angiitis of the central nervous system. Neurology 45:1462–1465
Engelter ST, Rueegg S, Kirsch EC et al (2002) CADASIL mimicking primary angiitis of the central nervous system. Arch Neurol 59:1480–1483
Ferris EJ, Levine HL (1973) Cerebral arteritis: classification. Radiology 109:327–341
Finelli PF, Onyiuke HC, Uphoff DF (1997) Idiopathic granulomatous angiitis of the CNS manifesting as diffuse white matter disease. Neurology 49:1696–1699
Fountain NB, Eberhard DA (1996) Primary angiitis of the central nervous system associated with cerebral amyloid angiopathy: report of two cases and review of the literature. Neurology 46:190–197
Fountain NB, Lopes MBS (1999) Control of primary angiitis of the CNS associated with cerebral amyloid angiopathy by cyclophosphamide alone. Neurology 52:660–662
Gallagher KT, Shaham B, Reiff A (2001) Primary angiitis of the central nervous system in children: 5 cases. J Rheumatol 28:616–623
Gertner E, Hamlar D (2002) Necrotizing granulomatous vasculitis associated with cocaine use. J Rheumatol 29:1795–1797
Giang DW (1994) Central nervous system vasculitis secondary to infections, toxins, and neoplasms. Semin Neurol 14:313–319
Giovanini MA, Eskin TA, Mukherji SK et al (1994) Granulomatous angiitis of the spinal cord: a case report. Neurosurgery 34:540–543
Glick R, Hoying J, Cerullo L et al (1987) Phenylpropanolamine: an over-the-counter drug causing central nervous system vasculitis and intracerebral hemorrhage (case report and review). Neurosurgery 20:969–974
Greco FA, Kolins J, Rajjoub RK et al (1976) Hodgkin's disease and granulomatous angiitis of the central nervous system. Cancer 38:2027–2032
Greenan TJ, Grossman RI, Goldberg HI (1992) Cerebral vasculitis: MR imaging and angiographic correlation. Radiology 182:65–72
Griffin J, Price DL, Davis L (1973) Granulomatous angiitis of the central nervous system with aneurysms on multiple cerebral arteries. Trans Am Neurol Assoc 98:145–148
Hajj-Ali RA, Villa-Forte AL, Abou-Chebel A et al (2000) Long term outcomes of patients with primary angiitis of the central nervous system (PACNS) (abstract). Arthritis Rheum 43 (Suppl 9):S162
Hajj-Ali RA, Furlan A, Abou-Chebel A et al (2002) Benign angiopathy of the central nervous system: cohort of 16 patients with clinical course and long-term follow-up. Arthritis Rheum 47:662–669
Harbitz F (1922) Unknown forms of arteritis with special reference to their relation to syphilitic arteritis and periarteritis nodosa. Am J Med 163:250
Harris KG, Tran DD, Sickels WJ et al (1994) Diagnosing intracranial vasculitis: the roles of MR and angiography. Am J Neuroradiol 15:317–330
Heiserman JE, Dean BL, Hodak JA et al (1994) Neurologic complications of cerebral angiography. Am J Neuroradiol 15:1401–1407
Houser OW, Baker HL Jr (1968) Fibromuscular dysplasia and other uncommon diseases of the cervical carotid artery: angiographic aspects. Am J Roentgenol Radium Ther Nucl Med 104:201–212
Johnson M, Maciunas R, Dutt P et al (1989) Granulomatous angiitis masquerading as a mass lesion: magnetic resonance imaging and stereotactic findings in a patient with occult Hodgkin's disease. Surg Neurol 31:49–53
Katsicas MM, Russo R, Taratuto A et al (2000) Primary angiitis of the central nervous system presenting as a mass lesion in a child. J Rheumatol 27:1297–1298
Kolodny EH, Rebeiz JJ, Caviness VS et al (1968) Granulomatous angiitis of the central nervous system. Arch Neurol 19:510–524
Koo EH, Massey EW (1988) Granulomatous angiitis of the central nervous system: protean manifestations and response to treatment. J Neurol Neurosurg Psychiatry 51:1126–1133
Kumar R, Wijdicks EF, Brown RD Jr et al (1997) Isolated angiitis of the CNS presenting as subarachnoid haemorrhage. J Neurol Neurosurg Psychiatry 62:649–651
Langford CA (2003) Vasculitis. J Allergy Clin Immunol 111: S602–S612

Lanthier S, Lortie A, Michaud J et al (2001) Isolated angiitis of the CNS in children. Neurology 56:837–842
Leeds NE, Goldberg HI (1971) Angiographic manifestations in cerebral inflammatory disease. Radiology 98:595–604
Lehrer H (1966) The angiographic triad in tuberculous meningitis. A radiographic and clinicopathologic correlation. Radiology 87:829–835
Lie JT (1992) Primary (granulomatous) angiitis of the central nervous system: a clinicopathologic analysis of 15 new cases and a review of the literature. Hum Pathol 23:164–171
Liem MD, Gzesh DJ, Flanders AE (1996) MRI and angiographic diagnosis of lupus cerebral vasculitis. Neuroradiology 38:134–136
Mackenzie RA, Forbes GS, Karnes WE (1981) Angiographic findings in herpes zoster arteritis. Ann Neurol 10:458–464
Mandybur TI, Balko G (1992) Cerebral amyloid angiopathy with granulomatous angiitis ameliorated by steroid-cytoxan treatment. Clin Neuropharmacol 15:241–247
Marazuela M, Garcia-Merino A, Yebra M et al (1989) Magnetic resonance imaging and angiography of the brain in embolic left atrial myxoma. Neuroradiology 31:137–139
Margolis MT, Newton TH (1971) Methamphetamine ("speed") arteritis. Neuroradiology 2:179–182
Matsell DG, Keene DL, Jimenez C et al (1990) Isolated angiitis of the central nervous system in childhood. Can J Neurol Sci 17:151–154
Merkel KH, Ginsberg PL, Parker JC Jr (1978) Cerebrovascular disease in sickle cell anemia: a clinical, pathological and radiological correlation. Stroke 9:45–52
Moore PM (1989) Diagnosis and management of isolated angiitis of the central nervous system. Neurology 39:167–173
Moore PM (1994) Vasculitis of the central nervous system. Semin Neurol 14:313–319
Moore PM (1995) Neurological manifestation of vasculitis: update on immunopathogenic mechanisms and clinical features. Ann Neurol 37:S131–S141
Moore PM, Cupps TR (1983) Neurological complications of vasculitis. Ann Neurol 14:155–167
Moore PM, Richardson B (1998) Neurology of the vasculitides and connective tissue diseases. J Neurol Neurosurg Psychiatry 65:10–22
Negishi C, Sze G (1993) Vasculitis presenting as primary leptomeningeal enhancement with minimal parenchymal findings. Am J Neuroradiol 14:26–28
Newman W, Wolf A (1952) Non-infectious granulomatous angiitis involving the central nervous system. Trans Am Neurol Assoc 77:114–117
Nishikawa M, Sakamoto H, Katsuyama J et al (1998) Multiple appearing and vanishing aneurysms: primary angiitis of the central nervous system. J Neurosurg 88:133–137
Nogueras C, Sala M, Sasal M et al (2002) Recurrent stroke as a manifestation of primary angiitis of the central nervous system in a patient infected with human immunodeficiency virus. Arch Neurol 59:468–473
Nurick S, Blackwood W, Mair WGP (1972) Giant cell granulomatous angiitis of the central nervous system. Brain 95:133–142
Oliveira V, Povoa P, Costa A et al (1994) Cerebrospinal fluid and therapy of isolated angiitis of the central nervous system. Stroke 25:1693–1695
Parisi JE, Moore PM (1994) The role of biopsy in vasculitis of the central nervous system. Semin Neurol 14:341–348
Rabinov KR (1963) Angiographic findings in a case of brain syphilis. Radiology 80:622–624
Ramos M, Mandybur TI (1975) Cerebral vasculitis in rheumatoid arthritis. Arch Neurol 32:271–275
Regan M, Haque U, Pomper M et al (2001) Central nervous system vasculitis as a complication of refractory dermatomyositis. J Rheumatol 28:207–211
Reik L, Grunnet ML, Spencer RP et al (1983) Granulomatous angiitis presenting as chronic meningitis and ventriculitis. Neurology 33:1609–1612
Reyes MG, Fresco R, Chokrovety S et al (1976) Virus-like particles in granulomatous angiitis of the central nervous system. Neurology 26:797–799
Riemer G, Lamszus K, Kschaber R et al (1999) Isolated angiitis of the central nervous system: lack of inflammation after long-term treatment. Neurology 52:196–199
Ritter MA, Dziewas R, Papke K et al (2002) Follow-up examinations by transcranial Doppler ultrasound in primary angiitis of the central nervous system. Cerebrovasc Dis 14:139–142
Rosenblum WI, Hadfield MG (1972) Granulomatous angiitis of the nervous system in cases of herpes zoster and lymphosarcoma. Neurology 22:348–354
Rumbaugh CL, Bergeron RT, Fang HC et al (1971) Cerebral angiographic changes in the drug abuse patient. Radiology 101:335–344
Schwab P, Lidov HGW, Schwartz RB (2003) Cerebral amyloid angiopathy associated with primary angiitis of the central nervous system: report of 2 cases and review of the literature. Arthritis Rheum 49:421–427
Scully R (1989) Case records of the Massachusetts General Hospital, case 8-1989: weekly clinicopathological exercises. N Engl J Med 320:514–524
Shoemaker EI, Lin ZS, Rae-Grant AD et al (1994) Primary angiitis of the central nervous system: unusual MR appearance. Am J Neuroradiol 15:331–334
Siva A (2001) Vasculitis of the nervous system. J Neurol 248:151–168
Siva A, Kantarci OH, Saip S et al (2001) Behset's disease: diagnostic and prognostic aspects of neurological involvement. J Neurol 248:95–103
Snyder BD, McClelland RR (1978) Isolated benign cerebral vasculitis. Arch Neurol 35:612–614
Stein RL, Martino CR, Weinert DM et al (1987) Cerebral angiography as a guide for therapy in isolated central nervous system vasculitis. J Am Med Assoc 257:2193–2195
Stone JH, Pomper MG, Roubenoff R et al (1994) Sensitivities of noninvasive tests for central nervous system vasculitis: a comparison of lumbar puncture, computed tomography, and magnetic resonance imaging. J Rheumatol 21:1277–1282
Trevor RP, Sondheimer FK, Fessel WJ et al (1972) Angiographic demonstration of major cerebral vessel occlusion in systemic lupus erythematosus. Neuroradiology 4:202–207
Trump BF, Berezesky IK, Laiho KU et al (1980) The role of calcium in cell injury (a review). Scan Electron Microsc 492:437–462
Vanderzant C, Bromberg M, MacGuire A et al (1988) Isolated small-vessel angiitis of the central nervous system. Arch Neurol 45:683–687
Vollmer TL, Guarnaccia J, Harrington W et al (1993) Idiopathic granulomatous angiitis of the central nervous system: diagnostic challenges. Arch Neurol 50:925–930

Walker RJ III, Gammal TE, Allen MB (1973) Cranial arteritis associated with herpes zoster. Case report with angiographic findings. Radiology 107:109–110

Woolfenden AR, Tong DC, Marks MP et al (1998) Angiographically defined primary angiitis of the CNS. Is it really benign? Neurology 51:183–188

Yasuda Y, Matsuda I, Kang Y et al (1993) Isolated angiitis of the central nervous system first presenting as intracranial hemorrhage during cesarean section. Intern Med 32:745–748

Younger DS, Calabrese LH, Hays AP (1997) Granulomatous angiitis of the nervous system. Neurol Clin 15:821–834

Zivkovic S, Moore PM (2000) Systemic and central nervous system vasculitides. Curr Treat Opt Neurol 2:459–472

21 Neuro-Psychiatric Systemic Lupus Erythematosus

BART J. EMMER, TOM W. J. HUIZINGA, and MARK A. VAN BUCHEM

CONTENTS

21.1 SLE and NPSLE

Systemic lupus erythematosus (SLE) is an autoimmune disease characterized by a relapsing and remitting course and symptoms based on multi-organ involvement. These symptoms are mainly caused by inflammation of connective tissues due to the presence of antibodies directed against various self-epitopes.

B. J. EMMER, MD, PhD; T. W. J. HUIZINGA, MD
Department of Radiology, Leiden University Medical Center, Albinusdreef 2, Postbus 9600, 2300 RC Leiden, The Netherlands
M. A. VAN BUCHEM, MD, PhD
Professor and Head Neuroradiology, Department of Radiology, Leiden University Medical Center, Albinusdreef 2, Postbus 9600, 2300 RC Leiden, The Netherlands

Reports on the prevalence of SLE range from 1:2000 to 1:4000 and estimations of the female to male ratio vary from 5:1 to 10:1. Systemic lupus erythematosus is more common in people of Hispanic, African, or Asian descent. (AINIALA et al. 2001; BREY et al. 2002; CERVERA et al. 2003). Genetic factors may contribute to the development of SLE as is suggested by the observed 25% concordance in identical twins (GILES and ISENBERG 2001).

Systemic lupus erythematosus has a wide variety of possible presentations and for classification purposes a patient is considered to have SLE if at least 4 of the 11 criteria listed in Table 21.1 are positive. The mortality in SLE has decreased over the last couple of decades. In a literature-based study by UROWITZ and GLADMAN (2000) published survival rates were collected from 1955 through 1999, showing an increase in 5-year survival from 50 to of 91%. A recent longitudinal study of 1000 patients over 10 years by (CERVERA et al. 2003) found a survival rate of 92%; however, with this increase in survival due to better treatment options, these studies also revealed increased morbidity due to serious side effects of drugs such as steroids and cytostatic agents.

21.1.2 NPSLE

Many SLE patients develop neurological or psychiatric symptoms during the course of the disease, with reported percentages as high as 75%. BREY et al. found a striking discrepancy between the percentage of SLE patients (28%) that met the accepted neurological criteria for the diagnosis of SLE based on current criteria by the American College of Rheumatology (TAN et al. 1982) and the percentage of SLE patients (80%) that met the more recently developed diagnostic criteria for neuropsychiatric (NP) syndromes associated with SLE using the neuropsychiatric SLE (NPSLE) case definitions (BREY et al. 2002; Table 21.2) In this context, diagnostic definitions for NPSLE as well as exclusion criteria have

Table 21.1 The "1997 revised" criteria (From Tan et al. 1982)

Malar rash	Fixed erythema, flat or raised, over the malar eminences, tending to spare to nasolabial folds
Discoid rash	Erythematous raised patches with adherent keratotic scaling and follicular plugging. Atrophic scarring may occur in older lesions
Photosensitivity	Skin rash as a result of unusual reaction to sunlight, by patient history or physician observation
Oral ulcers	Oral or nasopharyngeal ulceration, usually painless, observed by physician
Arthritis	Nonerosive arthritis involving two or more peripheral joints, characterized by tenderness, swelling, or effusion
Serositis	a) Pleuritis-convincing history of pleuritic pain or rubbing heard by a physician or evidence of pleural effusion OR b) Pericarditis-documented by ECG or rub or evidence of pericardial effusion
Renal disorder	a) Persistent proteinuria greater than 0.5 g per day or greater than 3+ if quantitation not performed b) Cellular casts: may be red cell, hemoglobin, granular, tubular, or mixed
Neurological disorder	a) Seizures, in the absence of offending drugs or known metabolic derangements, e.g., uremia, ketoacidosis, or electrolyte imbalance b) Psychosis, in the absence of offending drugs or known metabolic derangements, e.g., uremia, ketoacidosis, or electrolyte imbalance
Hematological disorder	a) Hemolytic anemia, with reticulocytosis, or b) Leukopenia, $<4000/mm^3$ total on two or more occasions, or c) Lymphopenia, $<1500/mm^3$ on two or more occasions d) Thrombocytopenia, $<100{,}000/mm^3$ in the absence of offending drugs)
Immunological disorder	Anti-DNA: antibody to native DNA in abnormal titer or anti-Sm: presence of antibody to Sm nuclear antigen or positive finding of antiphospholipid antibodies based on: 1) An abnormal serum level of IgG or IgM anticardiolipin antibodies 2) A positive test result for lupus anticoagulant using a standard method 3) A false-positive serological test for syphilis known to be positive for at least 6 months and confirmed by *Treponema pallidum* immobilization or fluorescent treponemal antibody absorption test. "Standard" methods should be used in testing for the presence of antiphospholipid
Antinuclear antibody	An abnormal titer of antinuclear antibody by immunofluorescence or an equivalent assay at any point in time and in the absence of drugs known to be associated with "drug-induced" lupus syndrome

been described. In patients with, for example, chorea, it is mandated that conditions such as Huntington disease and Wilson disease and medication associated with chorea be excluded (Huizinga et al. 2001; The American College Of Rheumatology 1999). Brey et al. also found a large contribution of NP manifestations to the overall SLE disease activity index (SLEDAI) and SLE damage index (SDI) suggesting that nervous system manifestations are an important source of both acute and chronic morbidity in SLE patients (Brey et al. 2002). The SLEDAI is a validated model of experienced clinicians' global assessments of disease activity in lupus. It represents the consensus of a group of experts in the field of SLE research (Bombardier et al. 1992). The SDI records damage occurring in patients with SLE regardless of its cause (Gladman et al. 1996).

The NPSLE patients can be subdivided into primary and secondary NPSLE. In 40% of cases NPSLE is the consequence of secondary causes such as metabolic derangement based on SLE damage to organs other than the brain or due to side effects of drug treatment. These conditions are known as secondary NPSLE. In the remaining 60% of cases the symptoms are ascribed to primary SLE involvement of the brain, which is referred to as primary NPSLE (Rood et al. 1999).

Primary NPSLE can be divided into focal and diffuse disease. The focal disease is strongly associated with the occurrence of thrombo-embolic events. Diffuse primary NPSLE is an elusive group of neurological, psychiatric, and cognitive symptoms (Bosma et al. 2002) comprising conditions such as aseptic meningitis, demyelination syndrome, seizures, cognitive dysfunction, headache, chorea, mood disturbances, myelopathy, cranial neuropathy, anxiety disorders, psychosis, and disorientation (Huizinga et al. 2001). Often no abnormalities are found on conventional neuro-imaging techniques in this group.

It is often unclear whether SLE patients with NP symptoms should be treated, and if so, what kind of treatment should be used. Diagnosing primary NPSLE is a dilemma since symptoms (Table 21.2) are non-specific and because a reliable diagnostic test is lacking. Despite the strict ACR case-definitions and the extensive research, primary NPSLE is still a diagnosis *per exclusionem*.

Table 21.2 The 1999 ACR standardized nomenclature system for NPSLE

Central nervous system	Peripheral nervous system
Aseptic meningitis	Acute inflammatory demyelinating polyradiculopathy (Guillain-Barré syndrome)
Cerebrovascular disease	Autonomic disorder, mononeuropathy (single or multiplex)
Demyelinating syndrome	Myasthenia gravis
Headache (including migraine and benign intracranial hypertension)	Neuropathy (cranial)
Movement disorder (chorea)	Plexopathy
Myelopathy	Polyneuropathy
Seizure disorders	–
Acute confusional state	–
Mood disorders	–
Psychosis	–
Anxiety disorder	–
Cognitive dysfunction	–

(The American College of Rheumatology nomenclature and case definitions for neuropsychiatric lupus syndromes 1999)

21.1.2.1 Pathology

Reports on histopathological findings in NPSLE are scarce. Bland vasculopathy of arterioles and capillaries is the most common finding and is associated with micro-infarction, most frequently observed in the cerebral cortex and brain stem. This vasculopathy is characterized by evidence of necrosis of the vessel wall, extravasations of fibrin and red blood cells, together with endothelial cell proliferation, hypertrophy, and the appearance of fibrin thrombi. Despite incidental perivascular cuffing of arterioles or venules, a true vasculitis, defined as nuclear debris and erythrocytes in the vessel wall, is not frequently demonstrated as a histological finding in NPSLE; however, very few studies are present from patients with acute symptomatology. So, the frequency of vessel involvement during acute symptoms in NPSLE is not exactly known. Rood et al. identified 65 case reports of patients with a histopathological description and acute symptoms in literature from 1966 to 1999 (Rood et al. 2001). In 20 cases there was infection, in 10 cases micro-infarcts and thrombo-embolic processes, and in 10 cases cerebral vasculitis. In conclusion, cerebral vasculitis is described in histopathological material obtained in patients with acute pathology. With regard to general histopathology studies, these series often describe patients with a history of NPSLE and thus the time course of the pathological changes with regard to symptomatology is difficult to assess. In such studies the presence of vasculitis is relatively rare (Ellis and Verity 1979; Hess 1997; Johnson and Richardson 1968; West 1994; Zvaifler and Bluestein 1982).

Although both inflammatory and thrombotic processes have been presumed to underlie the observed histological changes, the etiology of these findings is still unknown. Still, it is clear that complement, antibodies, thrombosis, and cytokines each have their part in the development of NPSLE.

Focal NPSLE can be explained by either a thrombotic event in a large vessel or by multiple events in small vessels. The first option is strongly associated with the presence of antiphospholipid antibodies (aPL). Antiphospholipid antibodies form a separate category within the group of auto-antibodies, and their presence may give rise to the development of thrombo-embolic disease, antiphospholipid syndrome (APS), cardiac lesions, fibromuscular dysplasia, vasculitis, and atherosclerosis. Antiphospholipid syndrome was first described in patients with SLE (secondary APS) but may occur in the absence of any other disorder (primary APS; Scolding and Joseph 2002). In the second option, vasculopathy of small vessels is the most likely cause. Thrombotic events, causing infarction with focal clinical signs, can be seen with conventional imaging techniques. On the other hand, when NP symptoms are due to events in small vessels, there often is a "clinico-radiological paradox", i.e., a lack of abnormalities on conventional MR images despite the presence of even severe symptoms.

It is much more difficult to incorporate the different observations in *diffuse* NPSLE into a single model. Vasculopathy is the most common abnormality at autopsy (Ellis and Verity 1979; Hess 1997; Johnson and Richardson 1968; West 1994). This vasculopathy can be caused by the presence of autoantibodies and/or circulating cytokines activating the endothelial vessel walls in the brain. (Belmont et al. 1996; Carvalho et al. 1999; Clancy et al. 2001; Hess 1997; Renaudineau et al. 2002). This process may induce activation of inflammatory cells leading to adherence of neutrophils and platelets to the activated vascular wall, occlusion of small vessels, and release of toxic mediators (Belmont et al. 1996). These changes may lead to hypoperfusion (Chen et al. 2002a,b; Colamussi et al. 1995; Emmi et al. 1993; Huang et al. 2002; Kao et al. 1999a; Nossent et al. 1991; Waterloo et al. 2001) and increased permeability of the blood-brain barrier (BBB). Antineuronal antibodies may gain access to the brain through the breached BBB (Rood et al. 2001; Zvaifler and Bluestein 1982) or they may develop *de novo* beyond the BBB in brain tissue (Rekvig and Nossent 2003). The activity of antineuronal antibodies may give rise to hypometabolism, neuronal loss, demyelination, and eventually atrophy (Bosma et al. 2000a,b; Brooks et al. 1997; Chinn et al. 1997; Griffey et al. 1990; Kao et al. 1999a,b; Otte et al. 1997; Sailer et al. 1997; Weiner et al. 2000b).

The mechanism of diffuse NPSLE probably also applies to cases with focal NPSLE without abnormalities on conventional imaging modalities. In these patients it is less likely that a thrombo-embolic process is the cause of the symptoms. In a large group of NPSLE patients markers indicating neuronal damage were markedly increased compared with SLE patients without NP symptoms (Trysberg et al. 2003). These findings agree with quantitative neuroimaging studies, showing loss of cerebral tissue in diffuse NPSLE (Bosma et al. 2000a,b). Furthermore, it has been shown in six patients that markers of neural damage normalize in CSF after treatment with cyclophosphamide (Trysberg et al. 2003).

21.1.2.2 Antibodies

Antibodies play a crucial role in the pathogenesis of SLE. A study by Arbuckle et al. describes the sequential development of autoantibodies years before SLE becomes clinically evident (Arbuckle et al. 2003). These authors suggest a model in which there are at least three phases. The first phase includes the asymptomatic persons without SLE autoantibodies. In the second phase, defined as *benign autoimmunity*, there are laboratory changes without corresponding clinical manifestations. Antinuclear, anti-Ro (intracytoplasmatic), Anti-La (lymphocytotoxic antibodies), or aPl antibodies are most likely to be present during this phase. The third phase, defined as *pathogenic autoimmunity*, is characterized by the presence of the more ominous autoantibodies anti-double-stranded DNA (anti-dsDNA), anti-Sm (intranuclear RNA molecules), and anti-nuclear ribonucleoprotein antibodies. During this stage prominent signs and symptoms appear.

The best proof that antibodies mediate pathology is the transfer of maternal autoantibodies crossing the placenta, causing neonatal lupus erythematosus (NLE). Given the fact that clinical signs and symptoms, such as cognitive deterioration, are extremely difficult to assess in newborns, neuroimaging studies have been performed. Neuroimaging abnormalities, similar to those seen in adults with NPSLE, have indeed been found. These abnormalities often resolve spontaneously after the maternal antibodies gradually disappear from the infant circulation. A correlation with clinical signs has not been observed in NLE (Prendiville et al. 2003).

In NPSLE, associations have been observed between NP symptoms and the presence of aPl antibodies as well as with anti-ribosomal-P protein antibodies (Baraczka et al. 2002; Sabet et al. 1998; Sanna et al. 2003b; Teh et al. 1993; Weiner et al. 2000a); however, these finding have been refuted as often as they have been confirmed and a clear correlation with NP symptoms remains to be established (Hanly et al. 1993; Tzioufas et al. 2000). More recently, neuronal antibodies have been found in NPSLE patients that act against the N-methyl-D-aspartate (NMDA) receptor NR2 (Kotzin and Kozora 2001). Activation of this receptor is known to play an important role in memory and cognitive function (Scherzer et al. 1998).

In addition to anti-endothelial antibodies (Belmont et al. 1996; Carvalho et al. 1999; Renaudineau et al. 2002), anti-cardiolipin antibodies have been implicated in activation of endothelial cells (Hess 1997). Furthermore, aPLs have been found to be associated with epilepsy (Herranz et al. 1994) as well with other CNS manifestations of SLE and MRI abnormalities (Sanna et al. 2003b; Toubi et al. 1995; Whitelaw et al. 1999). IgG and IgA (aCL) have been found to be associated with deterioration of cognitive function in SLE patients (Hanly et al. 1999; Menon et al. 1999).

Lai and Lan report intrathecal aPl antibody synthesis, suggesting an association with CNS involvement in a subset of patients (Lai and Lan 2000). Other authors have also proposed direct effects of aPL antibodies on CNS tissue, possibly by binding to neurons or glial cells and disrupting their function (Sanna et al. 2003a); however, these findings were not confirmed in another study (Jedryka-Goral et al. 2000).

21.1.2.3 Cytokines

Cytokines play an important role in activation and maintenance of the immune response (Bruyn 1995). Elevated levels of interferon (IFN) alpha have been found in SLE patients, and showed an association with psychotic episodes in SLE in a small group of patients (Shiozawa et al. 1992). These findings have recently been confirmed by the finding of a markedly increased expression of genes activated by interferon (alpha, beta, and gamma). This signature of elevated expression is found in 80% of SLE patients and seems to be related with the more severe forms of the disease involving multiple organs including the brain (Baechler et al. 2003).

Vallin and co-workers found that DNA and anti-dsDNA antibody immune complexes, both circulating in SLE patients, are capable of inducing production of IFN alpha (Vallin et al. 1999). IFN alpha induces B cells to differentiate into dendritic cells. Dendritic cells are professional antigen-presenting cells and stimulate T and B cells by presenting circulating apoptotic cells and nucleosomes in SLE as antigens to T cells (Blanco et al. 2001); thus, via the dendritic cells, IFN alpha maintains the immune reaction and causes elevated levels of DNA and anti-dsDNA antibody immune complexes in SLE.

21.1.2.4 Complement and Immune Complexes

The complement system plays an important role in inducing lysis in target cells, opsonization (coating) of target cells, and in attracting phagocytes. It can react directly with certain microorganisms or act together with antibodies to enhance phagocytosis. Decreases of complement level are associated with increased renal and hematological disease activity in SLE patients. Ho and co-workers also found a decrease in anti-dsDNA before SLE flares, with a frequent decrease during relapses, suggesting deposition in the tissue possibly together with complement (Ho et al. 2001a,b).

Pickering and Walport reviewed (a) the effects of rare genetic deficiencies in the complement C1q causing SLE, (b) SLE causing activation and consumption of C1q, and (c) the fact that autoantibodies against C1q are commonly found in SLE. Based on these observations the authors suggested that complement plays a beneficial role in SLE (Pickering and Walport 2000).

Observations in NLE have identified that maternal antibodies are able to induce the typical MR abnormalities. The mechanism by which antibodies mediate this phenomenon is unknown (Prendiville et al. 2003). One has to assume that in some way the BBB is affected by activation of endothelial cells. Subsequently, antibodies pass the BBB and lead to brain damage either by binding to cell surface receptors and subsequently affecting cell function or by inducing antibody-dependent cell-mediated cytotoxicity (ADCC). Alternatively, immune-complex deposition can lead to disturbance of the BBB; immune-complex deposition has indeed been found in the choroid plexus (Boyer et al. 1980). The choroid plexus has fenestrated capillaries in analogy to a glomerulus; however, *tight junctions* in the cerebral microvasculature, between endothelial cells as part of the BBB, are a unique feature and make it unlikely that immune complexes could be trapped there (Hess 1997).

As mentioned previously, true vasculitis, characterized by infiltration of the vessel wall by inflammatory cells, is found at autopsy in only 10% of patients with NPSLE, whereas vasculopathy of small vessels (without infiltration by inflammatory cells) is the most common finding in NPSLE (Ellis and Verity 1979; Hess 1997; Johnson and Richardson 1968; West 1994). Furthermore, the spectrum of symptoms of NPSLE is not reproduced by any of the other vasculitides. Activation of endothelium (Belmont et al. 1996) is possibly sufficient to permit passage of antibodies through the BBB, whereas inflammatory cells only pass in few cases.

It is likely that several pathways or mechanisms in the immune system lead to vascular edema and stroke as well as direct damage to the CNS via inflammatory mechanisms. The challenge remains to characterize the different lesions seen on MRI and elucidate the etiology and the evolution of these findings.

21.1.2.5 Treatment

The NPSLE patients with more severe manifestations, whether diffuse or focal, usually require high-dose corticosteroids. Patients with refractory or progressive symptoms benefit from intravenous pulse methylprednisolone or cytotoxic therapy. In patients with aPl antibodies and manifestations secondary to thrombosis, antiplatelet drugs and anticoagulation appear beneficial (Brown and Swash 1989; West 1996). An international survey confirmed that this is common practice among 59 SLE centers (Tincani et al. 1996).

Common pitfalls are: assessing whether psychosis is based on steroid side effects or based on SLE activity; assessing whether cognitive dysfunction and organic brain syndrome result from previous or acute disease activity; and assessing whether NP symptoms are due to infarctions related to APS or based on other autoimmune phenomena (West 1994). With the advent of advanced imaging techniques some headway has been made in filling these pitfalls, as discussed later in this chapter.

Experimental treatment of NPSLE includes high-dose chemotherapy with autologous stem-cell transplantation (Hermosillo-Romo and Brey 2002a,b; Traynor and Burt 1999).

In summary, anticoagulation is indicated in APS to prevent thrombotic events and corticosteroids can be used to lower inflammation and reduce the immune response. Immunosuppressive agents lower T- and B-cell responses as well as lower the levels of antibodies (Bruyn 1995). There is evidence that with reduction of mortality, the morbidity is increasing due to the negative long-term effects of treatment (Urowitz and Gladman 2000).

21.2 General Diagnostics

21.2.1 Serum

As is shown by items 10 and 11 in the ACR criteria (Table 21.1), laboratory investigations are an essential part of the evaluation of SLE patients (Hochberg 1997; Tan et al. 1982). The term antinuclear antibodies (ANAs) comprises all antibodies that are directed against components of cell nuclei. Examples of such antibodies are listed in Table 21.4. Although ANAs are sensitive for SLE they are not specific: most patients with ANAs do not have SLE, but most people with SLE have ANAs (Egner 2000). Also, "ANA-negative SLE" has been reported (Bohan 1979). Furthermore, drugs can induce development of ANAs. In about 10% of

Table 21.3 Symptomatic and immune modulating treatment of NPSLE manifestations (Hermosillo-Romo and Brey 2002a)

Neuropsychiatric manifestation	Symptomatically	Immune modulating treatment
Seizures	Antiepileptic therapy	Corticosteroids can be considered
Delirium	No specific symptomatic therapy	Effective treatment of extraneural disease
Psychosis	Antipsychotic medications	Effective treatment of extraneural disease
Cerebral vasculopathy	Anticoagulation or antiplatelet agents in selected cases	1. High-dose corticosteroids 2. Cytotoxic immunosuppressives 3. A combination of both
Stroke	1. Anticoagulation 2. Antiplatelet agents	Effective treatment of extraneural disease
Transverse myelopathy	No symptomatic treatment	High-dose corticosteroids in general with cytotoxic immunosuppressives
Cognitive dysfunction	No symptomatic treatment	Effective treatment of extraneural disease
Anxiety and depression	1. Psychotherapy 2. Cognitive behavior therapy 3. Supportive type therapy 4. Biofeedback 5. Pain control 6. Anti-depressive agents 7. Anxiolytics	Effective treatment of extraneural disease
Drug-induced aseptic meningitis	Withdrawal and avoidance of offending drugs	No specific immuno-modulating therapy Corticosteroids can be considered
Headaches	Migraine treatments Anti-platelet agents	Treatment of extraneural disease activity
Movement disorders	Dopamine antagonists	Corticosteroids with anticoagulation if they are related to antiphospholipid antibodies

Symptomatic treatment includes treatment of secondary causes, such as drugs; infections and metabolic problems related to kidney and liver dysfunction and electrolyte disturbances

Table 21.4 Frequency of serological positivity in SLE. ACA anticardiolipin antibody, dsDNA double-stranded DNA, ITP idiopathic thrombocytopenic purpura, MCTD mixed connective tissue disease, RNP ribonuclear protein (From Egner 2000)

Antibody target	Positive at any stage of the disease (any assay; %)	Possible clinical association
dsDNA	30–70	Nephritis, disease activity
Sm	20–40	Rarely seen outside SLE
RNP	40–60	MCTD/overlap features
Ro	10–15	Sjögren's skin involvement/congenital heart block
Ribosomal P0, P1, P2	5–10	Neuropsychiatric SLE, disease activity
Histone	30	Drug-induced SLE, idiopathic SLE, disease activity
ACA	40–50	Risk of thrombotic complications/fetal loss/ITP

SLE-like conditions, the disease is drug induced and potentially reversible. The presence of drug-induced ANAs is more common than the presence of SLE. Frequency and possible clinical associations of antibodies are listed in Table 21.4.

Auto-antibodies, including ANAs, are found in sera of SLE patients long before the diagnosis is made (Arbuckle et al. 2003); however, there is no single serological diagnostic test for detecting NPSLE and laboratory findings always have to be combined with neuroimaging techniques (Hanly 1998; Weiner et al. 2003).

Several studies were aimed at assessing correlations between the presence of antibodies and cognitive deficits or MRI findings in NPSLE. In some studies correlations were found between neuropsychiatric symptoms and the presence of anti-ribosomal-P protein antibodies in NPSLE (Teh et al. 1993; West et al. 1995) In other studies these findings were not found (Hanly et al. 1993).

The measurement of complement antigenic levels and functional activity in serum is commonly used as a marker of disease in SLE. During active SLE, serum complement activity is reduced. Typically C1q, C2, and C4 levels are low and especially in patients with severe disease levels of C3 are also low; however, in individual patients levels of C4 may also remain low when the SLE patient is well (Lloyd and Schur 1981; Pickering and Walport 2000).

Erythrocyte sedimentation rate is another sensitive but non-specific indicator of disease activity in SLE, and it is slow to reflect changes in disease activity. C-reactive protein (CRP) has a short half-life and rapidly reflects acute inflammation. A high CRP can distinguish bacterial infection from active SLE, where the CRP is usually low, although CRP may also be elevated in severe lupus serositis (Egner 2000).

Wais et al. found ongoing systemic immuno-inflammatory activity measured with a variety of cytokines, adhesion molecules, and other inflammatory markers in SLE patients. They also observed a correlation between these serological markers and renal disease activity in SLE patients; however, no correlations were found with mucocutaneous, musculoskeletal, or neurologic disease activity, suggesting different pathogenic mechanisms for these forms of SLE (Wais et al. 2003).

In conclusion, although in SLE patients increased concentrations of autoantibodies are observed during stages of active disease, the very frequent occurrence of serologically active but clinically quiescent disease does not justify treatment on the basis of rising titers. Moreover, it is uncertain if serological testing permits differentiating between NPSLE and other causes of neuropsychiatric symptoms. Therefore, it is crucial to interpret serological results in a clinical context.

21.2.2 Cerebrospinal Fluid

Routine cerebrospinal fluid (CSF) analysis is useful in all SLE patients with a change in neurological status. A major advantage of examining the CSF in SLE patients presenting with NP disease is that it permits excluding infections. Unspecific findings such as elevated white blood cells and protein occur in up to one-third of patients with active NPSLE (Hanly 1998; Mccune and Golbus 1988; West 1994); however, pleiocytosis in the absence of infection should raise the suspicion of acute NPSLE, requiring a more aggressive therapy (West 1994).

In a study by West et al. patients with diffuse or complex presentations were more likely to have elevated CSF index, oligoclonal bands, and CSF anti-neuronal antibodies (West et al. 1995). In a small group of patients with SLE psychosis Shiozawa et al. found elevated levels of interferon alpha in the CSF (Shiozawa et al. 1992).

In a recent study, significantly increased levels of cytokines, IL-6 and IL-8, were found in NPSLE patients as compared with SLE patients without cerebral involvement. In addition, increased concentrations of neuronal degradation products, neurofilament triplet protein (NFL), and glial fibrillary acidic protein (GFAP), were found in CSF. The NFL and GFAP had relatively high positive and negative predictive values for CNS involvement in SLE, suggesting that these markers could possibly be useful tools for diagnosis and monitoring of NPSLE patients (Trysberg et al. 2003).

In summary, CSF analysis can contribute to the diagnostic evaluation of NPSLE; however, additional longitudinal data are needed to confirm the specificity (86%) and sensitivity (100%) observed by West and colleagues when CSF analysis is used in combination with the determination of serum antiribosomal-P antibodies (West et al. 1995; West 1996).

21.2.3 Neuropsychiatric Testing

In an unselected group of SLE patients, using neuropsychiatric testing, unspecific defects in cognition were observed in 66% of patients. Cognitive impairment is not only found in 80% of NPSLE patients, but also in 42% of SLE patients with no prior CNS symptoms (Carbotte et al. 1986). The higher prevalence of cognitive impairment in NPSLE patients compared with SLE patients has been confirmed by some (Monastero et al. 2001) but not by others (Hanly et al. 1992). This discrepancy may be due to differences in patient selection and case definition, as is suggested by the wide range of prevalence (21–66%) of impaired cognition in other studies (Hanly and Liang 1997).

In two longitudinal studies, no relationship was observed between the degree of cognitive impairment and disease activity (Carlomagno et al. 2000; Waterloo et al. 2002). In another study, cognitive impairment was associated with more severe disease presentation, but not with specific organ involvement or organ damage (Gladman et al. 2000). Some authors observed a specific pattern of cognitive impairment in NPSLE, comprising loss of immediate memory, concentration or complex attention, and psychomotor speed (Fisk et al. 1993; Hanly and Liang 1997; Loukkola et al. 2003). In summary, NPT is a sensitive and inexpensive tool that permits detecting cognitive dysfunction in SLE patients (Bruyn 1995).

21.2.4 EEG and QEEG

Conventional EEG has a limited value for the diagnostic work-up of NPSLE patients. The non-specific finding of abnormal slow wave activity in about 20% of SLE patients suggests a global involvement of the brain (Bruyn 1995; Sibbitt et al. 1999); however, no correlations have been observed between conventional EEG and neuropsychological assessment. Waterloo et al. reported that sensitivity of EEG for brain involvement in SLE ranges from 33 to 85% (Waterloo et al. 1999). EEG is sensitive for seizure disorders, large lobar infarcts, CNS hemorrhage, and movement disorders.

Quantitative (QEEG) utilizes parametric statistics to compare EEG measures obtained from an individual patient with those obtained from an age-regressed database of normal individuals, and is free of cultural and ethnic biases. Reported sensitivity of QEEG is 87% and specificity is around 75% for detecting brain involvement in SLE. QEEG is more sensitive than EEG and QEEG abnormalities have been shown in 87% of definite NPSLE patients, 74% of probable NPSLE patients, and 28% of SLE without NP symptoms. In a study of 52 SLE patients by Ritchlin et al. QEEG was more sensitive than conventional MRI in detecting NP symptoms and was able to differentiate between different neuropsychiatric manifestations (Ritchlin et al. 1992); however, these results were achieved using extensive effort to prevent artifact selection during on-line registration and during off-line EEG epoch selection.

Although QEEG is more specific than EEG through its quantitative nature, it has a high false-positive rate. Also, it does not differentiate between active NPSLE and confounding factors such as idiopathic epilepsy, unrelated cognitive disorders, drug effects, primary affective disorders, and metabolic encephalopathy. Still, QEEG may contribute to diagnosing NPSLE by confirming the presence of a seizure disorder, determining brain abnormality when other methods fail, or confirming brain death (Bruyn 1995; Sibbitt et al. 1999).

21.3 Imaging Diagnostics

21.3.1 Computed Tomography

Computed tomography (CT) of the brain has been found to be abnormal in 29–59% of patients with NPSLE (Sibbitt et al. 1999). In a study by Gonzalez-Scarano, the most common CT finding in a series of 29 NPSLE patients was sulcal enlargement, either with or without ventricular enlargement, which was most prominent in patients with either psychosis or dementia. In addition, infarcts and intracranial hemorrhages were observed in this study (GONZALEZ-SCARANO et al. 1979). JACOBS and co-workers found no abnormalities on CT in a group of 13 NPSLE patients (JACOBS et al. 1988). Computed tomography is particularly insensitive for pathology underlying non-focal presentations such as seizures, confusional states, major depression, and cognitive disorders (SIBBITT et al. 1989); therefore, CT should only be considered as a primary approach when MRI is not tolerated, unavailable, or contraindicated (SIBBITT et al. 1999).

21.3.2 Digital Subtraction Angiography

Since a true CNS vasculitis is rare in NPSLE (ELLIS and VERITY 1979; HESS 1997; JOHNSON and RICHARDSON 1968; WEST 1994), digital subtraction angiography (DSA) has no place in the primary diagnostic evaluation of NPSLE. It is often normal in NPSLE and it is rarely necessary due to the availability of other vessel imaging modalities (SIBBITT et al. 1999); however, in the few cases where a true CNS vasculitis is suspected, DSA may still be indicated (POMPER et al. 1999; WASSERMAN et al. 2001). Still, due to its limited resolving power of about 500 μm, and since in CNS vasculitis vessels with a smaller diameter are affected, DSA has a limited sensitivity for detecting this condition (WASSERMAN et al. 2001; YUH et al. 1999a).

21.3.3 Single-Photon Emission Computed Tomography

Using single-photon emission computed tomography (SPECT), cerebral blood flow (CBF) can be measured following injection of radiolabeled tracers. The SPECT scans are often abnormal in SLE and NPSLE patients, indicating the presence of regional cerebral blood flow (rCBF) abnormalities. The most common finding in these patients is patchy hypoperfusion. HUANG and colleagues found the parietal lobe to be the most common and the cerebellum the least common location of hypoperfusion in a group of 78 NPSLE and SLE patients (HUANG et al. 2002). A correlation of left parietal and occipital hypoperfusion with cognitive deficits (short-term memory and visuospatial intelligence) has also been found (SABBADINI et al. 1999).

There is some controversy about the usefulness of SPECT in the evaluation of NPSLE patients. Some authors argue that SPECT is a good diagnostic tool, showing clear associations between SPECT abnormalities and clinical symptoms (CHEN et al. 2002b; HUANG et al. 2002; RUBBERT et al. 1993). Others, however, found no correlation between neuropsychiatric signs and SPECT, and feel that SPECT has no added value to other imaging techniques (EMMI et al. 1993; NOSSENT et al. 1991; OKU et al. 2003; WATERLOO et al. 2001). The non-specificity of SPECT is further illustrated by the following observations: firstly, it does not permit differentiating irreversible stroke from reversible neurological abnormalities; secondly, it cannot distinguish new brain lesions from old ones; thirdly, it is difficult to differentiate active NPSLE from confounding disorders such as chronic cognitive dysfunction, primary headache, primary seizures, primary depression, and established cerebrovascular disease (KOVACS et al. 1995).

In summary, hypoperfusion is a common finding on SPECT scans in patients with NPSLE. The SPECT is not useful in daily clinical practice and adds little to the diagnostic work-up of NPSLE patients due to low specificity of the observed abnormalities.

21.3.4 Positron Emission Tomography

Using positron emission tomography (PET), glucose uptake, brain oxygen consumption, and CBF can be measured. The PET examinations are often abnormal in patients with SLE, showing multiple focal defects in oxygen uptake, glucose uptake, and CBF (HOLMAN 1993; KAO et al. 1999a). Parieto-occipital hypometabolism is the most conspicuous finding in NPSLE patients with non-focal neurological and psychiatric symptoms (OTTE et al. 1997; WEINER et al. 2000b).

In SLE patients, PET may detect abnormalities when other imaging modalities fail to do so. In a group of SLE patients with normal MRI findings, KAO and co-workers found decreases in glucose metabolism and in regional CBF (rCBF) in patients with severe NPSLE, while normal glucose metabolism with decreases in rCBF were observed in SLE patients with and without NP symptoms (KAO et al. 1999a,b). In another study an increase in glucose metabolism was found in the striatum in a group of nine NPSLE patients. This was attributed to an inflammatory process based on neuronal antibodies directed against the caudate and subthalamic nuclei. It was suggested that this phenomenon may impair inhibitory signals in the brain, leading to diffuse symptoms, and notably chorea (De Jong et al. 1999).

Although PET is a sensitive technique to detect cerebral changes in NPSLE, it lacks specificity. Confounding disorders, such as primary headache, primary affective disorders, primary seizures, and non-SLE cognitive disorders may also give rise to abnormalities (Sibbitt et al. 1999). Furthermore, an anatomical image (MRI/CT) is required to identify obvious focal lesions or old lesions not related to the present condition which results in PET abnormalities. Based on these limitations combined with the limited availability of this technique, PET is not a routine investigation for clinical use in NPSLE patients (Kao et al. 1999b; Sibbitt et al. 1999).

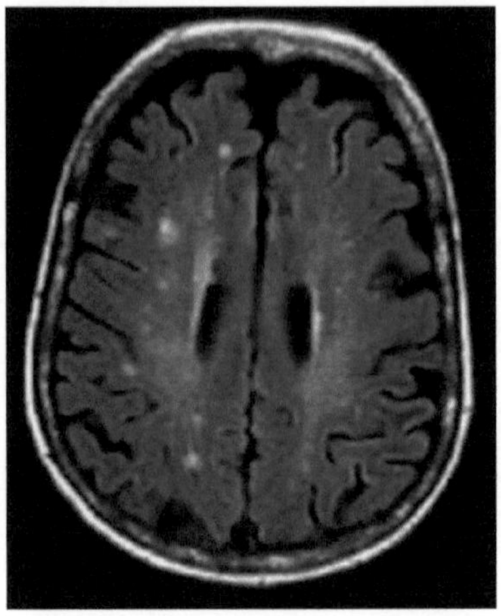

Fig. 21.1 Small punctate focal hyperintensities in the subcortical white matter on a fluid-attenuated inversion recovery (FLAIR) image in a 74-year-old patient with acute primary neuro-psychiatric systemic lupus erythematosus (NPSLE)

21.3.5 Conventional Magnetic Resonance Imaging

Magnetic resonance imaging (MRI) plays an important role in the diagnostic work-up of SLE patients with NP symptoms. The MRI may help differentiating secondary NPSLE from primary NPSLE by detecting abnormalities that are not directly caused by SLE involvement of the CNS such as brain abscesses, progressive multifocal leukoencephalopathy, and mycotic aneurysms (Sibbitt et al. 1999). Furthermore, MRI may reveal abnormalities in primary NPSLE. The most common MRI findings in NPSLE are small punctate focal hyperintensities [on T2-weighted or fluid-attenuated inversion recovery (FLAIR) images] in the subcortical white matter (WM; 15–60%; Fig. 21.1) and cerebral atrophy (Fig. 21.2). In addition, ventricular dilatation, cerebral infarcts (Fig. 21.3), periventricular and deep WM hyperintensities (Fig. 21.4), and gray matter hyperintensities have also been reported (Chinn et al. 1997; Fierro et al. 1999; Gonzalez-Crespo et al. 1995; Karassa et al. 2000; Sabbadini et al. 1999; Sibbitt et al. 1989; Sibbitt et al. 1999; Sibbitt Jr. et al. 2003). In NPSLE, abnormalities in the basal ganglia and infratentorial compartment are infrequently found, and when they are encountered they are not correlated with clinical activity (Gonzalez-Crespo et al. 1995; Hachulla et al. 1998; Ishikawa et al. 1994; Karassa et al. 2000).

Small focal WM hyperintensities are found mainly in subcortical WM, especially in the frontoparietal regions, but are also seen elsewhere in the brain (Chinn et al. 1997; Friedman et al. 1998; Ishikawa et al. 1994; Jacobs et al. 1988; Jarek et al. 1994; Mccune et al. 1988; Sibbitt et al. 1989; Sibbitt et al. 1994). Sometimes, these lesions extend in both gray and

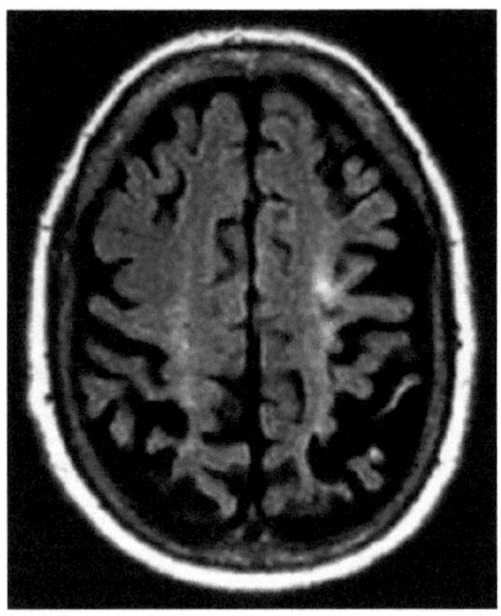

Fig. 21.2 Widening of sulci, indicative of cerebral atrophy in a 36-year-old patient with inactive chronic primary NPSLE

WM (Mccune et al. 1988; Moritani et al. 2001). The significance of focal WM lesions in NPSLE remains unclear, since WM abnormalities are also present in 20% of the normal population under 50 years, increasing to 90% for healthy subjects over 70 years (Yetkin et al. 1993).

Reports on the prevalence of global atrophy in NPSLE vary widely (11–82%) probably due to the subjective nature of the methods used for measuring global atrophy and differences in patient populations (Brooks et al. 1997; Davie et al. 1995; Fierro et al. 1999; Gonzalez-Crespo et al. 1995; Lim et al. 2000; Mccune et al. 1988; Sabbadini et al. 1999). In an

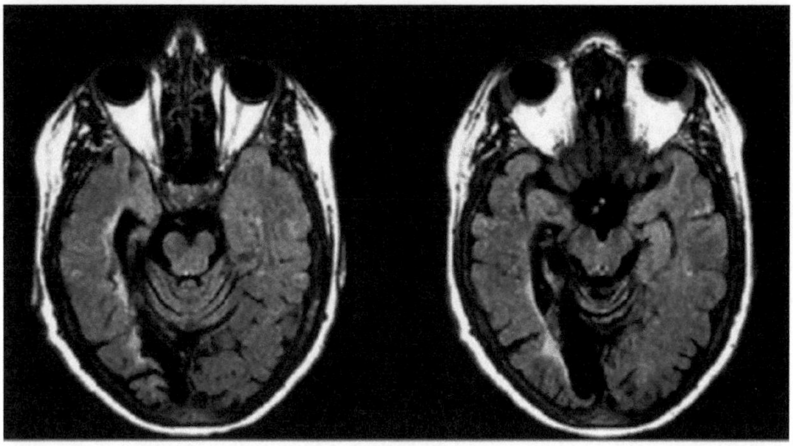

Fig. 21.3 Cerebral infarction in the posterior circulation in a 36-year-old patient with inactive chronic primary NPSLE

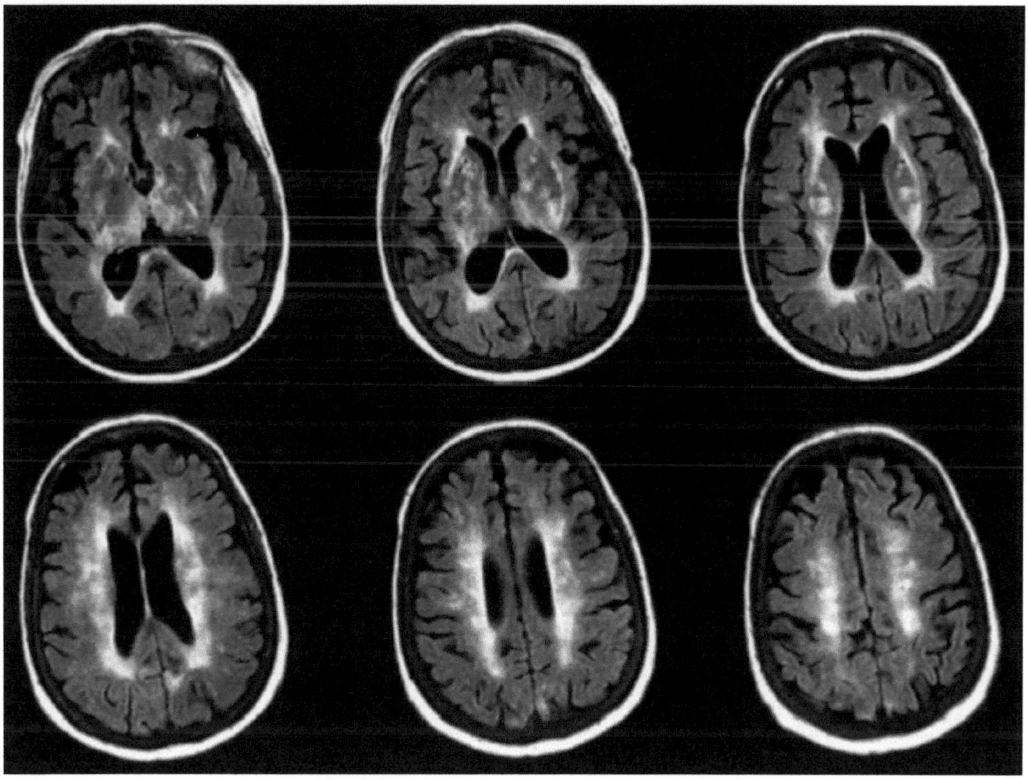

Fig. 21.4 Periventricular and deep white matter hyperintensities in a 55-year-old patient with active chronic primary NPSLE

unselected group of SLE patients, atrophy was only related with age and not with a peculiar clinical presentation of SL (Taccari et al. 1994).

Although in NPSLE patients MRI abnormalities are found more frequently than in SLE patients without NP symptoms, a considerable number of patients with florid NPSLE have no abnormalities on conventional MRI scans (Davie et al. 1995; Fierro et al. 1999; Gonzalez-Crespo et al. 1995; Ishikawa et al. 1994; Jacobs et al. 1988; Mccune et al. 1988;

Sabbadini et al. 1999; Sailer et al. 1997; Sanna et al. 2000). Reported estimates of normal brain appearance on MRI vary from 11 to 69% of NPSLE patients. In particular, conventional MRI tends to be normal in patients with diffuse, non-focal, neurological symptoms (Bell et al. 1991; Gonzalez-Crespo et al. 1995; Jacobs et al. 1988; Mccune et al. 1988; Sabbadini et al. 1999; Sailer et al. 1997; Sibbitt et al. 1989).

The question as to whether the clinical symptoms in NPSLE are caused by the observed abnormalities on MRI, is a challenging one (Jarek et al. 1994; Mccune et al. 1988). Among NPSLE patients without active NP symptoms chronic lesions may be observed in 25–50% of the cases. The prevalence of these lesions increases with increasing duration of disease and with a history of NPSLE (Brooks et al. 1997; Friedman et al. 1998; Hachulla et al. 1998; Jarek et al. 1994; Rozell et al. 1998). Acute lesions can sometimes be differentiated from chronic lesions by the lack of discrete borders, intermediate intensity on T2-weighted images, their intermediate size, their lacy and filamentous pattern, their peculiar location often following the gray–white matter junction along the sulci and gyri assuming a semilunate structure, the presence of overlying or adjacent gray matter hyperintensity, their possible resolution on follow-up studies, and enhancement following gadolinium administration (Mccune et al. 1988; Sibbitt et al. 1989; Sibbitt et al. 1995). Furthermore, active lesions in NPSLE are reported to be visible on T2-weighted images with increased signal intensity and can be located in both white and gray matter (Friedman et al. 1998; Rozell et al. 1998; Sibbitt et al. 1989; Sibbitt et al. 1995; Sibbitt et al. 1999). In particular, extensive bilateral WM abnormalities suggestive of edema can be found in cerebral hemispheres, brainstem, and cerebellum, and they may be associated with hypertension, benign intracranial hypertension (pseudotumor cerebri), and other clinical signs of active NPSLE (Sibbitt et al. 1989; Sibbitt et al. 1999). Acute lesions may have a good anatomical correspondence with newly acquired dysfunction and may be reversible with corticosteroid therapy. Furthermore, focal and punctuate high-intensity lesions in both white and gray matter have been found in patients with generalized seizures, and these lesions tend to resolve rapidly (Bell et al. 1991; Mccune et al. 1988; Sibbitt et al. 1989; Sibbitt et al. 1995; Sibbitt et al. 1999).

Associations have been found between the number of WM lesions and the presence of NP symptoms in SLE patients and disease indices for NPSLE and SLE (Sailer et al. 1997; Sanna et al. 2000; Sibbitt Jr. et al. 2003; Taccari et al. 1994); however, other studies found no association between small punctuate focal lesions in periventricular and subcortical WM and the presence of NP symptoms (Baum et al. 1993; Gonzalez-Crespo et al. 1995; Ishikawa et al. 1994; Jacobs et al. 1988; Sabbadini et al. 1999; Stimmler et al. 1993). Several studies have also reported reversible and irreversible lesions without clinical improvement (Bell et al. 1991; Gonzalez-Crespo et al. 1995; Griffey et al. 1990; Jacobs et al. 1988; Mccune et al. 1988; Sabbadini et al. 1999; Sibbitt et al. 1989; Stimmler et al. 1993). Reversible WM lesions were thought to represent edema, water filled dilated perivascular spaces, gliosis, demyelination, or tissue damage due to inflammatory vasculopathic insults to small vessels, resulting in breakdown of the BBB (Bell et al. 1991; Gonzalez-Crespo et al. 1995; Sabbadini et al. 1999; Sibbitt et al. 1989).

In another study, areas of increased signal, in subcortical WM, deep WM and gray matter did not improve after steroid treatment, suggesting (micro)infarcts or residual tissue injury (Bell et al. 1991; Gonzalez-Crespo et al. 1995; Hachulla et al. 1998; Jacobs et al. 1988; Provenzale et al. 1996; Sibbitt et al. 1989). Reversibility of gray matter lesions in association with clinical improvement has also been described in other studies (Aisen et al. 1985; Karassa et al. 2000; Mccune et al. 1988).

21.4 Advanced MRI Techniques

21.4.1 Relaxation Time Measurements

Several studies have shown that quantitative T2 measurements extend the utility and sensitivity of conventional MR imaging for evaluating NPSLE. The T2 relaxation time of white and gray matter is increased in active and chronic NPSLE patients (Miller et al. 1989; Petropoulos et al. 1999; Sibbitt et al. 1995). Furthermore, patients with diffuse neurological manifestations demonstrated a longer T2 in gray matter than other NPSLE patients, suggesting acute cerebral edema, associated with elevated disease activity (Sibbitt et al. 1995). In a study by Petropoulos et al., the authors also found a higher gray matter spin–spin T2 relaxation time in patients with severe NPSLE than in patients with mild NPSLE, indicating the presence of cerebral edema in patients with major active disease (Petropoulos et al. 1999). Cerebral edema could reflect the breakdown of the BBB in an area of focal injury, resulting in entrance of pathogenic antineuronal autoantibodies, and induce generalized cytotoxic cerebral edema (Sibbitt et al. 1995).

21.4.2 Magnetization Transfer Imaging

Magnetization transfer imaging (MTI) is a quantitative MRI technique: a technique aimed at providing meaningful gray values per pixel rather than providing images with useful contrasts (qualitative MRI techniques). In other words, MTI provides quantitative information on brain tissue that reflects its histological composition. In MTI this quantitative information is obtained by using a radio-frequency pre-pulse that reduces magnetization of the protons that are bound to macromolecules. Since in biological tissues there is a permanent exchange of protons between a compartment comprising these macromolecule-bound protons, and a compartment of free water protons, the reduced magnetization is transferred to the free water pool. In the free water pool the reduced magnetization can be measured, because the free water pool of protons is exploited in MRI to obtain tissue signal (Van Buchem and Tofts 2000). The amount of magnetization transfer between the two pools can be measured by performing an MRI sequence with and one without the saturation pre-pulse, by calculating the difference of the resulting images on a pixel-by-pixel basis, and by expressing that difference in a ratio, the magnetization transfer ratio (MTR).

The MTR is affected by tissue factors: the concentration; the surface chemistry; and the biophysical dynamics of macromolecules. In the brain MTR can be reduced due to dilution or destruction of macromolecules (Bosma et al. 2000b; Huizinga et al. 2001). Reduced MTR values have been observed in the brain in a number of neurodegenerative disorders, such as multiple sclerosis and Alzheimer's disease (Filippi et al. 2000; Van Buchem et al. 1998; Bozzali et al. 2001; Van Der Flier et al. 2002). In several studies it was demonstrated that MTR values better reflect the underlying histological changes than conventional MRI sequences. In addition, it was shown that MTR measurements are more sensitive to the presence of disease than conventional sequences, since abnormal MTR values can be observed in brain areas with a normal appearance on conventional MRI (Bosma et al. 2000b; Rovaris et al. 2000).

The MTR data can be analyzed regionally, by assessing the mean MTR in regions of interest, or it can be used to provide more global information on the brain. One way to obtain a more global MTR analysis of the brain is by generating MTR histograms of large tissue volumes, such as the whole brain. In normal individuals, MTR histograms of the brain are characterized by the presence of a single, sharp peak, indicating that the brain is homogeneous in terms of MTR characteristics.

Using MTR histogram analysis of the whole brain, Bosma and co-workers found differences between primary NPSLE patients without active NP symptoms at the time of scanning and without significant abnormalities on conventional MRI, on the one hand, and SLE patients without NP symptoms and normal controls, on the other. In NPSLE patients the histogram peak was lower and wider, which reflected loss of homogeneity in brain structure, probably due to demyelination (Bosma et al. 2000b). In another study by the same group, primary NPSLE patients were also shown to have abnormal MTR histograms during episodes of active NP symptoms. Furthermore, MTR histograms of NPSLE patients with past and active episodes of NP differed: in patients with active disease a shift of the histogram to higher values was observed. This shift was attributed to an early stage of demyelination that is characterized by breakdown of myelin molecules into multiple smaller fragments (Bosma et al. 2000a).

The MTR parameters showed no correlation with age, SLE duration, or time elapsed since the first occurrence of neuropsychiatric symptoms. This suggests that the damage detected by MTR is not accumulated in a gradually progressive way, but rather in a relapsing-remitting pattern. In other words, probably brain damage is acquired during the episodes of clinically active disease (Bosma et al. 2002).

Volumetric MTR parameters seem to reflect functionally relevant brain damage. Bosma and co-workers assessed correlations between volumetric MTR parameters and measures of clinical functioning in a group of primary NPSLE patients, again without significant abnormalities on conventional MRI. They found significant correlations between MTR parameters, on the one hand, and measures of cognitive, psychiatric, and neurological functioning, on the other (Bosma et al. 2002).

Demonstrating MTI differences between groups of patients does not imply that this technique contributes to diagnosing an individual new patient who is suspected to have the disease. In a study by Dehmeshki et al. multiple discriminant analysis (MDA) was used to improve classification of patients as active NPSLE, chronic NPSLE, non-NPSLE, multiple sclerosis, and healthy control based on MTR histograms. Using MDA, the conventional and arbitrary histogram descriptives, such as peak height and mean MTR, are no longer used, but the whole histogram shape is taken into account. In this preliminary study it was shown that combining MDA with MTR histogram analysis individual patients were classified correctly in almost all cases (Dehmeshki et al. 2002).

21.4.3 Magnetic Resonance Spectroscopy

Proton magnetic resonance spectroscopy (^{1}H-MRS) and phosphorus MRS (^{31}P-MRS) can be used to show a wealth of metabolic substances such as choline (Cho), N-acetylaspartic acid (NAA), creatine (Cr), lactate (Lac), inositol (Ins), glutamate (Glu), and glutamine (Gln). The MRS can reveal the presence of significant organic brain injury, anaerobic metabolism, and possibly the activity of NPSLE; however, it cannot be used to diagnose NPSLE (Sibbitt et al. 1999). A relationship between neurometabolite derangement and cognitive dysfunction in chronic NPSLE has been found (Bosma et al. 2002; Brooks et al. 1999).

One of the metabolites detected by ^{1}H-MRS is NAA, which can be used for detection and measurement of brain injury not detectable by other neuro-imaging methods. The NAA is located almost entirely in neurons and presents the highest peak in ^{1}H-MRS (Sibbitt et al. 1997; Sibbitt et al. 1999). Its function is unknown, but reduced levels have been found in many diseases, suggesting neuronal injury or death. The NAA is reduced in patients with a prior history of NPSLE as well as in patients with active NPSLE (Huizinga et al. 2001; Sibbitt et al. 1997). In NPSLE patients, NAA is reduced in normal-appearing WM, gray matter, and focal lesions (Axford et al. 2001; Brooks et al. 1997; Brooks et al. 1999; Chinn et al. 1997; Davie et al. 1995; Friedman et al. 1998; Handa et al. 2003; Leeds and Kieffer 2000; Sibbitt et al. 1994; Sibbitt et al. 1997).

The cause of decreased NAA levels in NPSLE is not clear. On the one hand, associations between IgG aPL and decreased levels of NAA have been observed, suggesting a thrombo-embolic origin (Sabet et al. 1998); on the other, NAA is also decreased in patients without signs of thrombo-embolic disease.

Cho is a neuronal metabolite and its peak reflects phosphocholine, glycerophosphocholine, and choline. Increased Cho may be a measure of membrane breakdown, myelinolysis, and infiltration of inflammatory cells (Chinn et al. 1997; Davie et al. 1995; Friedman et al. 1998; Lim et al. 2000). Elevated levels of Cho (Axford et al. 2001; Brooks et al. 1997; Lim et al. 2000; Sabet et al. 1998) have been found in NPSLE patients, suggesting disease activity or reactive brain inflammation; however, other studies do not confirm this observation (Davie et al. 1995; Sibbitt et al. 1994), but this can be attributed to the lack of acute lesions in the subjects enrolled.

The presence of Lac in the brain has not been observed in NPSLE (Brooks et al. 1997; Handa et al. 2003; Sibbitt et al. 1997). This could be due to the fact that the concentration of Lac is below the detection level of MRS (Soher et al. 1996); however, apart from cases with overt stroke, extensive anaerobic metabolism does not seem to be a fundamental characteristic of NPSLE. From this one can conclude that, although NPSLE may be primarily a disease of cerebral vascular injury, disturbed fluid dynamics and neurotoxin release may also be as important as ischemic processes (Handa et al. 2003; Sibbitt et al. 1997; Sibbitt et al. 1999). So, hypoperfusion, as detected by SPECT, may not be the primary process in NPSLE, but rather a secondary one.

^{31}P-MRS also provides a wealth of metabolic data; however, due to its limited availability and the preliminary nature of ^{31}P-MRS studies in NPSLE, it has still to be viewed as a research technique (Sibbitt et al. 1999). A good measure of tissue energetics can be obtained through ATP, phosphocreatine (PCr), and inorganic phosphate. Decreased levels of ATP and PCr have been found in deep WM in NPSLE patients. These abnormalities have been shown to be reversible with high-dose corticosteroid therapy (Griffey et al. 1990). In the same study, regions of the brain in some patients that were normal on conventional MRI demonstrated profound depletion of ATP and/or PCr on ^{31}P-MRS. Decreased high-energy phosphates in the brain of NPSLE patients may be a reflection of a diffuse metabolic derangement associated with SLE that is independent of the reversible high-intensity lesions present on MRI (Griffey et al. 1990).

21.4.4 Diffusion-Weighted Imaging

Diffusion-weighted imaging (DWI) is another quantitative MRI method. One of the quantitative parameters that can be derived from DWI is the apparent diffusion coefficient (ADC). The ADC reflects diffusivity of protons in tissue. In highly structured tissue, such as the brain, movement of protons is limited by multiple barriers, such as the myelin sheaths. In diseases that are associated with loss of tissue structure, such as demyelinative diseases, diffusivity of the brain tissue increases, which is reflected in elevated ADC values. On the other hand, abnormally decreased ADC values can also be encountered. Protons located in the interstitium experience more diffusivity than those located within the cells. Cytotoxic edema, which accompanies the early stage of a brain infarct, is characterized by an increase of the intracellular compartment at the expense of the extracellular compartment. Consequently, this gives rise to decreased diffusivity and ADC values.

Similar to MTR histograms, histograms can also be generated based on DWI studies. Bosma et al. performed DWI in primary NPSLE patients and healthy controls without significant abnormalities on conventional brain MRI (Bosma et al. 2003). The ADC histograms of NPSLE patients differed form those of controls. The histogram peak was lower and wider, and mean ADC values were higher in NPSLE patients, reflecting loss of uniformity and increase in brain diffusivity. In the same study, no abnormalities suggestive of cytotoxic edema were found. The observations from this study support the data from studies using MTR and MRS, in that in NPSLE structural damage is much more widespread than expected from conventional MRI.

Moritani et al. observed areas of hyperintensity on DWI and increased ADC representing vasogenic edema in a series of 20 SLE patients with neurological abnormalities. Some of these lesions resolved partially and some completely following treatment. In four patients, a hyperintense focus on DWI associated with a decreased ADC representing an acute infarction was observed (Moritani et al. 2001).

21.4.5 Perfusion-Weighted Imaging

Tracer bolus passage studies, such as perfusion-weighted imaging (PWI), allow mapping CBF without radiation exposure (Sibbitt et al. 1999). Borrelli et al. found 13 hypoperfused areas in 10 of 20 NPSLE patients using PWI; however, PWI showed fewer hypoperfused areas than did SPECT (43 hypoperfused areas in 17 of 20 patients; Borrelli et al. 2003). So far, PWI has been used little in NPSLE research; however, it has been suggested that in the diagnostic work-up PWI can exclude a CNS vasculitis (Yuh et al. 1999b).

References

The American College of Rheumatology (1999) Nomenclature and case definitions for neuropsychiatric lupus syndromes. Arthritis Rheum 42:599–608

Ainiala H, Loukkola J, Peltola J et al (2001) The prevalence of neuropsychiatric syndromes in systemic lupus erythematosus. Neurology 57:496–500

Aisen AM, Gabrielsen TO, McCune WJ (1985) MR imaging of systemic lupus erythematosus involving the brain. Am J Roentgenol 144:1027–1031

Arbuckle MR, McClain MT, Rubertone MV et al (2003) Development of autoantibodies before the clinical onset of systemic lupus erythematosus. N Engl J Med 349:1526–1533

Axford JS, Howe FA, Heron C, Griffiths JR (2001) Sensitivity of quantitative (1)H magnetic resonance spectroscopy of the brain in detecting early neuronal damage in systemic lupus erythematosus. Ann Rheum Dis 60:106–111

Baechler EC, Batliwalla FM, Karypis G et al (2003) Interferon-inducible gene expression signature in peripheral blood cells of patients with severe lupus. Proc Natl Acad Sci USA 100:2610–2615

Baraczka K, Lakos G, Sipka S (2002) Immunoserological changes in the cerebro-spinal fluid and serum in systemic lupus erythematosus patients with demyelinating syndrome and multiple sclerosis. Acta Neurol Scand 105:378–383

Baum KA, Hopf U, Nehrig C et al (1993) Systemic lupus erythematosus: neuropsychiatric signs and symptoms related to cerebral MRI findings. Clin Neurol Neurosurg 95:29–34

Bell CL, Partington C, Robbins M et al (1991) Magnetic resonance imaging of central nervous system lesions in patients with lupus erythematosus. Correlation with clinical remission and antineurofilament and anticardiolipin antibody titers. Arthritis Rheum 34:432–441

Belmont, Abramson SB, Lie JT (1996) Pathology and pathogenesis of vascular injury in systemic lupus erythematosus. Interactions of inflammatory cells and activated endothelium. Arthritis Rheum 39:9–22

Blanco P, Palucka AK, Gill M et al (2001) Induction of dendritic cell differentiation by IFN-alpha in systemic lupus erythematosus. Science 294:1540–1543

Bohan A (1979) Seronegative systemic lupus erythematosus. J Rheumatol 6:534–540

Bombardier C, Gladman DD, Urowitz MB et al (1992) Derivation of the Sledai-A disease: activity index for lupus patients. Arthritis Rheum 35:630–640

Borrelli M, Tamarozzi R, Colamussi P et al (2003) Evaluation with MR, perfusion MR and cerebral flowSPECT in NPSLE patients. Radiol Med (Torino) 105:482–489

Bosma GP, Rood MJ, Huizinga TW et al (2000a) Detection of cerebral involvement in patients with active neuropsychiatric systemic lupus erythematosus by the use of volumetric magnetization transfer imaging. Arthritis Rheum 43:2428–2436

Bosma GP, Rood MJ, Zwinderman AH et al (2000b) Evidence of central nervous system damage in patients with neuropsychiatric systemic lupus erythematosus, demonstrated by magnetization transfer imaging. Arthritis Rheum 43:48–54

Bosma GP, Middelkoop HA, Rood MJ et al (2002) Association of global brain damage and clinical functioning in neuropsychiatric systemic lupus erythematosus. Arthritis Rheum 46:2665–2672

Bosma GP, Huizinga TW, Mooijaart SP, van Buchem MA (2003) Abnormal brain diffusivity in patients with neuropsychiatric systemic lupus erythematosus. Am J Neuroradiol 24:850–854

Boyer RS, Sun NC, Verity A et al (1980) Immunoperoxidase staining of the choroid plexus in systemic lupus erythematosus. J Rheumatol 7:645–650

Bozzali M, Franceschi M, Falini A et al (2001) Quantification of tissue damage in AD using diffusion tensor and magnetization transfer MRI. Neurology 57:1135–1137

Brey RL, Holliday SL, Saklad AR et al (2002) Neuropsychiatric syndromes in lupus: prevalence using standardized definitions. Neurology 58:1214–1220

Brooks WM, Sabet A, Sibbitt WL et al (1997) Neurochemistry of brain lesions determined by spectroscopic imaging in systemic lupus erythematosus. J Rheumatol 24:2323–2329

Brooks WM, Jung RE, Ford CC et al (1999) Relationship between neurometabolite derangement and neurocognitive dysfunction in systemic lupus erythematosus. J Rheumatol 26:81–85

Brown MM, Swash M (1989) Systemic lupus erythematosus. In: Vinken PJ, Bruyn GW, Klawans HL (eds) Handbook of clinical neurology. Elsevier, Amsterdam, pp 369–385

Bruyn GA (1995) Controversies in lupus: nervous system involvement. Ann Rheum Dis 54:159–167

Carbotte RM, Denburg SD, Denburg JA (1986) Prevalence of cognitive impairment in systemic lupus erythematosus. J Nerv Ment Dis 174:357–364

Carlomagno S, Migliaresi S, Ambrosone L et al (2000) Cognitive impairment in systemic lupus erythematosus: a follow-up study. J Neurol 247:273–279

Carvalho D, Savage CO, Isenberg D, Pearson JD (1999) IgG anti-endothelial cell autoantibodies from patients with systemic lupus erythematosus or systemic vasculitis stimulate the release of two endothelial cell-derived mediators, which enhance adhesion molecule expression and leukocyte adhesion in an autocrine manner. Arthritis Rheum 42:631–640

Cervera R, Khamashta MA, Font J et al (2003) Morbidity and mortality in systemic lupus erythematosus during a 10-year period: a comparison of early and late manifestations in a cohort of 1000 patients. Medicine 82:299–308

Chen JJ, Shiau YC, Wang JJ et al (2002a) Abnormal regional cerebral blood flow in primary antiphospholipid antibody syndrome patients with normal magnetic resonance imaging findings. A preliminary report. Scand J Rheumatol 31:89–93

Chen JJ, Yen RF, Kao A et al (2002b) Abnormal regional cerebral blood flow found by technetium-99m ethyl cysteinate dimer brain single photon emission computed tomography in systemic lupus erythematosus patients with normal brain MRI findings. Clin Rheumatol 21:516–519

Chinn RJ, Wilkinson ID, Hall-Craggs MA et al (1997) Magnetic resonance imaging of the brain and cerebral proton spectroscopy in patients with systemic lupus erythematosus. Arthritis Rheum 40:36–46

Clancy R, Marder G, Martin V et al (2001) Circulating activated endothelial cells in systemic lupus erythematosus: further evidence for diffuse vasculopathy. Arthritis Rheum 44:1203–1208

Colamussi P, Giganti M, Cittanti C et al (1995) Brain single-photon emission tomography with 99mTc-HMPAO in neuropsychiatric systemic lupus erythematosus: relations with EEG and MRI findings and clinical manifestations. Eur J Nucl Med 22:17–24

Davie CA, Feinstein A, Kartsounis LD et al (1995) Proton magnetic resonance spectroscopy of systemic lupus erythematosus involving the central nervous system. J Neurol 242:522–528

de Jong BM, Pruim J, Sinnige LG et al (1999) Regional specific changes of cerebral metabolism in systemic lupus erythematosus identified by positron emission tomography. Eur Neurol 41:187–193

Dehmeshki J, van Buchem MA, Bosma GP et al (2002) Systemic lupus erythematosus: diagnostic application of magnetization transfer ratio histograms in patients with neuropsychiatric symptoms: initial results. Radiology 222:722–728

Egner W (2000) The use of laboratory tests in the diagnosis of SLE. J Clin Pathol 53:424–432

Ellis SG, Verity MA (1979) Central nervous system involvement in systemic lupus erythematosus: a review of neuropathologic findings in 57 cases, 1955–1977. Semin Arthritis Rheum 8:212–221

Emmi L, Bramati M, Cristofaro MT de et al (1993) MRI and SPECT investigations of the CNS in SLE patients. Clin Exp Rheumatol 11:13–20

Fierro B, Brighina F, Amico L et al (1999) Evoked potential study and radiological findings in patients with systemic lupus erythematosus. Electromyogr Clin Neurophysiol 39:305–313

Filippi M, Inglese M, Rovaris M et al (2000) Magnetization transfer imaging to monitor the evolution of MS: a 1-year follow-up study. Neurology 55:940–946

Fisk JD, Eastwood B, Sherwood G, Hanly JG (1993) Patterns of cognitive impairment in patients with systemic lupus-erythematosus. Br J Rheum 32:458–462

Friedman SD, Stidley CA, Brooks WM et al (1998) Brain injury and neurometabolic abnormalities in systemic lupus erythematosus. Radiology 209:79–84

Giles IP, Isenberg D (2001) Lupus in the family: analysis of a cohort followed from 1978 to 1999. Lupus 10:38–44

Gladman D, Ginzler E, Goldsmith C et al (1996) The development and initial validation of the systemic lupus international collaborating clinics American College of Rheumatology Damage Index for Systemic Lupus Erythematosus. Arthritis Rheum 39:363–369

Gladman D, Urowitz MB, Slonim D et al (2000) Evaluation of predictive factors for neurocognitive dysfunction in patients with inactive systemic lupus erythematosus. J Rheumatol 27:2367–2371

Gonzalez-Crespo MR, Blanco FJ, Ramos A et al (1995) Magnetic resonance imaging of the brain in systemic lupus erythematosus. Br J Rheum 34:1055–1060

Gonzalez-Scarano F, Lisak RP, Bilaniuk LT et al (1979) Cranial computed tomography in the diagnosis of systemic lupus erythematosus. Ann Neurol 5:158–165

Griffey RH, Brown MS, Bankhurst AD et al (1990) Depletion of high-energy phosphates in the central nervous system of patients with systemic lupus erythematosus, as determined by phosphorus-31 nuclear magnetic resonance spectroscopy. Arthritis Rheum 33:827–833

Hachulla E, Michon-Pasturel U, Leys D et al (1998) Cerebral magnetic resonance imaging in patients with or without antiphospholipid antibodies. Lupus 7:124–131

Handa R, Sahota P, Kumar M et al (2003) In vivo proton magnetic resonance spectroscopy (MRS) and single photon

emission computerized tomography (SPECT) in systemic lupus erythematosus (SLE). Magn Reson Imaging 21:1033–1037
Hanly JG (1998) Evaluation of patients with CNS involvement in SLE. Baillieres Clin Rheumatol 12:415–431
Hanly JG, Liang MH (1997) Cognitive disorders in systemic lupus erythematosus: epidemiologic and clinical issues. Ann NY Acad Sci 823:60–68
Hanly JG, Fisk JD, Sherwood G et al (1992) Cognitive impairment in patients with systemic lupus erythematosus. J Rheumatol 19:562–567
Hanly JG, Walsh NM, Fisk JD et al (1993) Cognitive impairment and autoantibodies in systemic lupus erythematosus. Br J Rheum 32:291–296
Hanly JG, Hong C, Smith S, Fisk JD (1999) A prospective analysis of cognitive function and anticardiolipin antibodies in systemic lupus erythematosus. Arthritis Rheum 42:728–734
Hermosillo-Romo D, Brey RL (2002a) Diagnosis and management of patients with neuropsychiatric systemic lupus erythematosus (NPSLE). Best Pract Res Clin Rheumatol 16:229–244
Hermosillo-Romo D, Brey RL (2002b) Neuropsychiatric involvement in systemic lupus erythematosus. Curr Rheumatol Rep 4:337–344
Herranz MT, Rivier G, Khamashta MA et al (1994) Association between antiphospholipid antibodies and epilepsy in patients with systemic lupus erythematosus. Arthritis Rheum 37:568–571
Hess DC (1997) Cerebral lupus vasculopathy. Mechanisms and clinical relevance. Ann NY Acad Sci 823:154–168
Ho A, Barr SG, Magder LS, Petri M (2001a) A decrease in complement is associated with increased renal and hematologic activity in patients with systemic lupus erythematosus. Arthritis Rheum 44:2350–2357
Ho A, Magder LS, Barr SG, Petri M (2001b) Decreases in anti-double-stranded DNA levels are associated with concurrent flares in patients with systemic lupus erythematosus. Arthritis Rheum 44:2342–2349
Hochberg MC (1997) Updating the American College of Rheumatology revised criteria for the classification of systemic lupus erythematosus. Arthritis Rheum 40:1725
Holman HR (1993) Functional imaging in systemic lupus erythematosus: an accurate indicator of central nervous system involvement? Arthritis Rheum 36:1193–1195
Huang WS, Chiu PY, Tsai CH et al (2002) Objective evidence of abnormal regional cerebral blood flow in patients with systemic lupus erythematosus on Tc-99m ECD brain SPECT. Rheumatol Int 22:178–181
Huizinga TW, Steens SC, van Buchem MA (2001) Imaging modalities in central nervous system systemic lupus erythematosus. Curr Opin Rheumatol 13:383–388
Ishikawa O, Ohnishi K, Miyachi Y, Ishizaka H (1994) Cerebral lesions in systemic lupus erythematosus detected by magnetic resonance imaging. Relationship to anticardiolipin antibody. J Rheumatol 21:87–90
Jacobs L, Kinkel PR, Costello PB et al (1988) Central nervous system lupus erythematosus: the value of magnetic resonance imaging. J Rheumatol 15:601–606
Jarek MJ, West SG, Baker MR, Rak KM (1994) Magnetic resonance imaging in systemic lupus erythematosus patients without a history of neuropsychiatric lupus erythematosus. Arthritis Rheum 37:1609–1613
Jedryka-Goral A, Zabek J, Wojciechowski B et al (2000) Evaluation of cerebrospinal fluid for the presense of anticardiolipin antibodies (aCL) in NP-SLE patients. Clin Rheumatol 19:306–310
Johnson GD, Richardson EP (1968) The neurological manifestations of systemic lupus erythematosus. Medicine (Baltimore) 47:337–369
Kao CH, Ho YJ, Lan JL et al (1999a) Discrepancy between regional cerebral blood flow and glucose metabolism of the brain in systemic lupus erythematosus patients with normal brain magnetic resonance imaging findings. Arthritis Rheum 42:61–68
Kao CH, Lan JL, ChangLai SP et al (1999b) The role of FDG-PET, HMPAO-SPET and MRI in the detection of brain involvement in patients with systemic lupus erythematosus. Eur J Nucl Med 26:129–134
Karassa FB, Ioannidis JP, Boki KA et al (2000) Predictors of clinical outcome and radiologic progression in patients with neuropsychiatric manifestations of systemic lupus erythematosus. Am J Med 109:628–634
Kotzin BL, Kozora E (2001) Anti-DNA meets NMDA in neuropsychiatric lupus. Nat Med 7:1175–1176
Kovacs JA, Urowitz MB, Gladman DD, Zeman R (1995) The use of single photon emission computerized tomography in neuropsychiatric SLE: a pilot study. J Rheumatol 22:1247–1253
Lai NS, Lan JL (2000) Evaluation of cerebrospinal anticardiolipin antibodies in lupus patients with neuropsychiatric manifestations. Lupus 9:353–357
Leeds NE, Kieffer SA (2000) Evolution of diagnostic neuroradiology from 1904 to 1999. Radiology 217:309–318
Lim MK, Suh CH, Kim HJ et al (2000) Systemic lupus erythematosus: brain MR imaging and single-voxel hydrogen 1 MR spectroscopy. Radiology 217:43–49
Lloyd W, Schur PH (1981) Immune-complexes, complement, and anti-DNA in exacerbations of systemic lupus-erythematosus (SLE). Medicine 60:208–217
Loukkola J, Laine M, Ainiala H et al (2003) Cognitive impairment in systemic lupus erythematosus and neuropsychiatric systemic lupus erythematosus: a population-based neuropsychological study. J Clin Exp Neuropsychol 25:145–151
McCune WJ, Golbus J (1988) Neuropsychiatric lupus. Rheum Dis Clin North Am 14:149–167
McCune WJ, MacGuire A, Aisen A, Gebarski S (1988) Identification of brain lesions in neuropsychiatric systemic lupus erythematosus by magnetic resonance scanning. Arthritis Rheum 31:159–166
Menon S, Jameson-Shortall E, Newman SP, Hall-Craggs MR et al (1999) A longitudinal study of anticardiolipin antibody levels and cognitive functioning in systemic lupus erythematosus. Arthritis Rheum 42:735–741
Miller DH, Johnson G, Tofts PS et al (1989) Precise relaxation time measurements of normal-appearing white matter in inflammatory central nervous system disease. Magn Reson Med 11:331–336
Monastero R, Bettini P, Del Zotto E et al (2001) Prevalence and pattern of cognitive impairment in systemic lupus erythematosus patients with and without overt neuropsychiatric manifestations. J Neurol Sci 184:33–39
Moritani T, Shrier DA, Numaguchi Y et al (2001) Diffusion-weighted echo-planar MR imaging of CNS involvement in systemic lupus erythematosus. Acad Radiol 8:741–753

Nossent JC, Hovestadt A, Schonfeld DH, Swaak AJ (1991) Single-photon-emission computed tomography of the brain in the evaluation of cerebral lupus. Arthritis Rheum 34:1397–1403

Oku K, Atsumi T, Furukawa S et al (2003) Cerebral imaging by magnetic resonance imaging and single photon emission computed tomography in systemic lupus erythematosus with central nervous system involvement. Rheumatology (Oxford) 42:773–777

Otte A, Weiner SM, Peter HH et al (1997) Brain glucose utilization in systemic lupus erythematosus with neuropsychiatric symptoms: a controlled positron emission tomography study. Eur J Nucl Med 24:787–791

Petropoulos H, Sibbitt WL, Brooks WM (1999) Automated T2 quantitation in neuropsychiatric lupus erythematosus: a marker of active disease. J Magn Reson Imaging 9:39–43

Pickering MC, Walport MJ (2000) Links between complement abnormalities and systemic lupus erythematosus. Rheumatology (Oxford) 39:133–141

Pomper MG, Miller TJ, Stone JH et al (1999) CNS vasculitis in autoimmune disease: MR imaging findings and correlation with angiography. Am J Neuroradiol 20:75–85

Prendiville JS, Cabral DA, Poskitt KJ et al (2003) Central nervous system involvement in neonatal lupus erythematosus. Pediatr Dermatol 20:60–67

Provenzale JM, Barboriak DP, Allen NB, Ortel TL (1996) Patients with antiphospholipid antibodies: CT and MR findings of the brain. Am J Roentgenol 167:1573–1578

Rekvig OP, Nossent JC (2003) Anti-double-stranded DNA antibodies, nucleosomes, and systemic lupus erythematosus: a time for new paradigms? Arthritis Rheum 48:300–312

Renaudineau Y, Dugue C, Dueymes M, Youinou P (2002) Antiendothelial cell antibodies in systemic lupus erythematosus. Autoimmun Rev 1:365–372

Ritchlin CT, Chabot RJ, Alper K et al (1992) Quantitative electroencephalography. A new approach to the diagnosis of cerebral dysfunction in systemic lupus erythematosus. Arthritis Rheum 35:1330–1342

Rood MJ, Breedveld FC, Huizinga TW (1999) The accuracy of diagnosing neuropsychiatric systemic lupus erythematosus in a series of 49 hospitalized patients. Clin Exp Rheumatol 17:55–61

Rood MJ, Haverman JF, van Duinen SG et al (2001) CNS involvement in systemic lupus erythematosus: a case with remarkable histopathological findings. Ann Rheum Dis 60:299–300

Rovaris M, Viti B, Ciboddo G et al (2000) Brain involvement in systemic immune mediated diseases: magnetic resonance and magnetisation transfer imaging study. J Neurol Neurosurg Psychiatry 68:170–177

Rozell CL, Sibbitt WL Jr, Brooks WM (1998) Structural and neurochemical markers of brain injury in the migraine diathesis of systemic lupus erythematosus. Cephalalgia 18:209–215

Rubbert A, Marienhagen J, Pirner K et al (1993) Single-photon-emission computed tomography analysis of cerebral blood flow in the evaluation of central nervous system involvement in patients with systemic lupus erythematosus. Arthritis Rheum 36:1253–1262

Sabbadini MG, Manfredi AA, Bozzolo E et al (1999) Central nervous system involvement in systemic lupus erythematosus patients without overt neuropsychiatric manifestations. Lupus 8:11–19

Sabet A, Sibbitt WL, Stidley CA et al (1998) Neurometabolite markers of cerebral injury in the antiphospholipid antibody syndrome of systemic lupus erythematosus. Stroke 29:2254–2260

Sailer C, Burchert W, Ehrenheim C et al (1997) Positron emission tomography and magnetic resonance imaging for cerebral involvement in patients with systemic lupus erythematosus. J Neurol 244:186–193

Sanna G, Piga M, Terryberry JW et al (2000) Central nervous system involvement in systemic lupus erythematosus: cerebral imaging and serological profile in patients with and without overt neuropsychiatric manifestations. Lupus 9:573–583

Sanna G, Bertolaccini ML, Cuadrado MJ et al (2003a) Central nervous system involvement in the antiphospholipid (Hughes) syndrome. Rheumatology (Oxford) 42:200–213

Sanna G, Bertolaccini ML, Cuadrado MJ et al (2003b) Neuropsychiatric manifestations in systemic lupus erythematosus: prevalence and association with antiphospholipid antibodies. J Rheumatol 30:985–992

Scherzer CR, Landwehrmeyer GB, Kerner JA et al (1998) Expression of N-methyl-D-aspartate receptor subunit mRNAs in the human brain: hippocampus and cortex. J Comp Neurol 390:75–90

Scolding NJ, Joseph FG (2002) The neuropathology and pathogenesis of systemic lupus erythematosus. Neuropathol Appl Neurobiol 28:173–189

Shiozawa S, Kuroki Y, Kim M et al (1992) Interferon-alpha in lupus psychosis. Arthritis Rheum 35:417–422

Sibbitt WR Jr, Sibbitt RR, Griffey RH et al (1989) Magnetic resonance and computed tomographic imaging in the evaluation of acute neuropsychiatric disease in systemic lupus erythematosus. Ann Rheum Dis 48:1014–1022

Sibbitt WR Jr, Haseler LJ, Griffey RH et al (1994) Analysis of cerebral structural changes in systemic lupus erythematosus by proton MR spectroscopy. Am J Neuroradiol 15:923–928

Sibbitt WR Jr, Brooks WM, Haseler LJ et al (1995) Spin-spin relaxation of brain tissues in systemic lupus erythematosus. A method for increasing the sensitivity of magnetic resonance imaging for neuropsychiatric lupus. Arthritis Rheum 38:810–818

Sibbitt WR Jr, Haseler LJ, Griffey RR et al (1997) Neurometabolism of active neuropsychiatric lupus determined with proton MR spectroscopy. Am J Neuroradiol 18:1271–1277

Sibbitt WR Jr, Sibbitt RR, Brooks WM (1999) Neuroimaging in neuropsychiatric systemic lupus erythematosus. Arthritis Rheum 42:2026–2038

Sibbitt WR Jr, Schmidt PJ, Hart BL, Brooks WM (2003) Fluid attenuated inversion recovery (FLAIR) imaging in neuropsychiatric systemic lupus erythematosus. J Rheumatol 30:1983–1989

Soher BJ, van Zijl PC, Duyn JH, Barker PB (1996) Quantitative proton MR spectroscopic imaging of the human brain. Magn Reson Med 35:356–363

Stimmler MM, Coletti PM, Quismorio FP Jr (1993) Magnetic resonance imaging of the brain in neuropsychiatric systemic lupus erythematosus. Semin Arthritis Rheum 22:335–349

Taccari E, Sili SA, Spadaro A et al (1994) Magnetic resonance imaging (MRI) of the brain in SLE: ECLAM and SLEDAI correlations. Clin Exp Rheumatol 12:23–28

Tan IL, Cohen AS, Fries JF et al (1982) The 1982 revised criteria for the classification of systemic lupus erythematosus. Arthritis Rheum 25:1271–1277

Teh LS, Hay EM, Amos N et al (1993) Anti-P antibodies are associated with psychiatric and focal cerebral disorders in patients with systemic lupus erythematosus. Br J Rheum 32:287–290

Tincani A, Brey R, Balestrieri G et al (1996) International survey on the management of patients with SLE. II. The results of a questionnaire regarding neuropsychiatric manifestations. Clin Exp Rheumatol 14 (Suppl 16):S23–S29

Toubi E, Khamashta MA, Panarra A, Hughes GR (1995) Association of antiphospholipid antibodies with central nervous system disease in systemic lupus erythematosus. Am J Med 99:397–401

Traynor AE, Burt RK (1999) Haematopoietic stem cell transplantation for active systemic lupus erythematosus. Rheumatology (Oxford) 38:767–772

Trysberg E, Nylen K, Rosengren LE, Tarkowski A (2003) Neuronal and astrocytic damage in systemic lupus erythematosus patients with central nervous system involvement. Arthritis Rheum 48:2881–2887

Tzioufas AG, Tzortzakis NG, Panou-Pomonis E et al (2000) The clinical relevance of antibodies to ribosomal-P common epitope in two targeted systemic lupus erythematosus populations: a large cohort of consecutive patients and patients with active central nervous system disease. Ann Rheum Dis 59:99–104

Urowitz MB, Gladman DD (2000) How to improve morbidity and mortality in systemic lupus erythematosus. Rheumatology (Oxford) 39:238–244

Vallin H, Perers A, Alm GV, Ronnblom L (1999) Anti-double-stranded DNA antibodies and immunostimulatory plasmid DNA in combination mimic the endogenous IFN-alpha inducer in systemic lupus erythematosus. J Immunol 163:6306–6313

van Buchem MA, Tofts PS (2000) Magnetization transfer imaging. Neuroimaging Clin N Am 10:771–788

van Buchem MA, Grossman RI, Armstrong C et al (1998) Correlation of volumetric magnetization transfer imaging with clinical data in MS. Neurology 50:1609–1617

van der Flier WM, van den Heuvel DMJ, Weverling-Rijnsburger AWE et al (2002) Magnetization transfer imaging in normal aging, mild cognitive impairment, and Alzheimer's disease. Ann Neurol 52:62–67

Wais T, Fierz W, Stoll T, Villiger PM (2003) Subclinical disease activity in systemic lupus erythematosus: immunoinflammatory markers do not normalize in clinical remission. J Rheumatol 30:2133–2139

Wasserman BA, Stone JH, Hellmann DB, Pomper MG (2001) Reliability of normal findings on MR imaging for excluding the diagnosis of vasculitis of the central nervous system. Am J Roentgenol 177:455–459

Waterloo K, Omdal R, Jacobsen EA et al (1999) Cerebral computed tomography and electroencephalography compared with neuropsychological findings in systemic lupus erythematosus. J Neurol 246:706–711

Waterloo K, Omdal R, Sjoholm H et al (2001) Neuropsychological dysfunction in systemic lupus erythematosus is not associated with changes in cerebral blood flow. J Neurol 248:595–602

Waterloo K, Omdal R, Husby G, Mellgren SI (2002) Neuropsychological function in systemic lupus erythematosus: a 5-year longitudinal study. Rheumatology (Oxford) 41:411–415

Weiner SM, Klein R, Berg PA (2000a) A longitudinal study of autoantibodies against central nervous system tissue and gangliosides in connective tissue diseases. Rheumatol Int 19:83–88

Weiner SM, Otte A, Schumacher M et al (2000b) Diagnosis and monitoring of central nervous system involvement in systemic lupus erythematosus: value of F-18 fluorodeoxyglucose PET. Ann Rheum Dis 59:377–385

Weiner SM, Otte A, Uhl M et al (2003) Neuropsychatric involvement in systemic lupus erythematosus. Part 2: Diagnostic and therapy. Med Klin 98:79–90 [in German]

West SG (1994) Neuropsychiatric lupus. Rheum Dis Clin North Am 20:129–158

West SG (1996) Lupus and the central nervous system. Curr Opin Rheumatol 8:408–414

West SG, Emlen W, Wener MH, Kotzin BL (1995) Neuropsychiatric lupus erythematosus: a 10-year prospective study on the value of diagnostic tests. Am J Med 99:153–163

Whitelaw DA, Spangenberg JJ, Rickman R et al (1999) The association between the antiphospholipid antibody syndrome and neuropsychological impairment in SLE. Lupus 8:444–448

Yetkin FZ, Fischer ME, Papke RA, Haughton VM (1993) Focal hyperintensities in cerebral white matter on MR images of asymptomatic volunteers: correlation with social and medical histories. Am J Roentgenol 161:855–858

Yuh WT, Ueda T, Maley JE (1999a) Perfusion and diffusion imaging: a potential tool for improved diagnosis of CNS vasculitis. Am J Neuroradiol 20:87–89

Yuh WT, Ueda T, Maley JE et al (1999b) Diagnosis of microvasculopathy in CNS vasculitis: value of perfusion and diffusion imaging. J Magn Reson Imaging 10:310–313

Zvaifler NJ, Bluestein HG (1982) The pathogenesis of central nervous system manifestations of systemic lupus erythematosus. Arthritis Rheum 25:862–866

22 Non-MS Inflammatory Diseases of the CNS: MR Features in Addition to the White Matter

Mario Mascalchi and Fabrizio Salvi

CONTENTS

22.1 Introduction

Many non-multiple sclerosis (MS) inflammatory diseases of the central nervous system (CNS) can cause a multifocal white matter damage of the brain similar to that of MS. In many of them, however, the damage is not confined to the white matter. Two of the latter conditions, namely systemic lupus erythematosus (SLE) and primary angiitis of the CNS, are dealt with in other chapters herein (Van Buchem: neuro-SLE; Okuda: primary angiitis of the CNS). Herein, we shall review the conventional MR imaging features of the CNS (brain, optic nerve and spinal cord) lesions besides white matter in some of the systemic vasculitis–including Behçet's disease, Sjögren syndrome and polyarteritis nodosa–which can help in the differential diagnoses of the white matter multifocal lesions (Miller et al. 1987). Other systemic angiitis including rheumatoid arthritis (Bekkelund et al. 1995), giant cell arteritis, and Wegener disease, albeit capable of producing brain damage, usually do not determine white matter changes and, consequently, will not be addressed. In addition, the CNS damage associated with vasculitis due to the use of illicit drugs such as amphetamines will not be reviewed. On the other hand, the MR findings that can be observed besides the white matter damage in antiphospholipid antibody syndrome will be reviewed. Finally, after a brief account on post-infective angiitis, we shall review the wide spectrum of lesions beyond the white matter in sarcoidosis.

Conventional brain MR imaging is here considered the usual protocol that includes T1-weighted, proton density-weighted and T2-weighted (with and without inversion recovery RF pulse to attenuate the CSF signal) sequences, T1-weighted images after administration of intravenous gadolinium chelates (at equilibrium) and MR angiography. In addition, the MR imaging findings in the optic nerve and spinal cord will refer to the usual techniques, namely T1-weighted and fat-suppressed T2-weighted images and contrast-enhanced, fat-suppressed T1-weighted sequences for the optic nerve, and T1-weighted, T2-weighted and contrast enhanced, T1 weighted sequences for the spinal cord.

M. Mascalchi, MD
Professor, Sezione di Radiodiagnostica, Dipartimento di Fisiopatologia Clinica, Università di Firenze, Viale Morgagni, 85, 50134 Firenze, Italy
F. Salvi, MD
Sezione di Radiodiagnostica, Dipartimento di Fisiopatologia Clinica, Università di Firenze, Viale Morgagni, 85, 50134 Firenze, Italy

22.2.1 Systemic Vasculitides

22.2.1.1 Behçet's Disease

Behçet's disease (BD) is a systemic inflammatory disease of unknown aetiology that typically affects young adults in Japan, the Middle East and the Mediterranean area (Inaba 1989) along the ancient Silk Route. Since there is no specific laboratory or pathological feature, the diagnosis of BD rests entirely on clinical findings and should satisfy the criteria fixed in 1989 by an international study group (Lancet). These include recurrent oral ulcerations, plus at least two of the following four features: recurrent genital ulcerations, uveitis, positive pathergy test, and one of the skin lesions among erythema nodosum, pseudofolliculitis and papulopustular lesions. Neurological complications of BD occur in 10–49% of cases, usually after other manifestations of the disease (Inaba 1989).

Brain

The most common MRI findings in BD are focal white matter and grey matter lesions in the cerebral hemispheres and brainstem that can enhance after intravenous contrast administration, when examined in the acute phase (Kocer et al. 1999; Cellerini et al. 2003). A predilection was noted for the mesodiencephalic junction, with a distribution pattern similar to that of the intra-axial veins, suggesting that in BD the vasculitis is predominantly perivenular (Kocer et al. 1999). In some instances, the mesodiencephalic lesion may present as a large pseudo-tumoral lesion that rapidly resolves after corticosteroids (Kermode et al. 1989) (Fig. 22.1). In a minority of patients intraparenchymal haemorrhagic lesions can be detected (Al Kawi 1991; Kocer et al. 1999), possibly reflecting a more necrotizing type of vasculitis, and these appear as hypointense areas due to deoxyhaemoglobin in the acute phase and due to haemosiderin in the chronic phase, when they are combined with overt atrophy (Fig. 22.2).

Thrombosis of the intracranial dural sinuses is another neurological presentation of BD and was emphasized as a common occurrence in one series (Wechsler et al. 1993). However, this was not confirmed in other series (Kocer et al. 1999; Cellerini et al. 2003). Interestingly, intracranial dural thrombosis generally affects younger individuals and does not occur in BD patients with multifocal brain lesions, and vice versa (Akman-Demir et al. 1999). The MRI features are similar to those in idiopathic intracra-

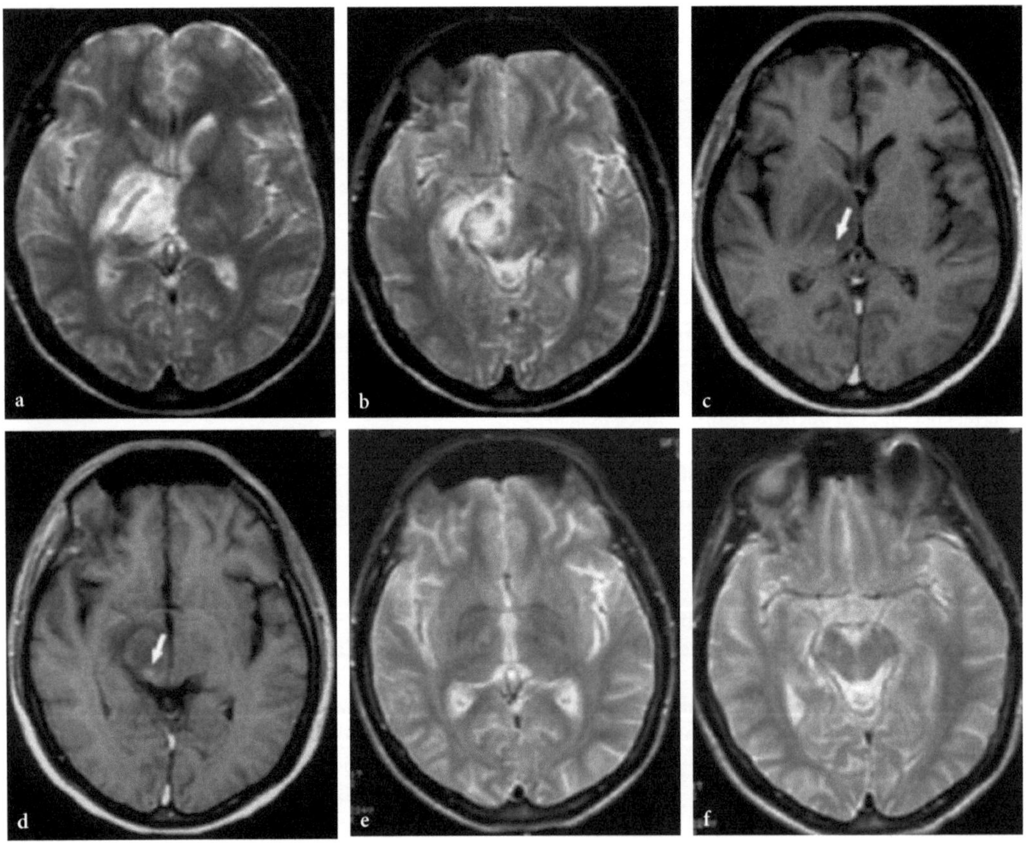

Fig. 22.1a–f. Behçet's disease. Large pseudotumoral mesodiencephalic lesion in a 34 year-old-man. Axial T2-weighted images at clinical presentation (**a, b**) show a large hyperintense lesion in the right thalamo-capsular region and cerebral peduncle. Axial T1-weighted images (**c, d**) after intravenous administration of a gadolinium chelate demonstrate two small peripheral foci of contrast enhancement within the lesion (*arrows* **a, b**) and mild mass effect (**b**). Axial T2-weighted images obtained 3 months after corticosteroid therapy (**e, f**) show almost complete resolution of the signal change.

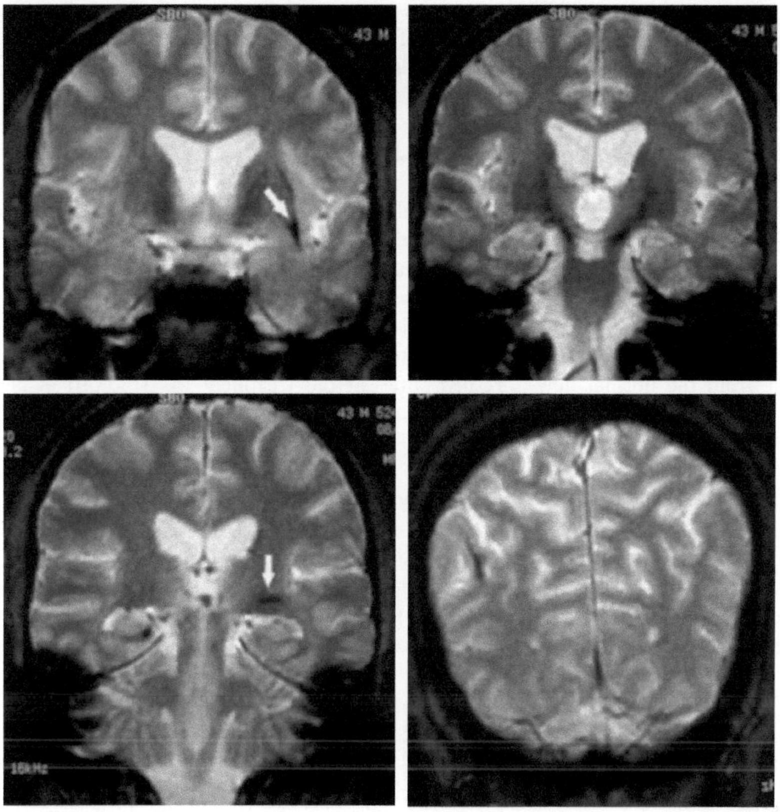

a b c d

Fig. 22.2a–d. Behçet's disease. Multiple intra-parenchymal haemorrhages in a 40-year-old woman. Coronal T2*-weighted images (**a–d**) obtained 7 years after clinical onset of neurological symptoms in a patient with BD demonstrate multiple hypointense foci in the subcortical white matter (*arrows* in **a, c** and **d**) consistent with old haemorrhagic lesions and thinning of the cerebral peduncles (**b**)

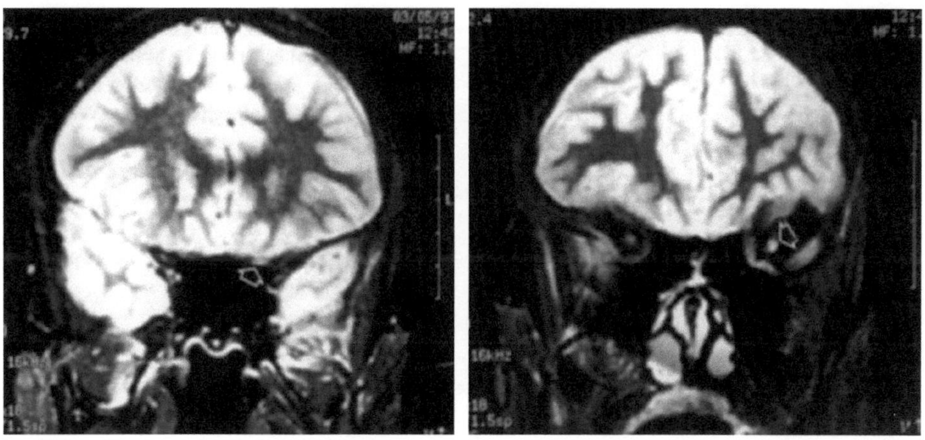

a b

Fig. 22.3a,b. Behçet's disease. Optic nerve damage in a 37-year-old woman. Coronal STIR images show hyperintensity and slight swelling of the left optic nerve (*arrows*) extending from the intracranial (**a**) to the mid-orbital (**b**) portion. Reprinted from Salvi et al. 1999 nial venous thrombosis (Condor and Jarosz 2002) (Fig. 22.3) and include intra-parenchymal haemorrhages with a lobar distribution, haemorrhagic infarcts in areas not corresponding to arterial territories, and signal changes in the thrombosed sinuses that are different depending on the time elapsed between thrombosis and imaging, the MR sequence and the field strength of the magnet. Combination of MR imaging and MR angiography is always recommended in the case of suspicion of dural sinus thrombosis, especially in the acute phase, when the thrombus may exhibit low signal in T2-weighted images due to deoxyhaemoglobin formation and hence be indistinguishable from the normal flow-related signal void.

Optic Nerve

BD can affect the optic nerve and represent the first clinical evidence of the disease (Salvi et al. 1999). The MR imaging features are similar to those of MS and other secondary vasculitis affecting the optic nerve (Sklal et al.1996) and are better appreciated with fat-suppressed T2-weighted images. They consist of increased signal intensity of one or both optic nerves (Fig. 22.4) and of contrast enhancement if the examination is performed in the acute phase (Kocer et al. 1999).

Spinal Cord

The spinal cord is involved in less than 20% of patients with BD and clinical signs of neurological involvement (Shakir et al. 1990). The cervical and thoracic segments can be affected, and MRI shows extensive lesions that exhibit contrast enhancement in the acute phase (Fig. 22.5) and almost completely resolve after steroid treatment (Mascalchi et al. 1998a; Kocer 1999).

22.2.1.2 Sjögren Syndrome

Primary Sjögren syndrome (SS) is most frequently a connective tissue disease (Lafitte 2002), and its diagnosis rests on the clinical findings of xerostomia and xerophthalmia, positive lacrimal or minor

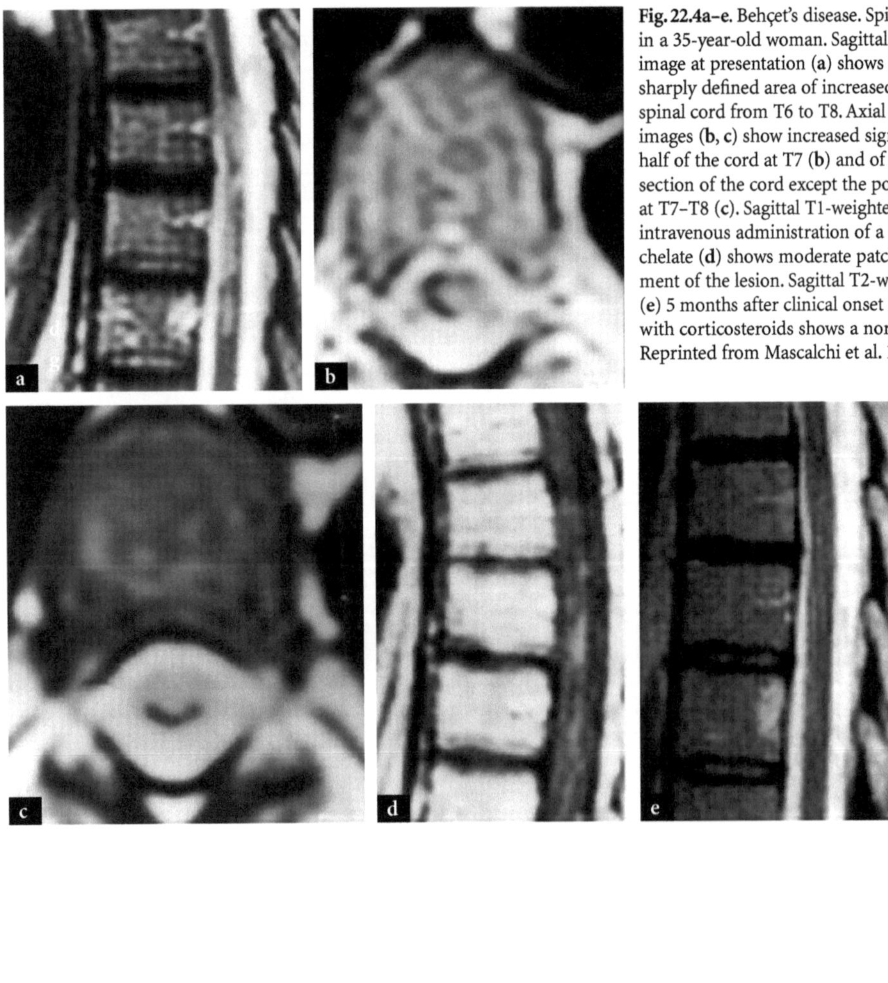

Fig. 22.4a–e. Behçet's disease. Spinal cord damage in a 35-year-old woman. Sagittal T2-weighted image at presentation (**a**) shows an irregular, sharply defined area of increased signal in the spinal cord from T6 to T8. Axial T2-weighted images (**b, c**) show increased signal of the left half of the cord at T7 (**b**) and of the entire cross-section of the cord except the posterior columns at T7–T8 (**c**). Sagittal T1-weighted image after intravenous administration of a gadolinium chelate (**d**) shows moderate patchy enhancement of the lesion. Sagittal T2-weighted image (**e**) 5 months after clinical onset and treatment with corticosteroids shows a normal spinal cord. Reprinted from Mascalchi et al. 1998a

a b c

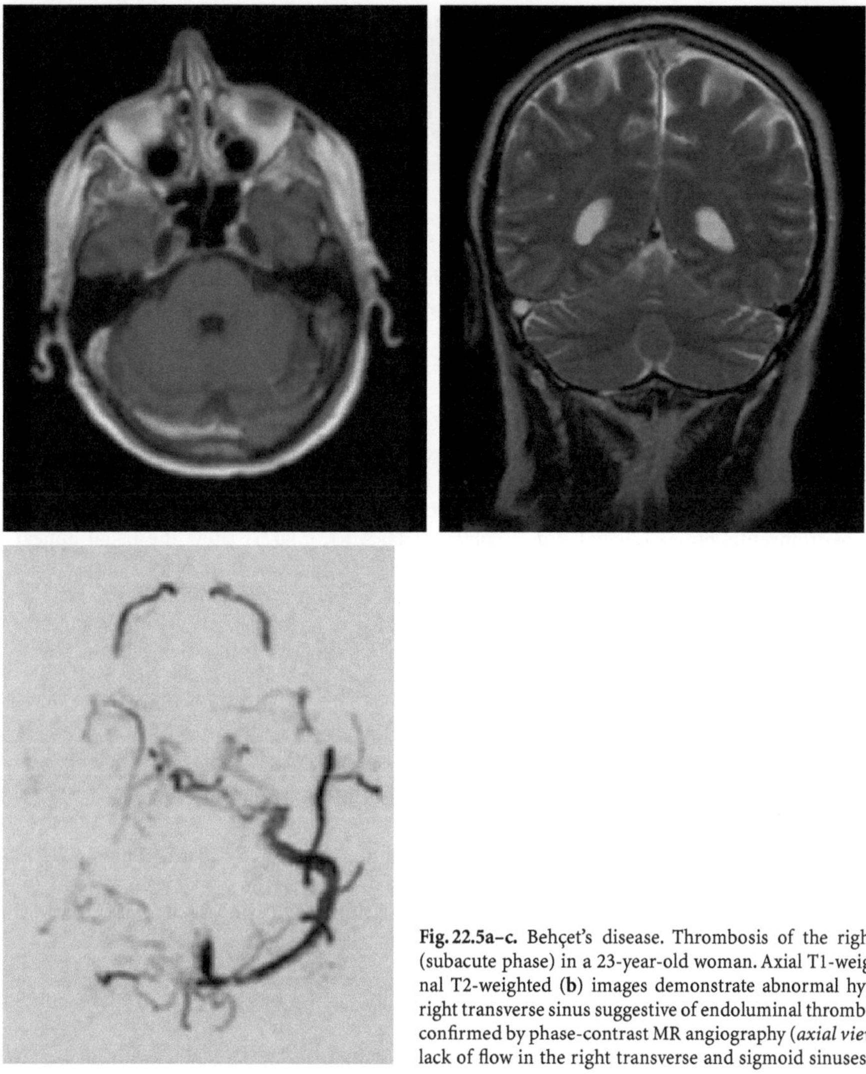

Fig. 22.5a–c. Behçet's disease. Thrombosis of the right transverse sinus (subacute phase) in a 23-year-old woman. Axial T1-weighted (**a**) and coronal T2-weighted (**b**) images demonstrate abnormal hyperintensity in the right transverse sinus suggestive of endoluminal thrombus. The diagnosis is confirmed by phase-contrast MR angiography (*axial view*) (**c**), which shows lack of flow in the right transverse and sigmoid sinuses

salivary gland biopsy and high titres of antinuclear and anti-SSA (Ro) and anti-SSB (La) antibodies. Neurological complications can occur in up to one-third of patients with primary SS, sometimes representing the clinical onset of the disease. Although peripheral nervous system involvement predominates (Lafitte et al. 2001), brain, optic nerve and spinal cord damage may be demonstrated by MRI.

Brain

Brain lesions in primary SS consist of nonspecific, multifocal white matter lesions that can be observed in patients with focal neurological deficit, psychiatric or cognitive dysfunction alone, or in absence of any clinical sign or symptom of CNS dysfunction (Alexander et al. 1988; Pierrot et al.1993; Lafitte 2002). No other brain lesion besides the multifocal white matter changes have so far been documented with MRI.

Optic Nerve

In primary SS, optic nerve involvement is distinctly rare and usually symptomatic (Tesar et al. 1992; Kadota et al. 2002). In the only reported case (Kadota et al. 2002), the MRI features were indistinguishable from those of other optic nerve vasculitis (Sklar et al. 1996)

Spinal Cord

Three variants can be recognized: (1) acute myelitis indistinguishable from acute transverse myelitis (Manabe et al. 2000; de Seze et al. 2001); (2) chronic myelitis similar to that observed in chronic MS (de Seze et al. 2001); and (3) tractopathy reflecting peripheral nervous involvement (Mori et al. 2001). The latter is the consequence of sensory neuronopathy and consists of diffuse hyperintensity of the posterior columns in T2*-weighted images of the spinal cord, better appreciated in the cervical segment. Also, this MRI finding is nonspecific and can be observed in other diseases causing chronic deafferentation such as Friedreich's ataxia (Mascalchi et al. 1994).

Interestingly, in many cases of primary SS the spinal cord damage is combined with optic nerve involvement (de Seze et al. 2001; Mochizuchi et al. 2000) featuring a neuromyelitis optica (Devic) syndrome as in other systemic vasculitides such as SLE.

22.2.1.3 Polyarteritis Nodosa

Polyarteritis nodosa (PAN) is a rare disease that affects middle-aged subjects and is characterised by focal, segmental necrotising vasculitis of small and medium-sized arteries. The nervous system is usually involved in the form of mononeuritis multiplex, but ischaemic or haemorrhagic strokes and subarachnoid haemorrhages secondary to rupture of aneurysms, which more commonly involve the renal, hepatic and visceral arteries, occur in 20–40% of patients, usually after the initial diagnosis is made (Reichhart et al. 2000)

Multifocal white matter lesions were observed in 18% of patients with PAN reviewed by Reichhart et al. (2000) (Fig. 22.6). No case of optic nerve or spinal cord damage has been reported so far.

Brain

Small infarcts in the deep cerebral hemisphere or brainstem related to thrombotic microangiopathy along penetrating arteries, rather than to vasculitis, are the most common MRI features besides white matter damage in PAN (Provenzale and Allen 1996; Reichhart et al. 2000).

Large infarcts and intra-parenchymal haemorrhages are less common (Provenzale and Allen 1996; Reichhart et al. 2000; De Reuck 2003). On conventional MRI, infarcts show the usual appearance of well-defined areas of increased signal in T2-weighted images, with a delay of several hours from the clinical onset (Fig. 22.6). Lesion contrast enhancement reflecting damage of the blood–brain barrier can be observed a few days after onset.

22.2.2 Antiphospholipid Antibody Syndrome

Antiphospholipid antibody syndrome (APS) is characterised by arterial or venous thrombosis and pregnant morbidity in the presence of anti-

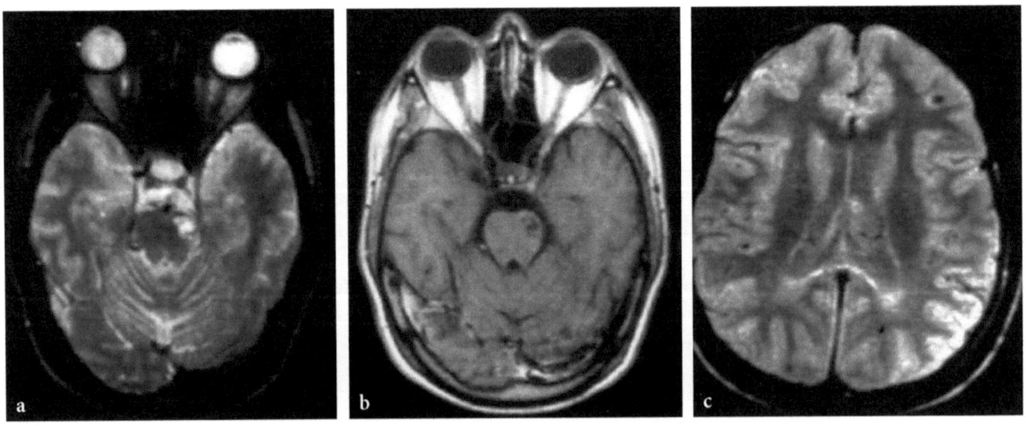

Fig. 22.6a–c. Polyarteritis nodosa. Midbrain infarct in an 18-year-old-man. Axial T2-weighted image (**a**) demonstrates an irregular but well-defined focal area of hyperintensity in the left midbrain 5 days after stroke. Axial T1-weighted image after intravenous administration of a gadolinium chelate (**b**) shows mild peripheral enhancement of the lesion. In axial proton density image (**c**), small hyperintense foci are visible in the peritrigonal white matter. The patient underwent catheter angiography, which enabled diagnosis of periarteritis nodosa by revealing a typical small aneurysm in the renal arteries

cardiolipin antibodies and/or lupus anticoagulant. Thrombocytopenia may be part of the syndrome (HARRIS 1986; TRENT et al. 1997; FUNAUCHI et al. 1997). APS can occur as either a primary disorder or be secondary to a connective tissue disease, most frequently SLE (PROVENZALE et al. 1996; SANNA et al. 2003).

APS is considered among the immunomediated non-MS diseases of the CNS but is not a vasculitis. In fact neuropathological examination indicates that the pathogenesis of the cerebral vasculopathy responsible for the cerebral white matter lesions is non-inflammatory and is associated with reactive endothelial hyperplasia and thrombosis of small arterioles (WESTERMAN et al. 1992). The clinical and laboratory diagnostic criteria were defined by an international committee (WILSON et al. 1999).

Recently, APS has emerged as an important cause of stroke in children and young adults, responsible for either arterial or venous thromboses (TAKANASHI et al. 1995; KIM et al. 2000; HELLER et al. 2003). Moreover, subclinical CNS involvement in the form of multifocal cerebral white matter lesions mimicking MS is demonstrated by MRI in up to about 40% of patients with primary and secondary APS (PROVENZALE et al. 1996; KIM et al. 2000) (Fig. 22.7).

Brain

Large and small infarcts in children and young adults show the usual appearance on conventional MRI (TAKANASHI et al. 1995; KIM et al. 2000) (Fig. 22.8). Also in the context of strokes in children, diffusion MR imaging has an established role for a more rapid detection of cerebral ischaemia (GADIAN et al. 2000).

Haemorrhagic infarcts and intra-parenchymal haemorrhages are demonstrated by conventional MRI as areas exhibiting low signal intensity in T2-weighted images, due to the paramagnetic properties of deoxyhaemoglobin in the acute phase, and high signal intensity in T1-weighted images, due to extracellular methaemoglobin in the subacute phase. Their identification should promote evaluation of the patency of the arterial or venous vessels with MR angiography, especially to rule out possible concomitant dural sinus thrombosis (KIM et al. 2000).

Cortical atrophy was reported as an additional finding in APS (KIM et al. 2000), but this is nonspecific, representing a possible effect of chronic steroid therapy as in SLE.

Optic Nerve

The MRI features of optic neuropathy in APS that is nonspecific resemble that in other form of "optic neuritis" (BESABS et al. 2001) (Fig. 22.7).

Spinal Cord

Spinal cord damage can be observed in patients with APS as primary clinical manifestation of the disease. In some instances it shows the typical MRI features of spinal cord infarction (HASEGAWA et al. 1993).

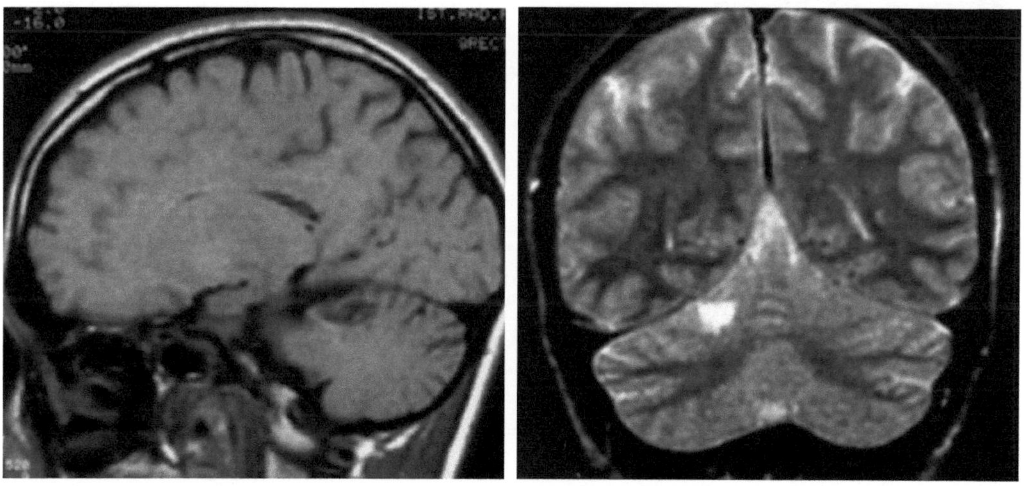

a b

Fig. 22.7a,b. Primary antiphospholipid syndrome. Cerebellar infarct in a 26-year-old woman. Sagittal T1-weighted (**a**) and coronal T2-weighted (**b**) images demonstrate a small focal area of signal change in the right cerebellar hemisphere in the territory of the right anterior cerebellar artery

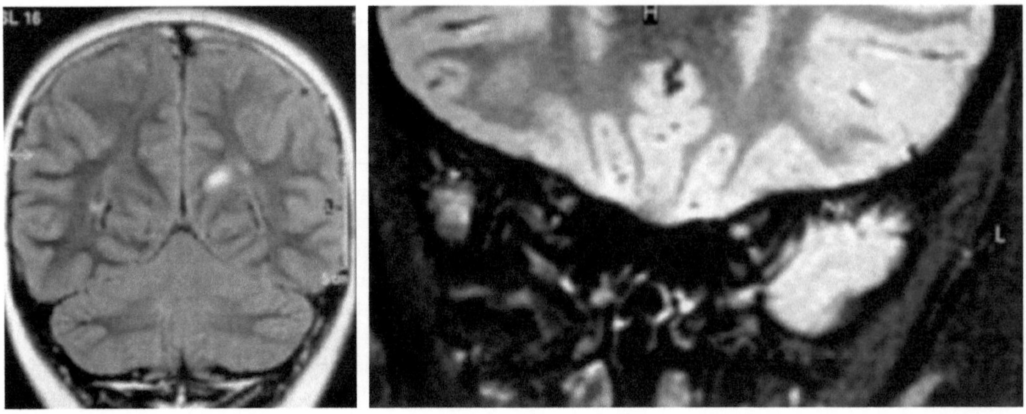

Fig. 22.8a,b. Primary antiphospholipid syndrome. White matter and optic nerve damage in an 8-year-old girl. Coronal proton density image (a) shows a focal white matter lesion in the left occipital lobe. Coronal STIR image (b) demonstrates hyperintensity of the left optic nerve in its posterior intraorbital portion

In other cases, the features are less distinctive and resemble those that can be observed in other systemic vasculitis.

22.2.3 Post-infective Angiitis

Although infective vasculitis can complicate the course of syphilis (meningovascular syphilis), tuberculosis (tuberculous meningitis), as well as fungal or bacterial (*H. influenzae*, staphylococcal, pneumococcal) meningeal infections, these conditions generally do not determine multifocal white matter damage and, as such, they will not be reviewed here. On the other hand, several viral infections–namely, chickenpox, measles, rubella and smallpox–can be followed by usually monophasic, multifocal white matter and grey matter damage (acute disseminated encephalomyelitis) that is addressed elsewhere in this book.

A peculiar case of post-infection vasculitis is the syndrome of herpes zoster ophthalmicus with delayed contralateral hemiparesis (Eidelberg et al. 1986). This association is rare and based upon the usual temporal evolution (first herpes ophthalmicus, second headache and hemiplegia) and the demonstration of viral particles in the smooth muscle cells of the media and varicella-zoster virus antigens in the media of the affected leptomeningeal vessels. Its pathogenesis is assumed to result from direct invasion of arterial walls via viral spread along the intracranial branches of the trigeminal nerve.

MR imaging demonstrates typical infarcted lesions with variable distribution in the anterior, middle and posterior cerebral arteries (Fig. 22.9).

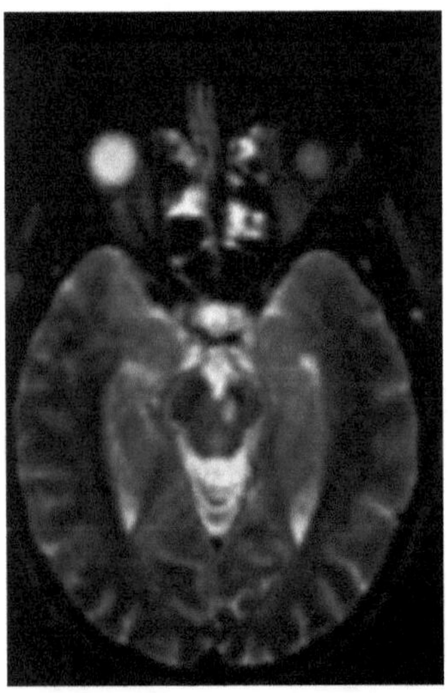

Fig. 22.9 Midbrain infarct due to zoster angiitis in a 42-year-old man. Axial T2-weighted image obtained 6 months after right hemiparesis, which came 3 weeks after left zoster ophthalmicus, shows a focal area of signal change and mild thinning of the left cerebral peduncle

22.2.4 Neurosarcoidosis

Sarcoidosis is a multisystem granulomatous disease, usually presenting with hilar adenopathy, pulmonary infiltration, and skin, eye and CNS involvement (Fig. 22.10). Very rarely, neurosarcoidosis may present

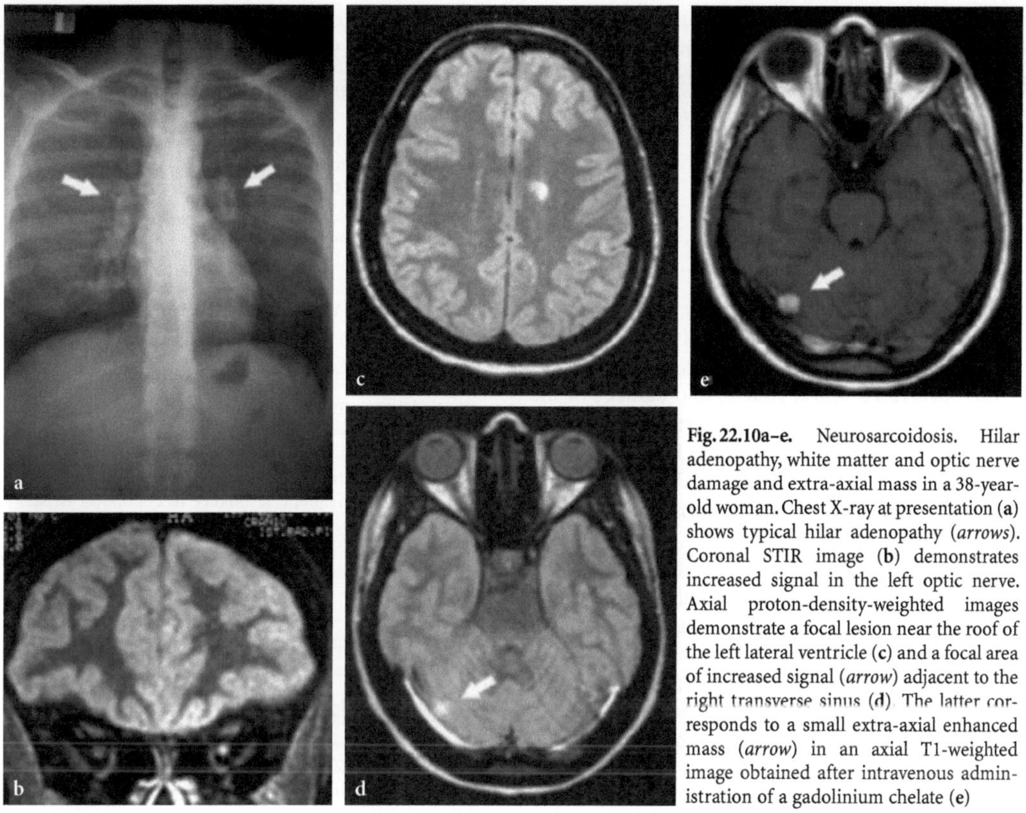

Fig. 22.10a–e. Neurosarcoidosis. Hilar adenopathy, white matter and optic nerve damage and extra-axial mass in a 38-year-old woman. Chest X-ray at presentation (**a**) shows typical hilar adenopathy (*arrows*). Coronal STIR image (**b**) demonstrates increased signal in the left optic nerve. Axial proton-density-weighted images demonstrate a focal lesion near the roof of the left lateral ventricle (**c**) and a focal area of increased signal (*arrow*) adjacent to the right transverse sinus (**d**). The latter corresponds to a small extra-axial enhanced mass (*arrow*) in an axial T1-weighted image obtained after intravenous administration of a gadolinium chelate (**e**)

in the absence of systemic involvement, and in such cases it requires biopsy for the diagnosis (Seltzer et al. 1991; Cipri et al. 2000; Bode et al. 2001). Most of the CNS lesions in sarcoidosis are markedly sensitive to steroids (Lexa and Grossman 1994). However, considering this phenomenon, an indirect clue of neurosarcoidosis can delay the correct diagnosis in patients presenting with other steroid-responsive lesions, in particular tumours including lymphoma and germ cell tumour (Mascalchi et al. 1998b).

Brain

Multifocal, cerebral white matter damage indistinguishable from that seen in MS is common in neurosarcoidosis (Miller et al. 1988; Lexa and Grossman 1994) (Fig. 22.10). Although not specific, a key feature indicating sarcoidosis as the possible underlying substrate of the white matter lesions is diffuse focal leptomeningeal or dural enhancement better demonstrated by MRI after intravenous contrast administration (Sherman and Sherry 1990; Khaw et al. 1991; Seltzer et al. 1991). Additional features that should raise suspicion of neurosarcoidosis include (Seltzer et al. 1991; Lexa & Grossman 1994): extra-axial contrast-enhancing masses mimicking meningioma (Fig. 22.10), intra-axial enhancing masses, periventricular enhancement, enlarged pituitary stalk, and enhancing nerve roots. All lesions, in particular their contrast enhancement, typically regress with steroid therapy (Lexa and Grossman 1994).

Optic Nerve

Optic nerve and chiasma are typical sites of CNS involvement in neurosarcoidosis (Bode et al. 2001; Carmody et al. 1994). Enlargement of optic nerve and chiasma, associated with signal changes (Fig. 22.10) and contrast enhancement, is seen in the acute phase, and this regresses with steroid treatment. Atrophic optic nerve is observed in the chronic phase.

Spinal Cord

Spinal cord involvement in neurosarcoidosis is extremely rare (Seltzer et al. 1991; Lexa and

Grossman 1994). In the few available descriptions it was associated with extensive intramedullary lesions exhibiting contrast enhancement and was difficult to differentiate from an intramedullary neoplasm.

22.3 Conclusions

In addition to the multifocal white matter damage mimicking MS in secondary vasculitis and APS, the lesions include infarcts, haemorrhages, thrombosis of the intracranial dural sinuses and damage of the optic nerve and spinal cord of uncertain pathophysiology. It is noteworthy that the MRI features of these lesions are specific, and, hence, the differential diagnosis relies completely on the integration of clinical and laboratory findings.

The spectrum of lesions in neurosarcoidosis is wide, but coexistence of multifocal cerebral white matter lesions with meningeal enhancement or intra-axial or extra-axial contrast-enhancing masses should raise suspicions that this condition is present. However, lacking systemic manifestations of the disease, diagnosis of neurosarcoidosis still requires biopsy.

References

Akman-Demir G, Sorderoglu P, Tasci B et al (1999) Clinical patterns of neurological involvement in Behçet's disease: evaluation of 200 patients. Brain 122:2171–2181

Alexander EL, Beall SS, Gordon B et al (1988) Magnetic resonance imaging of cerebral lesions in patients with Sjögren syndrome. Ann Intern Med 108:815–823

Al Kawi MZ, Bohlega S, Banna M (1991) MRI findings in neuroBehçet disease. Neurology 41:405–408

Angelini L, Rumi V, Nardocci N et al (1993) Hemidystonia symptomatic of primary antiphospholipid syndrome in childhood. Mov Disord 8:383–386

Bekkelund SI, Pierre-Jerome C, Husby G, Mellgren SI (1995) Quantitative cerebral MR in rheumatoid arthritis. AJNR Am J Neuroradiol 16:767–772

Besbas N, Anlar B, Apak A, Kansu T (2001) Optic neuropathy in primary antiphospholipid syndrome in childhood. J Child Neurol 16:690–693

Bode MK, Tikkakoski T, Tuisku S et al (2001) Isolated neurosarcoidosis–MR findings and pathologic correlation. Acta Radiol 42:563–567

Carmody RF, Mafee MF, Goodwin JA et al (1994) Orbital and optic pathway sarcoidosis: MR findings. AJNR Am J Neuroradiol 15:775–783

Cellerini M, Bartolucci M, Mortilla M et al (2003) MR imaging and proton MR spectroscopy of the brain in Behçet's disease. Riv Neuroradiol 16:267–274

Cipri S, Gambardella G, Campolo C et al (2000) Unusual clinical presentation of cerebral-isolated sarcoidosis. J Neurosurg Sci 44:140–144

Condor SEJ, Jarosz JM (2002) Magnetic resonance imaging of cerebral venous sinus thrombosis. Clin Radiol 57:449–461

De Reuck J (2003) Dorsal thalamic hemorrhage complicating polyarteritis nodosa: a clinico-pathologic case report. Acta Neurol Belg 103:40–42

De Seze J, Stojkovic T, Hachulla E et al (2001) Myelopathy-Sjogren's syndrome association: analysis of clinical and radiological findings and clinical course. Rev Neurol 157:669–678

Eidelberg D, Sotrel A, Horoupian DA et al (1986) Thrombotic cerebral vasculopathy associated with herpes zoster. Ann Neurol 19:7–14

Funauchi M, Hamada K, Enomoto H et al (1997) Characteristics of the clinical findings in patients with idiopathic thrombocytopenic purpura who are positive for anti-phospholipid antibodies. Intern Med 36:882–885

Gadian DG, Calamante F, Kirkham FJ et al (2000) Diffusion and perfusion magnetic resonance in childhood stroke. J Child Neurol 15:279–283

Galli M, Barbui T (2003) Antiphospolipid antibodies and thrombosis: strength of the association. Hematol J 4:180–186

Harris EN, Gharavi AE, Hughes GRV (1985) Antiphospholipid antibodies. Clin Rheum Dis 11:591–609

Hasegawa M, Yamashita J, Yamashima T et al (1993) Spinal cord infarction associated with primary antiphospholipid syndrome in a young child. Case report. J Neurosurg 79:447–450

Heller C, Heinecke A, Junker R et al (2003) Cerebral venous thrombosis in children. A multifactorial origin. Circulation 108:1362–1367

Kadota Y, Tokumaru AM, Kamakura K et al (2002) Primary Sjogren syndrome initially manifested by optic neuritis: MRI findings. Neuroradiology 44:338–41

Kermode AG, Plant GT, Mac Manus DG et al (1989) Behçet's disease with slowly enlarging midbrain mass on MRI: resolution following steroid therapy. Neurology 39:1251–1252

Khaw KT, Manji H, Britton J, Schon F (1991) Neurosarcoidosis–demonstration of meningeal disease by gadolinium-enhanced magnetic resonance imaging. J Neurol Neurosurg Psychiatry 54: 499–502

Kim JH, Choi CG, Choi SJ et al (2000) Primary antiphospholipid antibody syndrome: neuroradiologic findings in 11 patients. Korean J Radiol 1:5–10

Koçer N, Islak C, Siva A et al (1999) CNS involvement in neuro-Behçet syndrome: an MR study. AJNR Am J Neuroradiol 20:1015–1024

Inaba G (1989) Behçet disease. In: Vynken PJ, Bruyn GW, Klawans HL (eds) Handbook of clinical neurology, vol 12. Elsevier, Amsterdam, pp 593–610

International study group for Behçet's disease (1990) Lancet 335:1078-1080

Lafitte C (2002) Neuroradiological manifestations of primary Sjogren's syndrome. Rev Neurol 158:959–965

Lafitte C, Amoura Z, Cacoub P et al (2001) Neurological complications of primary Sjogren's syndrome. J Neurol 248:577–584

Lexa FJ, Grossman RI (1994) MR of sarcoidosis in the head and spine: spectrum of manifestations and radiographic

response to steroid therapy. AJNR Am J Neuroradiol 15:973–982
Manabe Y, Sasaki H, Marita H et al (2000) Sjogren's syndrome with acute transverse myelopathy as the initial manifestation. J Neurol Sci 176:158–161
Mascalchi M, Salvi F, Piacentini S, Bartolozzi C (1994) Friedreich's ataxia: MR findings involving the cervical portion of the spinal cord. AJR Am J Roentgenol 163:187–191
Mascalchi M, Cosottini M, Cellerini M et al (1998a) MRI of spinal cord involvement in Behçet's disease: case report. Neuroradiology 40:255–257
Mascalchi M, Roncaroli F, Salvi F, Frank G (1998b) Transient regression of intracranial germ cell tumor following steroid intravenous administration. J Neurol Neurosurg Psychiatry 64:670–672
Miller DH, Ormerod IEC, Gibson A et al (1987) MR brain scanning in patients with vasculitis: differentiation from multiple sclerosis. Neuroradiology 29:226–231
Miller DH, Kendall BE, Barter S et al (1988) Magnetic resonance imaging in central nervous system sarcoidosis. Neurology 38:378–383
Mochizuki A, Hayashi A, Hisahara S, Shoji S (2000) Steroid-responsive Devic's variant in Sjogren's syndrome. Neurology 54:1391–1392
Mori K, Koike H, Misu K et al (2001) Spinal cord magnetic resonance imaging demonstrates sensory neuronal involvement and clinical severity in neuronopathy associated with Sjogren's syndrome. J Neurol Neurosurg Psychiatry 71:488–492
Pierot L, Sauve C, Leger JM et al (1993) Asymptomatic cerebral involvement in Sjogren's syndrome: MRI findings in 15 cases. Neuroradiology 35:378–380
Provenzale JM, Allen NB (1996) Neuroradiologic findings in polyarteritis nodosa. AJNR Am J Neuroradiol 17:1119–1126
Provenzale JM, Barboriak DP, Allen NB, Ortel TL (1996) Patients with antiphospholipid antibodies: CT and MR findings of the brain. AJR Am J Roentgenol 167:1573–1578
Reichhart MD, Bogousslavsky J, Janzer RC (2000) Early lacunar strokes complicating polyarteritis nodosa. Thrombotic microangiopathy. Neurology 54:883–889
Reshef E, Greenberg SB, Jankovic J (1985) Herpes zoster ophthalmicus followed by contralateral hemiparesis: report of two cases and review of the literature. J Neurol Neurosurg Psychiatry 48:122–127
Salvi F, Mascalchi M, Malatesta R et al (1999) Optic neuropathy in Behçet's disease. Report of two cases. Ital J Neurol Sci 20:181–186
Sanna G, Bertolaccini ML, Cuadrado MJ et al (2003) Central nervous system involvement in the antiphospholipid (Hughes) syndrome. Rheumatology 42:200–213
Seltzer S, Mark AS, Atlas SW (1991) CNS sarcoidosis: evaluation with contrast-enhanced MR imaging. AJNR Am J Neuroradiol 12:1227–1233
Shakir RA, Sulaiman K, Kahn RA, Rudwan M (1990) Neurological presentation of Neuro-Behçet's syndrome: clinical categories. Eur Neurol 30:249–253
Sherman JL, Stern BJ (1990) Sarcoidosis of the CNS: comparison of unenhanced and enhanced MR images. AJNR Am J Neuroradiol 11:915–923
Sklar AM, Schatz NJ, Glaser JS et al (1996) MR of vasculitis-induced optic neuropathy. AJNR Am J Neuroradiol 17:121–128
Takanashi J, Sugita K, Miyazato S et al (1995) Antiphospholipid antibody syndrome in childhood strokes. Pediatr Neurol 13:323–326
Tesar JT, McMillan V, Molina R, Armstrong J (1992) Optic neuropathy and central nervous system disease associated with primary Sjogren's syndrome. Am J Med 92:686–692
Trent K, Neustater BR, Lottenberg R (1997) Chronic relapsing thrombotic thrombocytopenic purpura and antiphospholipid antibodies: a report of two cases. Am J Hematol 54:155–159
Wechsler B, Dell'Isola B, Vidailhet M et al (1993) MRI in 31 patients with Behçet's disease and neurological involvement: prospective study with clinical correlation. J Neurol Neurosurg Psychiatry 56:793–798
Westerman EM, Miles JM, Backonja M, Sundstrom WR (1992) Neuropathologic findings in multi-infarct dementia associated with anticardiolipin antibody. Evidence for endothelial injury as the primary event. Arthritis Rheum 35:1038–1042
Wilson WA, Gharavi AE, Koike T et al (1999) International consensus statement on preliminary classification criteria for definite antiphospholipid syndrome. Arthritis Rheum 12:1309–1311

23 White Matter Pathology in Systemic Immune-Mediated Diseases

MARCO ROVARIS and MASSIMO FILIPPI

CONTENTS

23.1 Introduction

Systemic immune-mediated diseases (SID) can affect the central nervous system (CNS), either as the onset clinical manifestation or as a late complication in the context of a multiple organ involvement (CALABRESE et al. 1997; FIESCHI et al. 1998). Among SID, systemic lupus erythematosus (SLE), Behçet disease (BD), small-vessel vasculitides (SVV) and primary antiphospholipid antibody syndrome (APS) may often have a flare-like clinical course which closely resembles that of multiple sclerosis (MS) and, therefore, be considered in the differential diagnosis of this latter condition.

Numerous studies reported that conventional, T2-weighted brain magnetic resonance imaging (MRI) is sensitive for detecting CNS lesions in patients with SID (MILLER et al. 1987; COBAN et al. 1996; LIEM et al. 1996; PROVENZALE and ALLEN 1996; GUMÀ et al. 1998; HACHULLA et al. 1998). A wide spectrum of non-specific MRI abnormalities has been described in these patients, including cerebral infarctions, brain atrophy, dural sinus thrombosis and, more rarely, hemorrhages or meningeal involvement. In a significant proportion of patients with SID, however, multiple brain white matter lesions mimicking those due to MS can be the only MRI-visible abnormalities (MILLER et al. 1987; NADEAU 1997; TRIULZI and SCOTTI 1998) (Fig. 23.1). Unfortunately, the limited pathological specificity of the latter findings hampers their diagnostic accuracy, as well as their prognostic value and relevance in the work-up of SID patients.

Quantitative MR-based techniques, such as magnetization transfer (MT) MRI, diffusion-weighted (DW) MRI and magnetic resonance spectroscopy (MRS), make it possible to obtain information about white matter damage with increased pathological specificity over T2-weighted sequences (MILLER et al. 2003). In addition, all these techniques have the ability to assess and quantify the extent of white matter pathology beyond the resolution of conventional MRI, e.g. in the so-called normal-appearing white matter (NAWM). NAWM pathology seems to be a relevant contributor to the neurological impairment in patients with MS (MILLER et al. 2003) and its accurate assessment might also be useful for the differential diagnosis between SID and other CNS diseases, as well as for a better understanding of the mechanisms leading to CNS dysfunction in the former conditions.

This chapter reviews the contributions of conventional and modern MRI techniques to the in vivo investigation of white matter pathology in SID.

23.2 Conventional MRI

Between 30% and 70% of patients with SLE develop neuropsychiatric complications (NSLE) during the course of the disease. In NSLE patients, brain MRI is abnormal in 40%–60% of cases (CSÉPÀNY et al. 2003; JENNINGS et al. 2004), but the observed findings are not disease-specific, the commonest being cerebral infarcts, brain atrophy and multiple, MS-like white matter lesions. The prevalence of brain MRI abnormalities in patients with BD and CNS involvement (NBD) varies between 30% and 86% (AKMAN-DEMIR et al. 1999; COBAN et al. 1996; GERBER et al. 1996; LEE

M. ROVARIS, MD; M. FILIPPI, MD
Neuroimaging Research Unit, Department of Neurology, Scientific Institute and University Ospedale San Raffaele, Milan, Italy

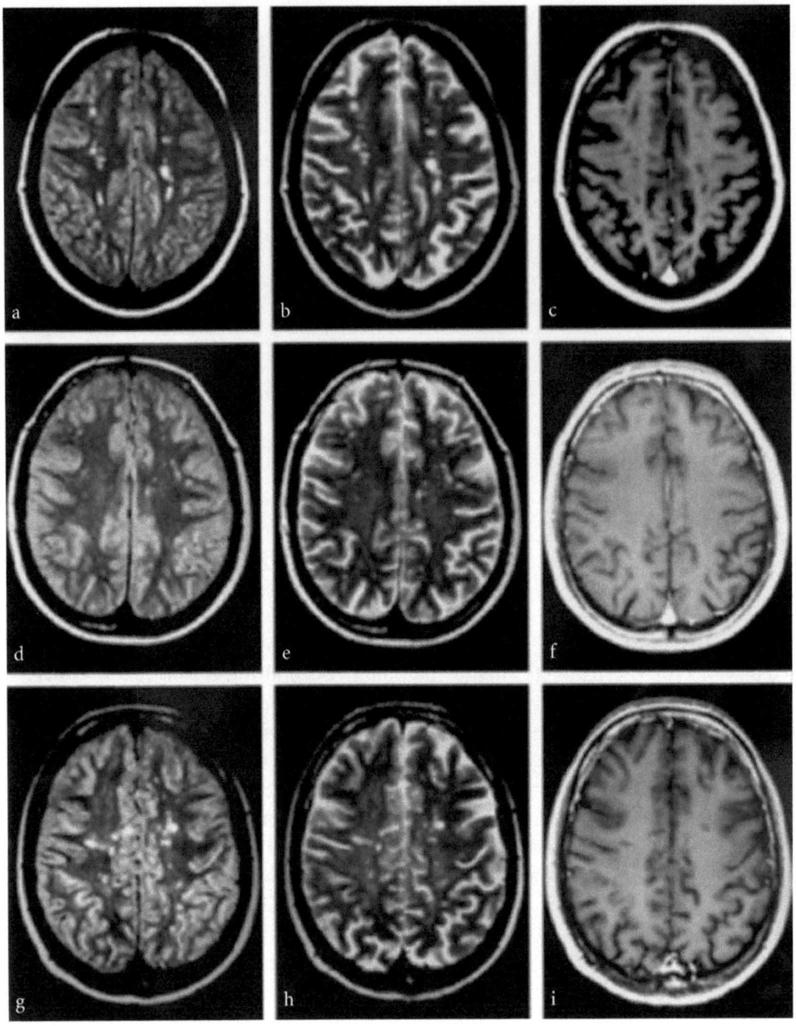

Fig. 23.1a–i. Axial proton density-weighted spin echo (**a, d, g**), T2-weighted spin echo (**b, e, h**) and post-contrast T1-weighted spin echo (**c, f, i**) images of the brain obtained from patients with NSLE (**a–c**), WG (**d–f**) and relapsing-remitting MS (**g–i**) just above the roof of the lateral ventricles. The pattern of T2-visible abnormalities is similar for the three patients, although fewer lesions can be seen on the images from the patient with WG (**d, e**) than on those from the patients with MS and NSLE. [Reproduced with permission from Rovaris et al. (2000b)]

et al. 2001). Most frequently, these abnormalities consist of brainstem and basal ganglia lesions that may shrink or disappear at follow-up (Lee et al. 2001). In 20%–40% of NBD cerebral white matter is diffusely involved (Akman-Demir et al. 1999; Lee et al. 2001). Among patients with SVV, only a minority of those with Wegener granulomatosis (WG) may show some degree of brain MRI abnormalities (Provenzale and Allen 1996), although the prevalence of clinical CNS involvement ranges between 22% and 54% of cases (Fieschi et al. 1998). Focal infarcts are the commonest MRI abnormalities described in APS, but brain atrophy and diffuse, T2-hyperintense white matter lesions can also be found in a high percentage of cases (Hachulla et al. 1998; Ijdo et al. 1999; Weingarten et al. 1997). Moreover, recent reports found that up to 20% of MS patients with brain MRI findings highly suggestive for this disease (Ijdo et al. 1999; Karussis et al. 1998) can be consistently positive for antiphospholipid antibodies, thus suggesting the possibility of a concomitant diagnosis of MS and APS.

It is worthy noting that, in SID patients, the use of fast fluid-attenuated inversion recovery (fFLAIR) sequences, which are known to be more sensitive than conventional T2-weighted MRI for detecting lesions in the brain of patients with inflammatory or demyelinating diseases of the CNS (Maubon et al. 1998), does not seem to increase the sensitivity of brain scanning for the detection of white matter abnormalities (Rovaris et al. 2000a). Among the potential explanations for this finding, the pathological heterogeneity of white matter damage in SID also has to be considered. Brain pathology in SID may range from inflammation to acute and chronic ischaemia, which can be secondary to vessel thrombosis or vasculitis. Small chronic infarcts can appear isointense to normal tissue on fFLAIR scans, and, therefore, go undetected when using this sequence.

White matter abnormalities detected on T2-weighted and post-contrast T1-weighted MRI of the brain have a limited diagnostic specificity for SID. Several studies (Boumpas et al. 1990; Deodhar et al. 1999; Mascalchi et al. 1998; Mok et al. 1998; Morrissey et al. 1993; Provenzale et al. 1994; Salmaggi et al. 1994; Yoshioka et al. 1996) have suggested that MRI abnormalities in the cord of patients with SID are well correlated with ongoing symptoms of myelopathy and that they can completely disappear after steroid or immunosuppressive treatment (Boumpas et al. 1990; Lee et al. 2001; Mascalchi et al. 1998; Rovaris et al. 2000c; Salmaggi et al. 1994; Yoshioka et al. 1996). On the other hand, spinal cord MRI abnormalities can be detected in up to 90% of MS patients (Lycklama à Nijeholt et al. 1998; Miller et al. 1998; Rocca et al. 1999), often without a concomitant clinical involvement, and the presence of such lesions may increase the confidence when diagnosing MS at its clinical onset (Fazekas et al. 1999). Against this background, the detection of MRI-visible white matter pathology in the cord might provide useful information for the work-up of patients with CNS disturbances, especially when a differential diagnosis between SID and MS has to be made. In a cross-sectional study of 44 patients with SID (Rovaris et al. 2002), of whom 48% had had clinical manifestations of CNS involvement, cervical cord MRI scans were always found to be normal, whereas brain MRI revealed white matter lesions in 52% of the cases. The application of standardized criteria for brain MR image interpretation (Barkhof et al. 1997), which were originally developed for predicting the evolution to established MS in patients at presentation with clinically isolated neurological syndromes suggestive of MS, yielded an accuracy of about 85% in differentiating SID from age-matched MS patients and, by using the presence or absence of cervical cord MRI lesions as a dichotomized criterion, a correct re-classification of 77% of MS patients and two SLE patients who were misclassified based upon their patterns of brain abnormalities was possible (Rovaris et al. 2002). The additional value of cord MRI in the differentiation of MS from SID and other neurological diseases of ischaemic etiology has been emphasized by another study (Bot et al. 2002), where asymptomatic cord lesions were found in 92% of MS and 6% of non-MS patients and the concomitant evaluation of both brain and cord MRI findings achieved a 95% diagnostic accuracy (Fig. 23.2). Both these studies (Bot et al. 2002; Rovaris et al. 2002) confirm that conventional MRI patterns of brain white matter damage related to SID do not have a clear-cut diagnostic value and they also underpin the importance of a careful interpretation

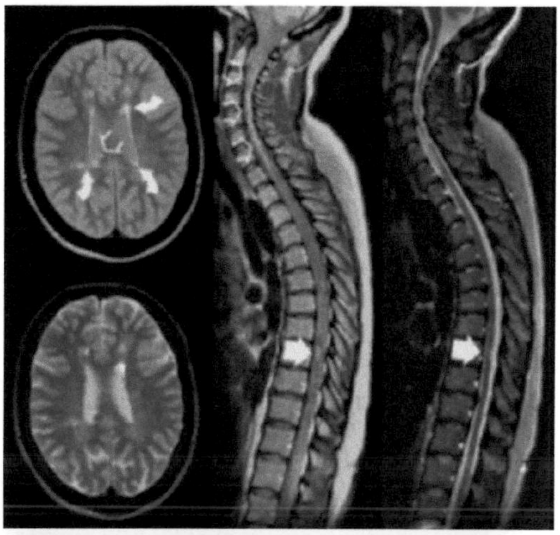
a

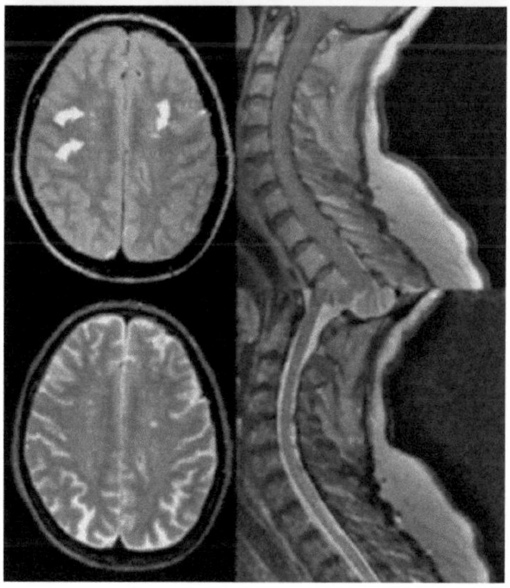
b

Fig. 23.2a,b. Brain and spinal cord MR images in a patient with MS (**a**) and in a patient with Sjögren disease associated with clinical CNS dysfunction (**b**). Brain images fulfill diagnostic criteria for MS in both cases. However, sagittal cord images reveal the presence of diffuse abnormalities in the cervical tract and one focal lesion in the thoracic tract of the patient with MS, whereas no abnormalities can be seen in the patient with Sjögren disease. [Reproduced with permission from Bot et al. (2002)]

of MRI findings based on a comprehensive image evaluation, which should consider, on the one hand, the radiologist's opinion and, on the other, the application of standardized criteria.

Several studies have investigated whether the conventional MRI patterns of white matter pathology in SID patients may correlate with their clinical or immunological status and, therefore, have a value as paraclinical outcomes to monitor the disease evolution.

The severity of neuropsychological dysfunction in SLE patients seems to be associated with the presence of cerebral infarcts (Waterloo et al. 2001) rather than with the overall burden of white matter lesions (Kozora et al. 1998; Sailer et al. 1997). The limited functional relevance of T2-visible white matter abnormalities is also consistent with their weak correlation with neuroimaging correlates of brain metabolisms (Sailer et al. 1997; Waterloo et al. 2001). On the other hand, however, it has been found (Bell et al. 1991; West et al. 1995) that NSLE patients with non-focal psychiatric symptoms more frequently show an MRI pattern of multiple white matter abnormalities and have higher titers of antineurofilament antibodies than those with focal CNS disturbances. Two recent studies of NSLE patients also reported a significant relationship of MRI findings with the presence of antiphospholipid antibodies (Csèpàny et al. 2003) and the levels of biochemical markers of axonal damage in the cerebrospinal fluid (Trysberg et al. 2003). These findings suggest that, in NSLE, different pathogenic mechanisms may be responsible for brain tissue damage, including both vasculopathic and immune-mediated neuronal injury, and underpin the need of MRI-derived measures with higher pathological specificity to monitor the disease course and its response to treatment. In patients with NBD, conventional MRI patterns of CNS involvement do not seem to have a clear-cut prognostic value (Akman-Demir et al. 1999; Lee et al. 2001), even though the presence of brainstem lesions, together with other clinical and laboratory characteristics, make it possible to identify those patients with a poorer clinical outcome (Akman-Demir et al. 1999). In a study of patients with SVV (Mattioli et al. 2002), the presence of multiple white matter MRI abnormalities was frequently associated with subclinical cognitive impairment. Admittedly, caution must be exercised when interpreting MRI data from the latter study (Mattioli et al. 2002), which were obtained from a small sample of patients. However, the observation that less than 15% of cognitively impaired SVV patients in this series had a normal brain MRI (Mattioli et al. 2002) may indicate that the presence of MRI-visible white matter lesions significantly increases the possibility for an SVV patient to have neuropsychological impairment.

23.3 Magnetization Transfer MRI

MT MRI has several advantages over conventional T2- and T1-weighted MRI for the in vivo structural investigation of CNS disorders. First, it provides information with a high pathological specificity. Low magnetization transfer ratio (MTR) indicates a reduced capacity of the molecules in the brain tissue matrix to exchange magnetization with the surrounding (MRI-visible) water molecules and is associated with severe demyelination and axonal loss (Brochet and Dousset 1999). Secondly, MT MRI enables us to assess the "invisible" disease burden in the normal-appearing brain tissue (NABT). Thirdly, MT MRI can provide, from a single procedure, multiple parameters influenced by both the MRI-visible and MRI-undetectable disease burden. They are obtained after the automated creation of MTR maps, where the signal intensity of each pixel represents its MTR value. The analysis can then be done on a region-of-interest (ROI) basis or more globally using MTR histograms (van Buchem et al. 1996).

An ROI-based study comparing MT MRI findings from 21 patients with MS and nine with SLE showed that the average MTR values of T2-visible white matter lesions and NAWM in the brain were significantly lower for the former group (Campi et al. 1996). In the same study, MTR values from the NAWM of SLE patients were found not to differ from those of healthy controls. Using histogram-based analysis, an MT MRI study of 44 patients with SID, of whom 15 with SLE, nine with NSLE, five with BD, nine with WG and six with APS, was also conducted (Rovaris et al. 2000b). Ten patients with MS served as a control group. T2-weighted brain MRI abnormalities were found in all MS cases and in 52% of patients with SID, for whom a white matter lesion pattern indistinguishable from that of MS was observed in 40% of cases. MS patients had significantly lower lesion MTR than SLE and WG patients; NSLE had significantly lower lesion MTR than SLE patients. MS patients had significantly lower average MTR values in the NABT than all SID but NSLE patients, who, in turn, had significantly lower average NABT MTR than SLE patients (Fig. 23.3). Both T2-weighted lesion volume and av-

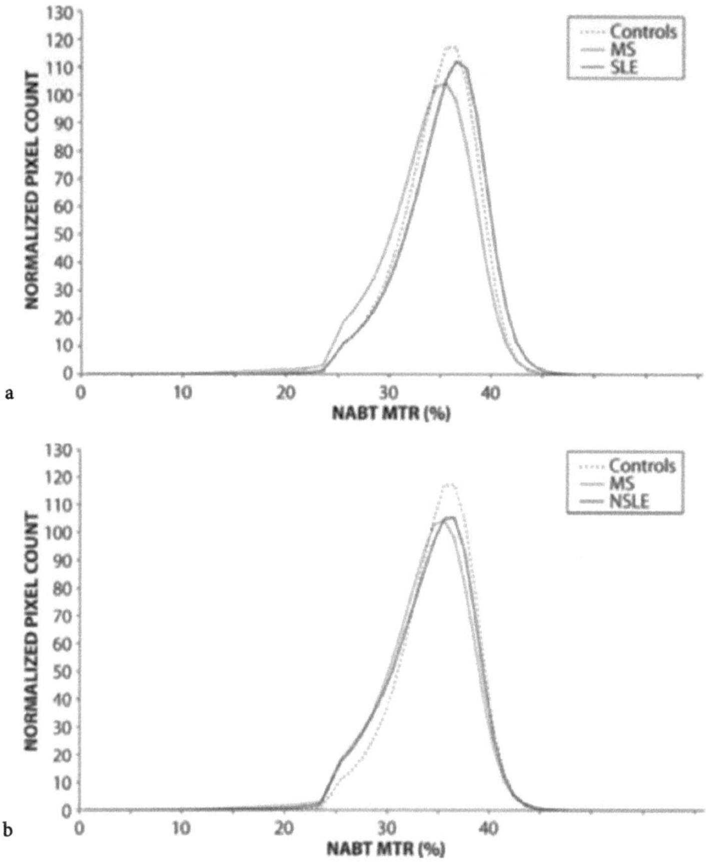

Fig. 23.3a,b. NABT MTR histograms from healthy controls, patients with relapsing-remitting MS, patients with SLE without clinical signs of CNS involvement (**a**) or patients with NSLE (**b**). For SLE patients, the shape of the histogram resembles that of healthy controls and average NABT MTR values are significantly higher than those of MS patients, whilst there are no significant differences between MS and NSLE patients in terms of NABT MTR histogram-derived metrics. [Reproduced with permission from Rovaris and Filippi (2003)]

erage lesion MTR fitted a multiparametric model significantly separating MS from SID patients, with a significantly higher risk of having MS with increasing lesion volume and decreasing lesion MTR values. No conventional or MT MRI-derived variables significantly separated MS patients as a group from NSLE patients. Similar results were obtained by Bosma et al. (2000a,b), who found that NSLE patients had significantly lower brain MTR histogram peak height than age-matched healthy controls and SLE patients without overt CNS involvement, independent of the presence of T2-visible white matter lesions. In patients during the acute stage of NSLE (Bosma et al. 2000b), the average MTR histogram peak height was found to be lower than that of patients with chronic inactive NSLE, SLE and MS. More recently, Bosma et al. (2002) also investigated the relationship between brain MTR histogram-derived quantities and clinical status in 24 patients with NSLE. Significant correlations were found between MTR histogram peak height and measures of neurologic, cognitive and psychiatric functioning, whereas no significant relationship was observed between MT MRI findings and NSLE patients' disease duration.

Available data show that the presence of CNS dysfunction in SLE is associated with a diffuse, MT MRI-detectable damage of the brain parenchyma, whereas this does not seem to be the case for other SID (Rovaris et al. 2000b). Such damage is probably primarily present in the NABT and does not greatly depend upon the burden of T2-visible white matter abnormalities. Indeed, the latter abnormalities can also be found in 30%–40% (Rovaris et al. 2000b; Bosma et al. 2000a,b) of SLE patients without overt CNS disturbances, but MTR histogram-derived quantities of these patients do not significantly differ from those of healthy controls. Moreover, when brain MTR histograms are obtained after the exclusion of pixels belonging to T2-visible lesions, the observed differences between NSLE patients and normal controls or patients with other SID do not change (Rovaris et al. 2000b). It remains to be established which is the causal relationship between the extent and nature of NSLE-related diffuse brain tissue damage and MT MRI-detectable abnormalities. The contribution of NAWM pathology appears to be relevant for a number of reasons. First, despite the concomitant finding of brain atrophy in NSLE (Bosma et al. 2000a,b), the magnitude of the decrease of brain MTR histogram peak height in comparison with SLE and healthy controls did not change when this metric was normalized for brain volume, thus suggesting that atrophy per se cannot explain the observed MT MRI abnormalities. Second, a preliminary, ROI-based study (Campi et al. 1996) did not find any difference in NAWM MTR values between SLE patients and age-matched healthy subjects. Third, on the one hand, macromolecules that contribute to the MT effect in the brain tissue are mainly cerebrosides and phospholipids, which are the major components of myelinated white matter tracts (Brochet and Dousset 1999), and, on the other, NAWM constitutes a great portion of the NABT. Thus, it is conceivable that changes in the MTR histogram characteristics of the latter compartment mainly depend upon diffuse, MRI-undetectable white matter abnormalities leading to demyelination and loss of axons. Admittedly, these speculations need to be confirmed by further studies with a separate analysis of white and gray matter MTR histograms in NSLE and other SID. Preliminary MT MRI data (personal observations, unpublished results) seem to suggest that normal-appearing gray matter damage, if any, is minimal in SID, independently of the presence of overt CNS involvement or T2-visible white matter abnormalities. This is in contrast with what has been found in MS patients, for whom gray matter damage seems to play a central role in the pathobiology of CNS dysfunction (Miller et al. 2003).

The potential usefulness of MT MRI as a paraclinical tool to monitor SID evolution is suggested by the ability of the technique to differentiate the active from the chronic stage of NSLE (Bosma et al. 2000b), as well as by the observed, significant association between volumetric MT MRI data and NSLE patients' clinical status (Bosma et al. 2002). As regards the application of MT MRI to the diagnostic work-up of SID patients with CNS disturbances, Bosma et al. (2000a) found nearly no overlap between the individual MTR histogram peak height values of NSLE patients and those of either SLE patients or healthy controls, yielding a 95% specificity in the diagnostic classification of subjects with a cut-off value of 96.8. When the multiparametric model proposed by Rovaris et al. (2000b) was used to classify patients with MRI-visible white matter abnormalities as MS or SID other than NSLE, 60% of patients with MS and 91% of those with SID were correctly classified. More recently (Rovaris et al. 2002), the value of brain MTR histogram-derived findings for the differential diagnosis between MS and SID other than NSLE in individual cases has been investigated. Only one SLE of 44 SID patients had an average brain MTR one standard deviation below the control group mean value, whereas this was the case for 33 of 64 MS patients (52%); the combined evaluation of cervical cord MRI and brain MT MRI findings made it possible to correctly classify as MS or SID all but one patient, supporting a more extensive use of these two techniques to differentiate between MS and SID when non-specific MRI abnormalities of brain white matter are detected. That MT MRI might serve as a diagnostic tool in the work-up of SLE patients has also been indicated by the preliminary results obtained by Dehmeshki et al. (2002), using a multivariate discriminant analysis approach.

23.4 Diffusion-Weighted MRI

Diffusion is the microscopic random translational motion of molecules in a fluid system. In the CNS, diffusion is influenced by the microstructural components of tissue, including cell membranes and organelles. The diffusion coefficient of biological tissues (which can be measured in vivo by MRI) is, therefore, lower than the diffusion coefficient in free water and, for this reason, is named apparent diffusion coefficient (ADC) (Le Bihan et al. 1986). Pathological processes which modify tissue integrity, thus resulting in a loss or increased permeability of "restricting" barriers, can determine an increase of the ADC. Since some cellular structures are aligned on the scale of an image pixel, the measurement of diffusion is also dependent on the direction in which diffusion is measured. As a consequence, diffusion measurements can give information about the size, shape, integrity and orientation of tissues (Le Bihan et al. 1991). A measure of diffusion which is independent of the orientation of structures is provided by the mean diffusivity (MD), the average of the ADCs measured in three orthogonal directions. A full characterization of diffusion can be obtained in terms of a tensor (Basser et al. 1994), a 3×3 matrix which accounts for the correlation existing between molecular displacement along orthogonal directions. From the tensor, it is possible to derive MD, equal to one third of its trace, and some other dimensionless indexes of anisotropy, such as fractional anisotropy (FA) (Basser and Pierpaoli 1996). Inflammation and demyelination have the potential to alter the permeability or geometry of structural barriers to water molecular diffusion in the brain white matter, thus leading to DW MRI-detectable changes. Recently, a preliminary, post mortem high field MRI study of the spinal cord of patients with MS (Mottershead et al. 2003) reported that myelin content and axonal density of the specimens correlated strongly with diffusion anisotropy, but only weakly with ADC values.

Available DW MRI studies of SLE patients (Moritani et al. 2001; Bosma et al. 2003; Jennings et al. 2003) reveal that areas with decreased ADC values, corresponding to T2-visible white matter lesions, can be seen in 10%–20% of patients (Moritani et al. 2001; Jennings et al. 2003), suggesting the presence of acute or subacute ischemic damage. Less frequently, ADC values can be increased within T2-isointense or slightly T2-hyperintense lesions (Moritani et al. 2001), indicating the presence of vasogenic edema or demyelination. Bosma et al. (2003), using a histogram analysis technique, found that the average ADC values in the brain of 11 NSLE patients were significantly higher than those of age-matched healthy controls, even though the visual inspection of DW images did not reveal other abnormalities than those visible on the corresponding T2-weighted MRI scans, i.e. subtle white matter hyperintensities, in about 50% of these patients. These data are consistent with those obtained using MT MRI (Rovaris et al. 2000b; Bosma et al. 2000a, b), indicating the presence of diffuse, structural brain damage. On the contrary, DW MRI studies of NBD (Hiwatashi et al. 2003; Kunimatsu et al. 2003) show that both acute and chronic white matter lesions have higher ADC values than the NABT areas, confirming the primarily inflammatory pathogenesis of white matter damage in this condition.

23.5 Magnetic Resonance Spectroscopy

MRS can complement conventional MRI in the assessment of patients with CNS disorders, by defining several chemical correlates of the pathological changes occurring within and outside T2-visible lesions (De Stefano and Federico 2001). Proton MRS of the brain at long echo times reveals major resonances from tetramethylamines [mainly from choline-containing phospholipids (Cho)], from creatine and phosphocreatine (Cr) and from N-acetyl groups [mainly N-acetyl-aspartate (NAA)]. Reduced N-acetyl aspartate (NAA) levels are associated with axonal dysfunction, while increased Cho, inositol and lactate concentrations are correlated with membrane turnover, possibly secondary to inflammation and demyelination (De Stefano and Federico 2001).

Partially conflicting results have been achieved by MRS studies of patients with SLE and CNS involvement (Davie et al. 1995; Chinn et al. 1997; Sibbitt et al. 1997; Sabet et al. 1998; Friedman et al. 1998; Lim et al. 2000; Handa et al. 2003). Sibbitt et al. (1997) found that lower NAA/Cr and higher lipid levels in the NAWM of patients with major symptoms of NSLE than in patients without or with minor CNS disturbances. Increased lipid levels were not associated with the presence of T2-visible white matter lesions. These findings have been confirmed by more recent studies (Lim et al. 2000; Handa et al. 2003). Other authors (Davie et al. 1995), however, failed to demonstrate significant correlations between MRS-derived measures and presence or severity of neuropsychiatric symptoms. In the latter study (Davie et al. 1995), the pattern of MSR abnormalities did not allow differentiation of SLE lesions from MS plaques. Sabet et al. (1998) investigated the MRS patterns of SLE patients with or without secondary APS. They found that the burden of T2-weighted MRI abnormalities and the severity of brain atrophy were significantly higher in SLE patients with APS than in those without. In addition, in SLE patients with APS, NAA/Cr levels were significantly decreased and Cho/Cr levels increased when compared to normal controls and patients without APS. These changes were present both within MRI-visible white matter lesions and in the NAWM. Interestingly, the results of a linear regression analysis showed that reduced NAA/Cr was more closely related to increased levels of IgG antiphospholipid antibodies (aPL) than the presence of APS. These data suggest that the presence of aPL indicates an increased risk for brain injury in SLE patients, independently of the development of concomitant APS. The presence of brain abnormalities at a microscopic level might be a consequence of direct, immune-mediated tissue damage secondary to SLE more than the result of diffuse ischemic injury due to APS. However, these findings may also be consistent with a direct interaction between IgG aPL and brain cells, leading to progressive tissue damage in SLE patients with aPL positivity, even when the clinical features of APS are absent. On the other hand, Friedman et al. (1998), in an MRI/MRS study of 42 patients with SLE, reported a significant association between small, focal white matter lesions and decreased NAA/Cr ratios, as well as between increased Cho/Cr ratios and cerebral infarctions, concluding that cerebrovascular abnormalities may be the basis of diffuse cerebral damage in NSLE, with small vessel injury as the major factor responsible for white matter axonal loss. Recently, an MRS study (Cellerini et al. 2003) of 17 BD patients has found that NAA/Cr and Cho/Cr levels in the NAWM do not differ between patients and age-matched healthy controls, nor between patients with and those without CNS disturbances. MR spectra from contrast-enhancing white matter lesions were also obtained in two cases, both in the acute phase and at follow-up, showing a normalization of NAA/Cr and Cho/Cr values after steroid therapy.

23.6 Conclusions

Conventional MRI can demonstrate the presence of white matter focal damage in the brain of patients with SID, but the observed patterns of T2-visible lesions have a limited diagnostic specificity, as well as a modest correlation with the clinical manifestations of CNS dysfunction related to these disorders. Available data underpin the need for developing standardized criteria for diagnostic image interpretation in the work-up of patients with SID, similar to what has been done for MS, with particular emphasis on cases at the onset of the neurological disturbances. The integration of brain scanning with imaging of the spinal cord might reasonably improve the diagnostic value of conventional MRI findings when a differential diagnosis between MS and SID has to be made.

Quantitative MR-based techniques seem to be able to contribute both to the in vivo investigation of white matter pathology in SID and to the diagnostic work-up of individual patients. The results of MT MRI, DW MRI and MRS studies of NSLE were all consistent with the presence of clinically relevant NAWM damage in this condition, whereas this does not seem to be the case for other SID. The pathogenesis of NAWM damage in NSLE might be secondary to both small-vessel ischemic injury and immune-mediated brain tissue disruption. The few available data obtained in patients with BD seem to indicate that the pathobiology of white matter damage in this condition is primarily inflammatory-based and limited to T2-visible abnormalities. Further multiparametric and longitudinal studies will probably allow us to better define the role of quantitative MR-based techniques for helping in the diagnostic work-up of SID, investigating the natural course of these diseases and, ideally, providing surrogate markers of disease evolution to monitor treatment efficacy in experimental trials.

References

Akman-Demir G, Serdaroglu P, Tasçi B and the Neuro-Behçet Study Group (1999) Clinical patterns of neurological involvement in Behçet's disease: evaluation of 200 patients. Brain 122:2171–2181

Barkhof F, Filippi M, Miller DH et al (1997) Comparison of MRI criteria at first presentation to predict conversion to clinically definite multiple sclerosis. Brain 120:2059–2069

Basser PJ, Pierpaoli C (1996) Microstructural features measured using diffusion tensor imaging. J Magn Reson B 111:209–219

Basser PJ, Mattiello J, Le Bihan D (1994) Estimation of the effective self-diffusion tensor from the NMR spin-echo. J Magn Reson B 103:247–254

Bell CL, Partington C, Robbins M et al (1991) Magnetic resonance imaging of central nervous system lesions in patients with lupus erythematosus. Correlation with clinical remission and antineurofilament and anticardiolipin antibody titers. Arthritis Rheum 34:432–441

Bosma GPT, Rood MJ, Zwinderman AH et al (2000a) Evidence of central nervous system damage in patients with neuropsychiatric systemic lupus erythematosus, demonstrated by magnetization transfer imaging. Arthr Reum 43:48–54

Bosma GPT, Rood MJ, Huizinga TWJ et al (2000b) Detection of cerebral involvement in patients with active neuropsychiatric systemic lupus erythematosus by the use of volumetric magnetization transfer imaging. Arthr Reum 43:428–2436

Bosma GPT, Middelkoop HAM, Rood MJ et al (2002) Association of global brain damage and clinical functioning in neuropsychiatric systemic lupus erythematosus. Arthr Reum 46:2665–2672

Bosma GPT, Huizinga TWJ, Mooijaart SP et al (2003) Abnormal brain diffusivity in patients with neuropsychiatric systemic lupus erythematosus. AJNR Am J Neuroradiol 24:850–854

Bot JCJ, Barkhof F, Lycklama à Nijeholt G et al (2002) Differentiation of multiple sclerosis from other inflammatory disorders and cerebrovascular disease: value of spinal MR imaging. Radiology 223:46–56

Boumpas DT, Patronas NJ, Dalakas MC et al (1990) Acute transverse myelitis in systemic lupus erythematosus: magnetic resonance imaging and review of the literature. J Rheumatol 17:89–92

Brochet B, Dousset V (1999) Pathological correlates of magnetization transfer imaging abnormalities in animal models and humans with multiple sclerosis. Neurology 53 [Suppl 3]:S12–S17

Calabrese LH, Duna GF, Lie T (1997) Vasculitis in the central nervous system. Arthritis Rheum 40:1189–1201

Campi A, Filippi M, Gerevini S et al (1996) Multiple white matter lesions of the brain. Magnetization transfer ratios in systemic lupus erythematosus and multiple sclerosis. Int J Neuroradiol 2:134–140

Cellerini M, Bartolucci M, Mortilla M et al (2003) MR imaging and proton MR spectroscopy of the brain in Behçet's disease. Rivista di Neuroradiologia 16:267–274

Chinn RJS, Wilkinson ID, Hall-Craggs MA et al (1997) Magnetic resonance imaging of the brain and cerebral proton spectroscopy in patients with systemic lupus erythematosus. Arthritis Rheum 40:36–46

Coban O, Bahar S, Akman-Demir G et al (1996) A controlled study of reliability and validity of MRI findings in neuro-Behçet disease. Neuroradiology 38:312–316

Csépàny T, Bereczki D, Kollar J et al (2003) MRI findings in central nervous system systemic lupus erythematosus are associated with immunoserological parameters and hypertension. J Neurol 250:1348–1354

Davie CA, Fenstein A, Kartsounis LD et al (1995) Proton magnetic resonance spectroscopy of systemic lupus erythematosus involving the central nervous system. J Neurol 242:522–528

Dehmeshki J, van Buchem MA, Bosma GPT et al (2002) Systemic lupus erythematosus: diagnostic application of magnetization transfer ratio histograms in patients with neuropsychiatric symptoms – initial results. Radiology 222:722–728

Deodhar AA, Hochenedel T, Bennett RM (1999) Longitudinal involvement of the spinal cord in a patient with lupus related transverse myelitis. J Rheumatol 26:446–449

De Stefano N Federico A (2001) Overview of magnetic resonance spectroscopy studies in white matter diseases other than multiple sclerosis. In: Filippi M, Arnold DL, Comi G (eds) Magnetic resonance spectroscopy in multiple sclerosis. Springer, Milan, pp 121-133

Fazekas F, Barkhof F, Filippi M et al (1999) The contribution of magnetic resonance imaging to the diagnosis of multiple sclerosis. Neurology 53:448–456

Fieschi C, Rasura M, Anzini A et al (1998) Central nervous system vasculitis. J Neurol Sci 153:159–171

Friedman SD, Stidley CA, Brooks WM et al (1998) Brain injury and neurometabolic abnormalities in systemic lupus erythematosus. Radiology 209:79–84

Gerber S, Biondi A, Dormont D et al (1996) Long-term MR follow-up of cerebral lesions in neuro-Behçet disease. Neuroradiology 38:761–768

Gumà A, Aguileira C, Acebes J et al (1998) Meningeal involvement in Behçet disease: MRI. Neuroradiology 40:512–515

Hachulla E, Michon Pasturel U, Leys D et al (1998) Cerebral magnetic resonance imaging in patients with or without antiphospholipid antibodies. Lupus 7:124–131

Handa R, Sahota P, Kumar M et al (2003) In vivo proton magnetic resonance spectroscopy (MRS) and single photon emission computerized tomography (SPECT) in systemic lupus erythematosus (SLE). Magn Reson Imaging 21:1033–1037

Hiwatashi A, Garber T, Moritani T et al (2003) Diffusion-weighted MR imaging of neuro-Behçet's disease: case report. Neuroradiology 45:468–471

Ijdo JW, Conti-Kelly AM, Greco P et al (1999) Anti-phospholipid antibodies in patients with multiple sclerosis and MS-like illnesses: MS or APS? Lupus 8:109–115

Jennings JE, Sundgren PC, Attwood J et al (2004) Value of MRI of the brain in patients with systemic lupus erythematosus and neurologic disturbance. Neuroradiology 461:15–21

Karussis D, Leker RR, Ashkenazi A et al (1998) A subgroup of multiple sclerosis patients with anticardiolipin antibodies and unusual clinical manifestations: do they represent a new nosological entity? Ann Neurol 44:629–634

Kozora E, West SG, Kotzin BL et al (1998) Magnetic resonance imaging abnormalities and cognitive deficits in systemic lupus erythematosus patients without overt central nervous system disease. Arthritis Rheum 41:41–47

Kunimatsu A, Abe O, Aoki S et al (2003) Neuro-Behçet's disease: analysis of apparent diffusion coefficients. Neuroradiology 45:524–527

Le Bihan D, Breton E, Lallemand D et al (1986) MR imaging of intravoxel incoherent motions: application to diffusion and perfusion in neurologic disorders. Radiology 161:401–407

Le Bihan D, Turner R, Pekar J et al (1991) Diffusion and perfusion imaging by gradient sensitization: design, strategy and significance. J Magn Reson Imaging 1:7–8

Lee SH, Yoon PH, Park SJ et al (2001) MRI findings in neuro-Behçet's disease. Clin Radiol 56:485–494

Liem MD, Gzesh DJ, Flanders AE (1996) MRI and angiographic diagnosis of lupus cerebral vasculitis. Neuroradiology 38:134–136

Lim K, Suh CH, Kim HJ et al (2000) Systemic lupus erythematosus: brain MR imaging and single-voxel hydrogen 1 MR spectroscopy. Radiology 217:43–49

Lycklama à Nijeholt GJ, van Walderveen MAA, Castelijns JA et al (1998) Brain and spinal cord abnormalities in multiple sclerosis. Correlation between MRI parameters, clinical subtypes and symptoms. Brain 121:687–697

Mascalchi M, Cosottini M, Cellerini M et al (1998) MRI of spinal cord involvement in Behçet disease: case report. Neuroradiology 40:255–257

Mattioli F, Capra R, Rovaris M et al (2002) Frequency and patterns of subclinical cognitive impairment in patients with ANCA-associated small vessel vasculitides. J Neurol Sci 195:161–166

Maubon AJ, Pothin A, Ferru JM et al (1998) Unselected brain 0.5 T MR imaging: comparison of lesion detection and characterization with three T2-weighted sequences. Radiology 208:671–678

Miller DH, Ormerod IEC, Gibson A et al (1987) MR brain scanning in patients with vasculitis: differentiation from multiple sclerosis. Neuroradiology 29:226–231

Miller DH, Grossman RI, Reingold SC et al (1998) The role of magnetic resonance techniques in understanding and managing multiple sclerosis. Brain 121:3–24

Miller DH, Thompson AJ, Filippi M (2003) Magnetic resonance studies of abnormalities in the normal appearing white matter and grey matter in multiple sclerosis. J Neurol 250:1407–1419

Mok CC, Lau CS, Chan EY et al (1998) Acute transverse myelopathy in systemic lupus erythematosus: clinical presentation, treatment and outcome. J Rheumatol 25:467–473

Moritani T, Shrier DA, Nugamuchi Y et al (2001) Diffusion-weighted echo-planar MR imaging of CNS involvement in systemic lupus erythematosus. Acad Radiol 8:741–753

Morrissey SP, Miller DH, Hermaszawski R et al (1993) Magnetic resonance imaging in the central nervous system in Behçet's disease. Eur Neurol 33:287–293

Mottershead JP, Schmierer K, Clemence M et al (2003) High field MRI correlates of myelin content and axonal density in multiple sclerosis. A post-mortem study of the spinal cord. J Neurol 250:1293–1301

Nadeau SE (1997) Diagnostic approach to central and peripheral nervous system vasculitis. Neurol Clin 15:759–777

Provenzale JM, Allen NB (1996) Wegener granulomatosis: CT and MR findings. AJNR Am J Neuroradiol 17:785–792
Provenzale JM, Barboriak DP, Gaensler EH et al (1994) Lupus-related myelitis: serial MR findings. AJNR Am J Neuroradiol 15:1911–1917
Rovaris M, Filippi M (2003) Magnetization transfer imaging. In: Filippi M., Comi G (eds) New frontiers of MR-based techniques in multiple sclerosis. Springer, Milan, p 19
Rocca MA, Mastronardo G, Horsfield MA et al (1999) Comparison of three MR sequences for the detection of cervical cord lesions in multiple sclerosis. AJNR Am J Neuroradiol 20:1710–1716
Rovaris M, Inglese M, Viti B et al (2000a) The contribution of fast-FLAIR MRI for lesion detection in the brain of patients with systemic autoimmune diseases. J Neurol 247:29–33
Rovaris M, Viti B, Ciboddo G et al (2000b) Brain involvement in systemic immune-mediated diseases: magnetic resonance and magnetisation transfer imaging study. J Neurol Neurosurg Psychiatry 68:170–177
Rovaris M, Viti B, Ciboddo G et al (2000c) Cervical cord magnetic resonance imaging in systemic immune-mediated diseases. J Neurol Sci 176:128–130
Rovaris M, Holtmannspotter M, Rocca MA et al (2002) Contribution of cervical cord MRI and brain magnetization transfer imaging to the assessment of individual patients with multiple sclerosis: a preliminary study. Mult Scler 8:52–58
Sabet A, Sibbitt WL Jr, Stidley CA, Danska J, Brooks WM (1998) Neurometabolite markers of cerebral injury in the antiphospholipid antibody syndrome of systemic lupus erythematosus. Stroke 29:2254–2260
Sailer M, Burchert W, Ehrenheim C et al (1997) Positron emission tomography and magnetic resonance imaging for cerebral involvement in patients with systemic lupus erythematosus. J Neurol 244:186–193
Salmaggi A, Lamperti E, Eoli M et al (1994) Spinal cord involvement and systemic lupus erythematosus: clinical and magnetic resonance findings in 5 patients. Clin Exp Rheumatol 12:389–394
Sibbit WL, Haseler LJ, Griffey RR et al (1997) Neurometabolism of active neuropsychiatric lupus determined with proton MR Spectroscopy. AJNR Am J Neuroradiol 18:1271–1277
Triulzi F, Scotti G (1998) Differential diagnosis of multiple sclerosis: contribution of magnetic resonance techniques. J Neurol Neurosurg Psychiatry 64 [Suppl 1]:S6–S14
Trysberg E, Nylen K, Rosengren LE et al (2003) Neuronal and astrocytic damage in systemic lupus erythematosus patients with central nervous system involvement. Arthr Reum 48:2710–2712
van Buchem MA, McGowan JC, Kolson DL et al (1996) Quantitative volumetric magnetization transfer analysis in multiple sclerosis: estimation of macroscopic and microscopic disease burden. Magn Reson Med 36:632–636
Waterloo K, Omdal R, Sjoholm H et al (2001) Neuropsychological dysfunction in systemic lupus erythematosus is not associated with changes in cerebral blood flow. J Neurol 248:595–602
Weingarten K, Filippi C, Barbut D et al (1997) The neuroimaging features of the cardiolipin antibody syndrome. Clin Imaging 21:6–12
West SG, Emlen W, Wener MH et al (1995) Neuropsychiatric lupus erythematosus: a 10-year prospective study on the value of diagnostic tests. Am J Med 99:153–163
Yoshioka H, Matsubara T, Miyanomae Y et al (1996) Spinal cord MRI in neuro-Behçet disease. Neuroradiology 38:661–662

White Matter Disorders Related with Aging

24 Neuroimaging of Normal Brain Aging

Giovanni B. Frisoni

CONTENTS

24.1 Introduction

Defining what is normal and abnormal in the aging brain is a problematic task, and defining normality and abnormality of the changes that the white matter is subject to is even more. Age-associated brain changes develop over a continuum and become symptomatic (for example with the development of memory disturbances) only after a given threshold is overcome, such that sub-threshold changes may be regarded as normal and above-threshold changes as abnormal while they actually are only different severity stages of the same pathophysiological process. To complicate things further, the symptomatic threshold of one type of age-associated lesions (say subcortical microvascular disease) is modulated by the presence and severity of lesions with a different pathophysiology (senile plaques and neurofibrillary tangles) that may also become symptomatic with a threshold effect. These are the main reasons why the clinical effect of age-associated white matter changes has been hotly debated in the last 20 years and the issue is still only partly resolved.

G. B. Frisoni, MD and Neurologist
Head, LENITEM - Laboratory of Epidemiology Neuroimaging & Telemedicine, IRCCS San Giovanni di Dio FBF - The National Center for Research and Care of Alzheimer Disease, Via Pilastroni 4, 25125 Brescia, Italy

24.2 Macrostructural Changes

24.2.1 Volume Changes

The volume of the white matter – relative to the intracranial volume – increases until middle age and decreases afterwards (Hildebrand et al., 1993). Guttmann et al. (1998) have measured white matter volume in 72 healthy volunteers aged between 18 and 81 years and found that the volume remained stable until around age 50, to decrease significantly afterwards: beginning at age 60, the proportion of persons with white matter volumes below 2 SD below the mean for 20-year-old subjects increased progressively and at age 80 none had volumes above such value (Guttmann et al., 1998). These findings have been confirmed by another MR-based structural study on the frontal lobe of 70 healthy men aged 19 to 76 years showing that white matter volume increased until age 44 years for the frontal lobes and age 47 years for the temporal lobes and then declined (Bartzokis et al., 2001). Based on personal data on 229 healthy subjects (71 men and 158 women) of 40 years of age and older, we have found a quadratic relationship of age with white matter volume with decrease starting around age 50 with no right-left difference. The relationship was quadratic in men and women, but white matter loss was more accentuated in men (Riello et al., 2005) (Fig. 24.1).

Other studies have suggested differential aging of the white matter in men and women. Murphy et al. (1996) have found that the effect of aging on the brain in men affects more the frontal and temporal lobes, and in women the parietal lobes and the hippocampus. This makes sense in view of the higher frequency of Alzheimer disease (affecting primarily the hippocampus) in women and of white matter disease such as subcortical vascular dementia (affecting mainly the frontal lobes) in men. Dubb et al. (2003) have carried out a sophisticated voxel based analysis of the callosum and found that the anterior part

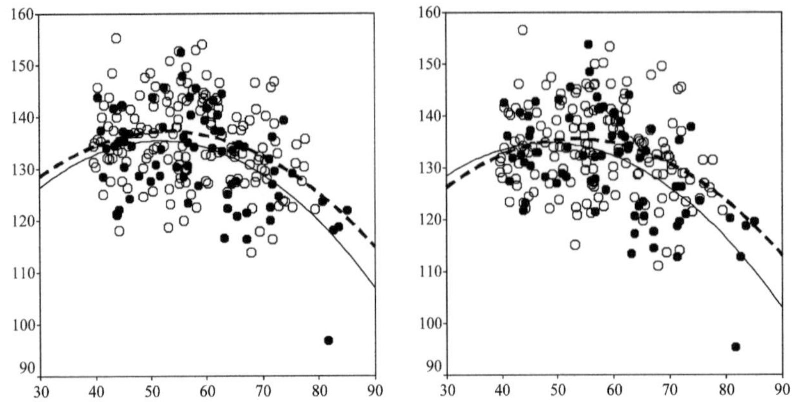

Fig. 24.1 Age effect on fractional white matter volumes in 71 healthy men (filled dots) and 158 women (*open dots*). Lines denote quadratic regression functions of white matter volumes on age in men (solid line) and women (*dashed line*) in the left hemisphere (left panel) and right hemisphere (*right panel*). From: RIELLO et al., 2005.

of the callosum (the splenium) contracts with age in men more than in women. The greater white matter loss in men might be related to vascular diseases and vascular risk factors, that are known to be more prevalent in men. The hypothesis is supported by observations indicating that hypertension is associated with smaller brain volumes (HEIJER et al., 2003; GOLDSTEIN et al., 2002).

A few studies have failed to find age-related white matter loss but all included few subjects above age 40 (GOOD et al., 2001; GUR et al.,1999).

The above findings on volumetric changes of the white matter are at odds with shrinkage of the gray matter, that starts much earlier, around age 20, suggesting that the neurobiological bases of the changes might be different.

Recently, a few studies have been carried out with prospective MR imaging showing brain tissue loss in cognitively normal persons with aging (RESNICK et al., 2003; SCAHILL et al., 2003; TANG et al., 2001). Few studies have disaggregated the effect of aging on the gray and white matter. Resnick and colleagues have quantified the scans of 92 non demented older adults between 59 and 85 years of age using scans taken at baseline and after 2 and 4 years (RESNICK et al., 2003). They found widespread white matter loss in the frontal, parietal, temporal, and occipital lobes between −0.43 and −0.58% per year in the subgroup of 24 healthy persons, while loss in those 68 with some medical problems was about 40% greater. Notably, gray matter loss had a more regional effect (greater loss in the parietal lobes) and was more affected by medical problems (about 100% greater in those with medical problems).

24.2.2 White Matter Hyperintensities

24.2.2.1 Morphologic Features

WMHs can be grouped according to morphologic features into smooth caps or halo, punctate, and confluent. The smooth caps and halo are located in the periventricular white matter adjacent to the ependimal layer. Caps are usually less than 10 mm thick, and the halo tends to be progressively thinner from anterior to posterior (Fig. 24.2).

Punctate and confluent lesions can be located in the periventricular or deep white matter (Fig. 24.2). Punctate hyperintensities are small (diameter less than 5 mm), round, with a regular boundary, and tend to be multiple in the same patient. Confluent lesions are larger than punctate (usually >5 mm), have irregular shape and boundaries, and seem to be originated by the confluence of smaller lesions. When periventricular, confluent lesions tend to be separated by the ventricles or the smooth periventricular halo by a more or less thin region of apparently normal white matter.

24.2.2.2 Pathophysiology

The ***periventricular caps or halo*** – which strictly speaking should not be called "lesions" – are symmetrical and can outline the ventricles more or less completely. A number of studies have shown that these hyperintensities develop as a consequence of

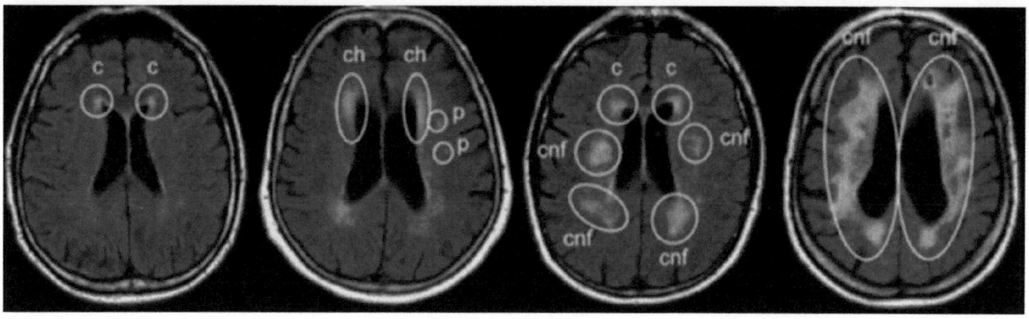

Fig. 24.2 Periventricular caps (*c*), caps and halo (*ch*), punctate (*p*) and confluent (*cnf*) hyperintensities of the white matter. Lacunar cavitations can be seen in (*D*) within the more severe confluent white matter hyperintensities.

local non vascular conditions including the loose network of myelinated fibers, the convergence of the flow of interstitial water to this area with large veins, and the frequently observed disruption of the ependymal layer (ependymitis granularis) (FAZEKAS et al., 1998a; SZE et al., 1986) (Table 24.1). Histopathological findings are disruption of the ependymal lining – which might lead to accumulation of CSF in the periventricular white matter – with a thin rim of subependymal gliosis and a wider, smooth band of white matter tissue with reduced staining for myelin around the lateral ventricles (FAZEKAS et al., 1998a; SZE et al., 1986) (Table 24.1). Notably, vascular arteriolar changes are absent (FAZEKAS et al., 1993). These hyperintensities have the same pathological substrate in cognitively normal persons and in patients with Alzheimer disease (Scheltens et al., 1995). In Alzheimer disease an additional pathogenetic mechanism might be the looser arrangement of fibers following cerebral atrophy (Fazekas et al., 1998a), as supported by the observation of a significant correlation between ventricular enlargement and the thickness of periventricular hyperintensity (FAZEKAS et al., 1996) (Table 24.1). The reported demyelination of the smooth caps and halo (SZE et al., 1986) might be due to chronic oedema, which has been shown to cause demyelination (FEIGIN & POPOFF, 1963).

Punctate hyperintensities can be associated with variable histopathologic correlates (FAZEKAS et al., 1998b), but most studies argue for perivascular tissue changes as the prevailing morphologic substrate (FAZEKAS et al., 1998a) (Table 24.1). Pathophysiological mechanisms include impaired diffusion of nutritional compounds through thickened vessel walls (KIRKPATRICK & HAYMAN, 1987; VAN SWIETEN et al., 1991), mechanic damage to the surrounding tissue by a water hammer effect of pulsating arterioles (AWAD et al., 1986) or both. Interestingly – and in agreement with epidemiological studies showing

Table 24.1. Pathophysiology and pathology of white matter hyperintensities.

	Primary cause	Predisposing factors	Pathophysiology	Pathology
Caps & halo	Non vascular	Loose network of myelinated fibers Convergence of interstitial water flow with large veins In Alzheimer's: looser arrangement of fibers following cerebral atrophy	Chronic oedema causing demyelination	Ependymitis granularis Subependymal gliosis Band with reduced staining for myelin (demyelination) Vascular arteriolar changes absent
Punctate	Vascular	Hypertension, diabetes, hypotension	Arteriolosclerosis > impaired diffusion of nutrients Water hammer effect	Enlargement of the perivascular space
	Unknown	Unknown	Unknown	No pathological findings
Confluent	Vascular	Hypertension, diabetes, hypotension	Chronic ischemia > reactive glial changes > breakdown of myelinated fibers > gliosis	Different degrees of gliosis, myelin loss, axonal rarefaction, and complete axonal loss

lack of progression over time – at least one study suggests that many punctate white matter hyperintensities are associated with no detectable changes on pathology (FAZEKAS et al., 1993) (Table 24.1). Whatever the pathophysiology, it needs to be stressed that punctate white matter hyperintensities usually do not represent lacunar infarcts (FAZEKAS et al., 1991).

Confluent hyperintensities are virtually always caused by chronic ischemia of white matter whose perfusion is provided by small arterioles with diameter smaller than 150 μm - the occlusion of arterioles larger than 400 μm leading to the development of lacunes (Fig. 24.3 and Table 24.1). It has been proposed that the first event following ischemia is reactive glial changes at the boundaries of the ischemic area, followed by breakdown of myelinated fibers within the area and finally gliosis (FAZEKAS et al., 1998a). Chronic ischemia is caused by vessel wall damage and abrupt changes of perfusion pressure. In hypertensive patients these are both common events, the latter being due to the hypertensive disease itself or by co-occurring hypotensive drug assumption (Fig. 24.3). The absence of significantly increased white matter changes in patients with dilatative cardiomyopathy argues against significant effects of perfusion pressure without a disturbed autoregulation or coexisting microvascular changes (SCHMIDT et al., 1991). Sometimes confluent lesions are categorized as early confluent and late confluent (or confluent *tout court*) based on the possibility to recognize the original lesions whose enlargement produces confluence (SCHMIDT et al., 2003); however, the pathophysiology is the same.

Unfortunately, conventional MRI techniques cannot separate the different degrees of white matter damage of gliosis, myelin loss, axonal rarefaction, and complete axonal loss. Recently, new techniques have been developed that allow to assess the microstructural integrity of the white matter with greater accuracy (see section on microstructural changes). The different microstructural severity within WMHs but also in the normally appearing white matter may explain the heterogeneity of clinical correlates of patients with WMHs and the relatively poor correlation between the extent of signal hyperintensities and neuropsychologic deficits.

24.2.2.3
Natural history and clinical correlates

A large epidemiological study using prospective MR scans has assessed the natural history of punctate and confluent WMHs (SCHMIDT et al., 2003) showing that punctate are not progressive while confluent hyperintensities have a striking tendency to progress over time. In the Austrian Stroke Prevention Registry, 296 persons aged 50 to 75 were scanned at baseline and after 6 years. Persons with no WMHs at baseline did not develop new lesions on follow-up and the volume change from baseline of persons with punctate hyperintensities (Fig. 24.4a) was on average 0.2 cm^3. On the contrary, persons with early confluent (Fig. 24.4b) and confluent lesions (Fig. 24.4c) had a lesion volume change of 2.7 and 9.3 cm^3.

This observation together with the notion that punctate hyperintensities can have no pathological substrate suggests that isolated punctate hyperintensities – even when multiple – may be benign and non progressive (FAZEKAS et al., 1993). However, recent findings seem to challenge this conclusion that will need to be addressed in further studies (MACLULLICH et al., 2004).

Population-based epidemiological studies indicate that WMHs are associated with poorer prevalent and

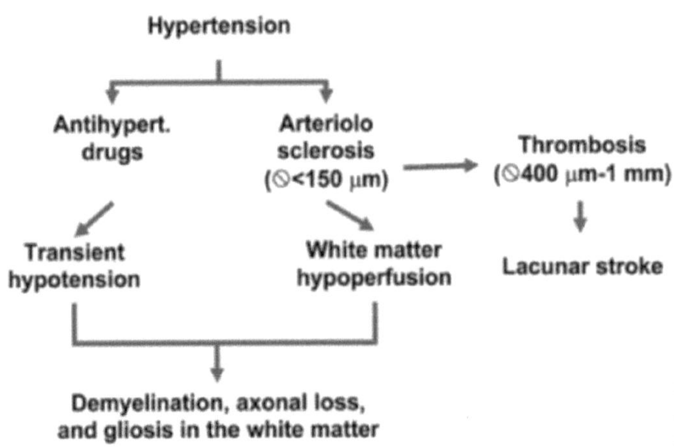

Fig. 24.3 Hypertension and hypotension in the pathophysiology of confluent white matter hyperintesities and lacunes.

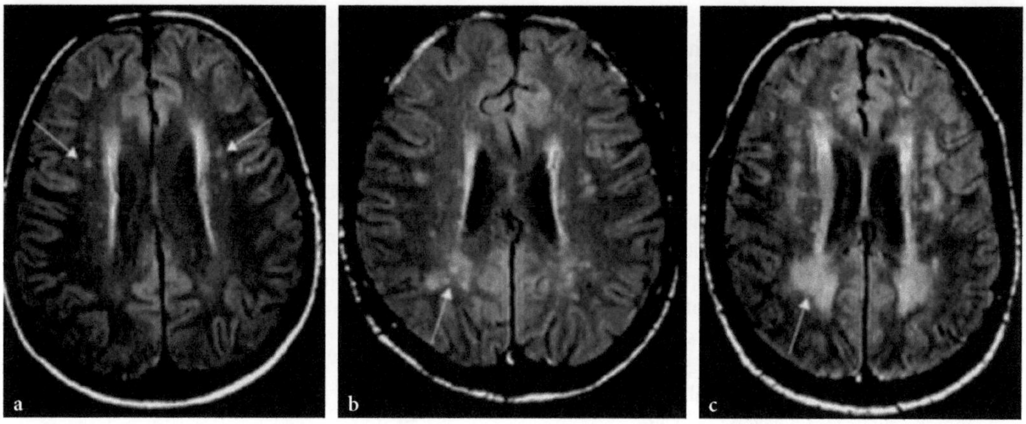

Fig. 24.4a–c Different morphologic features of white matter hyperintensities have different natural history. The volume change over 6 years of punctate hyperintensities (**a**), early confluent (**b**), and confluent lesions (**c**) was 0.2, 2.7, and 9.3 cm^3. From: Schmidt et al., 2003.

incident cognitive perfomance, psychomotor slowing, and balance disturbances in normal elderly persons. A relation has been found between age-related decline in intelligence and cerebral WMHs in healthy octogenarians (Garde et al., 2000). Sixty-eight healthy non-demented individuals were tested with the Wechsler adult intelligence scale at ages 50, 60, 70, and 80, and cerebral MRI was taken at age 80–82. Both periventricular and deep WMHs were significantly associated with decline in performance IQ from age 50 to age 80 years (bivariate correlation coefficients 0.32, p=0.009, and 0.28, p=0.02, respectively). However, despite the statistical significance, these results indicate that only about 10% of the variance of cognitive deterioration that develops over decades in the elderly is attributable to WMHs, implying that WMHs might be more relevant in persons whose cognitive deterioration develops over a shorter time span or – not mutually exclusively – that other factors (for example genetic factors or neurodegeneration) play a more relevant role. This finding has been more recently confirmed with data from the Rotterdam scan study that allowed to show increased risk for incident of dementia (hazard ratio of 1.7 for periventricular WMHs) (Prins et al., 2004) and greater cognitive deterioration (between −0.10 and −0.25 points of MMSE change per year) (De Groot et al., 2002), while silent lacunes in the white matter and basal ganglia have been found associated with grater risk of incident dementia (hazard ratio of 2.0) and decline of psychomotor speed (Vermeer et al., 2003).

Balance measures were investigated in over 700 community-dwelling older men and women in a Norwegian epidemiologic study. A summary of the balance measures was significantly related to WMHs even after adjustments for sex, race, age, cardiovascular disease, and hypertension (Tell et al., 1998). These epidemiological findings are credible in view of results obtained in clinical groups, where WMHs have been found associated with L-DOPA non-responsive parkinsonism (Zijlmans et al., 1995). While a relationship has been found between prevalent and progressive WMHs and refractory and relapsing late life depression (O'Brien et al., 1998; Taylor et al., 2003), a relationship has not yet been described in epidemiological populations.

It should be highlighted that to date there is no published evidence that the increase of size of confluent WMHs is associated with accelerated cognitive or psychomotor decline – which would be the final proof of causation.

24.3 Microstructural Changes

The macrostructural appreciation of WMHs through T2-weighted MR imaging reflects variable pathological substrates, ranging from increased water content to irreversible demyelination and axonal loss. Also, such an approach does not provide any hint about the status of the remaining apparently normal white matter. Recently developed techniques allow to better resolve the different degrees of anatomical damage that the white matter can be subjected to in aging.

Some studies have found that the aging-associated microstructural damage to the white matter is more marked in the frontal than other brain regions, both in the hemispheric white matter and in the corpus callosum (SULLIVAN & PFEFFERBAUM, 2003; SULLIVAN et al., 2001; O'SULLIVAN et al., 2001; CHUN et al., 2000; NUSBAUM et al., 2001; ABE et al., 2002). In a study by Sullivan and colleagues on 18 women and 31 men between 23 and 79 years of age (SULLIVAN et al., 2001), some measures of balance, gait, and motor performance were found to be significantly associated with fractional anisotropy (a measure of white matter tract disruption) in the splenium of the corpus callosum. Notably, the association of motor performance measures was stronger with fractional anisotropy than age, suggesting that white matter tract disruption might be the neurobiological basis of some motor deficits that develop in old age.

The study of age-associated microstructural changes of the white matter associated with aging is still in its infancy and more studies will be needed to understand their functional relevance both within and without obvious T2 changes.

References

Abe O, Aoki S, Hayashi N, Yamada H, Kunimatsu A, Mori H, Yoshikawa T, Okubo T, Ohtomo K (2002) Normal aging in the central nervous system: quantitative MR diffusion-tensor analysis. Neurobiol Aging 23:433–41

Awad IA, Johnson PC, Spetzler RF, Hodak JA (1986) Incidental subcortical lesions identified on magnetic resonance imaging in the elderly. II. Postmortem pathological correlations. Stroke 17:1090–7

Bartzokis G, Beckson M, Lu PH, Nuechterlein KH, Edwards N, Mintz J (2001) Age-related changes in frontal and temporal lobe volumes in men: a magnetic resonance imaging study. Arch Gen Psychiatry 58:461–5

Chun T, Filippi CG, Zimmerman RD, Ulug AM (2000) Diffusion changes in the aging human brain. AJNR Am J Neuroradiol 21:1078–83

De Groot JC, De Leeuw FE, Oudkerk M, Van Gijn J, Hofman A, Jolles J, Breteler MM (2002) Periventricular cerebral white matter lesions predict rate of cognitive decline. Ann Neurol 52:335–41

Dubb A, Gur R, Avants B, Gee J (2003) Characterization of sexual dimorphism in the human corpus callosum. Neuroimage 20:512–9

Fazekas F, Kleinert R, Offenbacher H, Payer F, Schmidt R, Kleinert G, Radner H, Lechner H (1991) The morphologic correlate of incidental punctate white matter hyperintensities on MR images. AJNR Am J Neuroradiol 12:915–21

Fazekas F, Kleinert R, Offenbacher H, Schmidt R, Kleinert G, Payer F, Radner H, Lechner H (1993) Pathologic correlates of incidental MRI white matter signal hyperintensities. Neurology 43:1683–9

Fazekas F, Kapeller P, Schmidt R, Offenbacher H, Payer F, Fazekas G (1996) The relation of cerebral magnetic resonance signal hyperintensities to Alzheimer's disease. J Neurol Sci 142:121–5

Fazekas F, Schmidt R, Scheltens P (1998a) Pathophysiologic mechanisms in the development of age-related white matter changes of the brain. Dement Geriatr Cogn Disord 9(Suppl 1):2–5

Fazekas F, Kleinert R, Schmidt R (1998b) The neuropathology of white matter changes in normal aging. In: Fazekas F, Schmidt R, Alavi A (eds) Neuroimaging of normal aging and uncommon causes of dementia. Current issues in neurodegenerative disorders. ICG Publications, Dordrecht, pp 27–46

Feigin I, Popoff N (1963) Neuropathological changes late in cerebral edema: the relationship to trauma, hypertensive disease and Binswanger's encephalopathy. J Neuropathol Exp Neurol 22:500–11

Garde E, Mortensen EL, Krabbe K, Rostrup E, Larsson HB (2000) Relation between age-related decline in intelligence and cerebral white-matter hyperintensities in healthy octogenarians: a longitudinal study. Lancet 356:628–34

Goldstein IB, Bartzokis G, Guthrie D, Shapiro D (2002) Ambulatory blood pressure and brain atrophy in the healthy elderly. Neurology 59:713–9

Good CD, Johnsrude IS, Ashburner J, Henson RN, Friston KJ, Frackowiak RS (2001) A voxel-based morphometric study of ageing in 465 normal adult human brains. Neuroimage 14:21–36

Gur RC, Turetsky BI, Matsui M, Yan M, Bilker W, Hughett P, Gur RE (1999) Sex differences in brain gray and white matter in healthy young adults: correlations with cognitive performance. J Neurosci 19:4065–72

Guttmann CR, Jolesz FA, Kikinis R, Killiany RJ, Moss MB, Sandor T, Albert MS (1998) White matter changes with normal aging. Neurology 50:972–8

Heijer T, Skoog I, Oudkerk M, de Leeuw FE, de Groot JC, Hofman A, Breteler MM (2003) Association between blood pressure levels over time and brain atrophy in the elderly. Neurobiol Aging 24:307–13

Hildebrand C, Remahl S, Persson H, Bjartmar C (1993) Myelinated nerve fibres in the CNS. Prog Neurobiol 40:319–84

Kirkpatrick JB, Hayman LA (1987) White-matter lesions in MR imaging of clinically healthy brains of elderly subjects: possible pathologic basis. Radiology 162:509–11

Murphy DG, DeCarli C, McIntosh AR, Daly E, Mentis MJ, Pietrini P, Szczepanik J, Schapiro MB, Grady CL, Horwitz B, Rapoport SI (1996) Sex differences in human brain morphometry and metabolism: an in vivo quantitative magnetic resonance imaging and positron emission tomography study on the effect of aging. Arch Gen Psychiatry 53:585–94

O'Brien J, Ames D, Chiu E, Schweitzer I, Desmond P, Tress B (1998) Severe deep white matter lesions and outcome in elderly patients with major depressive disorder: follow up study. BMJ 317:982–4

O'Sullivan M, Jones D, Summers P, Morris R, Williams S, Markus H (2001) Evidence for cortical "disconnection" as a mechanism of age-related cognitive decline. Neurology 57:632–8

Maclullich AM, Wardlaw JM, Ferguson KJ, Starr JM, Seckl JR, Deary IJ (2004) Enlarged perivascular spaces are associated with cognitive function in healthy elderly men. J Neurol Neurosurg Psychiatry 75:1519–23

Nusbaum AO, Tang CY, Buchsbaum MS, Wei TC, Atlas SW (2001) Regional and global changes in cerebral diffusion with normal aging. AJNR Am J Neuroradiol 22:136–42

Prins ND, van Dijk EJ, den Heijer T, Vermeer SE, Koudstaal PJ, Oudkerk M, Hofman A, Breteler MM (2004) Cerebral white matter lesions and the risk of dementia. Arch Neurol 61:1531–4
Resnick SM, Pham DL, Kraut MA, Zonderman AB, Davatzikos C (2003) Longitudinal magnetic resonance imaging studies of older adults: a shrinking brain. J Neurosci 23:3295–301
Riello R, Sabattoli F, Beltramello A, Bonetti M, Bono G, Falini A, Magnani G, Minonzio G, Piovan E, Alaimo G, Ettori M, Galluzzi S, Locatelli E, Noiszewska M, Testa C, Frisoni GB (2005) Brain volumes in healthy adults aged 40 years and over: a voxel based morphometry study. Aging Clin Exp Res, in press
Scahill RI, Frost C, Jenkins R, Whitwell JL, Rossor MN, Fox NC (2003) A longitudinal study of brain volume changes in normal aging using serial registered magnetic resonance imaging. Arch Neurol 60:989–94
Scheltens P, Barkhof F, Leys D, Wolters EC, Ravid R, Kamphorst W (1995) Histopathologic correlates of white matter changes on MRI in Alzheimer's disease and normal aging. Neurology 45:883–8
Schmidt R, Fazekas F, Offenbacher H, Dusleag J, Lechner H (1991) Brain magnetic resonance imaging and neuropsychologic evaluation of patients with idiopathic dilated cardiomyopathy. Stroke 22:195–9
Schmidt R, Enzinger C, Ropele S, Schmidt H, Fazekas F (2003) Progression of cerebral white matter lesions: 6-year results of the Austrian Stroke Prevention Study. Lancet 361:2046–8
Sullivan EV, Pfefferbaum A (2003) Diffusion tensor imaging in normal aging and neuropsychiatric disorders. Eur J Radiol 45:244–55
Sullivan EV, Adalsteinsson E, Hedehus M, Ju C, Moseley M, Lim KO, Pfefferbaum A (2001) Equivalent disruption of regional white matter microstructure in aging healthy men and women. Neuroreport 12:99–104
Sze G, De Armond SJ, Brant-Zawadzki M, Davis RL, Norman D, Newton TH (1986) Foci of MRI signal (pseudo lesions) anterior to the frontal horns: histologic correlations of a normal finding. AJR Am J Roentgenol 147:331–7
Tang Y, Whitman GT, Lopez I, Baloh RW (2001) Brain volume changes on longitudinal magnetic resonance imaging in normal older people. J Neuroimaging 11:393–400
Taylor WD, Steffens DC, MacFall JR, McQuoid DR, Payne ME, Provenzale JM, Krishnan KR (2003) White matter hyperintensity progression and late-life depression outcomes. Arch Gen Psychiatry 60:1090–6
Tell GS, Lefkowitz DS, Diehr P, Elster AD (1998) Relationship between balance and abnormalities in cerebral magnetic resonance imaging in older adults. Arch Neurol 55:73–9.
Vermeer SE, Prins ND, den Heijer T, Hofman A, Koudstaal PJ, Breteler MM (2003) Silent brain infarcts and the risk of dementia and cognitive decline. N Engl J Med 348:1215–22
van Swieten JC, van den Hout JH, van Ketel BA, Hijdra A, Wokke JH, van Gijn J (1991) Periventricular lesions in the white matter on magnetic resonance imaging in the elderly. A morphometric correlation with arteriolosclerosis and dilated perivascular spaces. Brain 114:761–74
Zijlmans JC, Thijssen HO, Vogels OJ, Kremer HP, Poels PJ, Schoonderwaldt HC, Merx JL, van 't Hof MA, Thien T, Horstink MW (1995) MRI in patients with suspected vascular parkinsonism. Neurology 45:2183–8

25 White Matter Abnormalities in Patients with Cerebrovascular Disease

Joao A. Gomes and Louis R. Caplan

CONTENTS

25.1 Introduction and Historical Background

Leukoaraiosis (LA) is a neologism coined in the late 1980s (Hachinski et al. 1987) from the Greek root *leuko-* (white), and the Greek adjective *araios* (rarefied), that was meant to represent a radiographic phenomenon rather than a distinct entity (Merino and Hachinski 2000). It represented an effort to further characterize the common finding of diffuse white matter changes observed in CT scan originally and subsequently on MRI in elderly individuals, particularly in those with cognitive impairment and vascular risk factors. As has been emphasized, it was to be a "*...neutral term, exact enough to define white-matter changes in the elderly or the demented, general enough that it serves as a description and a label, and demanding enough that it calls for a precise clinical and imaging description accompanied when possible by pathologic correlations*" (Hachinski et al. 1987).

J. A. Gomes, MD
Johns Hopkins Hospital, Neurocritical Care Division, Meyer 8-140, 600 N Wolfe St, Baltimore, MD, USA
L. R. Caplan, MD
Beth Israel Deaconess Medical Center, Harvard Medical School, 330 Brookline Avenue, Boston, MA, USA

Although patients with cerebrovascular disease may have white matter abnormalities related to large-vessel, embolic or ischemic-hypoxic etiologies, by far small-vessel disease is believed to be the most common substrate in cases of diffuse, bilateral, preferential white matter involvement. Therefore, we will concentrate our review on this topic.

Since the term leukoaraiosis was first introduced, much has been written on the subject and our understanding of white matter changes in the elderly has grown significantly. We shall review the current understanding of this phenomenon and the role that MRI technology plays in the characterization and research endeavors on this condition.

25.1.1 Historical Background

The study of white matter changes related to vascular etiologies has been plagued by much confusion of terms and unjustified assumptions. A brief, but thorough review of the history will help define some terms and hopefully establish a clear nomenclature.

Lacunes. From the Latin *lacuna* (a tiny hole or cavity), are small cavities within the substance of the brain associated with small perforating vessel disease ranging from 1–15 mm in size and most commonly located in the basal ganglia, internal capsule, corona radiata and brainstem. They were probably first described by Amedée Dechambre in 1838 (Dechambre 1838; Roman 2002) who concluded that "Lacunes result from liquefaction and partial re-absorption in the center of the [cerebral] softening..." (Roman 2002). In 1843 Durand-Fardel confirmed Dechambre's findings (Durand-Fardel 1843), and in 1894 Alzheimer and Binswanger described "arteriosclerotic brain atrophy", a condition characterized by multiple lacunar strokes involving the internal capsule, basal ganglia, and the white matter of the centrum ovale associated with arteriosclerosis of cerebral blood vessels (Alzheimer 1894; Binswanger 1894).

Pierre Marie provided the best clinicopathological correlation study of lacunes and dubbed the term *état lacunaire* to represent multiple, recurrent episodes of weakness in the elderly accompanied by pseudobulbar palsy, gait disturbance and incontinence (MARIE 1901).

It was CM Fisher who defined the nature and etiology of the vascular pathology causing lacunes, and described many clinical syndromes that can be readily diagnosed as lacunar (FISHER 1965, 1969; CAPLAN 2000).

Etat criblé. Dilatation of perivascular spaces around cerebral arterioles of elderly patients was first described by Durand-Fardel. Unfortunately, it has been a source of confusion with *état lacunaire* and should be reserved for the punctiform perivascular dilatation confined to the basal ganglia and the white matter that is frequently identified on MRI (ROMAN 2002).

Leukoaraiosis. This term has already been covered in Sect. 23.1. We just want to reiterate that it represents a descriptive term that literally means rarefaction of the white matter as seen on CT or MRI scans and is not a distinct entity by itself. More than likely many conditions lead to this state and the ultimate hope should be that "the eventual obsolescence of the term as labeling is replaced by understanding" (HACHINSKI et al. 1987).

The chronic white-matter abnormalities first described by Otto Binswanger (CAPLAN and SCHOENE 1978; CAPLAN 1995; BLASS et al. 1991). Binswanger sought to separate the pathological and clinical findings of syphilitic general paralysis from other conditions that caused mental and physical deterioration but had different pathologic and clinical findings. He was a very prominent German neuropathologist whose original article appeared in a weekly medical newspaper. Although Binswanger promised further reports of the pathology, apparently none were ever forthcoming. Alzheimer and Nissl, prominent students of Binswanger, later commented on the pathology of the condition that their teacher Binswanger described and emphasized chronic atrophy, gliosis and loss of myelin in the cerebral white matter. Olszewski, in a review of the history and pathology of the condition, used the term "subcortical arteriosclerotic encephalopathy" (OLSZEWSKI 1965).

More recently, a number of authors have reviewed the clinical and pathological findings in a series of cases of Binswanger disease (CAPLAN and SCHOENE 1978; BABIKIAN and ROPPER 1987; FISHER 1989; CAPLAN 1995).

Grossly visible in the cerebral white matter are confluent areas of soft, puckered, and granular tissue. These areas are patchy and emphasize the occipital lobes and periventricular white matter, especially anteriorly and close to the surface of the ventricles. The cerebellar white matter is also often involved. The ventricles are enlarged, and at times, the corpus callosum is small. The volume of white matter is reduced, but the cortex is generally spared. There are nearly always some lacunes. Microscopic study shows myelin pallor. Usually, the myelin pallor is not homogeneous, but islands of decreased myelination are surrounded by normal tissue. At times, the white-matter abnormalities are so severe that necrosis and cavitation occur. Gliosis is prominent in zones of myelin pallor. The walls of penetrating arteries are thickened and hyalinized but occlusion of the small arteries is rare. Occasional patients with Binswanger white-matter changes have had amyloid angiopathy as the underlying vascular pathology (GRAY et al. 1985; DUBAS et al. 1985; LOES et al. 1990; TOURNIER-LASSERVE et al. 1991; MAS et al. 1992). In these patients, arteries within the cerebral cortex and leptomeninges are thickened and contain a congophilic substance that stains for amyloid. Arteries within the white matter and basal ganglia are also concentrically thickened.

The clinical picture in patients with Binswanger white matter abnormalities is quite variable. Most patients have some abnormalities of cognitive function and behavior. Most often, patients become slow and abulic. Memory loss, aphasic abnormalities, and visuospatial dysfunction are also found. Pseudobulbar palsy, pyramidal signs, extensor plantar reflexes, and gait abnormalities are also common. The clinical findings often progress gradually or stepwise, with worsening within periods of days to weeks. Often, there are long plateau periods of stability of the findings (CAPLAN and SCHOENE 1978; CAPLAN 1995; BABIKIAN and ROPPER 1987). Many patients also have acute lacunar strokes.

25.2 Epidemiological Aspects of Leukoaraiosis

The prevalence of white matter changes (WMCs) on MRI in various population-based studies has ranged from 62% to 95% (VERMMER et al. 2002; LONGSTRETH et al. 1996; BRETELER et al. 1994; YLIKOSKI et al. 1995; LINDGREN et al. 1994; LIAO et al. 1997). In patients with vascular dementia WMCs are found in 80%, while subcortical changes are reported in 50% of such patients (GHIKA and BOGOUSSLAVSKY 1996). In Alzheimer disease the prevalence of WMCs varies between 26% and 70%, whereas subcortical changes are found in 20%–25% (MARTINEZ-LAGE and HACHINSKI 1998). The prevalence of LA in cognitive intact patients older than 60 years has been reported to range between 8% and 100% depending on the imaging method used (CT Vs. MRI) and the population studied (GHIKA and BOGOUSSLAVSKY 1996).

Stroke and LA share many risk factors. The effect of age has been shown repeatedly and consistently and is currently considered the most important risk factor for LA. In a CT study of WMCs in demented patients versus age- and sex-matched controls the mean age of subjects with LA was significantly higher (74.9 Vs. 70.5) (INZITARI et al. 1987). In another study, incidental subcortical lesions were identified on MRI in 51% of subjects between 41–60 years of age, while in individuals older than 60 years the prevalence of these lesions was an impressive 92% (AWAD et al. 1986).

Other associated factors include a prior history of stroke, hypertension, cardiac diseases, diabetes mellitus, smoking, lower income and education and possibly orthostatic hypotension and increased levels of fibrinogen and factor VIIc (INZITARI et al. 1987; LEYS et al. 1999; HÉNON et al. 1996; HIJDRA et al. 1990; ROMAN et al. 2002; BRETELER et al. 1994; RAIHA et al. 1993). Of these, hypertension and stroke have been the most consistent associations, particularly for subcortical rather than periventricular lesions (MERINO and HACHINSKI 2000). In the dementia study of the University of Western Ontario the prevalence of hypertension was twice as much in patients with LA than in LA-free subjects, whereas a previous stroke was four times more likely in patients with LA (INZITARI et al. 1987). This association is also true for asymptomatic patients in whom a prior history of brain ischemia and history of arterial hypertension are associated with an increase in the prevalence of incidental lesions in the white matter (AWAD et al. 1986).

Leukoaraiosis is also known to progress over time. In the Austrian stroke prevention study almost 18% of the subjects had progression of LA over a period of 3 years (SCHMIDT et al. 2002), while WHITMAN et al. (2001) documented a 1.1±1.8 cm^3 mean volume increase of LA over 4 years. The only factors that have been associated with the progression of LA include the degree of white matter hyperintensities and the presence of confluent lesions at baseline, as well as diastolic blood pressure (SCHMIDT et al. 2002, 2003; VELDINK et al. 1998).

25.3 Pathophysiology of Leukoaraiosis

Several theories try to explain the occurrence of white matter abnormalities in elderly individuals, but none has been conclusively proven (Table 23.1). Of these, chronic ischemia with incomplete infarction of the white matter is the most widely accepted (PANTONI and GARCIA 1997).

Table 25.1. Pathophysiology of white matter changes

Ischemia
Abnormalities in CSF circulation
White matter edema and blood–brain barrier abnormalities
Matrix metalloproteinases
Ischemic axonopathy
Apoptosis

Most of the blood supply to the white matter is through long perforating branches that originate from superficial vessels. These perforating arteries are small (average diameter 100–200 μm), arise at right angles and do not arborize (VAN DEN BERGH and VAN DER EECKEN 1968). The periventricular white matter is supplied by ventriculofugal vessels from subependymal arteries. Anastomoses between these two systems are rare (RAVENS 1974). This pattern of blood supply creates a border zone in the white matter that makes it prone to damage with reductions in cerebral blood flow.

It is believed that a myriad of risk factors lead to small vessel stenosis which, particularly in the presence of hypotension and hypoperfusion, results in chronic, recurrent ischemia of the susceptible white matter (PANTONI 2002). Impaired autoregulation (OHTANI et al. 2003), rheological factors (i.e. increased plasma viscosity) (CAPLAN 1995), and selective vulnerability of oligodendrocytes (TOMONAGA et al. 1982) may contribute to the ischemic damage.

Abnormalities in CSF circulation have also been implicated in the pathogenesis of LA (MURATA et al. 1981). In normal pressure hydrocephalus for instance, ventriculomegaly may raise the periventricular interstitial pressure causing ischemia. Ependymal dysfunction could also lead to CSF leakage and the formation of interstitial edema (ROMAN 1991).

It has been known for many years that conditions associated with chronic brain edema (i.e. tumors) may induce white matter abnormalities similar to those of LA (Feigin 1963). Chronic hypertension may lead to disruption of the blood–brain barrier resulting in increased interstitial fluid and protein content (Nag 1984). Abnormalities in the periventricular venules in patients with LA have also been documented (Moody et al. 1995), and may be another mechanism responsible for white matter edema.

Alterations in extracellular matrix metabolism with excess of macromolecules in patients with LA have been identified. A diffuse microglial inflammatory response was seen in patients with vascular dementia. These microglial cells and macrophages express high levels of matrix metalloproteinase 3 (MTP-3), similar to patients with ischemic stroke. Based on these findings, MTP-3-induced white matter abnormalities has been postulated as a pathogenic mechanism in LA (Rosenberg et al. 2001).

Another theory suggests that LA represents an ischemic axonopathy and that the primary inciting event is actually neocortical ischemia (Ball 2003). According to this, cortical hypoperfusion induces secondary axonal depletion (Ball 1988). Finally, apoptosis has also been implicated in the pathogenesis of LA (Brown et al. 2000). A preliminary report showed increased DNA fragmentation in oligodendrocytes in areas of LA, without evidence of necrosis, (Brown et al. 2000) further supporting apoptotic mechanisms.

25.4 Leukoaraiosis and Stroke Subtype

25.4.1 Leukoaraiosis and Lacunar Infarcts

Clinical, pathological, and imaging studies have reported the association between LA and lacunar strokes. By far, patients with lacunar infarcts have the highest frequency of subcortical and deep white matter changes of any stroke subtype, and the extent of these changes also seems to be more severe in this stroke category (Mäntylä et al. 1999). In a chronic progressive form of cerebrovascular disease, known to be highly associated with LA, up to 77.5% of the patients have been found to have evidence of small vessel disease and lacunar strokes (Domínguez et al. 2002). LA is also found more frequently in patients with deep infarcts (8%) than in those with cortical strokes (0.8%) (Bogousslavsky et al. 1987), and the progression of white matter changes is more pronounced in patients with lacunar infarcts (Boon et al. 1994).

While there is little doubt that there is a strong association between LA and lacunar strokes, the significance of this association is still unknown. Although small vessel disease is thought to be a pathological substrate in both conditions, it does not reconcile the fact that LA and lacunes are located in different vascular territories (basal ganglia and deep white matter for lacunes versus the territory of the superficial penetrating branches of large cerebral arteries in LA) (Furuta et al. 1991).

25.4.2 Leukoaraiosis and Large Artery Strokes

It is generally accepted that there is poor correlation between LA and territorial infarcts. Large vessel disease and cardioembolic sources were found in 7.5% and 5%, respectively, of a cohort of patients with chronic progressive cerebrovascular disease and LA (Domínguez et al. 2002). In another study, neither the degree of carotid stenosis, nor the presence of plaque ulceration were associated with LA (Streifler et al. 1995), and even though some degree of carotid artery atherosclerosis is frequently found at autopsy in patients with LA (Hijdra and Verbeeten 1991; Gupta et al. 1988), the diffuse white matter changes seem to correlate better with the degree of lipohyalinosis of the medullary arteries (Furuta et al. 1991).

25.4.3 Leukoaraiosis and Intracerebral Hemorrhage

There is emerging data that suggest that LA is a strong and independent risk factor for intracerebral hemorrhage (ICH). In hypertensive patients the coexistence of LA, lacunar infarcts, and ICH has been reported by various investigators (Chan et al. 1996; Tanaka et al. 1999). More than 90% of patients with post-stroke warfarin-related ICH (versus 48% of controls) have evidence of LA (Smith et al. 2002), independent of hemorrhage location (deep vs. lobar). The risk of developing ICH in this setting seems to be higher with increasing severity of white matter hyperintensities.

Microbleeds (as detected by T2*-weighted MRI sequences and thought to indicate advanced small vessel pathology) have also been correlated with the presence and severity of LA (Fig. 25.1), and seem to

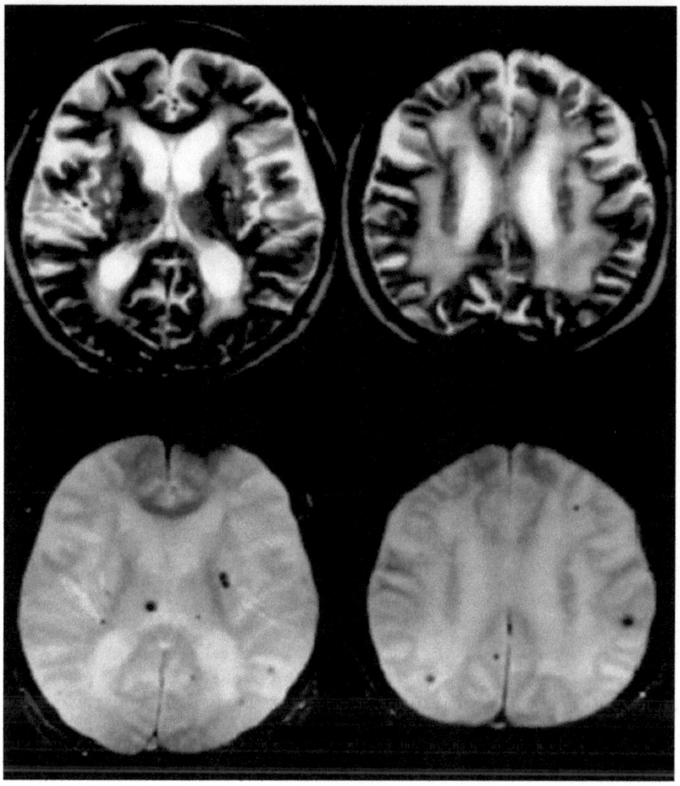

Fig. 25.1. T2-weighted (*top*) and T2*-weighted gradient echo (*bottom*) MRI. The upper panel shows extensive white matter hyperintensities, while the T2*-weighted images reveal associated microbleeds in a patient with Binswanger disease. [Taken with permission from HANYU et al. (2003)]

be associated with increased risk of ICH (KATO et al. 2002; HANYU et al. 2003). In a secondary stroke prevention study with oral anticoagulation, LA was associated with a six-fold increase in ICH, and the presence of severe white matter changes increased the risk of ICH 2.5 times compared to moderate LA scores (GORTER et al. 1999).

The implication of this relationship is two-fold. On the one hand, it supports the presence of a common underlying small vessel vasculopathy, and on the other, it raises the question whether LA should be considered a contraindication for long-term oral anticoagulation as it may offset any benefit derived from it. This issue remains unresolved.

23.4.4 Leukoaraiosis and Other Stroke Subtypes

Although various vasculitides and cerebroretinal vasculopathies are associated with diffuse changes in the cerebral white matter (CAPLAN 2000), we will focus on two entities that have received much attention in the literature recently, namely cerebral amyloid angiopathy and CADASIL (cerebral autosomal dominant arteriopathy with subcortical infarcts and leukoencephalopathy).

CADASIL. A small vessel arteriopathy caused by mutations in the *NOTCH3* gene on chromosome 19. Clinical manifestations include strokes, subcortical dementia, migraines with auras, and psychiatric disturbances in young to middle age adults (CAPLAN 2000; MAS et al. 1992; DAVOUS 1998), although an acute reversible encephalopathy has also been described (SCHON 2003).

Along with lacunar infarcts, the radiological hallmark of the disease is the presence of diffuse white matter changes that are hyperintense on T2-weighted MRI, and hypointense on T1-weighted images (CHABRIAT 1998). Two features seem to be relatively specific for this disorder, the involvement of subcortical U-fibers in the superior frontal and temporal regions, as well as prominent white matter involvement within the temporal poles and external capsules (AUER 2001; O'SULLIVAN et al. 2001). Although the onset and rate of progression of these white matter changes can be variable (DICHGANS 1999), by the age of 35 virtually all gene carriers will show evidence of white matter involvement on MRI.

Cerebral Amyloid angiopathy (CAA). Characterized by selective deposition of amyloid material in the cerebral vasculature in the absence of systemic amyloidosis. It preferentially involves the vessels that supply the cerebral cortex and the leptomeninges, for the most part sparing those of the basal ganglia and brainstem (Kase 1994). The amyloid deposition induces breakdown of the vessel wall with microaneurysm formation and fibrinoid necrosis (Mandybur 1986; Vonsattel et al. 1991), which predisposes primarily to ICH (usually located in cortico-subcortical regions), but also to cortical infarcts and leukoencephalopathy (Kase 1994).

The frequency of CAA increases steadily with advancing age, being found in approximately 5% of individuals in the seventh decade, but in over 50% of subjects over the age of 90 years (Vinters and Gilbert 1983). CAA also occurs with particularly high frequency in patients with Alzheimer disease (AD). In the Harvard Brain Tissue Resource Center 54% of brains with evidence of AD also had changes characteristics of CAA (versus 14% of brains without AD pathology) (Greenberg and Vonsattel 1997).

The high frequency of leukoaraiosis in patients with hereditary forms of CAA has been well documented. Individuals with the Dutch mutation usually present with ICH, cognitive decline, LA, and small ischemic infarctions (Wattendorff et al. 1995; Bornebroek et al. 1996). Patients with the Iowa mutation usually manifest an autosomal dominant progressive dementia, with no evidence of ICH, but extensive subcortical white matter changes with posterior predominance (Grabowski et al. 2001).

Similar white matter changes have also been documented in instances of sporadic CAA (the most common form of the disease) in radiological and pathological series (Gray et al. 1985; Loes et al. 1990; Hendricks et al. 1990), but the actual frequency of this finding is difficult to estimate accurately since brain biopsy is usually required to make the definitive diagnosis of amyloid angiopathy. This may be overcome in the near future as a promising amyloid-imaging agent in vivo was shown to specifically label amyloid deposits in transgenic mice (Bacskai et al. 2003).

The pathogenesis of these white matter changes in subjects with CAA is not completely understood. It is well known that white matter vessels do not show evidence of amyloid deposition, as there is an abrupt termination of such deposits as vessels leave the gray matter to enter the white matter (Fisher 1989). This finding has prompted most investigators to postulate white matter hypoperfusion related to obliteration of cortical vessel lumen, replacement of the vascular smooth muscle cell layer with impairment of vasomotor reactivity, and attenuation in increases of cerebral blood flow in response to pharmacologic or functional stimuli as the likely factors responsible for the changes seen in the white matter (Kase 1994; Greenberg 2002).

25.5 Magnetic Resonance Imaging of Leukoaraiosis

Conventional MRI is a very sensitive technique for detecting white matter abnormalities, and undoubtedly superior to CT scan. It not only helps define the full extent of white matter involvement, but also has a remarkable spatial resolution that allows the detection of small lesions. However, this enhanced sensitivity for disease processes involving the white matter also implies that in the majority of patients the white matter abnormalities are relatively non-specific.

There are certain changes observed in the white matter with advancing age that do not seem to correlate with brain dysfunction per se and are thought to represent normal ageing phenomena. Periventricular high signal areas called bands and caps are frequently found in the elderly and represent loss of ependymal lining and subependymal glia accumulation (Zimmerman et al. 1986; Scheltens et al. 1995). Similarly, dilatation of Virchow-Robin perivascular spaces can be mistaken for white matter abnormalities in T2-weighted images. They are usually found in the area of the basal ganglia and at the vertex, and can be easily differentiated by their very low CSF signal on T1-weighted and fluid-attenuated inversion recovery (FLAIR) images.

In patients who have cognitive and behavioral abnormalities as well as motor signs, there is a good correlation with the amount and type of white matter lesions. Irregular lesions that begin in the periventricular regions and extend into the corona radiata, lesions that begin within the corona radiata, and large lesions that begin or extend into the centrum semiovale are more important than periventricular rims that are diffuse. Smallness of the corpus callosum and relative paucity of white matter as well as ventricular enlargement are also often found in patients with neurological signs and cognitive abnormalities.

Many normal patients have periventricular smooth rims located around the frontal or occipital horns.

Most often, spin-echo (SE) sequences with a long TR and long TE (T2-weighted SE) are used to show white matter abnormalities. If intermediately long TEs (i.e. 40–60 ms) are employed, the lesions have a higher signal than CSF and the surrounding white matter, which improves their identification (proton-density images). Another MR sequence that is particularly suited for the identification of LA is FLAIR (Fig. 25.2). It uses a very long inversion time to suppress CSF, providing an even better contrast between white matter hyperintensities and CSF spaces. In the elderly, the homogenous low background signal allows for a dramatic demonstration of white matter abnormalities. As previously mentioned, it is the best sequence for separating lacunes, Virchow-Robin spaces and LA (Barkhof and Scheltens 2002).

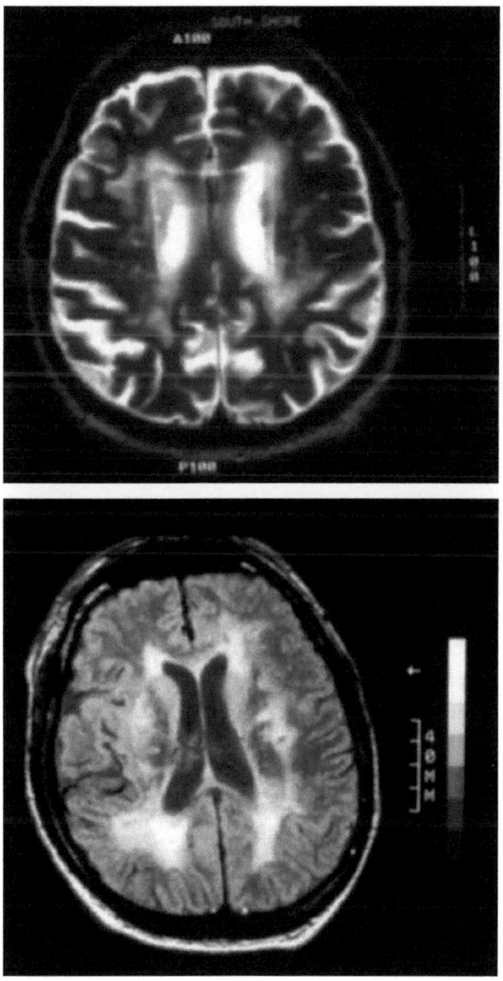

Fig. 25.2. T2-weighted (*top*) and FLAIR (*bottom*) images. The very long inversion time used in FLAIR images results in improved contrast between CSF spaces and white matter hyperintensities

A variety of scales have been proposed to rate the impact of white matter abnormalities. They have the advantage of providing a semiquantitative and standardized method for reporting LA, but are usually plagued with subjective interpretations and modifications which can lead to a high inter- and even intra-observer variability (Fazekas et al. 2002). Although no scale has been universally accepted, under the auspices of the European task force on age-related white matter changes a new rating scale was developed and validated for both CT and MRI. Five brain regions are rated following a four-point scale (frontal, parieto-occipital, infratentorial, cerebellar and temporal areas). Overall, it showed a good inter-rater reliability for MRI and moderate when CT was used (Wahlund et al. 2001) (Table 25.2, and Fig. 25.3).

The white matter abnormalities commonly found on MRI in the elderly are non-specific and tell the clinician little about their pathogenesis, other than to possibly suggest ischemia. Table 25.3 presents a clinicopathological classification of vascular dementia.

Table 25.2. The age-related white matter changes (ARWMC) scale for CT and MRI.

White matter lesions	
0	No lesions
1	Focal lesions
2	Beginning confluence of lesions
3	Diffuse involvement of the entire region with or without U fiber involvement
Basal ganglia lesions	
0	No lesions
1	1 focal lesion (≥5 mm)
2	> 1 focal lesion
3	Confluent lesions

Taken from Wahlund et al. (2001). The following areas are used for rating: frontal, parieto-occipital, temporal, infratentorial/cerebellum, and basal ganglia. Each hemisphere is rated separately.

25.5.1 Diffusion-Weighted and Diffusion Tensor Imaging

Diffusion-weighted imaging (DWI) has the ability to detect (even small) acute and subacute infarcts with great accuracy. It also permits the identification of ischemic lesions in otherwise asymptomatic

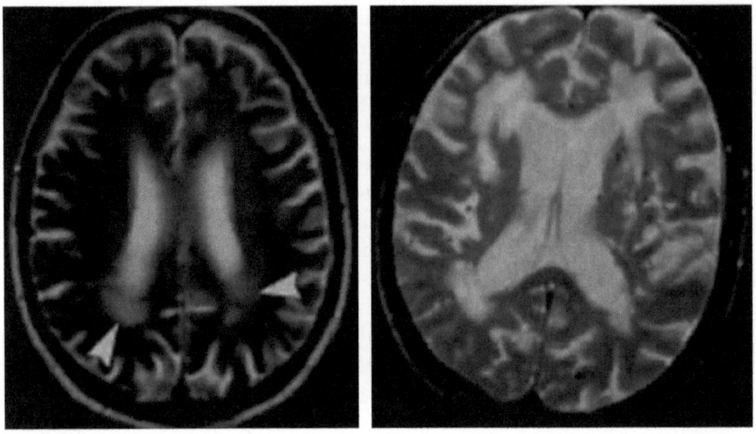

Fig. 25.3. ARWMC rating scale. *Left*, T2-weighted image showing a grade 2 rating score. *Right*, example of a grade 3 score. [Taken with permission from Wahlund et al. (2001)]

Table 25.3. Vascular dementia. [Modified with permission from Roman (2002)]

Large-vessel
- Multi-infarct dementia
- Strategic infarct dementia

Small vessel

Subcortical ischemic vascular dementia
- Binswanger's
- Lacunar dementia (état lacunaire)
- CADASIL

Cortical-subcortical
- Hypertensive and arteriolosclerotic angiopathy
- Cerebral amyloid angiopathies
- Venous occlusions
- Collagen-vascular diseases with dementia
- Other hereditary forms

Ischemic-hypoperfusive
- Diffuse anoxic-ischemic encephalopathy
- Selective vulnerability with restricted injury
- Border-zone infarction
- Incomplete white matter infarction

Hemorrhagic vascular dementia
- Traumatic subdural hematoma
- Subarachnoid hemorrhage
- Cerebral hemorrhage

individuals. Because of these, it may be useful in the longitudinal assessment of patients with LA to monitor the development of new ischemic lesions in the white matter.

In one study, more than one third of patients with vascular dementia associated with small vessel disease were found to have high-signal abnormalities on DWI suggestive of recent ischemia (Choi et al. 2000). In this study the mean apparent diffusion coefficient (ADC) was $0.71\pm0.15\times10^{-3}$ mm^2/S, the lesions were small (ranging from 0.07 to 2.40 ml), and located most commonly in the deep white matter. Remarkably, 20% of asymptomatic individuals had evidence of (silent) ischemia in the cerebral white matter, while some others had multiple small lesions suggesting either a proximal source of embolism or global hypoperfusion (Choi et al. 2000). The severity of LA also seems to correlate with a higher ADC value, and it has been suggested that DWI can be used to differentiate acute and chronic stroke lesions from LA (Helenius et al. 2002). Another potential advantage of this technique is the use of whole brain ADC histograms as a more reliable, quantitative tool to monitor disease progression at various time points (Mascalchi et al. 2002). Although promising, this needs to be further validated.

High *b* value diffusion MRI (high-*b* DWI), using *b* values >3000 s/mm^2, may be a more sensitive technique to identify disorders of myelin. In a small, preliminary study of two patients, high-*b* DWI was analyzed using the *q*-space approach (Fig. 25.4); a significant reduction in restricted diffusion (attributed to axonal loss and demyelination) much larger than the corresponding hyperintense lesions on T2-weighted or FLAIR images was observed. If corroborated, this finding would suggest that high-*b* DWI is a more sensitive technique for identifying early white matter changes, and that the extent of white matter abnormalities in these patients may be greater than currently assumed (Assaf et al. 2002).

The rate of diffusion of water molecules in normal white matter is not the same in all directions. In white matter tracts, the diffusion is less restricted along the long axis of the axons than across them. Diffusion tensor imaging (DT-MRI) measures the extent to which diffusion is directional (anisotropic), and the fractional anisotropy (FA) is an index of directionality of diffusion. Using this technique,

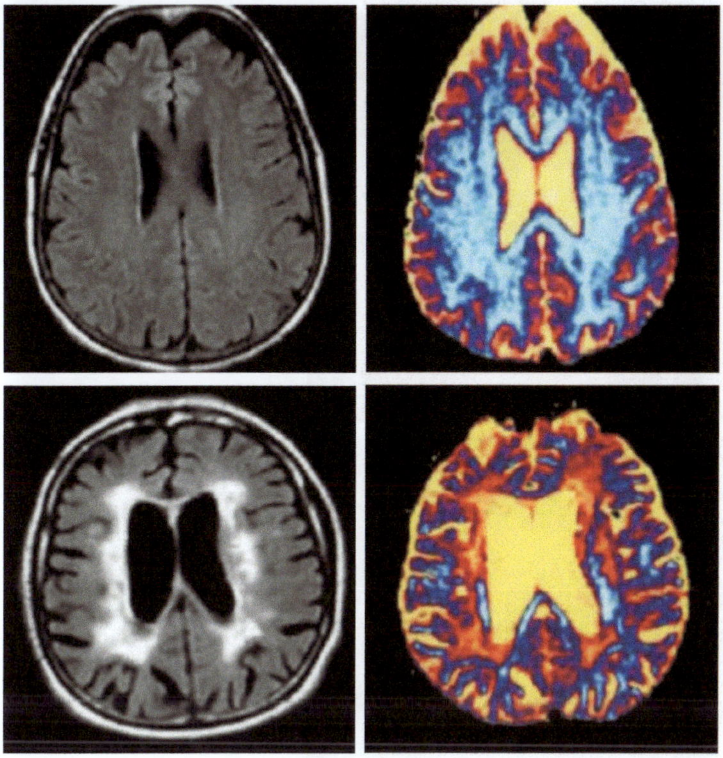

Fig. 25.4. FLAIR (*left*), and *q*-space probability (*right*) images of age-matched cognitively intact (*top*) and vascular dementia (*bottom*) subjects. Arbitrary units are used for the *q*-space probability image. In the subject with vascular dementia, this imaging modality reveals more extensive white matter abnormalities than those apparent in FLAIR MRI. [Taken from ASSAF et al. (2002) with permission]

JONES et al. (1999) found a characteristic pattern of moderate elevation in diffusion trace with a marked loss of FA in patients with LA. The authors postulated that these findings are consistent with the pathological correlate of axonal loss and gliosis commonly observed in LA, both of which would tend to result in decreased anisotropy. DT-MRI was also used to study the normal appearing white matter of patients with LA. Similar findings (increased mean diffusivity and decreased FA) were also found in white matter that appeared normal as assessed by T2-weighted images. Moreover, these subtle changes in DT-MRI correlated with cognitive dysfunction. The pathological substrate of this abnormality is unknown, but these findings also suggest that DT-MRI may be a more sensitive technique for the identification of early white matter changes in LA (O'SULLIVAN et al. 2001).

25.5.2 Magnetization Transfer MRI

Magnetization transfer (MT) is a technique used for tissue characterization. It measures the interaction between water protons bound to proteins and other macromolecules (such as those in myelin) and unbound tissue water protons. It has been extensively used in the characterization of multiple sclerosis lesions, and is believed to be more specific for white matter damage. This imaging modality has been applied to subjects with LA, and the MT ratios have been reported to be lower than that of normal white matter (38.6±4.5 and 47.3±2.1, respectively), but not nearly as low as in patients with frank demyelination (26.4±5.0). This finding has been attributed to a lesser extent to demyelination or ischemic damage, and more to increased water content (REIDEL et al. 2003).

In patients with dementia and LA, the mean MT ratio is also significantly lower than in non-demented patients with similar degrees of LA (37.4±1.5 versus 41.3±1.4), suggesting differences in the pathological substrate (Fig. 25.5). Moreover, the MT ratio of areas of periventricular hyperintensities correlates well with the mini-mental state examination score (HANYU et al. 1999). Taken together, these findings suggest that in patients with dementia and LA the white matter changes likely are more severe than in non-demented patients.

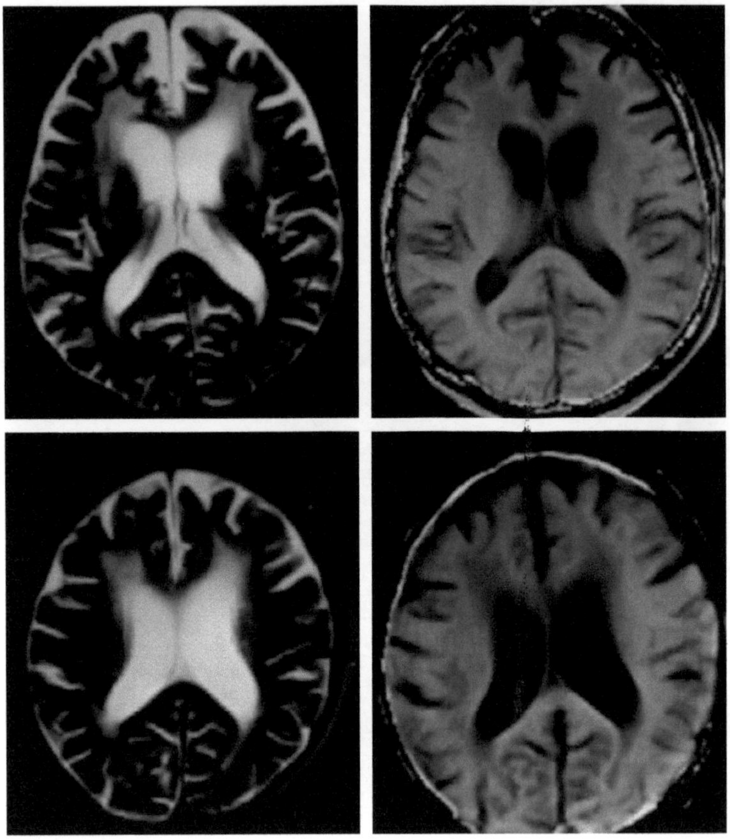

Fig. 25.5. T2-weighted MRI (*left*) and magnetization transfer ratio images (*right*) from age-matched normal (*top*) and demented (*bottom*) subjects. Even though the extent of white matter hyperintensities on T2-weighted images is similar in both subjects, the magnetization transfer images show more decreased intensity in the corresponding white matter of the demented patient. [Taken with permission from HANYU et al. (1999)]

25.5.3 Magnetic Resonance Spectroscopy

Proton magnetic resonance spectroscopic imaging (^{1}H-MRSI) reveals the distribution of the amino acid *N*-acetylaspartate (NAA) in the brain. NAA is exclusively found in neurons and is considered to be an indicator of neuronal density and metabolism. In patients with LA several interesting findings have been reported. First, decreased levels of NAA were found in the cortex independent of the amount of atrophy, and the frontal cortex NAA seemed to correlate inversely with the volume of white matter hyperintensities. These findings were quite unexpected and suggest that a subcortical injury could induce secondary changes in the cortex (CAPIZZANO et al. 2000).

Secondly and not surprisingly, decreased levels of NAA were found in these same patients, which is consistent with a greater susceptibility of the white matter to chronic ischemic changes. Thirdly, when patients with Alzheimer disease (AD) were compared with patients diagnosed with vascular dementia, they had a significantly lower NAA/creatine ratio in the hippocampus, suggesting that low hippocampal NAA may be relatively specific for AD and that it may help differentiate it from vascular dementia (CAPIZZANO et al. 2000; SCHUFF et al. 2003).

When otherwise healthy individuals with white matter lesions, controls, and patients with LA and dementia are compared, the NAA/creatine and NAA/choline ratios of the hyperintense white matter in asymptomatic individuals are virtually the same as those found in healthy controls. In demented patients with LA however, these ratios are reduced, suggesting chronic demyelination or ischemia. This technique may help identify clinically relevant white matter lesions and may also have a role in the diagnosis of vascular dementia.

25.5.4 Perfusion MRI

With recent advances in technique, it is now possible to calculate absolute regional cerebral blood flow (CBF) from MRI using an exogenous paramagnetic contrast agent with an accuracy and spatial resolution that is equal to or better than that of PET studies. Perfusion MRI has been applied to patients with LA in two settings. One has been to measure CBF and cerebral blood volume (CBV) in the actual area of white matter abnormalities. In one such study, the mean white matter CBF of regions of LA was reduced by almost 40% when compared to healthy controls, and this reduction was apparent in all regions of white matter (i.e. anterior, posterior, and superior). Interestingly, grey matter CBV in this same study was significantly increased in the LA group (Markus et al. 2000). The relevance of this finding is unknown at present, but further supports the notion of cortical dysfunction or injury triggered by subcortical insults.

The other setting in which perfusion MRI has been applied is in quantifying CBF in normal appearing white matter in patients with known LA. It has been found that CBF is significantly reduced in the periventricular white matter of these patients (17.9 vs 21.6 ml/100 g/min in controls). Such a reduction, however, was not found in the centrum semiovale (O'Sullivan et al. 2002). These findings support chronic hypoperfusion and ischemic damage with "incomplete infarction" as the underlying pathophysiologic mechanism in this condition. Perfusion MRI could also be used to identify areas of normal appearing white matter that are at risk by virtue of their decreased CBF value and potentially allow interventions that could prevent further injury.

References

Alzheimer A (1894) Die arteriosklerotische atropkie des gehirns. Neurol Zentralbl 13:765-768

Assaf Y, Mayzel-Oreg O, Gigi A et al (2002) High *b* value *q*-space-analyzed diffusion MRI in vascular dementia: a preliminary study. J Neurol Sci 203-204:235-239

Awad I, Spetzler R, Hodak J et al (1986) Incidental subcortical lesions identified on magnetic resonance imaging in the elderly. I. Correlation with age and cerebrovascular risk factors. Stroke 17:1084-1089

Babikian V, Ropper AH (1987) Binswanger disease: a review. Stroke 18:1-12

Bacskai BJ, Hickey GA, Skoch J et al (2003) Four-dimensional multiphoton imaging of brain entry, amyloid binding, and clearance of an amyloid- ligand in transgenic mice. PNAS 100:12462-12467

Ball MJ (1988) Ischemic axonopathy: further evidence that neocortical pathology accompanying cerebral hypoperfusion during systemic hypotension causes white matter rarefaction in the elderly and some people with Alzheimer dementia. J Neuropathol Exp Neurol 47:388

Ball MJ (2003) White matter lesions, dementia, and ischemic axonopathy. Alz Dis Assoc Dis 17:55

Barkhof F, Scheltens P (2002) Imaging of white matter lesions. Cerebrovasc Dis 13 [Suppl 2]:21-30

Binswanger O (1894) Die abgrenzung der allgemeinen progressiven paralyse. Berl Klin Wochenschr 31:1103-1105, 1137-1139, 1180-1186

Blass JP, Hoyer S, Nitsch R (1991) A translation of Otto Binswanger's article: the delineation of generalized progressive paralysis. Arch Neurol 48:961-972

Bogousslavsky J, Regli F, Uske A (1987) Leukoencephalopathy with ischemic stroke. Stroke 18:896-899

Boon A, Lodder J, Heuts-van Raak L et al (1994) Silent brain infarcts in 755 consecutive patients with a first-ever supratentorial ischemic stroke: relationship with index-stroke subtype, vascular risk factors, and mortality. Stroke 25:2384-2390

Bornebroek M, Hann J, van Buchem et al (1996) White matter lesions and cognitive deterioration in presymptomatic carriers of the amyloid precursor protein gene codon 693 mutation. Arch Neurol 53:43-48

Breteler MMB, Van Swieten JC, Bots MI et al (1994) Cerebral white matter lesions, vascular risk factors, and cognitive function in a population-based study: the Rotterdam study. Neurology 44:1246-1252

Brooks WM, Wesley MH, Kodituwakku PW et al (1997) 1H MRSI differentiates white matter hyperintensities in subcortical arteriosclerotic encephalopathy from those in normal elderly. Stroke 28:1940-1943

Brown WR, Moody DM, Thore CR, Challa VR (2000) Apoptosis in leukoaraiosis. Am J Neuroradiol 21:79-82

Capizzano AA, Schuff N, Amend DL et al (2000) Subcortical ischemic vascular dementia: assessment with quantitative MR imaging and ^{1}H MR spectroscopy. Am J Neuroradiol 21:621-630

Caplan LR (1995) Binswanger's disease revisited. Neurology 45:626-633

Caplan LR (2000) Caplan's stroke, 3rd edn. Butterworth-Heinemann, Boston

Caplan LR, Schoene W (1978) Subcortical arteriosclerotic encephalopathy (Binswanger disease): clinical features. Neurology 28:1206-1217

Chan S, Kratha K, Yoon SS et al (1996) Hilal, multifocal hypointense cerebral lesions on gradient-echo MR are associated with chronic hypertension. Am J Neuroradiol 17:1821-1827

Choi SH, Na DL, Chung CS et al (2000) Diffusion-weighted MRI in vascular dementia. Neurology 54:83-89
Davous P (1998) CADASIL: a review with proposed diagnostic criteria. Eur J Neurol 5:219-233
Dechambre A (1838) Mémoire sur la curabilité du ramollissement cerebral. Gaz Méd Paris 6:305-314
Domínguez RO, Marschoff ER, Serra JA et al (2002) Stroke vs. chronic progressive cerebrovascular disease: a magnetic resonance imaging study of symptomatic outpatients. J Neurol Sci 203/204:67-71
Dubas F, Gray F, Roullet E, Escourolle R (1985) Leukoencephalopathies arteriopathiques. Rev Neurol 141:93-108
Durand-Fardel M (1843) Traité du ramollissement du cerveau. Baillière, Paris
Fazekas F, Barkhof F, Wahlund LO et al (2002) CT and MRI rating of white matter lesions. Cerebrovasc Dis 13 [Suppl 2]:31-36
Fisher CM (1965) Lacunes, small deep cerebral infarcts. Neurology 15:774-784
Fisher CM (1969) The arterial lesions underlying lacunes. Acta Neuropathol 12:1-15
Fisher CM (1989) Binswanger's encephalopathy: a review. J Neurol 236:65-79
Furuta A, Ishii N, Nishihara Y et al (1991) Medullary arteries in aging and dementia. Stroke 22:442-446
Ghika J, Bogousslavsky J (1996) White matter disease and vascular dementia. In: Prohovnik I, Wade J, Knezevic S, Tatemichi T, Erkinjuntti T (eds) Vascular dementia: current concepts. Wiley, New York, pp 113-141
Gorter JW for the stroke prevention in reversible ischemia trial (SPIRIT), and European atrial fibrillation trial (EAFT) study groups (1999) Major bleeding during anticoagulation after cerebral ischemia. Neurology 53:1319
Grabowski TJ, Cho HS, Vonsattel JPG et al (2001) Novel amyloid precursor protein mutation in an Iowa family with dementia and severe cerebral amyloid angiopathy. Ann Neurol 49:697-705
Gray F, Dubas F, Roullet E et al (1985) Leukoencephalopathy in diffuse hemorrhagic cerebral amyloid angiopathy. Ann Neurol 18:54-59
Greenberg SM (2002) Cerebral amyloid angiopathy and vessel dysfunction. Cerebrovasc Dis 13 [Suppl 2]:42-47
Greenberg SM, Vonsattel JPG (1997) Diagnosis of cerebral amyloid angiopathy. Sensitivity and specificity of cortical biopsy. Stroke 28:1418-1422
Gupta SR, Naheedy MH, Young J et al (1988) Periventricular white matter changes and dementia. Clinical, neuropsychological, radiological, and pathological correlate. Arch Neurol 45:637-641
Hachinski V, Potter P, Merskey H (1987) Leuko-araiosis. Arch Neurol 44:21-23
Hanyu H, Asano T, Sakurai H et al (1999) magnetization transfer ratio in cerebral white matter lesions of Binswanger's disease. J Neurol Sci 166:85-90
Hanyu H, Tanaka Y, Shimizo S et al (2003) Cerebral microbleeds in Binswanger's disease: a gradient-echo T2*-weighted magnetic resonance imaging study. Neurosci Lett 340:213-216
Helenius J, Soinne L, Salonen O et al (2002) Leukoaraiosis, ischemic stroke, and normal white matter on diffusion-weighted MRI. Stroke 33:45-50
Hendricks HT, Franke CL, Theunissen PHMH (1990) Cerebral amyloid angiopathy: diagnosis by MRI and brain biopsy. Neurology 40:1308-1310
Hénon J, Godefroy O, Lucas Ch et al (1996) Risk factors ofr leuko-araiosis in stroke patients. Acta Neurol Scand 94:137-144
Hijdra A, Verbeeten B Jr (1991) Leukoaraiosis and ventricular enlargement in patients with ischemic stroke. Stroke 22:447-450
Hijdra A, Verbeeten B Jr, Verhulst JAPM (1990) Relationship of leuko-araiosis to lesion type in stroke patients. Stroke 21:890-894
Inzitari D, Diaz F, Fox A et al (1987) Vascular risk factors and leuko-araiosis. Arch Neurol 44:42-47
Jones Dk, Lythgoe D, Horsfield MA et al (1999) Characterization of white matter damage in ischemic leukoaraiosis with diffusion tensor MRI. Stroke 30:393-397
Kase CS (1994) Cerebral amyloid angiopathy. In: Kase CS, Caplan LR (eds) Intracerebral hemorrhage. Butterworth-Heinemann, Boston, pp 179-200
Kato H, Izumiyama K, Takahashi K et al (2002) Silent cerebral microbleeds on T2*-weighted MRI: correlation with stroke subtype, stroke recurrence, and and leukoaraiosis. Stroke 33:1536-1540
Leys D, Englund E, Del Ser T et al (1999) White matter changes in stroke patients: relationship with stroke subtype and outcome. Eur Neurol 42:67-75
Liao D, Cooper L, Cai J et al (1997) The prevalence and severity of white matter lesions, their relationship with age, ethnicity, gender, and cardiovascular risk factors: the ARIC study. Neuroepidemiology 16:149-162
Lindgren A, Roijer A, Rudling O et al (1994) Cerebral lesions on magnetic resonance imaging, heart disease, and vascular risk factors in subjects without stroke; a population-based study. Stroke 25:929-934
Loes DJ, Biller J, Yuh WTC et al (1990) Leukoencephalopathy in cerebral amyloid angiopathy: MR imaging in four cases. Am J Neuroradiol 11:485-488
Longstretch WT Jr, Manolio T, Arnold A et al (1996) Clinical correlates of white matter findings on cranial magnetic resonance imaging of 3301 elderly people: the cardiovascular health study. Stroke 27:1274-1282
Mandybur TI (1986) Cerebral amyloid angiopathy: the vascular pathology and complications. J Neuropathol Exp Neurol 45:79-90
Mäntylä R, Aronen HJ, Salonen et al (1999) Magnetic resonance imaging white matter hyperintensities and mechanism of ischemic stroke. Stroke 30:2053-2058
Marie P (1901) Des foyers lacunaires de disintegration et des differents autres états cavitaires du cerveau. Rev Méd 21:281-298
Markus HS, Lythgoe DJ, Ostegaard L et al (2000) Reduced cerebral blood flow in white matter in ischaemic leukoaraiosis demonstrated using quantitative exogenous contrast based perfusion MRI. J Neurol Neurosurg Psychiatry 69:48-53
Martinez-Lage P, Hachinski V (1998) Multi-infarct dementia. In: Barnett HJM, Mohr JP, Stein BM, Yatsu FM (eds) Stroke: pathophysiology, diagnosis and management. Churchill Livingstone, New York, pp 875-894
Mas JL, Dilouya A, de Recondo J (1992) A familial disorder with subcortical ischemic strokes, dementia, and leukoencephalopathy. Neurology 42:1015-1019
Mascalchi M, Moretti M, Della Nave R et al (2002) Longitudinal

evaluation of leukoaraiosis with whole brain ADC histograms. Neurology 59:938-940
Merino JG, Hachinski V (2000) Leukoaraiosis. Arch Neurol 57:925-926
Moody DM, Brown WR, Challa VR, Anderson RL (1995) Periventricular venous collagenosis: association with leukoaraiosis. Radiology 194:469-476
Murata T, Handa H, Mori K et al (1981) The significance of periventricular lucency on computed tomography: experimental study with canine hydrocephalus. Neuroradiology 20:221-227
Nag S (1984) Cerebral changes in chronic hypertension: combined permeability and immunohistochemical studies. Acta Neuropathol 62:178-184
O'Sullivan M, Summers PE, Jones DK et al (2001) Normal-appearing white matter in ischemic leukoaraiosis: a diffusion tensor MRI study. Neurology 57:2307-2310
O'Sullivan M, Lythgoe DJ, Pereira AC et al (2002) Patterns of cerebral blood flow reduction in patients with ischemic leukoaraiosis. Neurology 59:321-326
Ohtani R, Tomimoto H, Kawasaki T et al (2003) Cerebral vasomotor reactivity to postural change is impaired in patients with cerebrovascular white matter lesions. J Neurol 250:412-417
Olszewski J (1965) Subcortical arteriosclerotic encephalopathy. World Neurol 3:359-374
Pantoni L (2002) Pathophysiology of age-related cerebral white matter changes. Cerebrovasc Dis 13 [Suppl 2]:7-10
Pantoni L, Garcia J (1997) Pathogenesis of leukoaraiosis. Stroke 28:652-659
Raiha I, Tarvonen S, Kurki T et al (1993) Relationship between vascular factors and white matte low attenuation of the brain. Acta Neurol Scand 87:286-289
Ravens JR (1974) Anastomoses in the vascular bed of the human cerebrum. In: Cervós-Navarro J (ed) Pathology of cerebral microcirculation. De Gruyter; Berlin, pp 26-38
Reidel MA, Stippich C, Heiland S et al (2003) Differentiation of multiple sclerosis plaques, subacute ischemic cerebral infarcts, focal vasogenic oedema and lesions of subcortical arteriosclerotic encephalopathy using magnetization transfer measurements. Neuroradiology 45:289-294
Roman GC (1991) White matter lesions and normal-pressure hydrocephalus: Binswanger's disease or Hakim syndrome. Am J Neuroradiol 12:40-41
Roman GC (2002) On the history of lacunes, état criblé, and the white matter lesions of vascular dementia. Cerebrovasc Dis 13 [Suppl]:1-6
Roman GC, Erkinjuntti T, Wallin A et al (2002) Subcortical ischaemic vascular dementia. Lancet Neurol 1:426-436
Rosenberg GA, Sullivan N, Esiri M (2001) White matter damage is associated with matrix metalloproteinases in vascular dementia. Stroke 32:1162
Scheltens P, Barkhof F, Leys D et al (1995) Histopathological correlates of white matter changes on MRI in Alzheimer's disease and normal aging. Neurology 45:883-888
Schmidt R, Schmidt H, Kapeller P et al (2002) Evolution of white matter lesions. Cerebrovasc Dis 13 [Suppl 2]:16-20
Schmidt R, Enzinger C, Ropele S et al (2003) Progression of cerebral white matter lesions: 6-year results of the Austrian stroke prevention study. Lancet 361:2046-2048
Schuff N, Capizzano AA, Du AT et al (2003) Different patterns of N-acetylaspartate loss in subcortical ischemic vascular dementia and AD. Neurology 61:358-364
Smith EE, Rosand J, Knudsen KA et al (2002) Leukoaraiosis is associated with warfarin-related hemorrhage following ischemic stroke. Neurology 59:193-197
Streifler JY, Eliaziw M, Benavente OR et al (1995) Lack of relationship between leukoaraiosis and carotid artery disease. Arch Neurol 52:21-24
Tanaka A, Ueno Y, Nakayama Y et al (1999) Small chronic hemorrhages and ischemic lesions in association with spontaneous, intracerebral, hematomas. Stroke 30:1637-1642
Tomonaga M, Yamanouchi H, Tohgi H et al (1982) Clinicopathologic study of progressive subcortical vascular encephalopathy (Binswanger type) in the elderly. J Am Geriatr Soc 30:524-529
Tournier-Lasserve E, Iba-Zizen I-T, Romero N, Bousser M-G (1991) Autosomal dominant syndrome with stroke-like episodes and leukoencephalopathy. Stroke 22:1297-1302
Van den Bergh R, van der Eecken H (1968) Anatomy and embryology of cerebral circulation. Prog Brain Res 30:1-26
Veldink JH, Scheltens P, Jonker C et al (1998) Progression of cerebral white matter hyperintensities on MRI is related to diastolic blood pressure. Neurology 51:319-320
Vermeer SE, Koudstaal PJ, Oudrek M et al (2002) Prevalence and risk factors of silent brain infarcts in the population-based Rotterdam scan study. Stroke 33:21-25
Vinters HV, Gilbert JJ (1983) Cerebral amyloid angiopathy: incidence and complications in the aging brain. II. The distribution of amyloid vascular changes. Stroke 14:924-928
Vonsattel JP, Myers RH, Hedley-Whyte ET et al (1991) Cerebral amyloid angiopathy without and with cerebral hemorrhages: a comparative histological study. Ann Neurol 30:637-649
Wahlund LO, Barkhof F, Fazekas F et al (2001) A new rating scale for age-related white matter changes applicable to MRI and CT. Stroke 32:1318-1322
Wattendorff AR, Frangione B, Luyendijk W et al (1995) Hereditary cerebral hemorrhage with amyloidosis, Dutch type (HCHWA-D): clinicopathological studies. J Neurol Neurosurg Psychiatry 58:699-705
Whitman GT, Tang T, Lin A et al (2001) A prospective study of cerebral white matter abnormalities in older people with gait dysfunction. Neurology 57:990-994
Ylikoski A, Erkinjuntti T, Raininko et al (1995) White matter hyperintensities on the MRI in the neurologically nondemented elderly: analysis of cohorts of consecutive subjects aged 65 to 85 years living at home. Stroke 26:11781-11787
Zimmerman RD, Fleming CA, Lee BCP et al (1986) Periventricular hyperintensities as seen by magnetic resonance: prevalence and significance. AJNR 7:13-20

26 Neurodegenerative Diseases with Associated White Matter Pathology

Mario Mascalchi

CONTENTS

26.1 Introduction

Degenerative diseases of the central nervous system (CNS) comprise a variety of sporadic or inherited conditions characterized by progressive neuronal dysfunction and loss of unknown or incompletely known etiopathogenesis which typically are selective of some neuronal systems (Adams and Victor 1985). While the neuropathological hallmark of degenerative diseases of the CNS is a generally symmetric gray matter cortical or subcortical damage, white matter changes in the brain or spinal cord are increasingly recognized as a frequent magnetic resonance (MR) finding in most of them. In some instances they are apparent in the conventional MR examination and are useful diagnostic features, in other cases they are not visible in the conventional MR examination but can be demonstrated using non-conventional MR techniques.

Conventional MR imaging includes T1, proton density and T2 (with and without inversion recovery RF pulse to attenuate the CSF signal) weighted sequences. The non-conventional MR include proton MR spectroscopy (^{1}H-MRS), magnetization transfer imaging (MTI), and diffusion MR imaging.

^{1}H-MRS enables an in vivo biochemical characterization of operator selectable volume of interest through the evaluation of the absolute or relative concentrations of some proton containing metabolites such as *N*-acetyl-aspartate (NAA), which is a marker of neuronal integrity and function, creatine plus phosphocreatine (Cr), which are markers of cell density and energy state, choline-containing compounds (Cho), which are markers of membrane metabolism, myo-inositol (mI), which is a marker of glial cell density, and glutamine (Gln) and glutamate (Glu). Although in many ^{1}H-MRS studies of degenerative diseases of the CNS it was claimed that the volume of interest was placed in the cortical gray matter, with the current resolution of the single and multi-voxel techniques used for ^{1}H-MRS there is always partial volume with the white matter and the spectral findings variably reflect also white matter changes.

Magnetization transfer imaging (MTI) is based on the interaction between protons in a relatively free state and those in a restricted motion state and indirectly reflects the capacity of the molecules of the tissue matrix to exchange energy with the surrounding water molecules (McGowan et al. 1998). A decrease of the MT ratio usually indicates a damage of the tissue matrix.

Diffusion MR imaging exploits the sensitivity of MR to motion of water molecules and provides a sensitive tool to explore the integrity of tissue and

M. Mascalchi, MD
Professor, Sezione di Radiodiagnostica, Dipartimento di Fisiopatologia Clinica, Università di Firenze, Viale Morgagni, 85, 50134 Firenze, Italy

cellular barriers to water motion (Schaefer et al. 2000; Dong et al. 2004). The evaluation of maps of apparent diffusion coefficients (ADC) or mean diffusivity ($\overline{D}$) evaluation is emerging as a quantitative, reproducible, and sensitive method to assess white and gray matter brain diseases (Cercignani et al. 2000; Bozzali et al. 2001; Cercignani et al. 2003). In particular, analysis of the brain $\overline{D}$ can provide regional and global quantification not only of the macroscopic damage shown as areas of prolonged T2 but also of microscopic tissue damage which is not demonstrated by T2 weighted images. To this end, region of interest and histogram approaches are complementary. In fact, histogram analysis is intrinsically more powerful from a statistical point of view than region of interest analysis (Chun et al. 2000) and is more suited to evaluate diffuse pathological processes as those underlying degenerative diseases of the CNS (van Buchem 1999). On the other hand, the loss of spatial information associated to histogram analysis can be compensated using regions of interest analysis based on an a priori knowledge of the distribution of the pathological damage.

In this chapter we shall review the most frequent degenerative diseases of the CNS in which conventional and non-conventional MR studies have documented significant "macroscopic" or "microscopic" white matter changes.

26.2 Degenerative Dementias

26.2.1 Alzheimer Disease

Although the neuropathological hallmarks of Alzheimer disease (AD), namely intracellular neurofibrillary tangles and extracellular amyloid plaques, are observed in the cerebral gray matter, diffuse white matter damage which is related to microvascular pathology is demonstrated in the brains of AD patients (Brun and Englund 1986; Sjobeck et al. 2003). Moreover, Kril et al. (2002) observed that the degree of hippocampal neuronal loss and atrophy was similar in demented patients fulfilling the neuropathological criteria for small vessel disease dementia and AD, respectively. These data indicate that even on a pathological basis, a complete separation of AD from white matter damage due to vascular disease is not always possible.

26.2.1.1 Conventional MR

Proton density and T2 weighted images can show focal or diffuse white matter signal hyperintensity in patients with clinically probable AD (Fazekas et al. 1987). The most characteristic hyperintensities are symmetric and located along the cerebral periventricular regions or in the subcortical hippocampal and sylvian regions (Fazekas et al. 1987; Scheltens et al. 1990) (Fig. 26.1). Interestingly, de Leeuw et al. (2004) recently reported that white matter lesions were present on MR imaging in 29% of patients with a clinical diagnosis of probable AD and that there was a correlation between white matter signal changes, especially in the frontal and parieto-occipital regions, and hippocampal atrophy suggesting a relationship between vascular and typical AD pathology.

Although a loss of bulk of the white matter contributes to the pattern and progression of global and regional atrophy demonstrated by 3D T1 weighted images in cross-sectional and longitudinal studies in AD (Chan et al. 2001; Rusinek et al. 2003), most volumetric studies in AD measured the hippocampal formations alone (Jack et al. 2002; Dixon et al. 2002).

Voxel based morphometry (VBM) was introduced in 2000 as a new approach for global and regional estimation of brain volumes which is based on the statistical parametric mapping (SPM) soft-

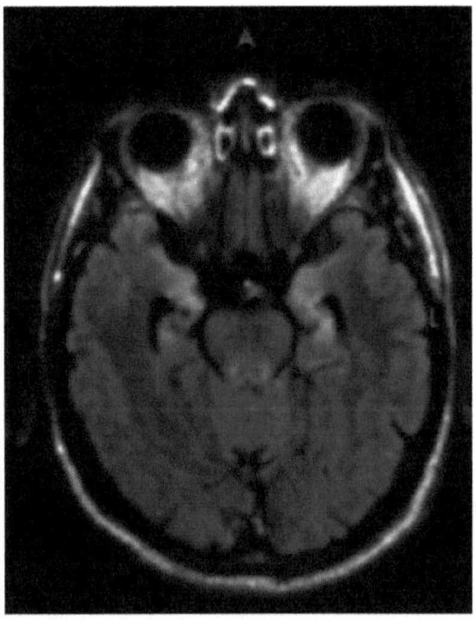

Fig. 26.1. Alzheimer disease. Axial T2 weighted FLAIR image shows symmetric hyperintensity in the hippocampus and subhippocampal white matter of a patient with probable AD

ware developed for nuclear medicine and functional MR techniques. SPM analysis combines a strong statistical power with an observer unbiased high resolution analysis (Ashburner and Friston 2000). Curiously, many studies employing VBM emphasized regional cortical gray matter loss (Baron et al. 2001; Frisoni et al. 2002; Karas et al. 2003), but none explored possible white matter volume changes in AD.

26.2.1.2 Non-conventional MR

26.2.1.2.1 ^{1}H-MRS

In degenerative diseases of the CNS, ^{1}H-MRS shows a decrease of the concentration of NAA or of the NAA/Cr ratio in the areas where there is the maximal neuronal damage and loss on neuropathological examination.

Spectroscopy was employed since the early 1990s in the evaluation of patients with clinical diagnosis of AD. Single voxels and MR spectroscopic imaging acquisitions were performed with volumes of interest placed in a number of sites, which included the occipital region (Shonk et al. 1995), the frontal region (Ernst et al. 1997), the parietal region (Schuff et al. 2002) the hippocampus (Dixon et al. 2002) the posterior cingulate (Kantarci et al. 2003) and the subcortical white matter (Catani et al. 2000).

The two main findings of ^{1}H-MRS in AD, essentially independent of the voxel locations, are a decrease of NAA concentration or NAA/Cr ratio and an increase of mI concentration or of the mI/Cr ratio, which can be expressed as NAA/mI ratio (Shonk et al. 1995). The sensitivity and the specificity of the two ^{1}H-MRS findings considered alone or combined for differentiation of mildly demented cases from age matched controls and for differentiation of AD from others dementias are high but not perfect (Shonk et al. 1995; Rapaport 2002; Catani et al. 2000). The decrease of NAA, NAA/Cr or NAA/mI correlate with the severity of the disease as judged based on the clinical and neuropsychological evaluation (Chantal et al. 2002; Waldman and Rai 2003), but its capacity to mark disease progression or cognitive decline in longitudinal studies is controversial (Jessen et al. 2001; Dixon et al. 2002).

This notwithstanding, ^{1}H-MRS was employed as a surrogate marker to evaluate the efficacy of a drug in a randomized clinical trial in patients with AD (Kishnan et al. 2003).

26.2.1.2.2 MTI

Bozzali et al. (2001) reported that the peak of the MT ratio histogram of the cerebral hemispheres and of the temporal lobes was reduced in patients with AD as compared to age matched healthy controls. Similar results in the whole brain, temporal and frontal lobes of patients with AD and mild cognitive impairment were reported in a study showing that the cognitive decline in these two categories of patients correlated with the relative peak height of the whole brain MT ratio histogram (van der Flier et al. 2002).

26.2.1.2.3 Diffusion MR

Two early studies of diffusion MR imaging in patients with clinical suspicion of AD employed the region of interest analysis in order to detect possible $\overline{D}$ changes in the cortical gray matter and subcortical white matter (Hanyu et al. 1998; Bozzao et al. 2001). Although both studies failed to demonstrate significant $\overline{D}$ changes in the hippocampi, one study (Hanyu et al. 1998) reported an increase of $\overline{D}$ and a decrease of anisotropy in the white matter of the temporal lobe which correlated with the clinical severity. Moreover, ADC perpendicular to the commissural fibers of the corpus callosum was increased and anisotropy decreased in patients with AD, the latter correlating with the mini-mental state examination score (Hanyu et al. 1999). Subsequent studies with diffusion tensor imaging confirmed the increase of $\overline{D}$ and the reduction of the fractional anisotropy in the association white matter tracts but not in the internal capsule of patients with clinical diagnosis of AD (Rose et al. 2000; Bozzali et al. 2002). Moreover, a strong correlation was reported between the score at the mini-mental state examination and an average overall white matter $\overline{D}$ and fractional anisotropy (Bozzali et al. 2002). Using histogram analysis after segmentation of the gray and white matter based on different FA, Bozzali et al. (2001) confirmed the increase of $\overline{D}$ in the cerebral white matter and cortical gray matter in patients with AD.

Interestingly, loss of anisotropy of the frontal white matter was found to increase with age and to correlate with neuropsychological evidence of cognitive decline in normal aging (O'Sullivan et al. 2001).

26.2.2
Fronto-temporal Dementia (FTD)

FTD comprises a variety of inherited or sporadic conditions characterized by progressive mental impairment and frontal lobe behavioral symptoms (The Lund and Manchester Group 1994). An immunohistochemistry-based classification of this group of diseases has been proposed, separating those associated with abnormal deposits of tau protein (tauopathies) from the others (Lowe 1998).

26.2.2.1
Conventional MR

T1, proton density and T2 weighted images show a variable combination of cortical atrophy and white matter signal changes in the frontal and temporal regions in pathologically proven cases of FTD (Savoiardo and Grisoli 2001) (Fig. 26.2). The more distinctive features as compared to AD are the frontal involvement and the asymmetric distribution. In a recent whole brain and regional volumetric study (Chan et al. 2001) a more heterogeneous progression rate of atrophy (annual volume loss from 0.3% to 8 %) was observed in patients with clinical diagnosis of FTD than in patients with AD (from 0.5% to 4.7%).

26.2.2.2
Non-conventional MR

Presently, no study addressed possible diffusion or MT ratio changes in FTD.

26.2.2.2.1
^{1}H-MRS

In a relatively large study comparing the MRS findings in the frontal and temporo-parietal cortical gray matter of two groups of patients with FTD and AD and a control group, Ernst et al. (1997) observed a significant reduction of NAA and increase of mI concentrations in the frontal lobe of patients with FTD but not of patients with AD. A distinct increase of lactate was seen in the frontal lobe of three out of 14 FTD patients. Using MRS data alone, 92% of the FTD patients were correctly differentiated from AD patients and control subjects.

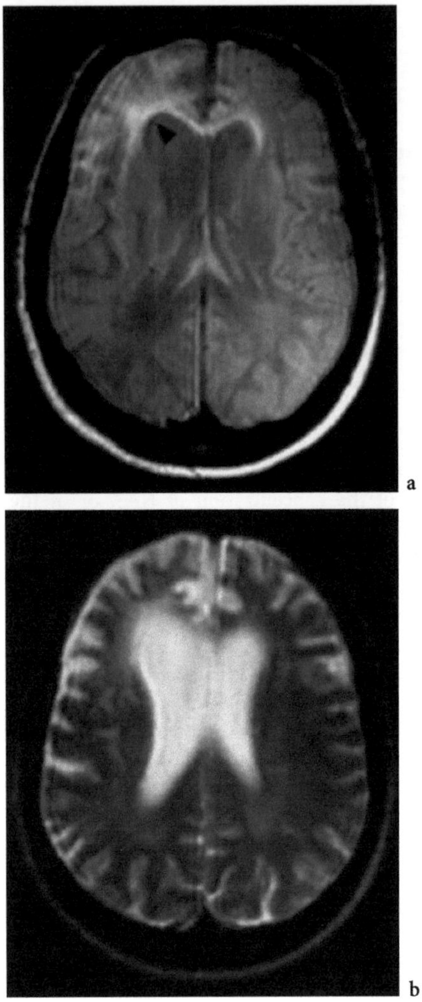

Fig. 26.2a,b. Fronto-temporal dementia. Axial proton density (**a**) and T2 weighted (**b**) images show asymmetric atrophy of the frontal lobes which is accompanied by diffuse hyperintensity of the subcortical white matter more evident in proton density image (*arrowhead*) in a patient with sporadic FTD

26.3
Degenerative Ataxias

Degenerative ataxias are a variety of inherited or sporadic diseases sharing the clinical features of progressive gait and coordination disturbances. In the last decade many of the genetic abnormalities underlying inherited ataxias were discovered and molecular screening tests are now available (Subramony and Filla 2001) with improved diagnostic accuracy and better genotype/phenotype correlation. The neuropathological examination shows three main patterns of distribution of loss of bulk and neurodegeneration, namely olivopontocerebellar atrophy (OPCA), spinal atrophy (SA) and cortical cerebellar atrophy (CCA) (LOWE et al. 1997). Each pattern is observed in either sporadic and genetically defined disease. Olivopontocerebellar degeneration is a neuropathological process characterized by neuronal loss, gliosis, wallerian degeneration and ultimately atrophy of the inferior olives, pons, middle cerebellar peduncles and cerebellum. Myelin stains demonstrates diffuse white matter damage in the brainstem and cerebellum with sparing of the corticospinal tracts and of the superior cerebellar peduncles. In SA the pathological hallmark is neuronal loss and shrinkage in the Clarke column of the spinal cord and in the spinal ganglion cells with macroscopic degeneration of the spinocerebellar and gracilis and cuneatus tracts of the spinal cord which is better appreciated on myelin stains. Secondary neuronal loss in the brainstem predominantly involves the accessory cuneate and gracile nuclei of the medulla. The cerebellar cortex is spared but there is cell loss in the dentate nuclei. In CCA, diffuse loss of Purkinje cells in the ganglial layer of the cerebellar cortex is the main pathological finding with secondary loss of cells in the inferior olives. White matter is macroscopically spared.

26.3.1
Conventional MR

The features of OPCA on conventional MRI were defined using subjective evaluation of morphology and signal intensity of the brainstem and cerebellum (SAVOIARDO et al. 1990; ORMEROD et al. 1994). In particular, SAVOIARDO et al. (1990) reported in sporadic and inherited OPCA characteristic thinning of the ventral pons and diffusely increased signal intensity of the brainstem, middle cerebellar peduncles and cerebellar white matter in proton density weighted images with sparing of the corticospinal tracts and of the superior cerebellar peduncles (Fig. 26.3). The signal changes are far less apparent in T2 weighted images (Fig. 26.3). They were observed in advanced but not in early cases of SCA1 and SCA2 (MASCALCHI et al. 1998; GIUFFRIDA et al. 1999) and were not reported in other studies of patients with inherited or sporadic OPCA (WULLNER et al. 1993; ORMEROD et al. 1994), conceivably also reflecting the subjectivity of the visual evaluation.

Conventional MRI using manual or semiautomatic measurements of the morphology or volume of the cerebellum, brainstem and cervical spinal cord demonstrates the three neuropathological patterns in vivo (WULLNER et al. 1993; MASCALCHI et al. 1994; BURK et al. 1996; KLOCKGETHER et al. 1998). In particular, using an array of area and linear measurements, WULLNER et al. (1993) defined the morphometric criteria for an in vivo diagnosis of OPCA, SA and CCA based on the distribution of atrophy. Recently the technique of VBM was applied to the evaluation of the distribution and severity of the atrophic changes in a genetically determined variant of OPCA, namely spinocerebellar ataxia type 2 (BRENNEIS et al. 2003). Significant white matter loss in the cerebellar hemispheres, pons, and midbrain was accompanied with supratentorial cortical and subcortical grey matter atrophy.

MRI studies in patients with SA pointed out marked atrophy of the spinal cord and medulla (WULLNER et al. 1993) which in FA are combined to symmetric signal changes of the posterior and lateral columns of the cervical spinal cord on T2 or T2* weighted images (MASCALCHI et al. 1994) (Fig. 26.4). This feature is not specific and can be observed in other conditions including combined sclerosis due to vitamin B12 deficiency. At variance with OPCA and CCA, atrophy of the brainstem and cerebellum is not remarkable in SA (WULLNER et al. 1993).

In CCA conventional MRI shows atrophy of the cerebellar vermis and hemisphere with normal brainstem volume and no signal changes (WULLNER et al. 1993).

MR imaging based morphometry measurements or subjective evaluation of brainstem and cerebellar atrophy were analyzed with respect to disease duration in two studies (BURK et al. 1996; GIUFFRIDA et al. 1999) and no correlation was found in either SCA1 or SCA2. In a recent study using voxel based morphometry, BRENNEIS et al. (2003) found a correlation between atrophy of the cerebellar hemispheres and severity of cerebellar symptoms in nine patients with SCA2.

26.3.2
Non-conventional MR

26.3.2.1
^{1}H-MRS

MRS studies in patients with degenerative ataxias included relatively small numbers of patients (DAVIE et al. 1995; MASCALCHI et al. 1998, 2002; BOESCH et al. 2001). They consistently reported

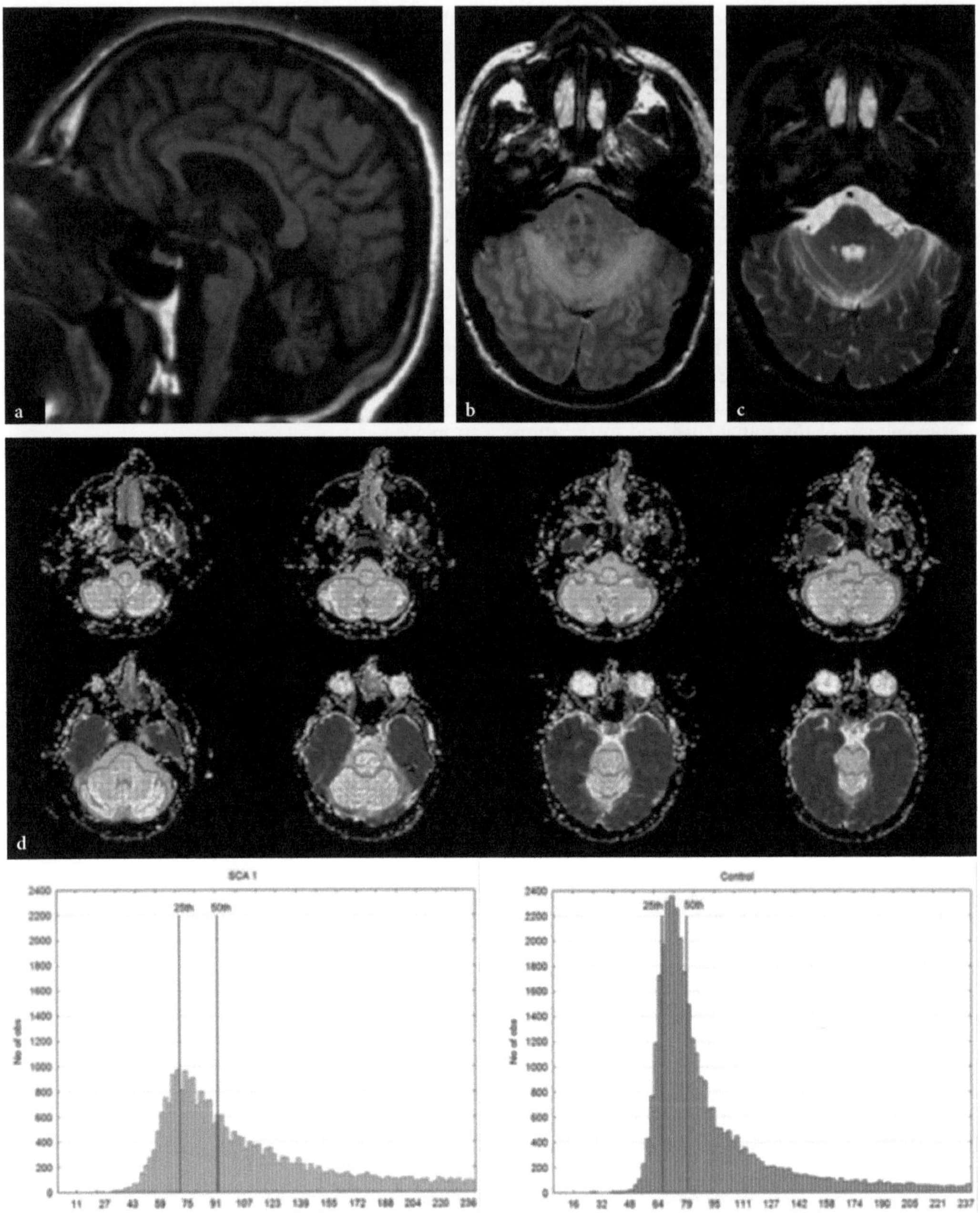

Fig. 26.3a–f. Olivopontocerebellar atrophy. Sagittal T1 weighted image (**a**) shows characteristic thinning of the ventral pons and widening of the IV ventricle in a patient with sporadic OPCA. Axial proton density (**b**) image in another patient with sporadic OPCA shows diffuse mild hyperintensity of the brainstem and cerebellar white matter sparing the corticospinal tracts ("*cross sign*"). The signal changes are far less evident on the corresponding T2 weighted image (**c**). Maps of mean diffusivity obtained in a patient with familial OPCA due to SCA2 (**d**) in which the posterior cranial fossa spaces (*shaded areas*) are manually segmented. Histograms of the posterior cranial fossa mean diffusivity derived from (**d**) after application of a threshold value to eliminate the CSF in the same patient (**e**) and in a healthy control (**f**). The histograms represent the mean diffusivity of the brainstem and cerebellum and demonstrate a modification of the shape of the histogram and an increase (rightward shift) of the 25th (69 vs 65 $10^{-5}mm^2/s$) and 50th (92 vs 78 $10^{-5} mm^2/s$) percentile values in the patient as compared to the control

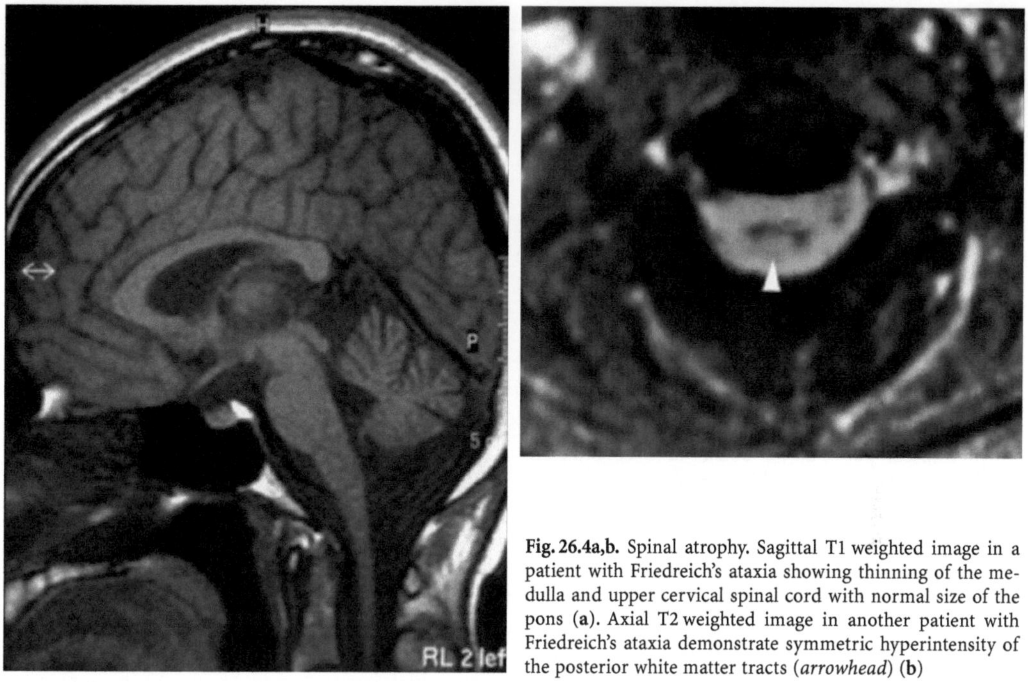

a b

Fig. 26.4a,b. Spinal atrophy. Sagittal T1 weighted image in a patient with Friedreich's ataxia showing thinning of the medulla and upper cervical spinal cord with normal size of the pons (**a**). Axial T2 weighted image in another patient with Friedreich's ataxia demonstrate symmetric hyperintensity of the posterior white matter tracts (*arrowhead*) (**b**)

a decrease of the concentration of NAA or of the NAA/Cr ratio in the deep cerebellum and pons of patients with sporadic or inherited OPCA, SA, and CCA. A reduction of Cho/Cr ratio in the same sites was observed in OPCA patients only (Mascalchi et al. 1998, 2002). Lactate peaks were occasionally observed in OPCA patients (Boesch et al. 2001; Mascalchi et al. 2002). In OPCA a correlation with the severity of the clinical deficit was observed for the reduction of the NAA/Cr ratio in the pons but not for the atrophy measurements (Mascalchi et al. 2002).

26.3.2.2 MTI

To date, no study with MT has focused on patients with degenerative ataxia.

26.3.2.3 Diffusion MR

$\overline{D}$ maps of the brainstem and cerebellum were obtained in a series of patients with degenerative ataxias with the aims of evaluating whether the diffusion changes match the distribution of neuropathological findings and correlate with the degree of neurological deficit (Della Nave et al. 2004).

The patients were representative of the different types of degenerative ataxias and were classified based on the MRI morphometry data in OPCA, SA, and CCA. The inclusion of patients with genetically proven spinocerebellar ataxia type 1 and 2 (SCA1 and SCA2) but without overt brainstem and cerebellar atrophy gave the opportunity to evaluate the pathological process leading to OPCA in a relatively early phase. Region-of-interest analysis showed a significant increase of $\overline{D}$ in the middle cerebellar peduncles, medulla, pons, and peridentate white matter of our patients with OPCA due to SCA1 and SCA2. Interestingly, similar findings were observed in patients with SCA1 and SCA2 without overt atrophy changes. Histogram analysis confirmed differences between SCA1 or SCA2 patients (OPCA or undefined) and controls for the 25th and 50th percentiles of the brainstem and cerebellum $\overline{D}$ (Fig. 26.3). However, only in SCA1 and SCA2 patients with OPCA, the brainstem and cerebellar $\overline{D}$ were combined with increase of the cerebral $\overline{D}$. This result is consistent with the development of supratentorial changes in the advanced phases of OPCA (Klockgether et al. 1998; Giuffrida et al. 1999). Although the exact pathological correlate of increase of the $\overline{D}$ in the brainstem and the cerebellum cannot be established, it presumably reflects the wallerian degeneration of the white matter observed in OPCA. More speculative is the significance of the mild changes in the supratentorial compartment. The region-of-interest analysis of $\overline{D}$ in our SA patients matched the above changes showing a significant increase in the medulla only. In agreement with the substantial paucity of the brainstem and cerebellar changes in SA, the histogram and volume analysis failed to show significant changes in the infratentorial compartment. The diffuse mild increase of the brainstem and cerebellar $\overline{D}$, possibly reflecting a microscopic damage of the cerebellar brainstem tracts and the normal cerebral $\overline{D}$, are consistent with the neuropathological description of CCA.

In the relatively large group of patients with olivopontocerebellar degeneration due to SCA1 and SCA2, i.e., including patients with OPCA and undefined morphological pattern, we observed a correlation between the median value of the brainstem and cerebellum $\overline{D}$ histogram and with an index of brainstem and cerebellar atrophy.

26.4 Motor Neuron Disease

This is a neurodegenerative condition characterized by dysfunction and loss of upper and lower motor neurons that are variably combined producing a spectrum of clinical syndromes from primary lateral sclerosis (PLS), in which a selective damage of the upper motor neuron occurs, to progressive spinal muscular atrophy, in which the damage is restricted to the spinal cord motor neurons (Chan et al. 1999). More frequently, the clinical signs of upper and lower motor neurons are observed altogether in the patient at a certain point in the disease course and this condition is termed amyotrophic lateral sclerosis (ALS).

Upper motor neuron damage implies a wallerian degeneration of the corticospinal tracts which can be tracked from the precentral gyrus to the lateral and anterior columns of the spinal cord (Lowe et al. 1997).

26.4.1 Conventional MR

Proton density and T2 weighted images show abnormally increased signal of the corticospinal tracts in the brains of patients with ALS and PLS (Goodin et al. 1988; Marti-Fabregas et al. 1990). The signal changes in the spinal cord are better demonstrated using axial T2* weighted gradient echo images in the cervical spine (Mascalchi et al. 1995).

The advent in the clinical protocols of turbo spin-echo (TSE) sequences and in particular the FLAIR TSE in which the normal parieto-pontine tract appears relatively hyperintense to the surrounding white matter, especially at the level of the internal capsule and cerebral peduncles, required redefinition of the diagnostic value of this feature. Hecht et al. (2001) reported that the hyperintensity of the corticospinal tracts in FLAIR images is distinctly abnormal when observed in the subcortical precentral gyrus, the centrum semiovale, the crus cerebri, the pons, and medulla oblongata (Fig. 26.5). Moreover, quantitative studies demonstrated that even in the internal capsule the pyramidal tract signal in FLAIR images is higher in patients with ALS and PLS as compared to healthy controls. Zhang et al. (2003) reported a sensitivity of 56% and specificity of 94% of hyperintensity of the subcortical white matter on FLAIR images for the diagnosis of ALS. The same study reported a 74% sensitivity and 67% specificity for evidence of a dark line along the posterior rim of the precentral gyrus which is assumed to reflect a T2 shortening effect due to excessive iron deposition, fibrillary gliosis, and macrophage infiltration. Follow-up examinations demonstrated that both corticospinal tract hyperintensity and the cortical rim hypointensity were unchanged (Hecht et al. 2001; Zhang et al. 2003).

26.4.2 Non-conventional MR

26.4.2.1 ^{1}H-MRS

^{1}H-MRS studies in patients with motor neuron disease predominantly employed single voxels located in the motor cortex and subcortical white matter (Kalra et al. 1998; Chan et al. 1999; Bowen et al. 2000; Sarchielli et al. 2001). Using a semiquantitative approach and a long TE acquisition, Chan et al. (1999) found that the NAA/Cr ratio in the precentral region enabled separation of patients with ALS and PLS from healthy controls and that the spectroscopic were more sensitive than the conventional MR imaging findings (Fig. 26.5). A correlation between the decrease of the NAA concentration in the precentral region and the severity of the neurological deficit was reported in two studies (Bowen et al. 2000; Sarchielli et al. 2001). Similar ^{1}H-MRS findings were observed when the

a

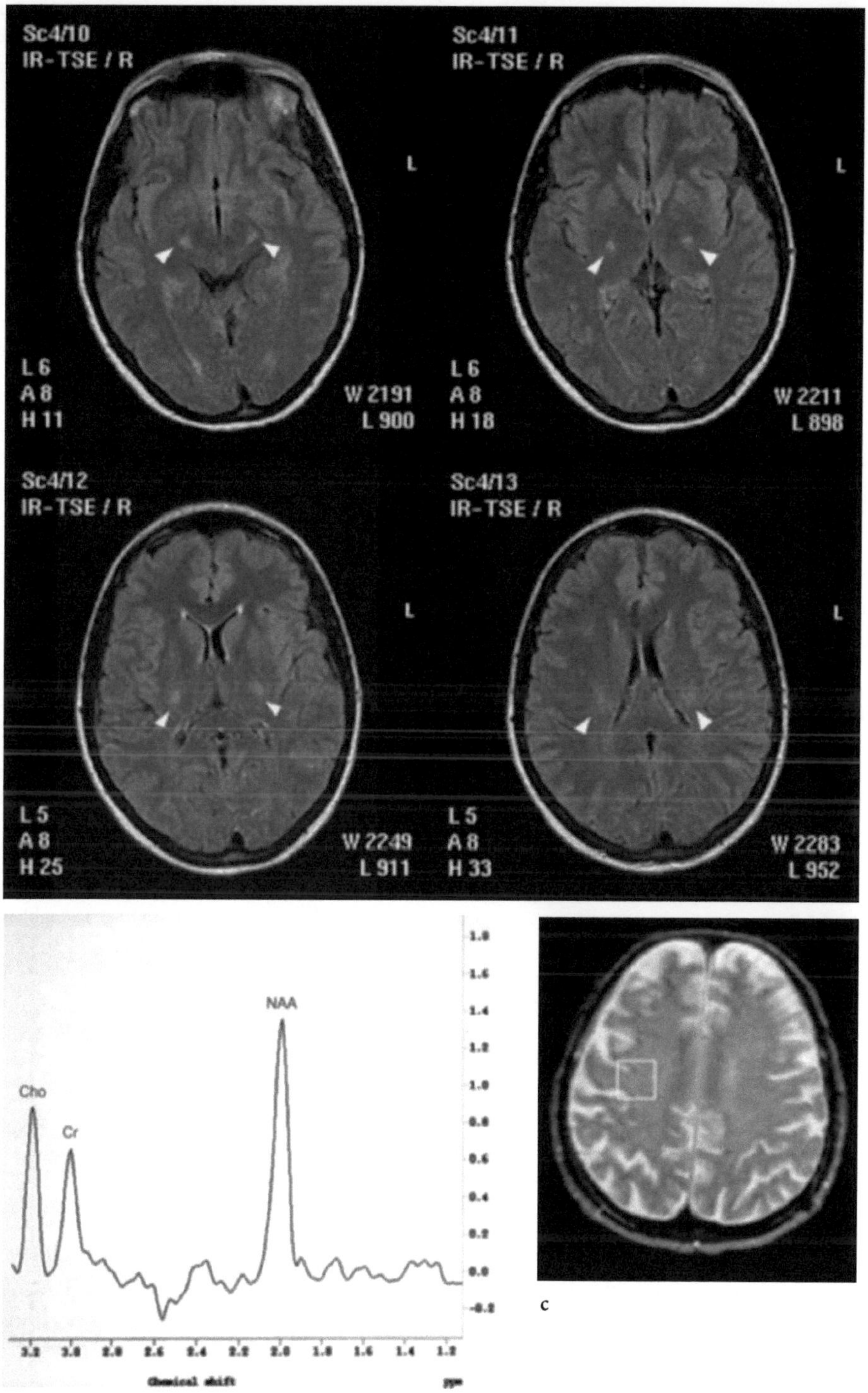

b

c

Fig. 26.5a–c. Axial T2 weighted FLAIR images (**a**) in a patient with ALS show symmetric areas of hyperintensity of the corticospinal tracts (*arrowheads*) which can be tracked from the subcortical white matter (*bottom right*) to the cerebral peduncles (*top left*). Single voxel proton MR spectroscopy of the motor cortex and subcortical white matter in a patient with ALS (**b**) and a healthy control (**c**) showing a decrease of the NAA peak in (**b**) volume of interest was placed in the brainstem pontomedullary region and medulla (Cwik et al. 1998; Pioro et al. 1999). With employment of short TE techniques some additional features of the ^{1}H-MRS changes of upper motor neuron dysfunction were recognized. Thus, an increase of Gln+Glu/Cr ratio was observed in the medulla, suggesting a role for Glu excitotoxicity in the ALS pathogenesis (Pioro et al. 1999), and increase of the concentration of the Cho and myo-inositol was reported in the precentral region (Bowen et al. 2000). In a longitudinal MRS imaging study a progressive decrease of the NAA, Cr and Cho concentrations were observed in the motor region, but not in non-motor regions (Suhy et al. 2002).

Kalra et al. (1998, 2003) evaluated with a volume of interest placed in the precentral region the response of treatment with new drugs in patients with upper motor neuron disease and documented a positive response to riluzole whereas gabapentin had no effect on the decline of the NAA/Cr ratio.

26.4.2.2 MTI

Kato et al. (1997) reported a significant decrease of the MT ratio in the posterior limb of the internal capsule of patients with upper motor neuron dysfunction. The MT change was present also in patients without signal changes on conventional MR imaging.

26.4.2.3 Diffusion MR

The strong diffusion anisotropy of the normal corticospinal fibers and the occurrence of anterograde degeneration in cases of MND and PLS justified investigation of the potential of diffusion MR imaging for the diagnosis of motor neuron disease. In a diffusion tensor MR imaging study including patients with clinically definite, probable and possible ALS, Ellis et al. (1999) observed a significant increase in the mean diffusivity and decrease of the fractional anisotropy along the corticospinal tracts. The mean diffusivity correlated with the disease duration, whereas the fractional anisotropy correlated with measures of disease severity. In a recent diffusion tensor MR imaging study Ulug et al. (2004) observed an increase of the mean diffusivity of the internal capsules in patients with primary lateral sclerosis which was highly correlated with a decrease of fractional anisotropy. Finally, fractional anisotropy was decreased in the corticospinal tract in patients with ALS before clinical onset of signs of upper motor neuron deficit (Sach et al. 2004), thus contributing to earlier diagnosis of MND.

26.5 Conclusions

Conventional MR imaging can show macroscopic white matter signal changes in degenerative diseases of the CNS which are a useful diagnostic tool for FTD, OPCA, SA, and PLS/ALS.

Non-conventional MR, including DTI, MT and ^{1}H-MRS, demonstrates abnormalities of the white matter in almost every degenerative disease of the CNS. These white matter changes are variably correlated to the severity of the clinical deficit and are currently evaluated as markers of disease progression and possible surrogate markers in pharmacological trials.

References

Adachi M, Hosoya T, Yamaguchi K et al (2000) Diffusion- and T2 weighted MRI of the transverse pontine fibers in spinocerebellar degeneration. Neuroradiology 42:803-809

Adams RD, Victor M (1985) Degenerative diseases of the nervous system. In: Adams RD, Victor M (eds) Principles of neurology, 3rd edn. McGraw Hill, New York, pp 859-901

Ashburner J, Friston KJ (2000) Voxel-based morphometry - the methods. Neuroimage 11:805-821

Baron JC, Chetelat G, Desgranges B et al (2001) In vivo mapping of gray matter loss with voxel-based morphometry in mild Alzheimer's disease. Neuroimage 14:298-309

Boesch SM, Schoecke M, Burk K et al (2001) Proton magnetic resonance spectroscopic imaging reveals differences in spinocerebellar ataxia types 2 and 6. J Magn Reson Imaging 13:553-559

Bozzali M, Franceschi M, Falini A et al (2001) Quantification of tissue damage in AD using diffusion tensor and magnetization transfer MRI. Neurology 57:1135-1137

Bozzali M, Falini A, Franceschi M et al (2002) White matter damage in Alzheimer's disease assessed in vivo using diffusion tensor magnetic resonance imaging. J Neurol Neurosurg Psychiatry 72:742-746

Bozzao A, Floris R, Baviera ME et al (2001) Diffusion and perfusion MR imaging in cases of Alzheimer's disease: correlations with cortical atrophy and lesion load. AJNR Am J Neuroradiol 22:1030-1036

Bowen BC, Pattany PM, Bradley WG et al (2000) MR imaging and localized proton spectroscopy of the precentral gyrus in amyotrophic lateral sclerosis. AJNR Am J Neuroradiol 21:647-658

Brenneis C, Bosch SM, Schocke M et al (2003) Atrophy pattern in SCA2 determined by voxel-based morphometry. Neuroreport 14:1799-1802

Brun A, Englund E (1986) A white matter disorder in dementia of the Alzheimer's type. Ann Neurol 19:253-262

Burk K, Abele M, Fetter M et al (1996) Autosomal dominant cerebellar ataxia type I. Clinical features and MRI in families with SCA1, SCA2 and SCA3. Brain 119:1497-1505

Catani M, Mecocci P, Tarducci R et al (2000) Proton magnetic resonance spectroscopy reveals similar white matter biochemical changes in patients with chronic hypertension and early Alzheimer's disease. J Am Geriatr Soc 50:1707-1710

Cercignani M, Iannucci G, Rocca MA et al (2000) Pathologic damage in MS assessed by diffusion-weighted and magnetization transfer MRI. Neurology 54:1139-1144

Cercignani M, Bammer R, Soriani MP et al (2003) Inter-sequence and inter-imaging unit variability of diffusion-tensor MR imaging histogram-derived metrics of the brain in healthy volunteers. AJNR Am J Neuroradiol 24:638-643

Chan S, Shungu DC, Douglas-Akinwande A et al (1999) Motor neuron diseases: comparison of single-voxel proton MR spectroscopy of the motor cortex with MR imaging of the brain. Radiology 212:763-769

Chan D, Fox NC, Jenkins R et al (2001) Rates of global and regional cerebral atrophy in AD and frontotemporal dementia. Neurology 57:1756-1763

Chantal S, Labelle M, Bouchard RW et al (2002) Correlation of regional proton magnetic resonance spectroscopic metabolic changes with cognitive deficits in mild Alzheimer's disease. Arch Neurol 59:955-962

Chun T, Filippi CG, Zimmerman RD et al (2000) Diffusion changes in the aging human brain; AJNR Am J Neuroradiol 21:1078-1083

Cwik VA, Hanstock CC, Allen PS et al (1998) Estimation of brainstem neuronal loss in amyotrophic lateral sclerosis with in vivo proton magnetic resonance spectroscopy. Neurology 50:72-77

Davie CA, Barker GJ, Webb S et al (1995) Persistent functional deficit in multiple sclerosis and autosomal dominant cerebellar ataxia is associated with axonal loss. Brain 118:1583-1592

De Leeuw FE, Barkhof F, Scheltens P (2004) White matter lesions and hippocampal atrophy in Alzheimer's disease. Neurology 62:310-312

Della Nave R, Foresti S, Tessa C et al (2004) ADC mapping of neurodegeneration in the brainstem and cerebellum of patients with progressive ataxias. NeuroImage (in press)

Dixon RM, Bradley KM, Budge MM et al (2002) Longitudinal quantitative proton magnetic resonance spectroscopy of the hippocampus in Alzheimer's disease. Brain 125:2332-2341

Dong Q, Welsh RC, Chevenert TL et al (2004) Clinical applications of diffusion tensor imaging. J Magn Reson Imaging 19:6-18

Ellis CM, Simmons A, Jones DK et al (1999) Diffusion tensor MRI assesses corticospinal tract damage in ALS. Neurology 53:1051-1058

Ernst T, Chang L, Melchor R (1997) Frontotemporal dementia and early Alzhiemer's disease: differentiation with frontal lobe H1 MR spectroscopy. Radiology 203:829-836

Fazekas F, Chawluk JB, Alavi A et al (1987) MR signal abnormalities at 1.5 T in Alzheimer's dementia and normal aging. AJNR Am J Neuroradiol 8:421-426

Frisoni GB, Testa C, Zorzan A et al (2002) Detection of grey matter loss in mild Alzheimer's disease with voxel based morphometry. J Neurol Neurosurg Psychiatry 73:657-664

Giuffrida S, Saponara R, Restivo DA et al (1999) Supratentorial atrophy in spinocerebellar ataxia type 2: MRI study of patients. J Neurol 246:383-388

Goodin DS, Rowley HA, Olney RK (1988) Magnetic resonance imaging in amyotrophic lateral sclerosis. Ann Neurol 23:418-420

Hanyu H, Sakurai H, Iwamoto T et al (1998) Diffusion-weighted MR imaging of the hippocampus and temporal lobe white matter in Alzheimer's disease. J Neurol Sci 156:195-200

Hanyu H, Asano T, Sakurai H et al (1999) Diffusion-weighted and magnetization transfer imaging of the corpus callosum in Alzheimer's disease. J Neurol Sci 167:37-44

Hecht MJ, Fellner F, Fellner C et al (2001) MRI-FLAIR images of the head show corticospinal tract alterations in ALS patients more frequently than T2, T1- and proton density-weighted images. J Neurol Sci 186:37-44

Hecht MJ, Fellner F, Fellner C et al (2002) Hyperintense and hypointense MRI signals of the precentral gyrus and corticospinal tract in ALS: a follow-up examination including FLAIR images. J Neurol Sci 199:59-65

Jack CR, Dickson DW, Parisi JE et al (2002) Antemortem MRI findings correlate with hippocampal neuropathology in typical aging and dementia. Neurology 58:750-757

Jessen F, Block W, Traber F et al (2001) Decrease of N-acetylaspartate in the MTL correlates with cognitive decline of AD patients. Neurology 57:930-932

Kalra S, Cashman NR, Genge A et al (1998) Recovery of N-acetylasparetate in corticomotor neurons of patients with ALS after riluzole therapy. Neuroreport 9:1757-1761

Kalra S, Cashman NR, Caramanos et al (2003) Gabapentin therapy for amyotrophic lateral sclerosis: lack of improvement in neuronal integrity shown by MR spectroscopy. AJNR Am J Neuroradiol 24:476-480

Kantarci K, Reynolds G, Petersen RC et al (2003) Proton MR spectroscopy in mild cognitive impairment and Alzheimer's disease: comparison of 1.5 and 3 T. AJNR Am J Neuroradiol 24:843-849

Karas GB, Burton EJ, Rombouts SARB et al (2003) A comprehensive study of gray matter loss in patients with Alzheimer's disease using optimized voxel-based morphometry. Neuroimage 18:895-907

Kato Y, Matsumura K, Kinosada Y et al (1997) Detection of pyramidal tract lesions in amyotrophic lateral sclerosis with magnetization-transfer measurements. AJNR Am J Neuroradiol 18:1541-1547

Klockgether T, Skalej M, Wedekind D et al (1998) Autosomal dominant cerebellar ataxia type I. MRI-based volumetry of posterior fossa structures and basal ganglia in spinocerebellar ataxia types 1, 2 and 3. Brain 121:1678-1693

Kril JJ, Patel S, Harding AJ et al (2002) Patients with vascular dementia due to microvascular pathology have significant hippocampal neuronal loss. J Neurol Neurosurg Psychiatry 72:747-751

Krishnan KRR, Charles HC, Doraiswamy PM et al (2003) Randomized, placebo-controlled trial of the effects of Donezepil on neuronal markers and hippocampal volumes in Alzheimer's disease. Am J Psychiatry 160:2003-2011

Lowe J (1998) Establishing a pathological diagnosis in degenerative dementias. Brain Pathol 8:403-406

Lowe J, Lennox G, Leigh PN (1997) Disorders of movement

and system degeneration. In: Graham DL, Lantos PL (eds) Greenfield's neuropathology, 6th edn, vol 2. Arnold, London, pp 281-366

Marti-Fabregas J, Pujol J (1990) Selective involvement of the pyramidal tract on magnetic resonance imaging in primary lateral sclerosis. Neurology 40:1799-1800

Mascalchi M, Salvi F, Piacentini S et al (1994) Friedreich 's ataxia: MR findings involving the cervical portion of the spinal cord. AJR 163: 187-191

Mascalchi M, Salvi F, Valzania F et al (1995) Cortico-spinal tract degeneration in motor neuron disease: report of two cases. AJNR Am J Neuroradiol 16:878-880

Mascalchi M, Tosetti M, Plasmati R et al (1998) Proton magnetic resonance spectroscopy in an Italian family with spinocerebellar ataxia type 1. Ann Neurol 43:244-252

Mascalchi M Cosottini M, Lolli F et al (2002) MR spectroscopy of the cerebellum and pons in patients with degenerative ataxia. Radiology 223:371-378

McGowan FC, Filippi M, Campi A (1998) Magnetization transfer imaging: theory and application to multiple sclerosis. J Neurol Neurosurg Psychiatry 64 [Suppl]:23-32

Pioro EP, Majors AW, Mitsumoto H et al (1999) 1H-MRS evidence of neurodegeneration and excess glutamate+glutamine in ALS medulla. Neurology 53:71-79

Ormerod IEC, Harding AE, Miller DH et al (1994) Magnetic resonance imaging in ataxic disorders. J Neurol Neurosurg Psychiatry 57:51-57

O'Sullivan M, Jones DK, Summers PE et al (2001) Evidence for cortical "disconnection" as a mechanism of age-related cognitive decline. Neurology 57:632-638

Rapaport SI (2002) Hydrogen magnetic resonance spectroscopy in Alzheimer's disease. Lancet Neurol 1:82

Rose SE, Chen F, Chalk JB et al (2000) Loss of connectivity in Alzheimer's disease: an evaluation of white matter tract integrity with colour coded MR diffusion tensor imaging. J Neurol Neurosurg Psychiatry 69:528-530

Rusinek H, de Santi S, Frid D et al (2003) Regional brain atrophy rate predicts future cognitive decline: 6-year longitudinal MR imaging study of normal aging. Radiology 229:691-696

Sach M, Winkler G, Glauche V et al (2004) Diffusion tensor MRI of early upper motor neuron involvement in amyotrophic lateral sclerosis. Brain 127:340-350

Sarchielli P, Pelliccioli GP, Tarducci R et al (2001) Magnetic resonance imaging and 1H magnetic resonance spectroscopy in amyotrophic lateral sclerosis. Neuroradiology 43:189-197

Savoiardo M, Grisoli M (2001) Imaging dementias. Eur Radiol 11:484-492

Savoiardo M, Strada L, Girotti F et al (1990) Olivopontocerebellar atrophy: MR diagnosis and relationship to multisystem atrophy. Radiology 174:693-696

Schaefer PW, Grant PE, Gonzalez RG (2000) Diffusion-weighted MR imaging of the brain. Radiology 217:331-345

Scheltens P, Barkof F, Algra J et al (1990) White matter hypeintensities on magnetic resonance in Alzheimer's disease and normal aging. Neurobiol Aging 11:263-264

Schuff N, Capizzano AA, Du AT et al (2002) Selective reduction of N-acetylaspartate in medial temporal and parietal lobes in AD. Neurology 58:928-935

Shonk TK, Moats RA, Gifford P et al (1995) Probable Alzheimer's disease: diagnosis with proton MR spectroscopy. Radiology 195:65-72

Sjobeck M, Haglund M, Persson A et al (2003) Brain tissue microarrays in dementia research: white matter microvascular pathology in Alzheimer's disease. Histopathology 23:290-295

Subramony SH, Filla A (2001) Autosomal dominant spinocerebellar ataxia ad infinitum? Neurology 56:287-289

Suhy J, Miller RG, Rule R et al (2002) Early detection and longitudinal changes in amyotrophic lateral sclerosis by 1H MRSI. Neurology 58:773-779

The Lund and Manchester Groups (1994) Clinical and neuropathological criteria for frontotemporal dementia. J Neurol Neurosurg Psychiatry 57:416-418

Ulug AM, Grunewald T, Lin MT et al (2004) Diffusion tensor imaging in the diagnosis of primary lateral sclerosis. J Magn Reson Imaging 19:34-39

Van Buchem MA (1999) Magnetization transfer: applications in neuroradiology. J Comput Assist Tomogr 23 [Suppl 1]: S9-S18

Van der Flier WM, van den Heuvel DMJ, Weverling-Rijnsburger AWE et al (2002) Cognitive decline in AD and mild cognitive impairment is associated with global brain damage. Neurology 59:874-879

Waldman AD, Rai GS (2003) The relationship between cognitive impairment and in vivo metabolite ratios in patients with clinical Alzheimer's disease and vascular dementia: a proton magnetic resonance spectroscopy study. Neuroradiology 45:507-512

Wullner U, Klockgether T, Petersen D (1993) Magnetic resonance imaging in hereditary and idiopathic ataxia. Neurology 43:318-326

Zhang L, Ulug AM, Zimmerman RD et al (2003) The diagnostic utility of FLAIR imaging in clinically verified amyotrophic lateral sclerosis. J Magn Reson Imaging 17:521-527

White Matter Changes Secondary to Other Conditions

27 Viral and Non-Viral Infections in Immunocompetent and Immunocompromised Patients

Vincent Dousset

CONTENTS

V. Dousset
Professor of Radiology, Université Victor Segalen Bordeaux 2, CHU de Bordeaux -Hôpital Pellegrin, Place Amélie-Raba Léon, 33076 Bordeaux, France

27.1 Introduction

Infectious diseases affecting humans have greatly decreased in the past decades thanks to the antibiotics and the level of hygiene in current life. However, the CNS must be seen as a potential target from many external organisms that have the ability to produce severe diseases with striking symptoms.

Imaging technology, CT and especially MRI, have led to an enhanced ability to characterize infectious processes. MRI techniques such as fast imaging T2-weighted images and fluid-attenuated inversion-recovery (FLAIR) make it possible to depict lesions in the brain, spinal cord, and the meninges. More recently, techniques such as diffusion weighted imaging (DWI) and magnetic resonance spectroscopy, have been applied to inflammatory and infectious lesions, bringing new capabilities for in vivo characterization (Zimmerman 2000; Lai et al. 2002; Cecil and Lenkinski 1998; Burtscher and Holtas 1999). They have an impact on making the positive diagnosis and for the understanding of the disease process.

The appearance of inflammatory lesions is the mirror of multiple factors, including the type of infectious organism, mode of spread, target and host response.

Infections can spread to the CNS in three ways:

- Hematogenously, either through the choroid plexus or through the blood–brain barrier (BBB). It is now the most frequent origin of infection in the CNS
- Direct spread from adjacent structures, such as the sinuses, nasopharynx, or mastoid air cells
- Retrograde axoplasmic flow along cranial or peripheral nerves by some viral agents such as herpes

The imaging features of CNS infections can be classified by the organisms, the location of the lesion and the host response.

- The organisms include viruses, mycotic agents, parasites, bacteria and prions (Gray et al. 2004)
- The location of the lesions might be one or several of the following: CSF, meninges, parenchyma, arteries, veins, cranial cavities (sinuses, mastoid). It is of importance in an imaging study to look at all these locations
- The host response:
  1. Immunocompetent patients (child and adults): the response is immunologic and most often symptoms and in vivo images are related to the host response rather than to the infectious agent itself. This means that common imaging features are present for several organisms, making the specific diagnosis somewhat difficult. There is now more evidence for a strong role in the individual genetic background for the development of an organism in the CNS. Not only prions develop in susceptible individuals, but many more organisms are probably infective for some individuals and not others. A transient decrease in the level of immunity may also be responsible for disease development
  2. Immunocompromised patients: this group includes several causes such as HIV infection – which, without treatment leads to deep immunodeficiency – anticancer chemotherapy, diabetes mellitus, long-term steroid administration and, more rarely, congenital immunodeficiency. In these patients, opportunistic agents develop, meaning that these germs might be present in non-immunocompromised people without the ability to develop (Post et al. 1986). HIV has infected more than 60 million people in the world, with 26 million in Africa. In the CNS of HIV-positive patients, some numerous and very specific agents may develop: the HIV virus itself, *Toxoplasma gondii*, JC virus, tuberculosis, cytomegalovirus (CMV), and *Cryptococcus* are the most frequent (Gray et al. 2004). CNS type-B lymphoma can also develop. In immunocompromised non-HIV patients, agents such as *Candida albicans*, mucormycosis or *Nocardia* may become pathogenic for the CNS
  3. Newborns: during birth and for a few weeks after, babies might be affected by infectious agents that are present in the mother's birth canal: herpes type 2, *Listeria monocytogenes*, and urinary germs such as *E. coli*, *Proteus*, or *Candida albicans*
  4. Embryo and fetus: several agents may develop that can lead to death of the embryo or to fetus CNS malformations. The most frequent agents are *Toxoplasma gondii*, and CMV, rubella, herpes or HIV viruses (Osborn and Byrd 1991)
  5. Finally, the immunologic system may be the origin of CNS manifestations, due to systemic infections of which agents promote a cross-reaction with some constitutive proteins of the CNS cells. The organism is usually absent from the CNS. The most sensitive targets are the myelin proteins, leading to acute disseminated encephalomyelitis (ADEM). This includes cross-reaction to viruses or bacteria following systemic infection or vaccination. Vasculitis may also be of immunologic origin in response to a systemic organism, leading to cerebral infarct. It is also possible to include in this group some granulomatous diseases, which produce normal immunologic-cell abnormal collection in the CNS, mostly in the meninges, facial cavities or cavernous sinus, e.g., inflammatory pseudotumor and sarcoidosis

We now will describe the infections by the type of organisms affecting the CNS: viruses and prions, bacteria, parasites, fungi, and granulomatous or immunologic reaction. The immunologic state of the host and the location will be discussed in each chapter.

27.2 Viral Infections

The two main features are meningitis and encephalitis. Neurological symptoms will depend on the location of the organism.

Meningitis due to viruses, a frequent infectious disease of immunocompetent hosts, has few imaging manifestations. The role of CT or MRI is questionable – waiting for imaging modalities may unnecessarily delay the time for lumbar puncture and treatment. Enhancement of meninges is rare.

Viral encephalitis is usually associated with seizure or reduced consciousness or focal symptoms such as motor or sensory deficits. Mild mass effect may be seen during the acute phase of encephalitis. Enhancement is often absent early on during the course of acute encephalitis, with sometimes an enhancement of the adjacent leptomeninges.

27.2.1 Viruses in Immunocompetent Patients

Some viruses may affect both immunocompetent and immunocompromised patients, children, adults or neonates. They belong to the groups of herpes viruses, enteroviruses and arboviruses.

27.2.1.1 Herpes Viruses

Herpes viruses are DNA viruses, and many can cause CNS infections in humans, including herpes simplex viruses 1 and 2, varicella-zoster virus, the Epstein-Barr virus, and cytomegalovirus (CMV) (Tien et al. 1993; Bonthius and Karacay 2002).

- **Herpes simplex virus 1** is the most common cause of sporadic viral meningoencephalitis. Clinical manifestations include fever, headache, neck stiffness, seizures, focal deficits, and depressed mental state. Because acyclovir therapy is safe, it is recommended that the drug be given on the basis of clinical findings. Encephalitis results from reactivation of latent viral infection of the gasserian (fifth cranial nerve) ganglion. From here, the infection spreads to the parenchyma. The virus has a predilection for the medial area of the temporal lobes, the frontal lobes and the insular lobes (Fig. 27.1). On CT, low densities are seen on affected areas. There is no enhancement, only the adjacent meninges may show some congestive changes, with very little contrast-agent uptake. On MRI, hyperintensities are encountered in the temporal, frontal or insular areas, and the bilateral nature of the process is frequent. Initially, the infection may appear unilateral on imaging studies, but over time, involvement of the contralateral temporal and frontal lobes will become apparent
- **Herpes simplex virus 2** is the most common cause of neonatal encephalitis. Infection occurs when the fetus passes through the birth canal of a mother who has genital herpes. Imaging findings reflect rapid brain destruction. Rare observations have been made on adults with extension to the spinal cord

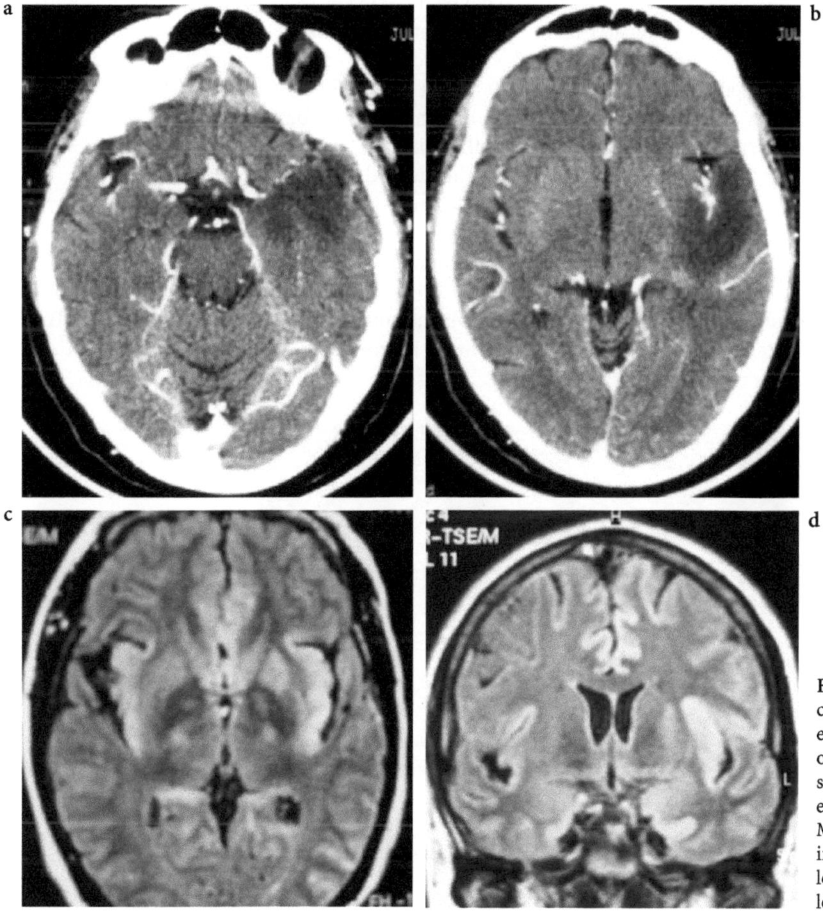

Fig. 27.1a–d Herpes encephalitis. **a, b** Contrast-enhanced CT. Low density of the temporal and insular lobes without focal enhancement. **c, d** Flair MR imaging. High signal intensities in both insular lobes and in both temporal lobes

- ***Varicella-zoster virus*** produces two distinct clinical syndromes, chicken pox and herpes zoster. Diffuse encephalitis is a rare complication of chicken pox, but it is more common in adults. It is usually mild. Herpes zoster may lead to an involvement of peripheral and cranial nerves. The affected cranial nerve will appear edematous and swollen, and it will enhance at MR imaging with gadolinium. Herpes zoster may also produce small vessel vasculitis, leading to cerebral infarcts
- ***CMV*** in adults is seen almost exclusively in immunocompromised patients. However, CMV is the most common cause of congenital encephalitis. It produces massive brain destruction during the first trimester. Infections acquired in the second trimester produce cortical dysplasia
- ***Epstein-Barr virus*** has been linked to diverse entities, such as Guillain-Barré syndrome, and lymphoma in patients with AIDS. About 5% of the patients with infectious mononucleosis develop an acute, usually self-limited encephalomyelitis. This disorder may be responsible for hyperintensities on T2-weighted images in the deep supratentorial gray matter and central gray matter of the spinal cord. Rapid resolution of the lesions has been reported in this disease
- ***Human herpes virus-6*** has been identified as a cause of encephalitis and febrile seizure (Bonthius and Karacay 2002)

27.2.1.2 Enterovirus

Enterovirus may be responsible for meningitis and, rarely, for encephalitis (Zimmerman 2000). In the latter, the spinal cord, medulla, pons, mesencephalon, the dentate nucleus of the cerebellum, and occasionally the thalamus may be affected. These structures appear hyperintense on T2-weighted images (Fig. 27.2).

The location in the rhombencephalon and mesencephalon is also the predilection of the bacteria *Listeria monocytogenes*.

27.2.1.3 West Nile Virus

This virus has emerged in the United States as a new etiologic pathogen causing encephalitis (Bonthius and Karacay 2002).

27.2.2 Viruses in Immunocompromised Patients

The CNS of immunocompromised patients may be affected by the same viruses that affect immunocompetent patients. Additionally, other viruses only develop in immunocompromised patients (Post et al. 1986; dal Canto 1997). The HIV virus that causes the depletion in immunity may be responsible for encephalitis. Another virus, JC virus, can also cause multifocal encephalitis with destruction of oligodendrocytes.

27.2.2.1 HIV Encephalitis

HIV-1 is the human RNA retrovirus that causes AIDS. The brain is one of the most commonly affected or-

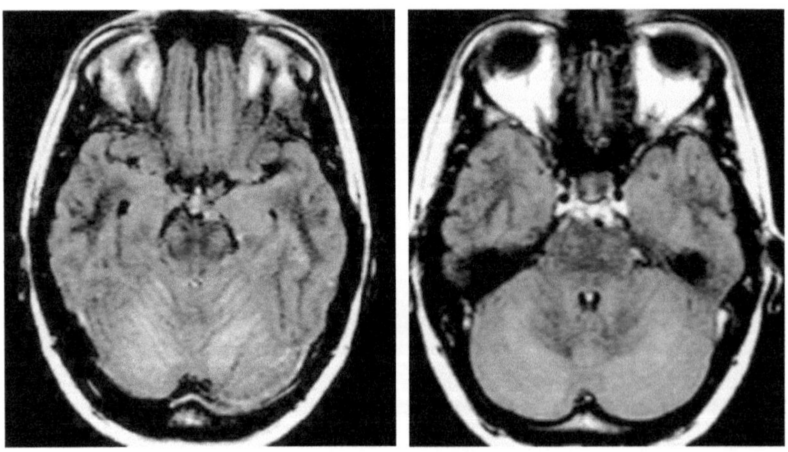

Fig. 27.2 Viral cerebellitis due to enterovirus. Flair MR imaging showing high signal intensities of the cerebellar cortex

gans. Almost all patients have the HIV virus in the CNS, and 10–15% may develop a decrease in mental status or dementia.

It has been described that the primary infection to HIV may lead to focal abnormal deep white matter spots recognized as hyperintensities on T2-weighted images (Trotot and Gray 1997). This is a nonspecific sign that should be taken cautiously, since it is very frequent in many other conditions such as aging, high blood pressure, tobacco, and diabetes mellitus. The brain parenchyma is one of the sites of residency of the HIV virus for several years. During the phase of latency, before the patient starts to have AIDS, it has been shown that some degree of atrophy may occur. When immunodepression is becoming stronger, the HIV virus itself causes subacute progressive encephalitis. The organism replicates within multinuclear giant cells and macrophages in the white matter (Dal Canto 1997). There is atrophy, water accumulation in the interstitium, slight demyelination, but no inflammatory changes.

The most common finding is generalized atrophy on CT or MR without focal abnormalities (Fig. 27.3a). Some degree of non-atrophic brain shrinkage is caused by systemic effects of the disease. In severe cases, diffuse symmetric hyperintensity is seen in the supratentorial white matter, predominantly in the periventricular region (Fig. 27.3b, c). Mass effect and enhancement are absent (Fig. 27.3d). On T1-weighted images, the white matter appears almost normal or slightly hypointense.

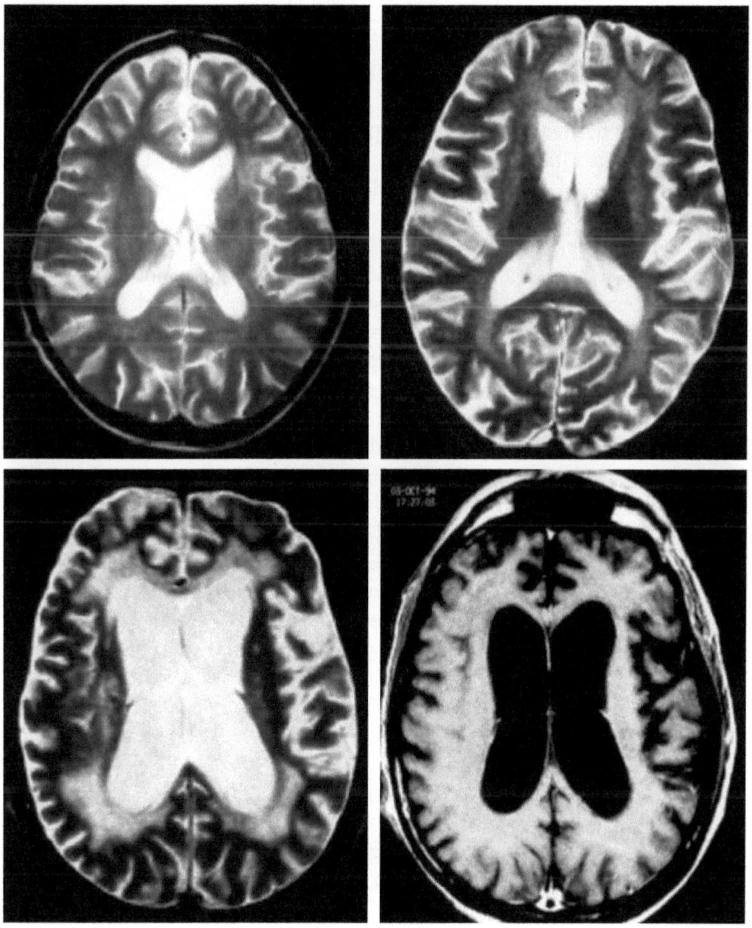

a b c d

Fig. 27.3a–d HIV encephalitis. **a** T2 MR imaging. Slight parenchymal atrophy and ventricular enlargement. **b** T2 MR imaging. Parenchymal atrophy, ventricular enlargement, bilateral and symmetrical deep white matter abnormal high signal intensities. **c** T2 MR imaging. Severe parenchymal atrophy, severe ventricular enlargement, bilateral and symmetrical deep white matter abnormal high signal intensities. **d** Gadolinium-enhanced MR imaging. Same patients as **c**. No gadolinium uptake. No noticeable changes on T1-weighted images

27.2.2.2
Progressive Multifocal Leukoencephalopathy

Progressive multifocal leukoencephalopathy (PML) is caused by a papovavirus—the JC virus. This virus is ubiquitous in the adult population. It is present in lymph nodes, and it has been suggested that it resides in the kidneys. When a deep immunodepression is present, usually with blood CD4 cells below 100/mm^3, the virus infects the myelin-producing oligodendrocytes, which results in severe demyelination with little inflammatory reaction. Patients complain of focal and progressive neurological impairment, with motor or visual function loss or cerebellar syndrome. Demyelination starts at the subcortical white matter, in the U-fibers (Fig. 27.4a–c). Areas of demyelination are seen as hyposignal on T1-weighted images, with a high signal on T2-weighted images and FLAIR images, without mass effect or enhancement (Fig. 27.4d–f) (Post et al. 1986; Dousset et al. 1997). There is always a strong correlation between the symptoms and the location of the abnormalities on MRI.

In the past, PML was inevitably fatal, with death occurring within 6–12 months of the onset. The administration of drugs developed to treat HIV, such as protease inhibitors, can cause, in some cases, a stabilization of the lesions produced by PML, probably by improving the function of the immune system. Additionally, the incidence of PML, around 5% before the development of antiretroviral drugs, has dropped significantly (Gray et al. 2003).

27.2.2.3
Cytomegalovirus Infection

CMV infection in immunocompromised patients leads to ventriculitis and leptomeningitis. Ventriculitis is diagnosed on MRI by the presence of enhancement of ventricle surfaces. The differential diagnosis is subependymal lymphoma.

27.3
Prion Diseases

A group of CNS diseases called transmissible spongiform encephalopathies (TSE) is characterized by spongiform degeneration of neurons in the cortex and subcortical nuclei. It is known to be transmissible since the 1920s, when it was observed that humans in Borneo eating the CNS of defeated warriors were affected by a fatal dementia called kuru. Several human and animal diseases produce this distinctive pattern, including kuru, bovine spongiform encephalopathy (mad cow disease) and scrapie (sheep and goat). There are four forms of TSE, according to the way of contamination:

- **Sporadic Creutzfeldt-Jakob disease** (CJD), the most frequent (80%) has a spontaneous and sporadic origin. However, tissues from those patients may transmit the disease to other humans when injected or grafted
- **Heritable TSE** affects families and is known as Gerstmann-Sträussler disease and fatal familial insomnia
- **Acquired TSE** is of medical transmission, when patients are grafted with contaminated tissues from infected donors: blood transfusion, pituitary extracts, dura mater, and corneal transplantation
- **Variant CJD** (vCJD) is believed to affect patients who have eaten meat from bovine spongiform encephalopathy-infected cattle. The epidemic has affected mostly the UK, with more than a hundred deaths and France with at least four deaths since 1996. The epidemia has stopped.

This classification shows the role of an infectious agent that becomes pathogenic in particular genetic settings. Prusiner and others have partially elucidated the origin of TSE (Prusiner 1987). Although still controversial, transmissible agents are likely to be proteins called prions. The normal protein PrP^c becomes pathogenic when beta-pleated, thus becoming insoluble and resistant to heat, and is called PrP^{res}. PrP^{res} is capable of inserting itself into the cell membrane of neurons and inducing their own reproduction. It accumulates in the CNS and is neurotoxic. This results in death of groups of neurons within the brain (Gray et al. 2004).

Patients with CJD usually present late in life (>50 years of age) with rapid onset of dementia and myoclonic jerks (Martindale et al. 2003). Most patients are dead within a year of the onset of symptoms.

MRI is becoming a technique of choice for diagnostic orientation. The earliest MRI signs are symmetric basal ganglia and cortical hyperintensities on FLAIR and/or DWI (Fig. 27.5a, b) (Collie et al. 2001). In the clinical setting, these MRI signs are quite specific, although not constant. In most cases, the MRI abnormalities of CJD are bilateral and symmetric, but they may be unilateral. Bilateral hyperintensity of the basal ganglia may be seen on top of the basilar artery infarct, deep venous thrombosis, in acute ex-

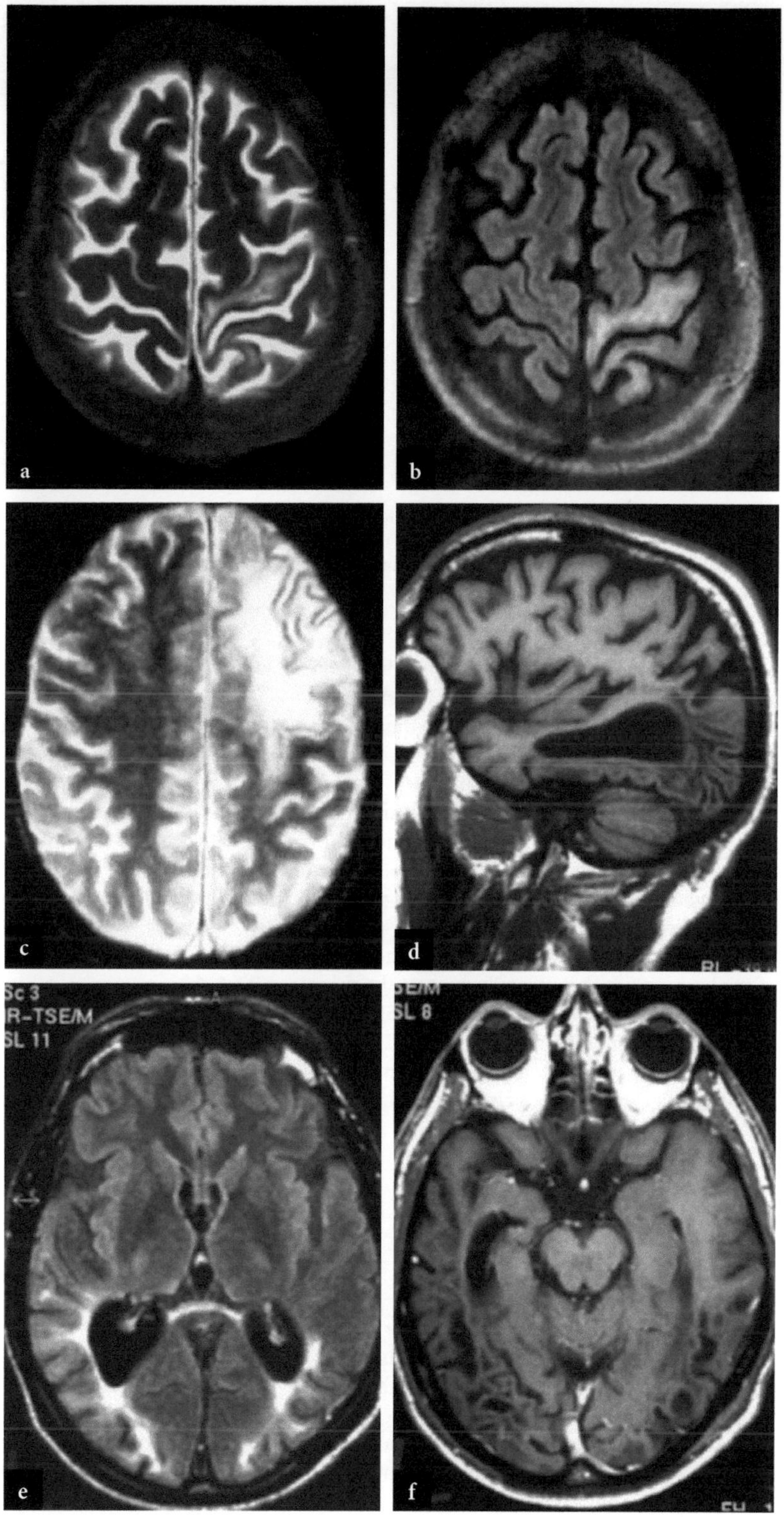

Fig. 27.4 a–f. Progressive multifocal leukoencephalopathy (PML). **a** T2 MR imaging. High signal intensity of arcuate fibers under the frontal motor cortex in an HIV-infected man complaining of right-hand paresis. **b** Flair MR imaging. Same patient as in **a**. The abnormality is more conspicuous than in part **a**. The cortex is spared. **c** T2 MR imaging. Evolution of PML on the same patient as in **a** and **b**. Subcortical high signal intensity extending into the frontal white matter. No mass effect. **d** T1 sagittal MR imaging. PML of the occipital lobe of an HIV patient with bilateral visual loss. Atrophy and low signal intensity of occipital-lobe white matter indicating destruction of the axonal fibers. **e** Flair MR imaging. Bilateral high signal intensity of the subcortical occipital white matter. **f** Gadolinium-enhanced MR imaging. No uptake of gadolinium

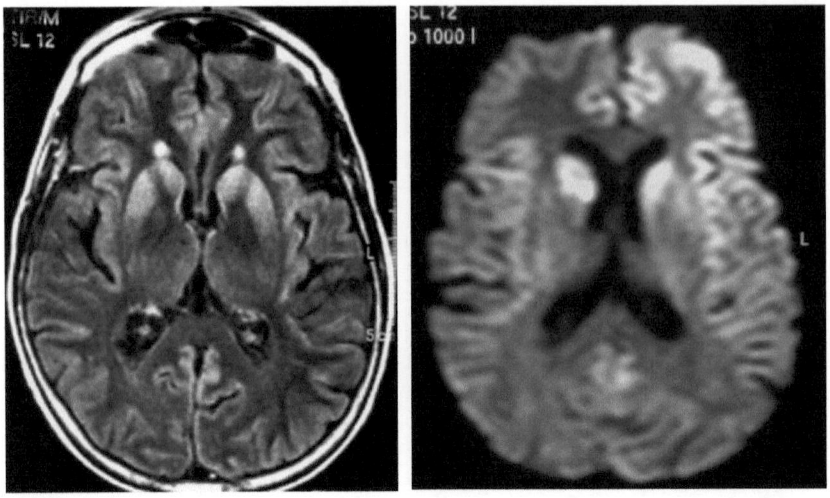

Fig. 27.5a,b Creutzfeldt-Jakob disease. **a** Flair MR imaging. Bilateral and symmetrical high signal intensity of the striatum from the basal ganglia. **b** Diffusion (b=1,000 mm^2/s, trace image) MR imaging. High signal intensity of the two caudate nuclei and high signal intensity of the left frontal and insular cortex

position to toxics, and in metabolic disorders such as Wernicke's encephalopathy. Usually the clinical setting is far different from CJD, making those diagnoses very unlikely.

Variant CJD shows a peculiar MRI sign, with high signal intensity in the pulvinar of the thalami (Collie et al. 2003). This "pulvinar sign" is, however, sometimes seen on sporadic CJD. Lately, atrophy and white matter high signal intensities are present on MRI studies.

Electric encephalograms may reveal the presence of triphasic waves that strongly suggest the disease. This sign is, however, of low sensitivity. CSF might be normal or with increased proteins. The 14-3-3 protein might be suggestively high although not specific. In vCJD, the search for the PrP^{res} protein includes biopsy of lymphoid organs or tonsils.

27.4 Bacterial Infections

Many bacteria may enter the CNS either hematogenously or by contiguity from the paranasal sinuses, the inner and middle ear or through a traumatic or surgical opening in the dura (Zimmerman 2000). The infection may affect one or several compartments of the brain at the same time: subdural (empyema) or CSF spaces (meningitis) and the brain parenchyma (encephalitis followed by a circumscribed abscess). Arteries, veins and perivascular Virchow-Robin spaces contribute to the spread of the bacteria from one compartment to another. Furthermore, acute or rapidly progressive thromboses of these vessels lead to additional abnormalities. The infection may also reach the surface of the endothelial wall causing the so-called distal mycotic aneurysms (see section 4.6) that have a high risk of rupture.

27.4.1 Bacteria

Staphylococci and ***streptococci pneumonia*** spread to the CNS either by a hematogenous path or via adjacent cranial structures.

Meningococci follow a hematogenous path and produce acute meningitis with high risk of death.

Koch bacilli causing tuberculosis (TB) usually is of hematogenous origin, leading to acute or subacute meningitis, and/or brain abscesses. TB affects many people worldwide, in underdeveloped countries, including patients with AIDS.

Nocardia affects immunocompromised patients (AIDS or others) and causes many brain abscesses, usually contemporary with chest infection.

Listeria monocytogenes may affect newborns or patients eating a high amount of bacteria in contaminated foods. The distribution of *Listeria* is usually the meninges and/or the rhombencephalon (brain stem and cerebellum), where it produces microabscesses (Maezawa et al. 2002; Gray et al. 2004).

E. coli or ***Proteus,*** bacteria of urinary origin, can cause brain abscesses in neonates.

Tropheryma whippelii causing Whipple disease is a rare infection, usually, but not constantly, encountered in patients with digestive malabsorption. It may appear as small lesions disseminated throughout the entire CNS with a predilection for gray matter (cortex, nuclei) (Gray et al. 2004).

Treponema pallidum causing syphilis is becoming a very rare cause of CNS infection. It produces mostly chronic meningitis, and, in a few cases, granulomatous reactions have been described along the cranial nerves.

Borrelia burgdorferi transmitted to humans by insect bytes causes Lyme disease. Involvement of spinal or cranial nerve roots is frequent. An immunological process leading to the involvement of the white matter resembling MS is much rarer.

27.4.2 Clinical and Imaging Features

Systemic signs of infection (e.g., fever and leukocytosis) may be present. Signs of CNS contamination include one or several of the following: neck stiffness and photophobia when meninges are affected, seizures and focal deficit or cerebellar signs when the parenchyma is involved.

Imaging features reflect the host reaction and are of variable appearance according to the type and location of the bacteria. Imaging techniques such as FLAIR and DWI, including the calculation of apparent diffusion coefficient (ADC) maps, are now used routinely in the indication of inflammatory CNS diseases. On DWI, purulent material is usually hyperintense and the decreased ADC shows the restriction of water motion (Desprechins et al. 1999; Lai et al. 2002). ADC helps in differentiating brain abscesses from CNS tumors. Indeed, necrotic debris from CNS tumors such as glioblastoma or metastases has variable and heterogeneous intensities and usually an increased ADC. There are, of course, some overlaps, especially in parasitic toxoplasmic abscesses or in punctured bacterial abscesses that may show increased ADC. MR spectroscopy, which is less routinely used, reveals the presence of amino acids from extracellular proteolysis and bacterial metabolism (fermentation products), including succinate, acetate, leucine, valine, and alanine, which are not seen in necrotic neoplasms (Lai et al. 2002; Cecil and Lenkinski 1998; Burtscher and Holtas 1999).

27.4.3 Bacterial Meningitis

The diagnosis is confirmed with lumbar puncture, and imaging does not play a primary role in the detection or treatment of this disorder. It is recommended to treat the patients as early as possible, without waiting for unnecessary imaging modalities. CT may be used to exclude increased intracranial pressure prior to lumbar puncture—only when there are clinical doubts. Meningitis without parenchyma involvement has a normal appearance on CT and MR T2-weighted images.

FLAIR imaging might be helpful in the diagnosis of meningitis, if the clinical presentation is not straightforward. It shows diffuse subarachnoid hyperintensity, while the CSF in the ventricles is dark (Fig. 27.6). However, there are three differential diagnoses when the subarachnoid space appears bright on Flair: (1) a CSF flow artifact, (2) a subarachnoid hemorrhage, (3) a hyperoxygenation such as during 100% oxygen supplementation for anesthesia or during a status epilepticus.

In bacterial meningitis, contrast-agent enhancement in the CSF space can be present, although it is unusual when the parenchyma is not involved. Tuberculous meningitis may be seen as an enhancement in the cisterna and along the sylvian fissures. CSF space enhancement may also evoke granulomatous diseases.

27.4.4 Subdural Empyema

Subdural empyema may be the result of direct spread of infection from the paranasal sinuses or the middle ear, or it can be of hematogenous origin or follow meningitis or cerebritis, through the venous structures. Subdural empyema produces an acute progressive syndrome characterized by fever and rapid development of neurologic abnormalities

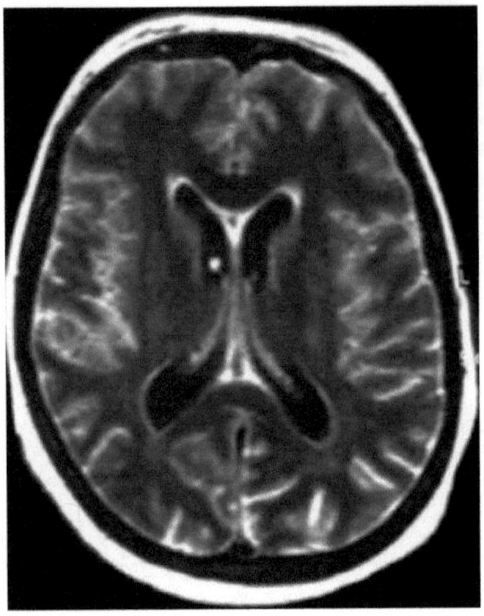

Fig. 27.6 Viral meningitis. Flair MR imaging. High signal intensity of the sub-arachnoid CSF space

(e.g., seizure and hemiparesis) (Rich et al. 2000). A complete imaging study of the brain and cranial structures is compelling in cases of subdural empyema. Subdural empyema produces brain complications by retrograde venous thrombosis that leads to cortical venous stasis with marked cortical swelling and brain abscesses.

Subdural empyema can be difficult to detect, particularly on unenhanced CT images (Fig. 27.7). The collection is typically narrow. There is disproportionate mass effect, with diffuse swelling of the hemisphere adjacent to the collection (Zimmerman 2000). The cortex may appear thickened because of venous stasis. There might be evidence of sinusitis or mastoiditis.

On MR images, the subdural collection is more conspicuous, particularly on FLAIR images, where it appears hyperintense to adjacent brain. On DWI, the content may appear bright, and the ADC values low (Fig. 27.7d). MR spectroscopy reveals the presence of amino acids. Contrast-enhanced CT and MR images reveal thin enhancement of the deep and superficial membranes of the subdural empyema (Fig. 27.7b, c).

27.4.5 Brain Abscesses

An abscess is the result of the host defense against bacteria, which initially produce a diffuse cerebritis or encephalitis. Macrophages produce a true collagenous capsule that marks the passage from cerebritis to the abscess phase. On CT, the capsule may appear with a slight increased density. Contrast enhancement with iodine contrast agents takes a regular ring appearance (Fig. 27.7b). The capsule made of fibrin and collagen has a typical appearance on MRI: low signal intensity on T2-weighted images and FLAIR, and ring enhancement with gadolinium (Fig. 27.7c). Additionally, on FLAIR and T2-weighted images, vasogenic edema appears as a high signal intensity infiltrating the white matter (Zimmerman and Weingarten 1991).

The central necrotic region is hyperintense on FLAIR images, and isointense to CSF on T2-weighted images. On diffusion imaging the center appears bright, which may be due to "T2 shine-through" effects. On ADC maps, the central necrotic material is hypointense, due to the restriction of water motion, because the water molecules move slowly in the dense abscess content, made of thick proteins and mucus (Fig. 27.7d). In at least two circumstances, the ADC may be increased: in toxoplasmic abscesses and in bacterial abscesses that have been punctured. Nevertheless, the decreased ADC values help to differentiate from brain necrotic tumors or metastases, which have increased ADC values. In brain abscesses, MR spectroscopy with long TR sequences reveals the presence of amino acids that are the proteolytic breakdown and fermentation products unique to bacterial infection. Enhancement will persist for up to 8 months.

A peculiar feature of brain abscesses is the miliary (Fig. 27.8). It may happen following the hematogenous spread of TB or *Nocardia*. Innumerable, small abscesses are present in the parenchyma.

27.4.6 Mycotic Aneurysms

Intracranial infectious aneurysms are important features that are not rare. They usually occur in patients with staphylococcal endocarditis and are called "mycotic" aneurysms (Phuong et al. 2002). They also develop in intravenous drug abusers (Tunkel and Pradhan 2002). Their imaging presentation is usually a small mass in the subarachnoid space near the cortex with strong enhancement. They may rupture, leading to subarachnoid hemorrhage with high risk of death. They also can be revealed by focal infarcts or seizures (Fig. 27.9). Note that stroke may occur without infective aneurysms in patients with valve endocarditis (Anderson et al. 2003). Non-ruptured aneurysms may disappear under antibiotics. Ruptured and sometimes non-ruptured aneurysms need endovascular treatment or surgical clipping.

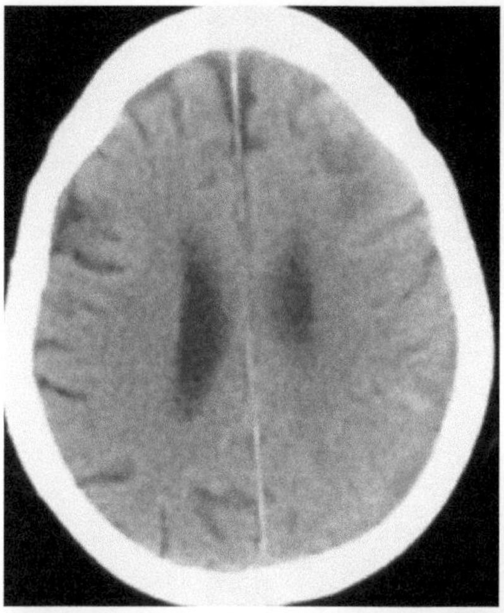

a

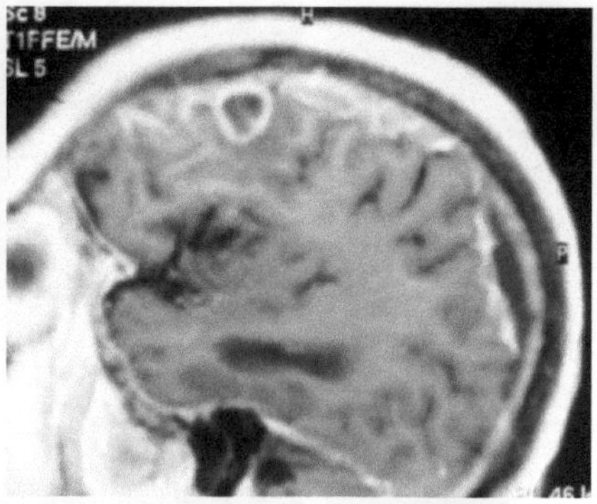

c

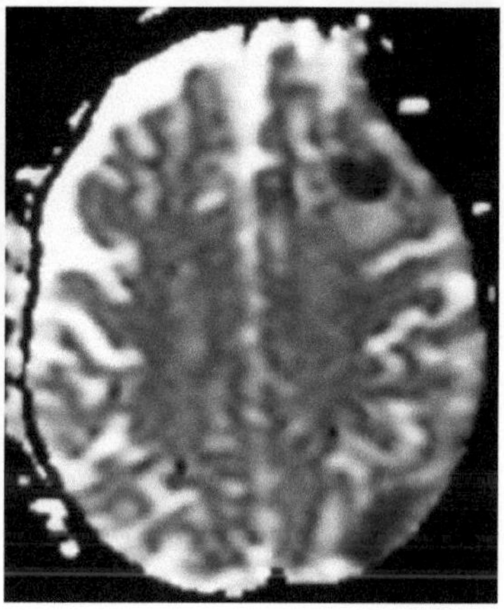

d

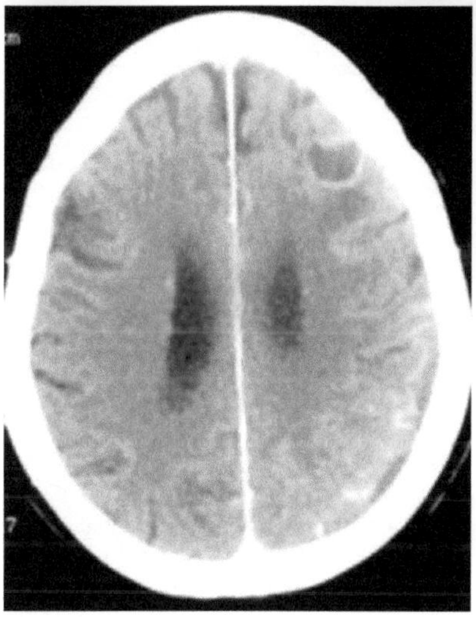

b

Fig. 27.7a–d. Subdural empyema and brain abscess. **a** CT without contrast media. A careful analysis shows a focal low density in the left frontal lobe and a lack of visibility of the parietal gyri. **b** Contrast-enhanced CT. Ring enhancing lesion of the left frontal lobe and enhancement of the meninges. **c** Sagittal contrast-enhanced MR imaging. Focal lesion of the frontal lobe and subdural collection. **d** Diffusion MR imaging: Apparent diffusion coefficient (ADC) map. The frontal lobe and meninges lesions show a restriction of water diffusion (low signal intensity). This is consistent with an infectious origin

27.5 Parasitic Infections

The most common parasitic infections that affect the CNS are (Chang et al. 1991; Gray et al. 2004):

- Protozoal infections:
  a) Amebiasis
  b) Cerebral malaria
  c) Toxoplasmosis that develops in the CNS of HIV-infected patients
  d) Trypanosomiasis
- Metazoal infections:
  a) Neurocysticercosis (*Taenia solium) from pork*
  b) Hydatidosis *(Taenia echinococcus / Echinococcus granulosus)* from dogs, responsible for hydatid cysts
  c) Echinococcus multilocularis (*Taenia multilocularis*) from foxes
  d) Toxocariasis (*Toxocara canis* and *Toxocara cati*), which may produce visceral larva migrans and CNS manifestations in children
  e) Paragonimiasis (*Paragonimus westermani*) from infected crabs or crayfish

Other parasitic infections including sparganosis, trichinosis (*Trichinella spiralis*), strongylosis, schistosomiasis may also develop in the CNS.

The three taenias, responsible for neurocysticercosis, hydatidosis and *Echinococcus multilocularis*, produce cystic lesions. A cystic wall is completely different from the capsule of a brain abscess. The cystic wall has a parasitic origin, whereas the cap-

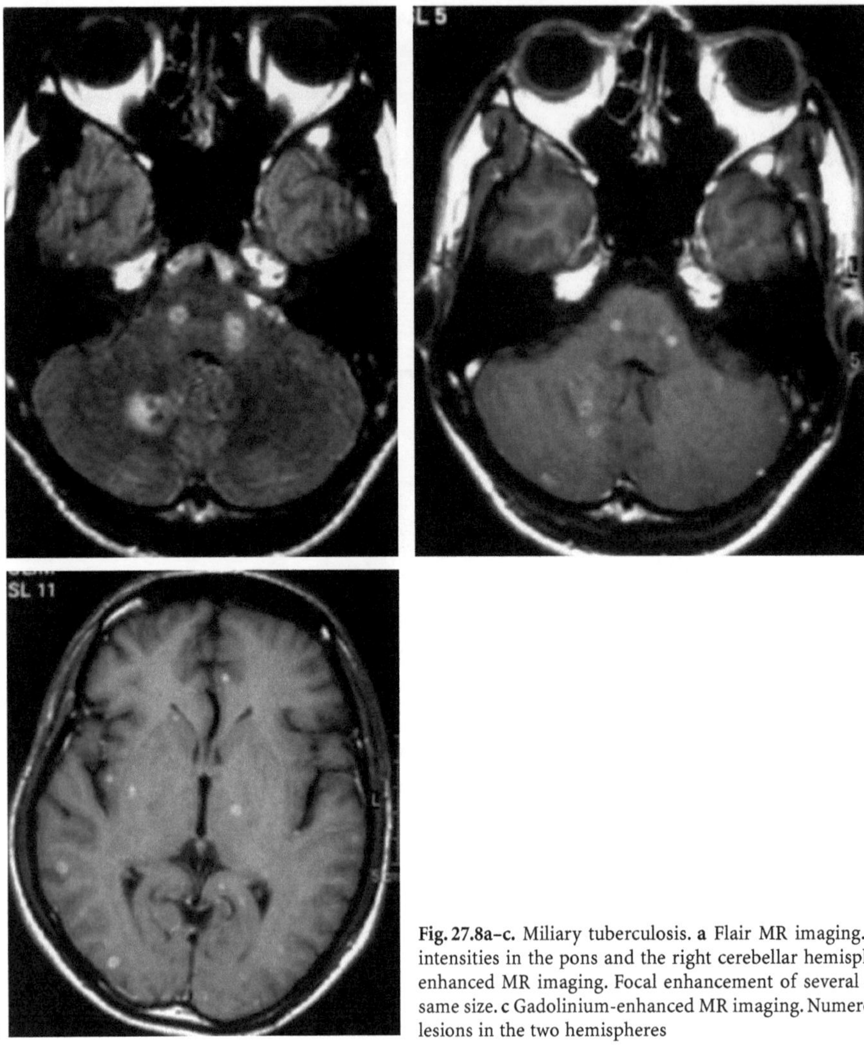

Fig. 27.8a–c. Miliary tuberculosis. **a** Flair MR imaging. Several high signal intensities in the pons and the right cerebellar hemisphere. **b** Gadolinium-enhanced MR imaging. Focal enhancement of several small lesions of the same size. **c** Gadolinium-enhanced MR imaging. Numerous small enhancing lesions in the two hemispheres

sule of an abscess has a host origin. The cystic wall is not detectable by the host immunologic system till the larva dies. The symptoms often arise after the death of the parasite, when the host response can occur. However, the location of the cyst may be also responsible for symptoms such as seizures, mass effect or CSF occlusion, before the death of the parasite.

27.5.1 Cysticercosis (*Taenia solium*)

Cysticercosis is the most common parasitic infection of the CNS and is endemic in all countries, particularly in Latin America (Gray et al. 2004). The larvae enter the intestinal wall and develop in the brain, the subarachnoid space, or the ventricles (del Brutto et al. 2001). Once the scolex is established, it makes itself immunologically invisible to the host and, consequently, incites no inflammatory reaction. Live cysts are isointense to CSF with all pulse sequences. No enhancement is seen within the cyst wall while the organism is alive (Fig. 27.10). The scolex may be seen as a 2-4 mm mural nodule in the cyst wall. There is no associated edema.

When the organism dies, an inflammatory granulomatous response occurs. The clinical manifestations are seizures or focal deficits. The wall enhances, and there is associated vasogenic edema (Fig. 27.10a,

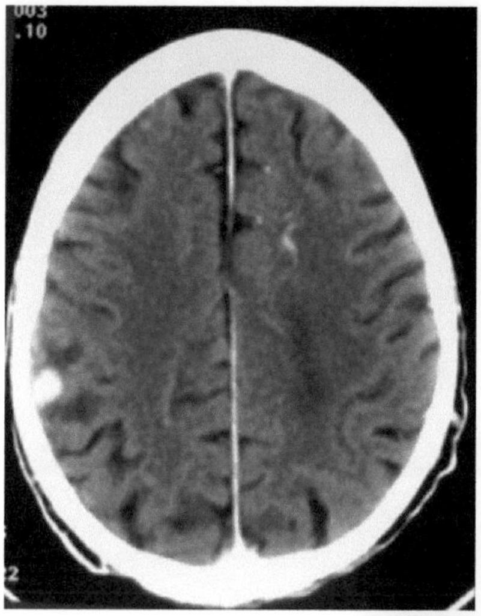
a
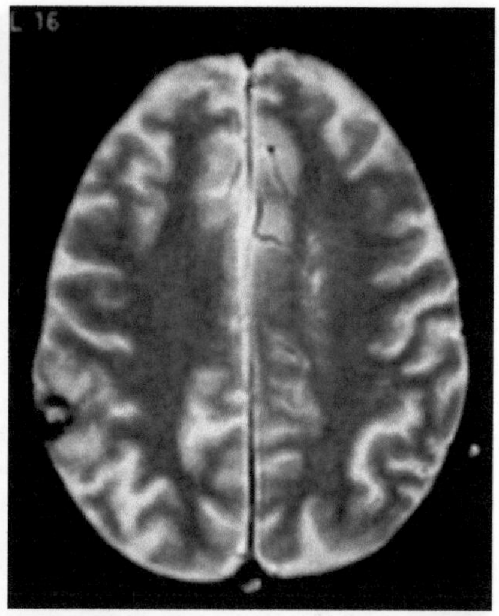
b
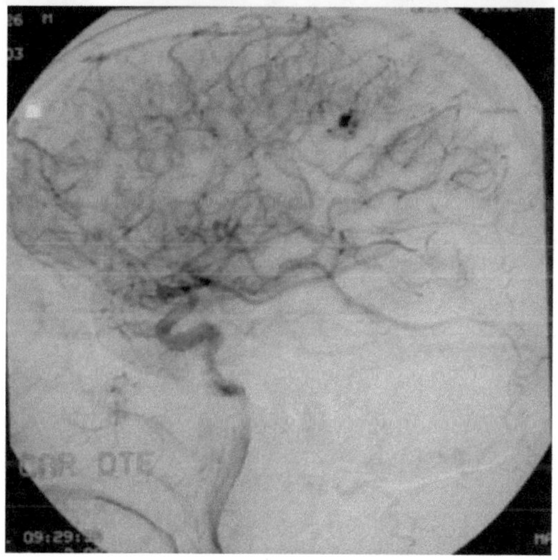
c

Fig. 27.9a–c. Mycotic aneurysm. **a** Contrast-enhanced CT. Small enhancing lesion adjacent to the right parietal cortex. Note the incidental finding of a venous angioma on the left hemisphere. **b** T2* MR imaging. Presence of magnetic susceptibility, probably due to hemosiderin surrounding the mycotic aneurysm. **c** Selective right carotid-artery angiogram. The small mycotic aneurysm appears filled by the contrast agent on an anterior parietal branch of the middle cerebral artery

c, h). The dead cyst commonly calcifies (Fig. 27.10f). Patients treated with praziquantel may develop acute symptoms because of the simultaneous death of all live cysts (Fig. 27.10c). Subarachnoid cysts may often produce secondary obstructive hydrocephalus (Fig. 27.10d, e).

27.5.2 Hydatid Cysts (*Echinococcus granulosus*)

Human *Echinococcus granulosus* contamination occurs by accidental ingestion of contaminated dog feces. The disease is endemic in the Mediterranean regions, the Middle East, and Latin America. The most common sites of development in humans are the liver, lung and bone. The brain is affected in less than 5% of patients. It is usually a single, unilocular and quite large cyst. When the cyst ruptures, it produces an inflammatory reaction.

27.5.3 *Echinococcus multilocularis*

This is a rare parasitic infection that usually has a fatal issue. The cysts are recognizable by their resemblance to wine grapes.

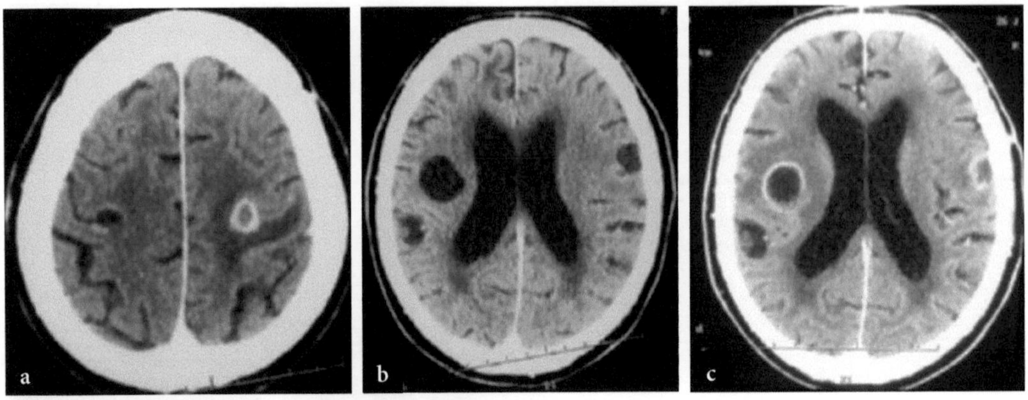

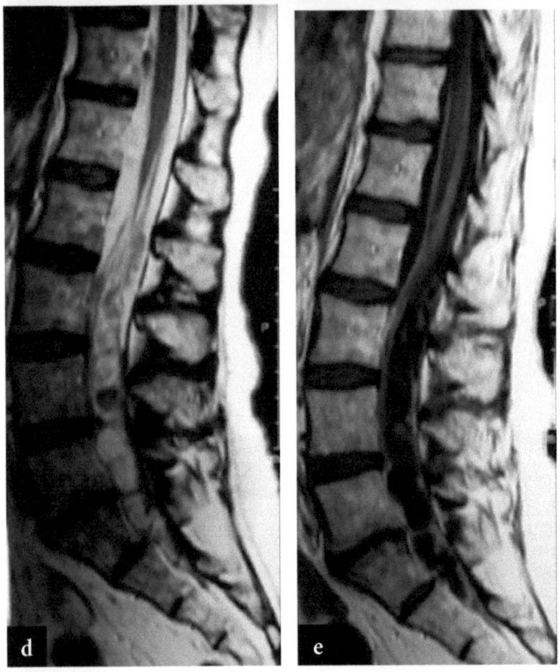

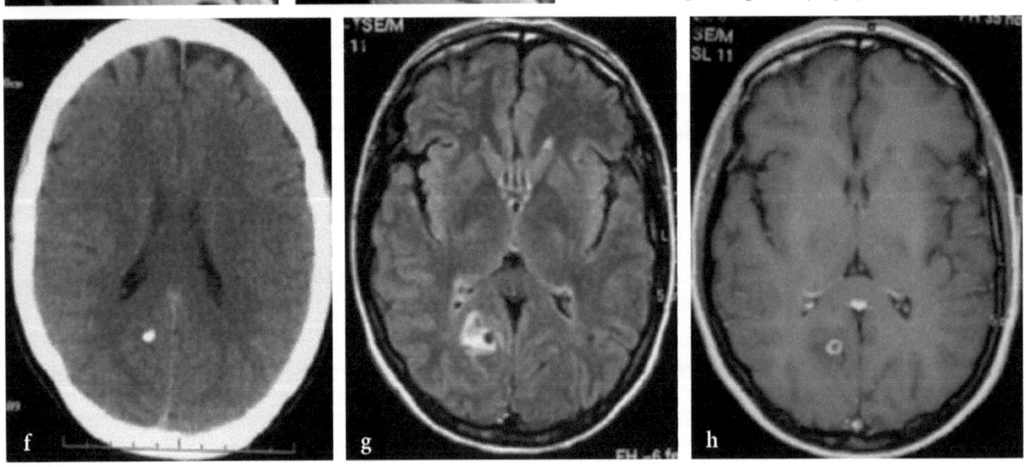

Fig. 27.10a–h. Cysticercosis. **a** Contrast-enhanced CT. Patient with right arm seizure. Focal ring enhancing lesion in the left frontal cortex. On the right hemisphere, presence of a cystic lesion with a high density on the margin representing a cysticercosis cyst. **b** Contrast-enhanced CT. Same patient. Three other non-enhancing cystic lesions in the brain parenchyma. **c** Contrast-enhanced CT. The same patient 3 weeks after praziquantel antibiotic. Simultaneous death of all live cysts leading to a ring enhancement of the cystic walls. **d** Sagittal T2 MR imaging. Cysticercosis cysts in the CSF of the cauda equina. **e** Gadolinium-enhanced MR imaging. The cystic walls enhance in the CSF of the cauda equina. **f** CT without contrast agent. Focal high density of the right subcortical occipital lobe corresponding to a calcification. **g** Flair MR imaging. High signal intensity corresponding to edema surrounding the low signal intensity calcification. **h** Gadolinium-enhanced MR imaging. Small and unique ring-enhancing lesion corresponding to a dying cyst

27.5.4 Toxoplasmosis

Toxoplasma gondii is distributed worldwide and infects more than 500 million humans (Ramsey and Dean 1997). It does not cause clinical intracranial infection in immunocompetent hosts, and, consequently, was rarely seen prior to the onset of the AIDS epidemia. However, toxoplasmosis may infect the embryo, producing diffuse necrotic lesions of the cortex, cerebral malformations and intracranial calcifications, especially in the periventricular regions (Gray et al. 2004).

Toxoplasmosis is the most common cerebral mass lesion encountered in the HIV-positive patient (Ramsey and Dean 1997). This is the first diagnosis to evoke when CNS manifestations occur with rapid progression in HIV-infected patients. The imaging appearance might be ubiquitous, but the antibiotic treatment is very efficient. Thus, AIDS patients with rapid CNS manifestations should be treated for toxoplasmosis regardless of the imaging features. The diagnosis might be reconsidered if the treatment is inefficient. With HAART (highly active antiretroviral therapy) treatment, the incidence of toxoplasmosis has dropped (Gray et al. 2003). Now, toxoplasmosis is encountered in patients who are unaware of their viral status for HIV. It is not rare that patients presenting inaugural seizures and several brain lesions are positive for HIV. This diagnosis must be evoked by the radiologist.

Although largely identical to an abscess, the lesion is not encapsulated, which accounts for the histologic classification of encephalitis rather than abscess (Zimmerman 2000; Gray et al. 2004). In the majority of cases, multiple mass lesions are present, and they may be located anywhere within the brain. The basal ganglia and the cortical-subcortical junction are more affected.

The imaging findings in the beginning include a mass effect with or without a slight, not well-demarcated, contrast enhancement (Fig. 27.11a). Later, the enhancement is quite similar to an abscess, like a ring (Fig. 27.11c, d). The central necrosis is typically hyperintense on FLAIR and T2-weighted images. DWI reveals heterogeneous intensity (Fig. 27.11e), and the ADC is usually increased. Hemorrhage is not present at the time of initial diagnosis. Signs of hemorrhage are present when the patient is treated with antibiotics. High signal intensity from methemoglobin is seen on non-enhanced T1-weighted images, leading to confirmation of the diagnosis in patients under treatment (Fig. 27.11f).

In patients who are not improving with antibiotics, the diagnosis of toxoplasmosis must be reconsidered, with the primary goal of differentiating toxoplasmosis from lymphoma. Although it is rare, lymphoma is the second most common causes of mass lesions in patients with AIDS (Ramsey and Dean 1997). Lymphoma lesions are usually single and located in the deep gray and white matter (basal ganglia and corpus callosum). Lymphoma is often hypointense on T2-weighted images. There is mild, adjacent edema, with a mass effect lower than expected. Enhancement is usually diffuse but may be of a ring appearance, especially when the lesion is superior to 3.5 cm. Single photon emission CT (SPECT) with radioactive thallium can be used to confirm the diagnosis of lymphoma prior to therapy. Inflammatory lesions, including toxoplasmosis, are negative on SPECT, while lymphoma uptakes the radioactive thallium. When the diagnosis cannot be established non-invasively, biopsy is necessary. Non-Hodgkin lymphoma type B is the most common. Its outcome is, unfortunately, fatal.

27.5.5 *Toxocara canis* and *Toxocara cati* Infections

These are dog and cat nematodes. Human infection occurs by accidental ingestion of their eggs passed from pet animals. The liver, lung and peritoneum are most frequently involved. They produce focal lesions in the white matter, which spontaneously resolve. Vasculitis or granulomas around the larvae may form in the parenchyma (Fig. 27.12a, b) (Dousset et al. 2003). The death of the parasite in the brain is followed by a non-encapsulated granulomatous reaction (Gray et al. 2004).

27.6 Mycotic Infections

CNS fungal infections are possible in exposed populations such as immunocompromised patients with AIDS, leukemia, diabetes mellitus, renal diseases, those under aggressive chemotherapy and in intravenous drug abusers with unsterilized materials (Harris and Enterline 1997).

The most frequent fungal infections are: cryptococcosis due to *Cryptococcus neoformans*, aspergillosis, mucormycosis, candidiasis and histoplasmosis. They are responsible for meningitis in infections

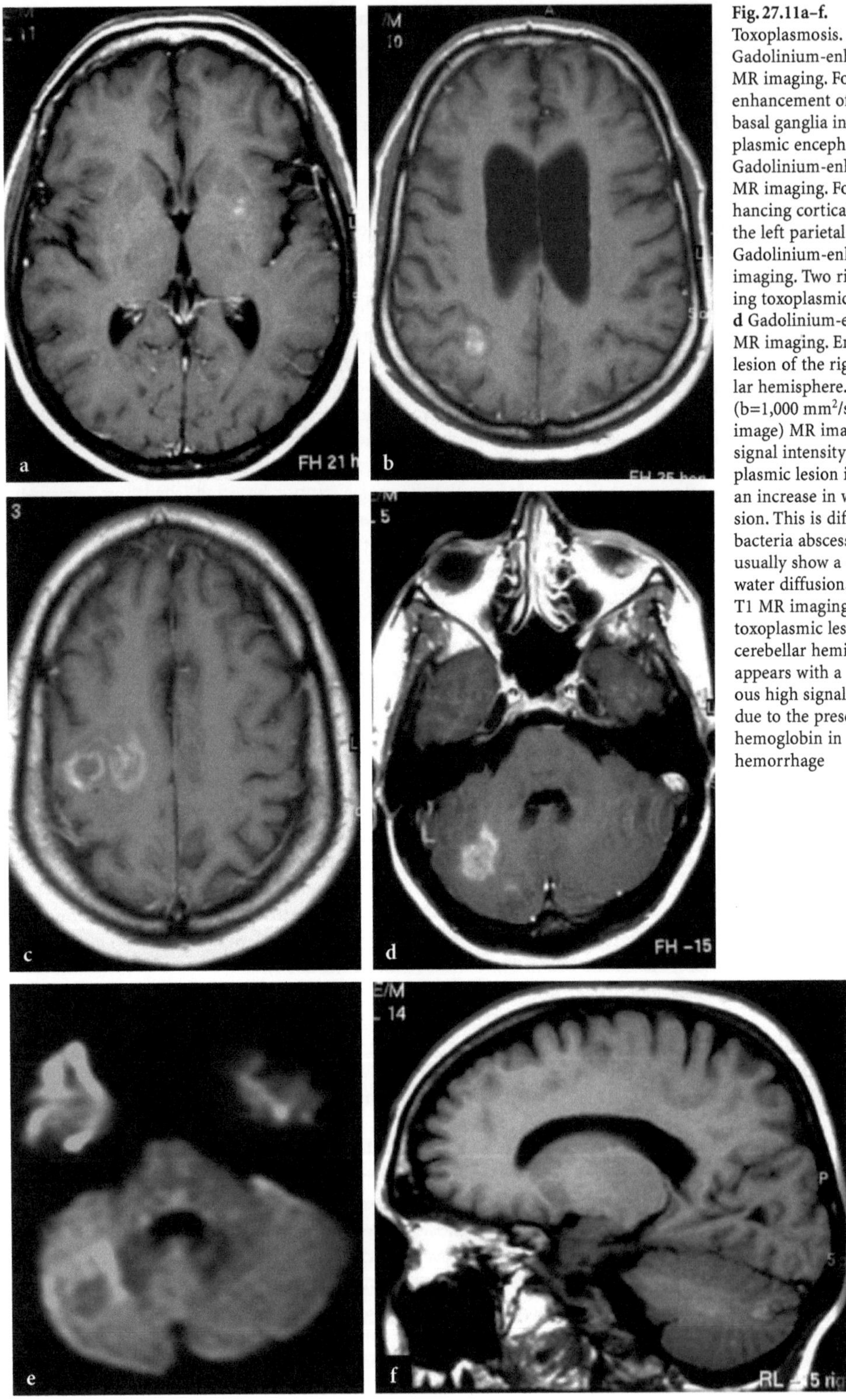

Fig. 27.11a–f. Toxoplasmosis. **a** Gadolinium-enhanced MR imaging. Focal slight enhancement of the left basal ganglia in toxoplasmic encephalitis. **b** Gadolinium-enhanced MR imaging. Focal enhancing cortical lesion of the left parietal cortex. **c** Gadolinium-enhanced MR imaging. Two ring-enhancing toxoplasmic lesions. **d** Gadolinium-enhanced MR imaging. Enhancing lesion of the right cerebellar hemisphere. **e** Diffusion ($b=1,000\ mm^2/s$, trace image) MR imaging. Low signal intensity in the toxoplasmic lesion indicating an increase in water diffusion. This is different from bacteria abscesses, which usually show a decrease in water diffusion. **f** Sagittal T1 MR imaging. Treated toxoplasmic lesion of the cerebellar hemisphere that appears with a spontaneous high signal intensity due to the presence of methemoglobin in subacute hemorrhage

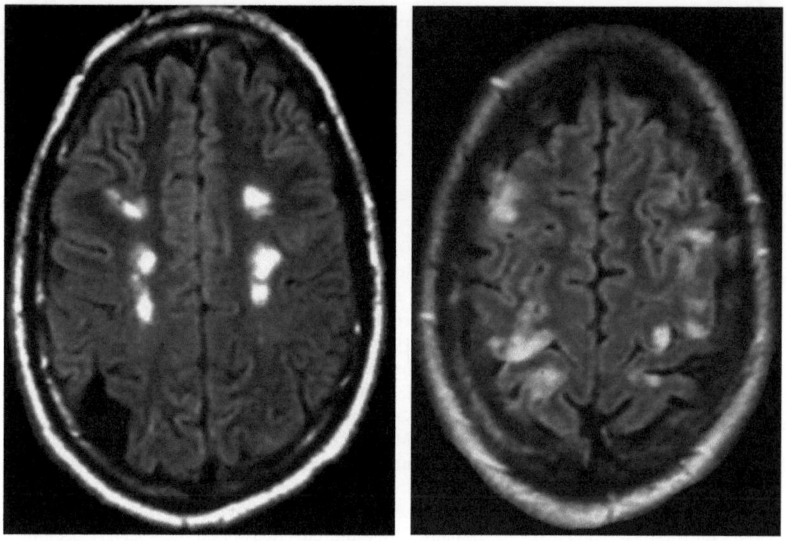

Fig. 27.12a, b. Toxocariasis. Flair MR imaging. Several lesions of the subcortical white matter (**a**) and of the cortex (**b**). The imaging findings are not sufficient to make the diagnosis, which requires blood serology for *Toxocara canis* or *Toxocara cati*

by the smallest fungi like *Cryptococcus neoformans* or small to extensive infarcts following occlusion of the vessels by bigger fungi such as *Aspergillus* and *Candida*.

27.6.1 Cryptococcosis

The patient usually presents with a meningoencephalitis (Harris and Enterline 1997). The infection is fatal without appropriate treatment using amphotericin B. Lumbar puncture is the single most useful test. After reaching the CSF, the organisms may extend along the perforating arteries in the perivascular Virchow-Robin spaces. The signal intensity is similar to the cerebrospinal fluid. Cerebral edema rarely occurs.

27.6.2 Aspergillosis

It is relatively rare in the AIDS population, but is more common in patients under corticosteroids. The organisms invade the lung parenchyma and spread hematogenously. Aspergillus may reach the CNS via direct spread from the paranasal sinuses or orbits. Aspergillus abscesses have a nonspecific appearance.

27.6.3 Mucormycosis

Most CNS mucormycosis-infected patients are diabetic, drug abusers, or patients receiving long-term antibiotics and corticosteroids. It has a secondary focus in skin, nasal mucosa and lungs. Rhinocerebral mucormycosis is a common feature. It provokes necrosis and vasculitis with hemorrhage.

27.7 Granulomatous Infections and Immunoreactive Diseases

27.7.1 Granulomatous Infections

Granulomas correspond to cellular mass with T-cells, macrophages and histiocytes without liquefied necrotic debris. Caseous ("cheesy") necrosis is typical of tuberculous granulomas.

Granulomatous infections can result from diverse pathogens, including bacteria (*Mycobacterium*, *Nocardia*, *Actinomyces*, spirochetes), fungi (aspergillosis or mucormycosis), and parasites. Sarcoidosis is an idiopathic granulomatous disease that most commonly affects young, otherwise healthy adult patients (Ulmer and Ester 1991). Most granulomatous infections affect the meninges. The brain parenchyma might be involved, usually by the spread of the granuloma along the perivascular Virchow-Robin spaces. Inflammatory pseudotumors may also affect the cavernous sinuses, the orbits and, rarely, the hypophysis sellae.

CT or MRI features of granulomatous meningitis are cisternal enhancement, usually following the vessel routes. Thus, contrast-enhanced images are critical in establishing the diagnosis of granulomatous meningitis. Basal meningitis often leads to hydrocephalus. There is often compromise of the vascular system, with secondary infarction or hemorrhage. The combination of hydrocephalus and deep infarction in a young adult should, therefore, always raise the suspicion of granulomatous meningitis (Zimmerman 2000).

The differential diagnosis of granulomatous infectious meningitis is neoplastic carcinomatous meningitis (Aparicio and Chamberlain 2002). It has a predilection for the retro-cerebellar cisterns. Sarcoidosis has a predilection for the suprasellar cistern, often producing thickening of the pituitary stalk (Ulmer and Ester 1991). Enhancement along the course of the cranial nerves is characteristic of sarcoidosis but can also be seen in lymphoma.

27.7.2 Vasculitis

Vasculitis may be the result of direct spread from the leptomeninges along the perivascular spaces or direct invasion and growth within the lumen of the vessel. It also can be the result of an immune reaction at the endothelial level, without infectious agents. Infarcts occur in the deep gray matter or in the cortex.

27.7.3 Acute Disseminated Encephalomyelitis

Acute disseminated encephalomyelitis is an autoimmune disorder that is similar to multiple sclerosis, except that it is monophasic (Talbot et al. 2001). Acute disseminated encephalomyelitis occurs with a latency of 1 week to several weeks after viral exposure or vaccination. In most of the cases, multiple lesions are present at the same time in the white matter, affecting the gray matter in at least one-third of cases. The disease may produce multifocal demyelination similar to viral encephalitis or multiple sclerosis. Enhancement is inconstant, although frequent. In most cases, improvement is good under steroids. Death is possible in the most severe cases.

References

Anderson DJ, Goldstein LB, Wilkinson WE et al (2003) Stroke location, characterization, severity, and outcome in mitral vs aortic valve endocarditis. Neurology 61:1341–1346

Aparicio A, Chamberlain MC (2002) Neoplastic meningitis. Curr Neurol Neurosci Rep 2:225–235

Bonthius DJ, Karacay B (2002) Meningitis and encephalitis in children. An update. Neurol Clin 20:1013–1038

Burtscher IM, Holtas M (1999) In vivo proton MR spectroscopy of untreated and treated brain abscesses. AJNR Am J Neuroradiol 20:1049–1053

Cecil KM, Lenkinski RE (1998) Proton MR spectroscopy in inflammatory and infectious brain disorders. Neuroimaging Clin N Am 8:863–880

Chang KH, Cho YS, Hesselink JR et al (1991) Parasitic diseases of the central nervous system. Neuroimaging Clin N Am 1:159–178

Collie DA, Sellar RJ, Zeidler M et al (2001) MRI of Creutzfeldt-Jakob disease: imaging features and recommended MRI protocol. Clin Radiol 56:726–739

Collie DA, Summers DM, Sellar RJ et al (2003) Diagnosing variant Creutzfeldt-Jakob disease with the pulvinar sign: MR imaging findings in 86 neuropathologically confirmed cases. AJNR Am J Neuroradiol 24:1560–1569

Dal Canto MC (1997) Mechanisms of HIV infection of the central nervous system and pathogenesis of AIDS-dementia complex. Neuroimaging Clin N Am 7:231–242

Del Brutto OH, Rajshekhar V, White AC Jr et al (2001) Proposed diagnostic criteria for neurocysticercosis. Neurology 57:177–183

Desprechins B, Stadnik T, Koerts G et al (1999) Use of diffusion-weighted MR imaging in differential diagnosis between intracerebral necrotic tumors and cerebral abscesses. AJNR Am J Neuroradiol 20:1252–1257

Dousset V, Armand JP, Lacoste D et al (1997) Magnetization transfer study of HIV encephalitis and progressive multifocal leukoencephalopathy. AJNR Am J Neuroradiol 18:895–901

Dousset V, Sibon I, Menegon P (2003) Cerebral vasculitis due to Toxocara canis (or catis) origin. J Radiol 84:89–91

Gray F, Chretien F, Vallat-Decouvelaere AV et al (2003) The changing pattern of HIV neuropathology in the HAART. J Neuropathol Exp Neurol 62:429–440

Gray F, de Girolami U, Poirier J (2004) Basic neuropathology, 4th edn. Elsevier, Philadelphia

Harris DE, Enterline DS (1997) Fungal infections of the central nervous system. Neuroimaging Clin N Am 7:187–198

Lai PH, Ho JT, Chen WL et al (2002) Brain abscess and necrotic brain tumor: discrimination with proton MR spectroscopy and diffusion-weighted imaging. AJNR Am J Neuroradiol 23:1369–1377

Maezawa Y, Hirasawa A, Abe T et al (2002) Successful treatment of listerial brain abscess: a case report and literature review. Intern Med 41:1073–1078

Martindale JL, Geschwind MD, Miller BL (2003) Psychiatric and neuroimaging findings in Creutzfeldt-Jakob disease. Curr Psychiatry Rep 5:43–46
Osborn RE, Byrd SE (1991) Congenital infections of the brain. Neuroimaging Clin N Am 1:105–118
Phuong LK, Link M, Widjdicks E (2002) Management of intracranial infectious aneurysms: a series of 16 cases. Neurosurgery 51:1145–1151
Post MJD, Sheldon JJ, Hensley GT et al (1986) Central nervous system disease in acquired immunodeficiency syndrome: prospective correlation using CT, MR imaging, and pathologic studies. Radiology 158:141–148
Prusiner SB (1987) Prions and neurodegenerative disease. N Engl J Med 317:1571–1581
Ramsey RG, Dean AD (1997) Central nervous system toxoplasmosis. Neuroimaging Clin N Am 7:171–186
Rich PM, Deasy NP, Jarosz JM (2000) Intracranial dural empyema. Br J Radiol 73:1329–1336
Talbot PJ, Arnold D, Antel JP (2001) Virus-induced autoimmune reactions in the CNS. Curr Top Microbiol Immunol 253:247–271
Tien RD, Felsberg GJ, Osumi AK (1993) Herpes virus infections of the CNS: MR findings. AJR Am J Roentgenol 161:167–176
Trotot PM, Gray F (1997) Diagnostic imaging contribution in the early stages of HIV infection of the brain. Neuroimaging Clin N Am 7:243–260
Tunkel AR, Pradhan SK (2002) Central nervous system infections in injection drug users. Infect Dis Clin North Am 16:589–605
Ulmer JL, Elster AD (1991) Sarcoidosis of the central nervous system. Neuroimaging Clin N Am 1:141–150
Zimmerman RD (2000) Infection. Proceedings of the Radiologic Society of North America Annual meeting RSNA categorial course in diagnostic radiology: neuroradiology. pp 45–63
Zimmerman RD, Weingarten KW (1991) Neuroimaging of cerebral abscess. Neuroimaging Clin N Am 1:1–16

28 Neoplastic Disorders

Alberto Bizzi, Bianca Pollo, and Carlo Marras

CONTENTS

28.1 Introduction

The American Cancer Society estimates that in the United States 16,800 new diagnosed intracranial neoplasms were diagnosed in 1999, more than double the number of diagnosed cases of Hodgkin's disease and over half the number of cases of melanoma (DeAngelis 2001). A large number of intracranial tumours arise from brain tissue while others arise from meninges (meningiomas) and hematopoietic tissue (lymphomas). Metastases to the brain are even more common: more than 100,000 patients per year die with symptomatic intracranial metastases. Incidence rates have a first peak before 10 years of age, then they decline to increase again after 25 years of age, and decline again only after 85 years of age. Data from the last three decades are showing that brain-tumour incidence increases with age through life. In the last three decades, the incidence of primary brain tumours has increased in Europe, Japan and the United States among people older than 65 years. However, this increase in rates is not real but it is attributed to improvements in management of common illnesses and better diagnostic workup of elderly patients.

This chapter will focus on the histopathology, biology, and imaging of the morphologic, metabolic and physiopathologic features of brain tumours, with particular attention to the most common type of primary intra-axial tumours: the glioma.

28.2 Neuropathology

The 2000 World Health Organization (WHO) classification of tumours of the nervous system is the most comprehensive to date, and it has received a large consensus among neuropathologists. It divides brain tumours into seven large categories: tumours arising from neuroepithelial tissue; from peripheral nerves; from the meninges; lymphomas and hematopoietic neoplasms; germ cell tumours; tumours of the sellar region and metastatic tumours. A simplified version of the WHO classification (Kleihues 2000) is presented on Table 28.1.

Among tumours of neuroepithelial tissue, the gliomas are by far the most common and best known. Gliomas include tumours arising from neoplastic transformation of astrocytes, oligodendrocytes, mixed gliomas and glial tumours of uncertain origin. The group of neuroepithelial tumours comprise also ependymomas, neuronal and mixed neuronal–glial tumours (as ganglioglioma), and embryonal tumours (as medulloblastoma). Much evidence has been recently reported in support of the hypothesis that brain tumours arise by transformation of proliferating neural stem cells. Neural stem cells are able to self-renew and differentiate into neurons and glia. Other masses may arise from normal constituents of the brain, such as hamartomas, or from embryologically misplaced tissues such as teratomas, dermoids and germinomas.

A. Bizzi, MD
B. Pollo, MD
C. Marras, MD
Department of Neuroradiology, Istituto Nazionale Neurologico "Carlo Besta", Via Caloria 11, 20133 Milan, Italy

Table 28.1 WHO Classification of Tumours of the Nervous System (modified from Kleihues and Cavenee 2000)

Tumour of Neuroepithelial Tissue	code
Astrocytic Tumours	
Diffuse astrocytoma	9400/3°
Fibrillary astrocytoma	9420/3
Protoplasmic astrocytoma	9410/3
Gemistocytic astrocytoma	9411/3
Anaplastic astrocytoma	9401/3
Glioblastoma	9440/3
Giant cell glioblastoma	9441/3
Gliosarcoma	9442/3
Pilocytic astrocytoma	9421/1
Pleomorphic xanthoastrocytoma	9424/3
Subependymal giant cell astrocytoma	9384/1
Oligodendroglial Tumours	
Oligodendroglioma	9450/3
Anaplastic oligodendroglioma	9451/3
Mixed Gliomas	
Oligoastrocytoma	9382/3
Anaplastic oligoastrocytoma	9382/3+
Ependymal Tumours	
Ependymoma	9391/3
Anaplastic ependymoma	9392/3
Myxopapillary ependymoma	9394/1
Subependymoma	9383/1
Choroid Plexus Tumours	
Choroid Plexus Tumours	9390/0
Choroid plexus carcinoma	9390/3
Glial Tumours of Uncertain Origin	
Astroblastoma	9430/3
Gliomatosis cerebri	9381/3
Choroid glioma of the third ventricle	9444/1
Neuronal and Mixed Neuronal-Glial Tumours	
Gangliocytoma	9492/0
Dysembryoplastic neuroepithelial tumour	9413/0
Ganglioglioma	9505/1
Central neurocytoma	9506/1
Paraganglioma of the filum terminale	8680/1
Neuroblastic Tumours	
Pineal Tumours	
Embryonal Tumours	
Ependymoblastoma	9392/3
Medulloblastoma	9470/3
Supratentorial primitive neuroectodermal tumour (PNET)	9473/3
Tumours of Peripheral Nerves	
Schwannoma	
Neurofibroma	9540/0
Malignant Peripheral Nerve Sheath Tumour (MPNST)	9540/3
Tumours of the Meninges	
Tumours of Meningothelial Cells	
Mesenchymal, Non-meningothelial Tumours	
Primary Melanocytic Lesions	
Lymphomas and Hematopoietic Neoplasm	
Germ Cell Tumours	
Germinoma	9064/3
Embryonal carcinoma	9070/3
Teratoma	9080/1
Mixed germ cell tumours	9085/3
Tumours of the Sellar Region	
Craniopharyngioma	9350/1
Metastatic Tumours	

Gliomas are classified by their histologic features, according to the presumptive "cell of origin," differentiation and malignancy grade. At the current state of knowledge, cytogenesis is more a theoretical concept than a definitive basis for tumour classification. In the near future the further discovery of molecular and cytogenetic features will form the basis of more objective tumour classification.

Age of the patient and anatomic location are also very important diagnostic and prognostic criteria. According to the WHO system or the St. Anne-Mayo system, glial tumours are graded on the basis of the most malignant area identified on the histopathologic specimens (Fig. 28.2.1). Fibrillary (grade II) astrocytoma is characterised by increased cellularity, with a monomorphic population of cells infiltrating the neuropil. Anaplastic (grade III) astrocytoma is characterised by nuclear polymorphism and mitoses. The presence of microvascular proliferation and necrosis are features of the (grade IV) glioblastoma. They can arise either alone (primary glioblastoma) or from a preexisting low-grade glioma (secondary glioblastoma). All gliomas are histologically and genetically heterogeneous. When a small specimen is taken for histopathology, it could not reflect the most malignant biology of the entire tumour. Among low grade astrocytomas the fibrillary (WHO grade II) must be distinguished from more benign tumours such as pilocytic astrocytoma (WHO I) and pleomorphic xanthoastrocytoma (WHO grade II). While fibrillary astrocytomas have a tendency to change their biologic behaviour with time and evolve into high-grade gliomas, the latter two types maintain a benign prognosis despite the presence of contrast enhancement on CT and MR imaging. The radiologist must be able to recognise promptly these true benign enhancing tumours!

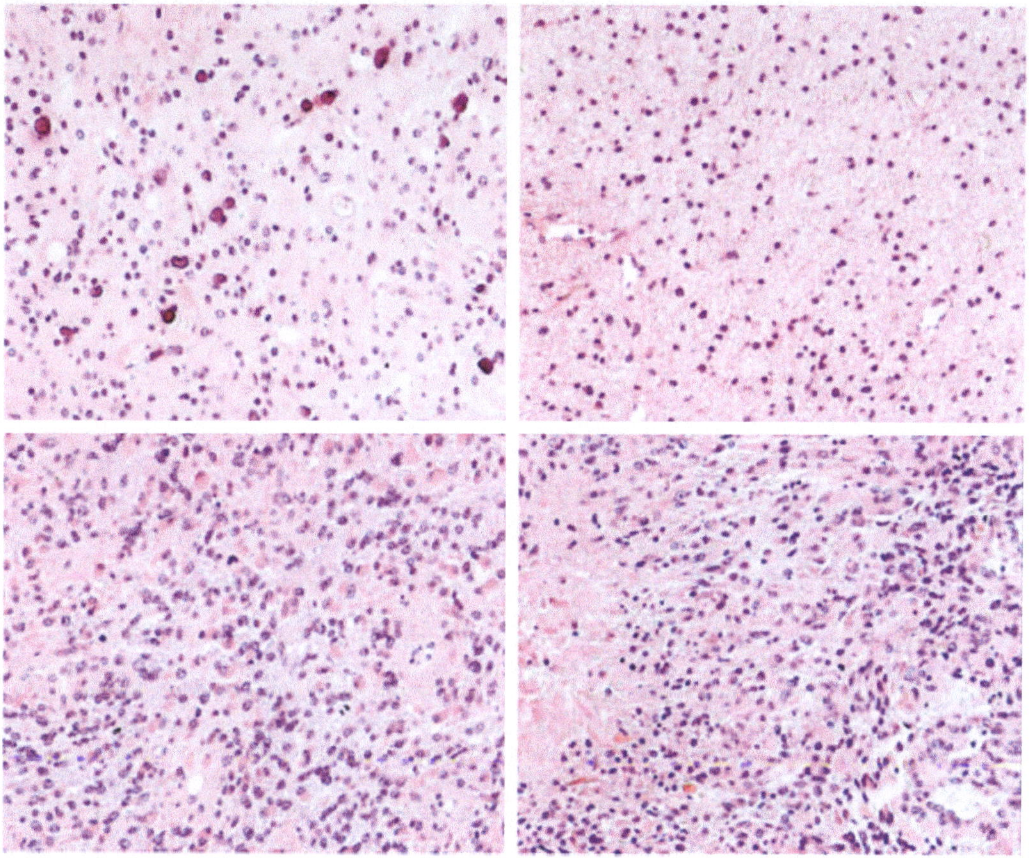

Fig. 28.2.1a–d. Histopathological features of WHO II, III and IV gliomas (haematoxylin-eosin stainings). Presence of cells with round nuclei, small branching vessels and microcalcifications are typical features of WHO II oligodendroglioma (**a**). Presence of mature astrocytes with fibrillary prolonging, low cellularity, small vessels and absence of mitoses are characteristic features of WHO II fibrillary astrocytoma (**b**). In contrast to grade II astrocytoma, higher cellularity, greater nuclear pleomorphism and scattered mitoses are seen in WHO III anaplastic astrocytoma (**c**). The MIB-1 labelling index is usually greater than 3% in grade III. The WHO system assigns a malignant glioma to WHO IV glioblastoma (**d**) when necrosis and microvascular proliferations are also present. In the left side of this section, palisading of small undifferentiated cells surround necrosis, while vascular proliferations in the viable part of the tumour are on the right lower corner of the picture

Oligodendrogliomas are tumours originating from oligodendrocytes or their precursors. Oligoastrocytomas have composite histologic features, reflecting both oligodendrocytic and astrocytic cells. With the recognition that these tumours may be particularly sensitive to chemotherapy, neuropathologists have made a greater effort to identify them. The recent demonstration that many oligodendrogliomas and oligoastrocytomas have deletion of 1p and 19q chromosomes, and that these molecular changes are linked to chemosensitivity (Smith et al. 2000), has enhanced the efforts to identify them. An estimate suggests that they represent approximately 20% of glial neoplasms (Fortin et al. 1999). Oligodendrogliomas are moderately cellular and composed of monotonous round, homogeneous nuclei with a clear cytoplasm. They have a dense network of branching capillaries. It is not rare for oligodendrogliomas to bleed, and they may present as an intracranial haemorrhage. Additional features include microcalcifications and macrocalcifications, and mucoid/cystic degeneration. The appearance of significant mitotic activity, prominent microvascular proliferation or necrosis indicates progression to high-grade oligodendroglioma (WHO grade III). Oligodendrogliomas grow diffusely in the cortex and white matter. Circumscribed leptomeningeal infiltration may induce a marked desmoplastic reaction.

The median survival of patients with low-grade astrocytomas is 5 years. However, the range of survival is broad and unpredictable (BAUMAN et al. 1999). Most patients die from progression to high-grade glioma. Studies of patients with oligodendrogliomas reported a median survival of about 10 years. A recent series of 106 patients yielded a median survival of 16 years (OLSON et al. 2000), probably due to earlier diagnosis after the advent of MRI.

28.3 Conventional MR Imaging

In the last three decades the development of more sophisticated and advanced imaging techniques has led to improved diagnostic accuracy. CT and MR imaging enable doctors to diagnose brain tumours that previously might have been incorrectly diagnosed as strokes, senile dementia, multiple sclerosis or other neurologic disorders. The sensitivity of MR imaging to detect intracranial neoplasms is very high, and it has been generally recognised as the imaging study of choice. When a large lesion is detected, this is the first question to be answered: "Is it a tumour?" The recognition of mechanical effects and structural deformities that can be explained as infiltration of brain tissue or growth of the lesion are summarised in one sentence: "There is a mass." The second question is: "What type of tumour is it?" Characterisation of the lesion includes distinction between intra-axial and extra-axial masses. The former is growing from inside, infiltrates and swells the brain tissue. The latter is growing from cells that are outside of the brain tissue, such as meninges (meningioma), nerve sheaths (schwannoma, neurofibroma), hypophysis (adenoma and craniopharyngioma), pineal gland (pineocytoma, pineoblastoma), germ cells (germinoma, teratoma, dermoid, epidermoid). Other tumours such as lymphoma and metastasis can grow as extra-axial as well as intra-axial masses.

The multiplanar capability of MR imaging has certainly improved our ability to localise a lesion and make that distinction. Unfortunately, the progress of MR imaging in specificity of brain tumour evaluation still has not paralleled its gains in sensitivity and anatomic localisation. Notwithstanding, MR imaging provides significant information about intrinsic tissue characterisation that the radiologist should exploit for determining tumour type and biological grade. The ability of MRI to discriminate differences in tissue by variations in signal intensities with multiple contrast techniques (i.e., T1, T2, PD, diffusion) parallels at least gross pathology examination in the majority of cases. The identification of haemorrhagic or necrotic components within the tumour is an important diagnostic and prognostic sign. The association of cysts with certain neoplasms may be helpful for the diagnosis and for planning surgical approach. The presence of fat (hyperintense on T1-weighted images) is specific for certain neoplasms: teratoma, dermoid, lipoma). There are clues and tricks that aid in the diagnosis of fat in tumours. One clue is the recognition of "chemical shift artefact" that is an artefact displayed as signal void at fat–water interfaces and hyperintensity at water–fat interfaces, along the frequency-encoding axis. One trick is the use of fat-selective suppression methods. The recognition of anomalous blood vessels within a presumed neoplasm is another important prognostic sign, because it is diagnostic of a high-grade tumour.

28.3.1 Growth and Signal Intensity Patterns

A very important distinction is made evaluating signal changes at the boundary of the mass: some intra-axial CNS tumours are relatively discrete; others are infiltrative. A discrete mass will show a defined transition zone between the lesion and the presumed adjacent brain tissue. An infiltrating mass will have a smoother and ill-defined transition zone with areas with subtle signal abnormalities in the presumed adjacent normal brain tissue. Most CNS tumours express one of these two growth patterns. A list of intra-axial brain tumours subdivided according to their prevalent growth pattern is reported in Table 28.2.

Table 28.2 A list of brain tumours divided according to infiltrative or circumscribed pattern of growth

Infiltrative	Circumscribed
Diffuse astrocytoma (WHO II)	Pilocytic astrocytoma
Oligodendroglioma (WHO II)	Ganglion cell tumour
Anaplastic astrocytoma (WHO III)	Pleomorphic xanthoastrocytoma
Glioblastoma multiforme (WHO IV)	Ependymoma
Gliomatosis cerebri	Dysembryoplastic neuroepithelial tumour (DNET)
Primary central nervous system lymphoma	Central neurocytoma Subependymoma Choroid plexus papilloma and carcinoma

The characteristic appearance of an astrocytoma (WHO grade II) is that of a diffuse, non-enhancing mass that is hypointense on T1-weighted images and hyperintense on PD-weighted and T2-weighted images. The hallmark of an astrocytoma is that of a highly infiltrative and non-destructive neoplasm with radiologically distinct borders. In young adults an astrocytoma frequently involves the fronto-insular-temporal crossroad (Fig. 28.4.1). Oedema is virtually absent. In those astrocytomas that infiltrate the cortex, the use of fluid attenuated inversion recovery (FLAIR) images better outlines the mass against normal brain cortex, disclosing abnormal signal that reaches the surface of the brain. The distinction between astrocytoma and oligodendrogliomas is often difficult: signal intensity pattern and location are not distinguishing features. The presence of intra-tumoral haemorrhages and/or areas of cystic degeneration in a well-demarcated benign-appearing mass are suggestive of oligodendroglioma. The occasional finding of scalloping in the overlying calvaria is suggestive of a relatively slow-growing mass. Calcification is more common in oligodendroglioma than astrocytoma, but it is not diagnostic (Fig. 28.4.2). Contrast enhancement is usually mild and poorly defined. It is found in nearly half the cases of low-grade oligodendroglioma (Lee and van Tassel 1989).

28.3.2 Blood–Brain Barrier Integrity Evaluation

The next step in evaluating the signal features of a mass is whether there are signs of blood–brain barrier disruption and immaturity. The brain interstitium is highly dependent on a constant internal milieu. The concept of blood–brain barrier was postulated by Goldmann in 1913 and only later confirmed by electron microscopy studies in 1960. Cerebral endothelial cells have highly differentiated features: tight junctions, continuous basement membranes,

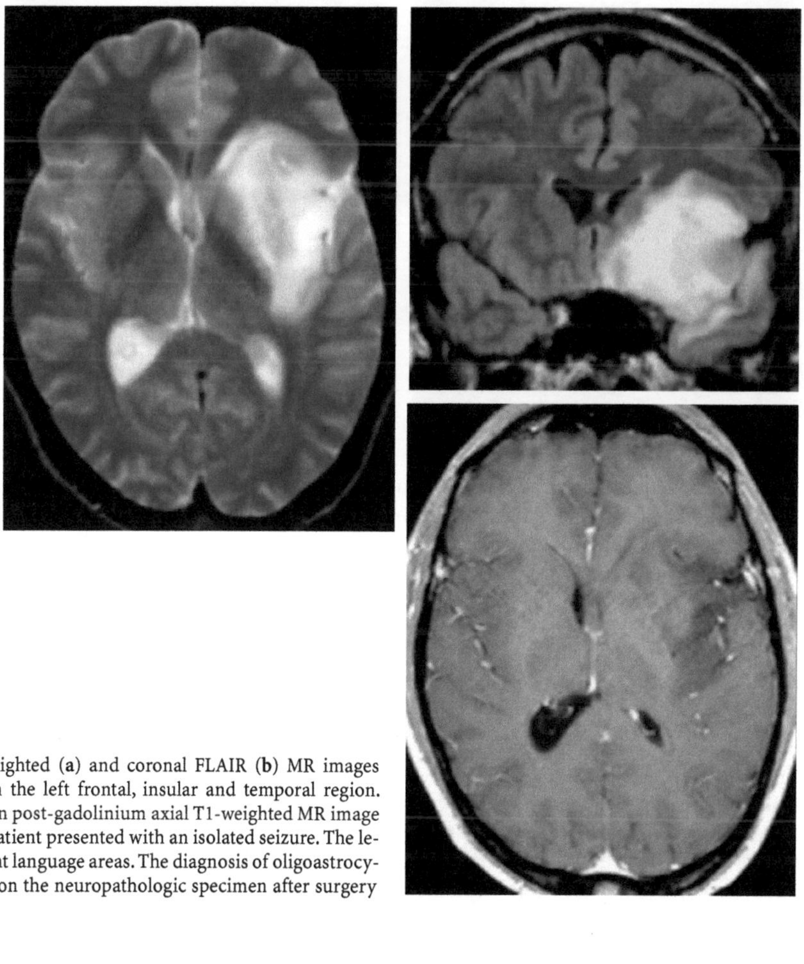

a b c

Fig. 28.4.1a–c. Axial T2-weighted (**a**) and coronal FLAIR (**b**) MR images showing a mass located in the left frontal, insular and temporal region. There is no enhancement on post-gadolinium axial T1-weighted MR image (**c**). The 33-year-old male patient presented with an isolated seizure. The lesion is very close to eloquent language areas. The diagnosis of oligoastrocytoma (WHO II) was made on the neuropathologic specimen after surgery

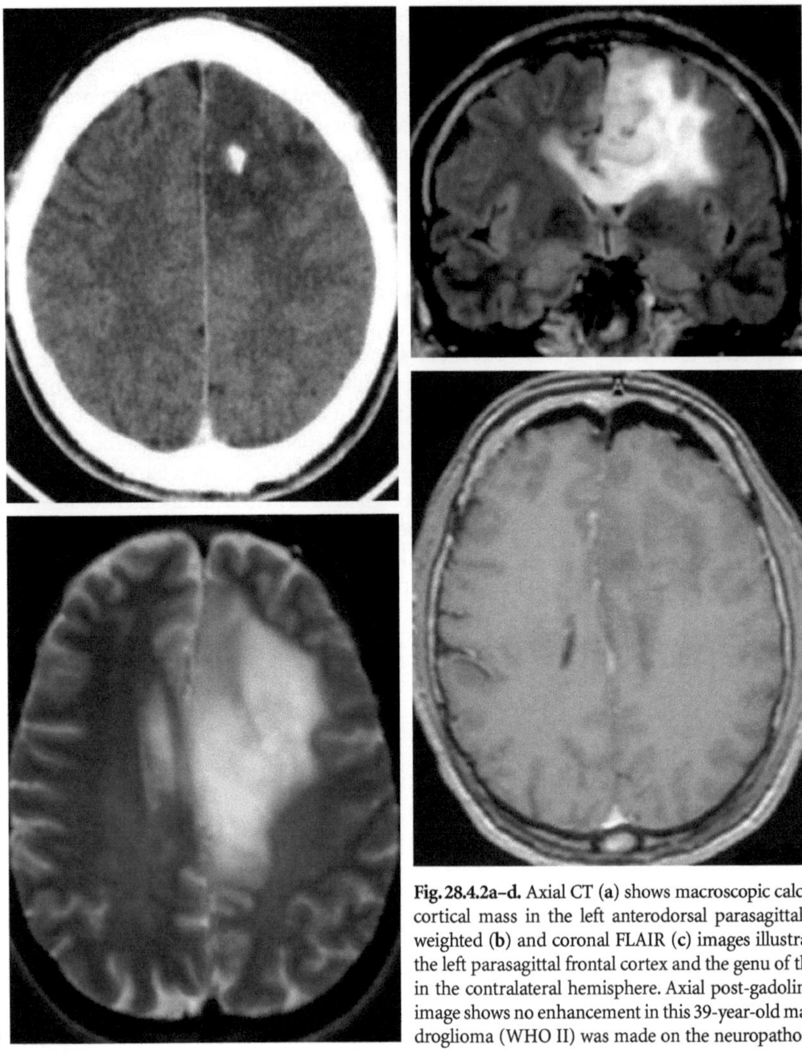

a b c d

Fig. 28.4.2a–d. Axial CT (**a**) shows macroscopic calcifications within a hypodense cortical mass in the left anterodorsal parasagittal frontal cortex. Axial SE T2-weighted (**b**) and coronal FLAIR (**c**) images illustrate a mass that has infiltrated the left parasagittal frontal cortex and the genu of the corpus callosum extending in the contralateral hemisphere. Axial post-gadolinium SE T1-weighted (**d**) MR image shows no enhancement in this 39-year-old male. The diagnosis of oligodendroglioma (WHO II) was made on the neuropathologic specimen after surgery

narrow intercellular gaps and a paucity of pinocytosis. Endothelial cells are also closely enveloped by astrocytic foot processes. Altogether, these structures form a continuous wall that prevents undesired protein molecules from diffusing from the bloodstream into the interstitium. The capillaries are impermeable to intravascularly injected contrast agents in normal brain and areas of intact blood–brain barrier.

Most discrete intra-axial masses show typically intense "enhancement" after injection of contrast agents, with only few exceptions. The presence of enhancement is not necessarily a sign of poor prognosis in this group. There is a long list of circumscribed masses that show variable degrees of enhancement: pilocytic astrocytoma (Fig. 28.4.3), pleomorphic xanthoastrocytoma (Fig. 28.4.4), subependymal giant cell astrocytoma, dysembryoplastic neuroepithelial tumour (DNET), ganglioglioma, central neurocytoma. It is mandatory to recognise these tumours that have a benign prognosis.

On the other hand, diffuse infiltrating neoplasms start showing scattered signs of enhancement when they are shifting to a higher grade of malignancy. Evidence of blood–brain barrier immaturity often correlates with shorter survival and shorter time to recurrence after surgery. This is particularly true for astrocytoma. Enhancement is present in over 95% of glioblastoma, in over 60% of anaplastic astrocytoma and in less than 10% of grade II astrocytoma. The presence of tumour capillaries deficient in blood–

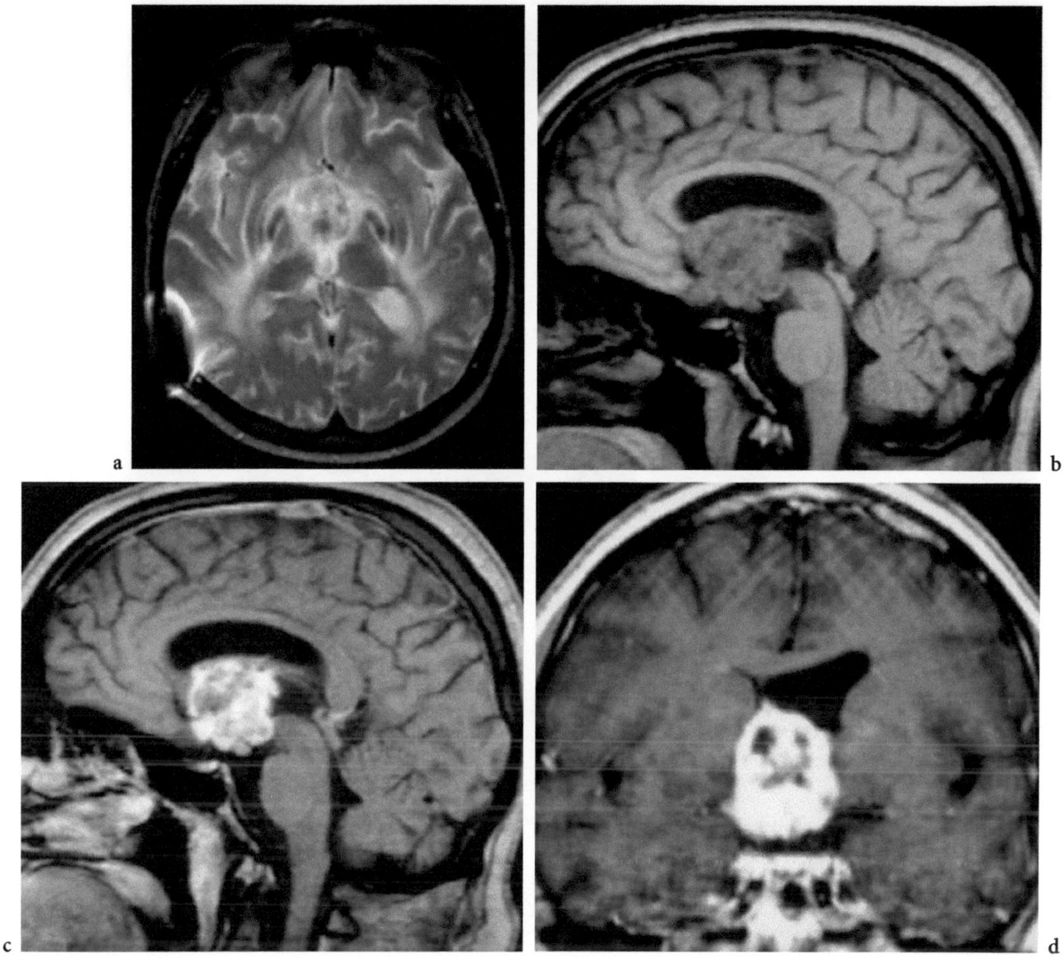

Fig. 28.4.3 a–d Axial (**a**) SE T2-weighted and sagittal (**b**) SE T1-weighted MR images showing a round mass in the third ventricle. Sagittal (**c**) and coronal (**d**) post-gadolinium SE T1-weighted MR images show enhancement in this 21-year-old male. The mass caused obstruction of the foramen of Monro with moderate dilatation of the lateral ventricles. A ventriculoperitoneal shunt was placed before surgery to decompress the ventricles. The diagnosis of pilocytic astrocytoma (WHO I) was made on the neuropathologic specimen after surgery

brain barrier constituents in zones where angiogenesis is most active, rather than destruction of the blood–brain barrier is the most likely explanation for tumour enhancement in glioma. Enhancement is almost always present in metastasis and meningioma. The former enhances since its own capillaries do not have tight junctions and continuous basement membranes. Metastases usually grow at the grey–white matter junction and tend to cavitate when the blood supply becomes insufficient, causing nutrient depletion, and a necrotic core develops. Metastasis is the second most common tumour of the brain, accounting for 30% of intracerebral tumours. In order of prevalence, the most common primary sites are: bronchogenic carcinoma (50%), breast (20%), colon and rectum (15%), kidney (10%) and melanoma (10%). In about 40% of intracerebral metastasis cases the primary location is unknown at time of diagnosis. In one-third of these cases, the primary site remains unknown despite extensive work-up. Metastases usually present as a ring-enhancing mass lesion (Fig. 28.4.5). They must be differentiated from glioblastoma, lymphoma and abscess.

Meningiomas are generally slow-growing tumours originating from meningothelial arachnoid cap cells. They virtually always enhance, because their capil-

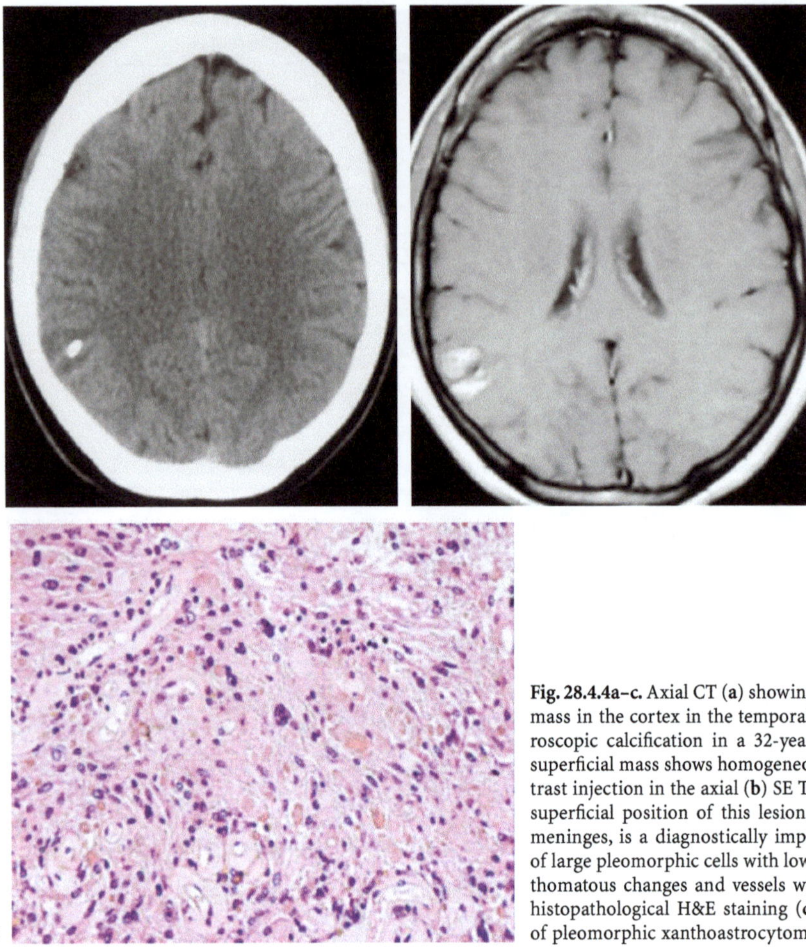

Fig. 28.4.4a–c. Axial CT (**a**) showing a small, round hypodense mass in the cortex in the temporal-parietal region with macroscopic calcification in a 32-year-old female. The discrete, superficial mass shows homogeneous enhancement after contrast injection in the axial (**b**) SE T1-weighted MR image. The superficial position of this lesion, often invading the leptomeninges, is a diagnostically important feature. The finding of large pleomorphic cells with low mitotic activity, focal xanthomatous changes and vessels with hyalinized walls on the histopathological H&E staining (**c**) confirmed the diagnosis of pleomorphic xanthoastrocytoma (WHO I)

laries do not have a blood-brain barrier. They are easier to diagnose since they are extra-axial masses that imprint the brain. They account for about 20% of intracerebral tumours. Those with low risk of recurrence and aggressive growth may displace the adjacent brain tissue without inducing any signal change in the brain tissue. The appearance of T2-weighted signal abnormality in the adjacent brain tissue suggests a more aggressive type of meningioma, and this aspect is often observed in "atypical" meningiomas). The hyperintensity is due to the formation of vasogenic oedema with diffusion of serum proteins, probably induced by the metalloproteinases. These proteins are endopeptidases that can degrade the extracellular matrix, break the basal membrane and alter the blood-brain barrier. Thus, they can play a role in tumour invasion and oedema (Nordqvist et al. 2001; Paek et al. 2002).

28.3.3 Tumour Size and Survival

Measuring a mass is often considered a secondary task for most radiologists. However, it is important for evaluating tumour growth and response to multiple treatment strategies. Assessing prognostic variables, tumour size, in particular, is essential to ongoing clinical trials. Patients likely to benefit from a given treatment can be included, while those who may not could avoid receiving related toxicities. The ideal measuring technique should be accurate, easy and low time-consuming to perform, allowing low intra-observer and inter-observer variations. It's intuitive that a three-dimensional (3D) volumetric measurement method obtained calculating tumour size on all sections would be more accurate than 1D or 2D methods obtained on a single selected section.

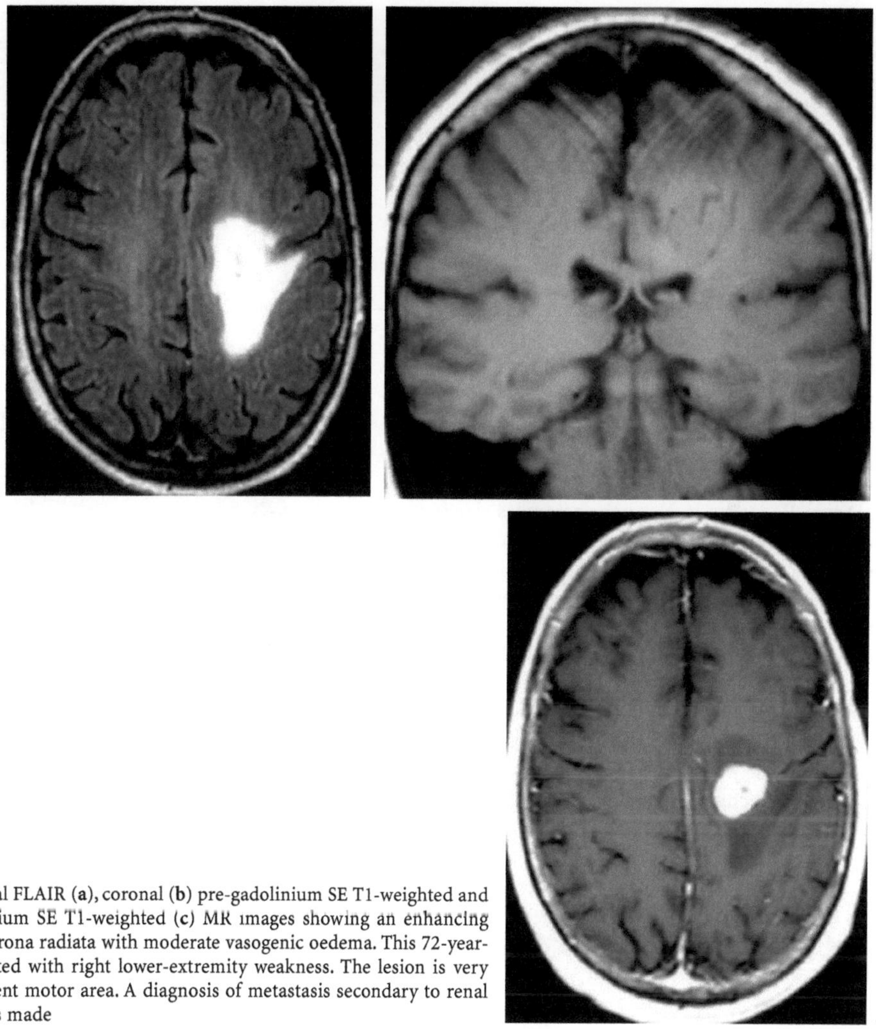

Fig. 28.4.5a–c. Axial FLAIR (a), coronal (b) pre-gadolinium SE T1-weighted and axial post-gadolinium SE T1-weighted (c) MR images showing an enhancing mass in the left corona radiata with moderate vasogenic oedema. This 72-year-old female presented with right lower-extremity weakness. The lesion is very close to the eloquent motor area. A diagnosis of metastasis secondary to renal cell carcinoma was made

However, it is time-consuming. Most internationally accepted protocols devised to standardise response assessment in solid tumours and in supratentorial glioma advise using one-dimensional or two-dimensional measurement of tumour size. The 1D technique measures the longest diameter through the enhancing area on the slice showing the largest area of enhancement. The 2D technique measures the 1D measurement multiplied by the longest perpendicular diameter to this through the area of enhancement. Both techniques are indirect measures of tumour bulk and have largely been adopted on the basis of neoplasms' roughly spherical shape. While this may be the case for most soft-tissue neoplasms, high-grade gliomas are very infiltrating, heterogeneous lesions with irregular shape. Warren et al. investigated whether 3D rather than 1D or 2D measurements better correlated with responses to treatment in 32 children with primary brain tumours (Warren et al. 2001). They found little difference in the detection of partial responses to treatment, although the results suggested volumetric estimates agreed more closely with clinical estimates of progression-free survival than either 1D or 2D measures.

The prognosis of many systemic solid tumours is inversely related to the size of the original lesion. This is not often the case for brain tumours. The low predictive value of size in high-grade glioma has important implications also to justify indication of surgical cytoreduction. Factors such as age, histologic grade and preoperative Karnofsky performance status can exert a fourfold change in survival, and the potential benefit of surgery cannot compensate for a difference of this magnitude. In the literature there are few studies that have determined the relationship between tumour size and prognosis in primary brain tumours. Most of them have evaluated the enhancing component of the mass on T1-weighted MR images of high-grade glioma (Reeves and Marks 1979; Chow et al. 2000; Warren et al. 2001). The findings of these few studies are inconsistent. In 1979 Reeves and Marks (1979) found that lesion size did not predict survival in a population of 56 glioblastoma multiforme (GBM). In 2000 Chow et al. found that enhancing tumour size at the time of recurrence diagnosis was significant for predicting survival following intra-arterial chemotherapy in a population of 41 recurrent high grade glioma (Chow et al. 2000). These controversial results might be due to inherent errors of the 1D and 2D methods. Nevertheless, mass size (or volume) will remain one of the most accessible pieces of information provided by neuroimaging. What the neuro-oncologist really needs to know is whether there is evidence of response to chemotherapy in a defined population. For example, if only smaller tumours respond, the maximum size we should treat with a specific chemotherapy protocol has to be determined. These considerations emphasize the need of optimising a standard, accurate, fast and possibly automated technique to include reliable tumour size as an outcome measure.

28.4 MR Spectroscopic Imaging

The excellent soft-tissue contrast of MR makes it the modality of choice for evaluation of mass lesions in the brain. A conventional MR imaging study confirms the presence of an abnormality, determines the location and apparent size of the tumour and assesses the integrity of the blood–brain barrier. In most medical centres neurosurgeons and neuro-oncologists make their management decisions or plan their therapeutic intervention after carefully reviewing anatomical MR images. Although this may be adequate for some lesions, it is recognised that conventional MRI has several limitations: it cannot distinguish tumour from oedema, since they both appear bright on T2-weighted images. It cannot accurately define the boundary that separates infiltrating tumour from adjacent functional reactive brain tissue; and it cannot rank in order of malignancy the zones of a heterogeneous tumour.

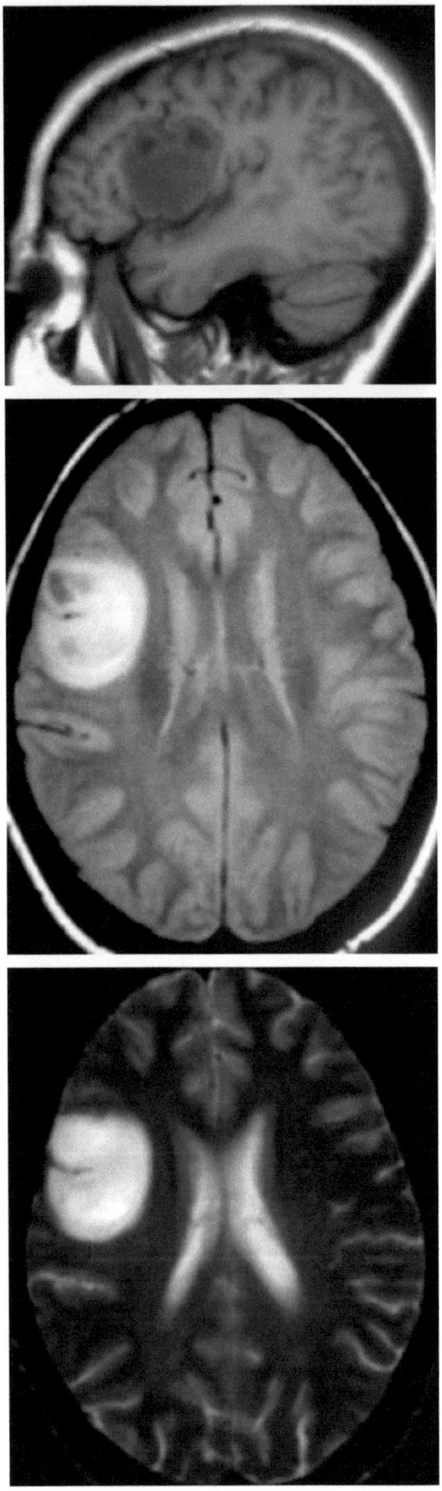

a b c

Fig. 28.7.1 a–c ▷▷

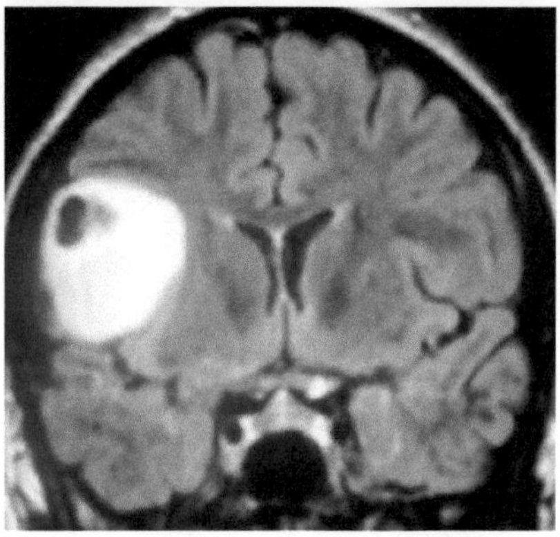
d

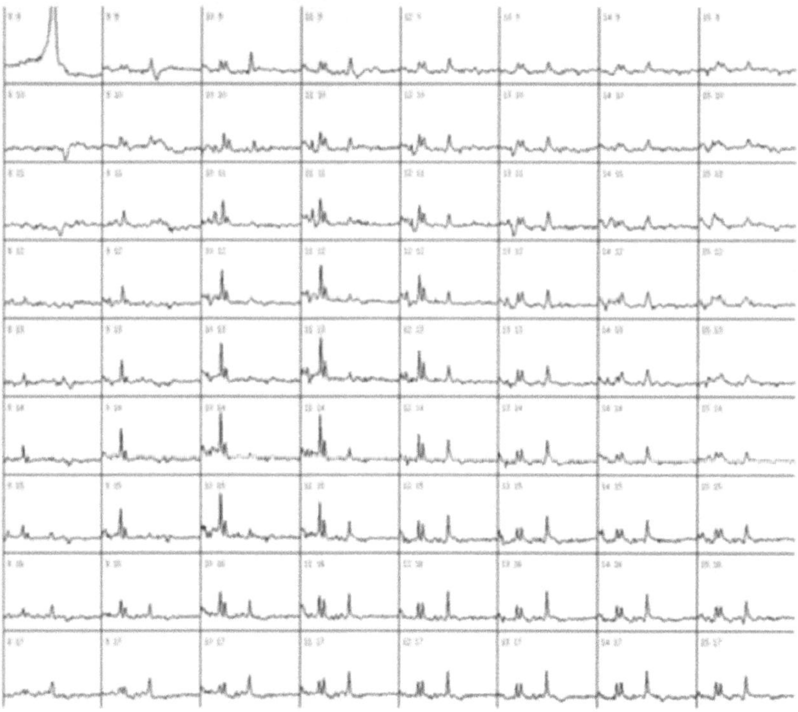
e

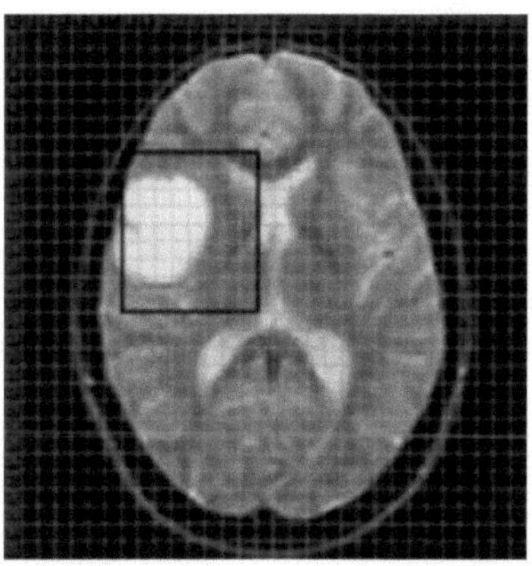
f

Fig. 28.7.1a–f. Sagittal SE T1-weighted (**a**), axial SE PD-(**b**) and T2-weighted (**c**) and coronal FLAIR (**d**) MR images showing a well-defined mass in the right inferior frontal and insular region of this 21-year-old female presenting with headache on Christmas Day. A small cystic component is seen in the right superior quadrant of the spherical mass. There was no enhancement after I .V. injection of contrast medium (picture not shown). H-MRSI (**e**) (multivoxel PRESS sequence; TR/TE=1,500/136 ms; 32×32 matrix; FOV=200×200×20 cm^3) shows a homogeneous metabolic lesion with borders well-defined by T2-weighted MR signal abnormalities. The spectra show moderate choline signal elevation with mild signal loss of creatine and NAA. Normal metabolic profile is seen in spectra outside the T2-signal abnormality. The volume of spectra displayed (**e**) are indicated in the reference T2-weighted MR image. The suspected diagnosis of fibrillary astrocytoma (WHO II) was confirmed on the neuropathologic specimen after surgery

Proton MR spectroscopic imaging (^{1}H-MRSI) is a technique that combines the excellent spatial localisation capabilities of MRI with the chemical information of MR spectroscopy. Since the chemical environment influences the resonant frequency of the atomic nuclei, protons from different compounds have different chemical shifts and appear as distinct peaks in the acquired MR spectrum. The main peaks observed in the healthy human brain at field strengths of 1.5 T or 3.0 T are, in order of resonance, myo-inositol (3.55 ppm), choline (3.2 ppm), creatine (3.02 ppm), glutamine and glutamate (2.1 ppm) and N-acetylaspartate (NAA) at 2.02 ppm. NAA is found in neurons, axons and dendrites; creatine (Cr) is found in neurons and glia; choline (Cho) is a building block of cellular membranes. Additional peaks may appear in pathologic areas of the brain: lactate (1.44 ppm) is a sign of hypoxia or necrosis; mobile lipids (1.4 ppm and 0.9 ppm) are found in areas of necrosis.

A multitude of ^{1}H-MRS studies have been published in the literature in the last 15 years (Bruhn et al. 1989; Alger et al. 1990; Demaerel et al. 1991; Fulham et al. 1992; Negendank 1992; Preul et al. 1996; de Edelenyi et al. 2000; Tamiya et al. 2000). These studies have consistently shown that choline signal is elevated in all tumour types because of altered membrane metabolism (Podo 1999; Ackerstaff et al. 2003). Choline signal increases with cellular density, and, according to some authors, also correlates with cellular proliferative activity (Ki-67) (Shimizu et al. 2000; Tamiya et al. 2000). NAA signal loss occurs following substitution of neurons and its prolonging by neoplastic-cell invasion. Changes in creatine signal may vary with the tendency towards a mild increase in low-grade astrocytomas and depletion in the most undifferentiated types.

Several hypotheses have been tested by multiple investigators. The hypothesis that accumulation of lactate may correlate with tumour grade was one of the first investigated. As originally described by Warburg, neoplastic cells may develop bioenergetic aberrations such as elevated anaerobic glycolysis (Warburg 1956). This phenomenon is mainly characteristic of higher grade tumours that have lost aerobic cell respiration, with their metabolism depending mostly on inefficient "anaerobic glycolysis" with relatively higher production of lactate. ^{1}H-MRS studies have shown that lactate accumulation may occur in gliomas; however, it is found only in a minority of tumours, irrespective of grade (Alger et al. 1990). This disappointing finding can be explained with the consideration that efficient lactate clearance in the venous blood stream can prevent lactate accumula-

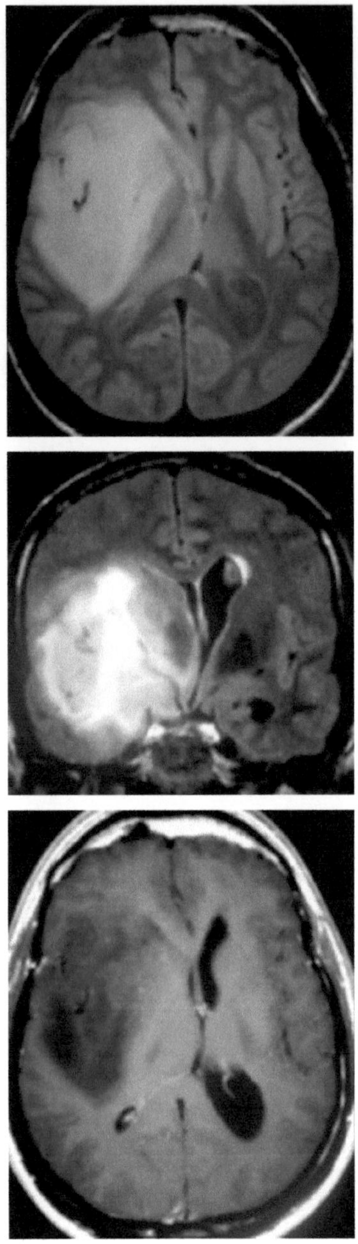

a

b

c

Fig. 28.7.2 a–c ▷▷

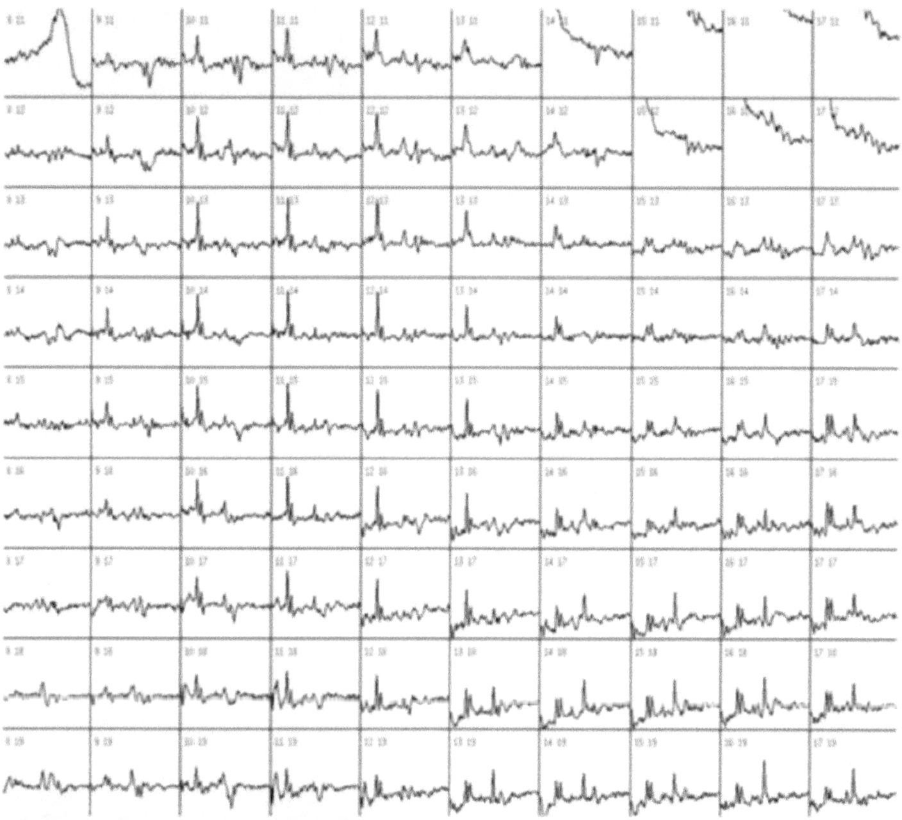

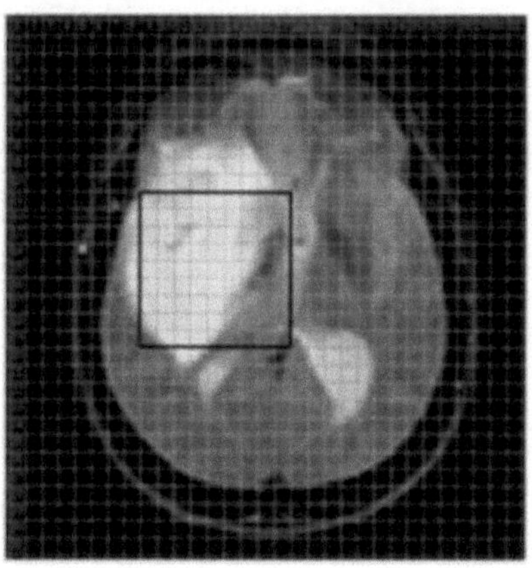

d

Fig. 28.7.2a–d. Axial SE PD-weighted (**a**) and coronal FLAIR (**b**) MR images showing a mass located in the right inferior frontal, temporal and insular region of this 47-year-old male. There is a moderate mass effect, with shifting over the midline. There was no enhancement after I.V. injection of contrast medium on SE T1-weighted MR image (**c**). H-MRSI (**d**) (multivoxel PRESS sequence; TR/TE=1,500/136 ms; 32×32 matrix; FOV=200×200×20 cm3) shows a homogeneous metabolic lesion with borders well-defined by T2-weighted MR signal abnormalities. The spectra show marked choline signal elevation with moderate loss of creatine and almost complete depletion of NAA. There is mild lactate accumulation in a few voxels in the centre of the mass. There is no accumulation of lipids. The volume of spectra displayed (**d**) are indicated in the reference T2-weighted SE MR image. The diagnosis of anaplastic astrocytoma (WHO III) was confirmed on the neuropathologic specimen after surgery tion. Increased lactate is often found within necrotic pseudocysts and in areas of the tumour where venular outflow is obstructed. Lactate is sometimes detected inside a cyst or a necrotic core of glioblastoma and metastasis.

The choline signal has become a novel, important biochemical indicator of tumour progression (FULHAM et al. 1992) and response to therapy (BIZZI et al. 1995). Precursors and catabolites of phospholipid metabolism are altered in tumours. The "choline peak" detected by clinical ^{1}H-MRS is composed of free choline and several choline-containing compounds, such as phosphocholine (PC) and phosphoethanolamine (PE), glycerol 3-phosphocholine (GPC) and glycerol 3-phosphoethanolamine (GPE). Elevation of intracellular phosphomonoesters (PME) PC and PE suggests enhanced cell-membrane synthesis, cellular growth and nutritional state, while increased phosphodiesters (PDE), GPC and GPE represent altered rates of membrane synthesis, catabolism and metabolic turnover. Diverse molecular alterations such as oncogene expression and malignant transformation arrive at common endpoints in choline phospholipid metabolism. They often determine a shift in GPC and PC that results in increasing PC/GPC ratio and total choline-containing metabolite level. Experimental data suggest that increased PC/GPC is primarily related to malignant degeneration. Conversely, reduced PC/GPC is related to growth arrest (BHAKOO et al. 1996). Extract studies have also shown that PC elevation is likely related to malignancy, since it is found at a twofold greater level in high-grade glioma compared with low-grade and normal tissue (USENIUS et al. 1994). Therefore, MRS appears to be more sensitive to up-regulation of the anabolic pathway than to acceleration of catabolic pathways.

In vivo ^{1}H-MRSI has shown that choline signal is increased in the solid portion of brain tumours. One study in 18 glioma patients demonstrated a significant linear correlation between normalised choline (nCho) signal and cell density, not with proliferative index (GUPTA et al. 2000). In the same study a significant inverse linear correlation between cell density and apparent diffusion coefficient (ADC) measured by diffusion MR was also demonstrated. Choline is consistently low in areas of necrosis. A progressive increase in choline signal as a tumour undergoes malignant degeneration has been reported (TEDESCHI et al. 1997). The finding of elevated choline signal in the enhancing rim of a mass does not allow solving the differential diagnosis between GBM, metastases or lymphomas. On the contrary, the identification of high choline in the T2-weighted hyperintense peri-

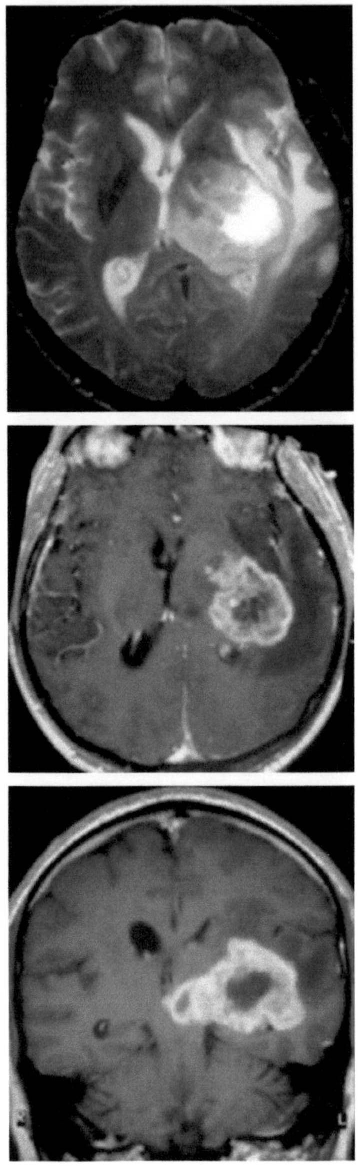
a
b
c

Fig. 28.7.3 a–c ▷▷

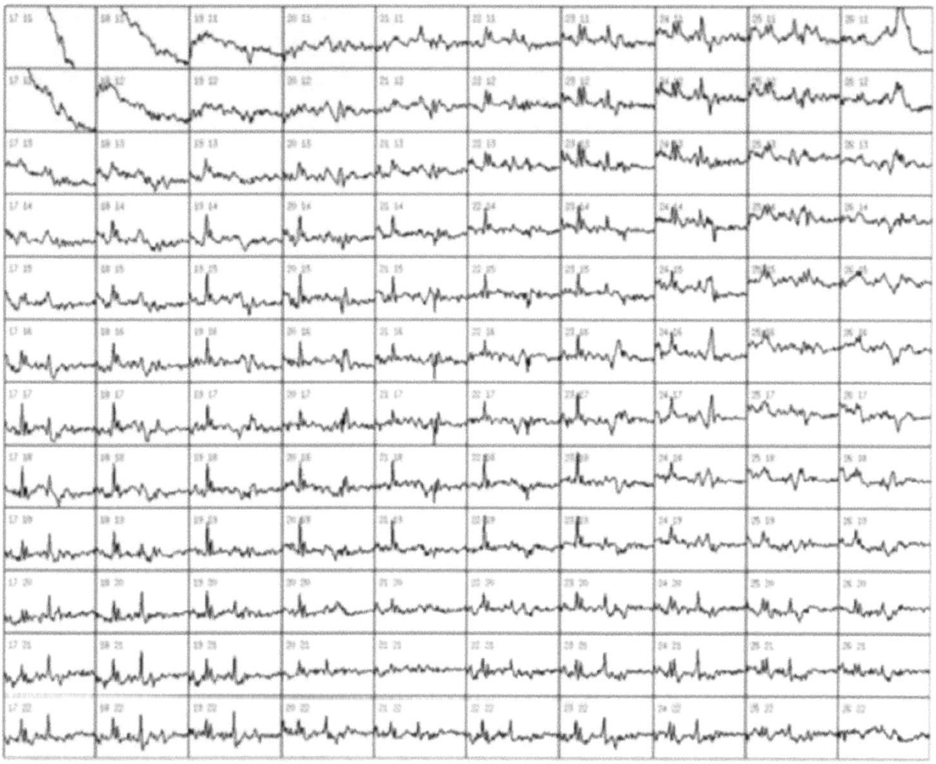

d 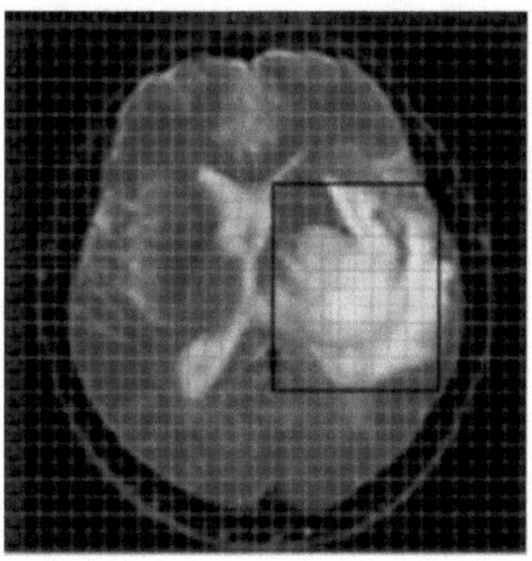

Fig. 28.7.3a–d. Axial SE T2-weighted (**a**) MR image shows a heterogeneous mass in the left basal ganglia, temporal and insular region. Axial (**b**) and coronal (**c**) post-contrast SE T1-weighted MR images show a thick ring of enhancement with a hypointense, likely necrotic, core in this 58-year-old male. There is marked mass effect with shifting over the midline. ^{1}H-MRSI (d) (multivoxel PRESS sequence; TR/TE=1,500/136 ms; 32×32 matrix; FOV=200×200×20 cm3) shows a heterogeneous metabolic lesion with borders ill-defined by T2-weighted MR signal abnormalities. The spectra show marked choline signal elevation with almost complete depletion of NAA and creatine. In the core of the lesion, there are a few voxels with lactate accumulation and others on the right with lipid accumulation. The latter are evidence supporting necrosis. The volume of spectra displayed (**d**) are indicated in the reference T2-weighted SE MR image. The diagnosis of WHO IV glioblastoma multiforme was confirmed on neuropathologic examination enhancing area is suggestive of GBM rather than metastases (LAW et al. 2002).

The finding of abnormal elevated MRS signals resonating at 1.4 ppm and 0.9 ppm indicates presence of lipid droplets in areas of extracellular necrosis (ZOULA et al. 2003). Mobile lipids are often found in the necrotic core of GBM, lymphomas and metastases (KUESEL et al. 1994; POPTANI et al. 1995; SIJENS et al. 1996). Primary cerebral lymphoma in immunocompetent patients mimics the infiltrative behaviour of glial neoplasms. The recognition of lymphoma is difficult with conventional MRI, and it has important diagnostic and therapeutic implications, since chemotherapy and radiotherapy are the treatment of choice and surgery is not effective. The demonstration of high choline with massively elevated lipid resonances associated with absent creatine and NAA signals is the hallmark of cerebral lymphoma (BIZZI et al. 1995; HARTING et al. 2003), but it is not found in all cases. Lipids can also be found in large amounts in areas that have been treated with radiotherapy and have evolved into areas of delayed radiation necrosis.

Questions remain whether ^{1}H-MRSI is a useful technique to determine in vivo the histopathological grade of gliomas. Most multivoxel (^{1}H-MRSI) studies have shown that higher grade tumours have a tendency to show higher choline levels compared with low-grade tumours (FULHAM et al. 1992; PREUL et al. 1996; LI et al. 2002). This is especially true if the voxel with the maximum Cho/NAA ratio is considered in the analysis. In the evaluation of tumour grade we believe that the multivoxel (2D and 3D MR spectroscopic imaging; LI et al. 2002) is superior to the single-voxel technique for at least three reasons. Spectroscopic imaging evaluates spatial heterogeneity, offers a definition of the macroscopic boundary of the mass and is less subjected to partial volume effects. Spectroscopic imaging is helpful in characterising areas with T2-weighted signal hyperintensity: it can point to areas of higher cellular density and it can distinguish areas with prevalent vasogenic oedema from areas with neoplastic invasion or necrosis.

However, in the individual case, assignment of grade becomes difficult, mainly because of overlapping between grade II and III. The biology of glioma during the progression from diffuse astrocytoma to anaplastic then glioblastomas is a spectrum. In neuropathology the arbitrary separation in grades is practical due to clear and simple histopathological criteria that can be applied by all medical centres. So far, with MR spectroscopy it has not been possible to set cut-off ratios that could be reliably used and compared by multiple groups.

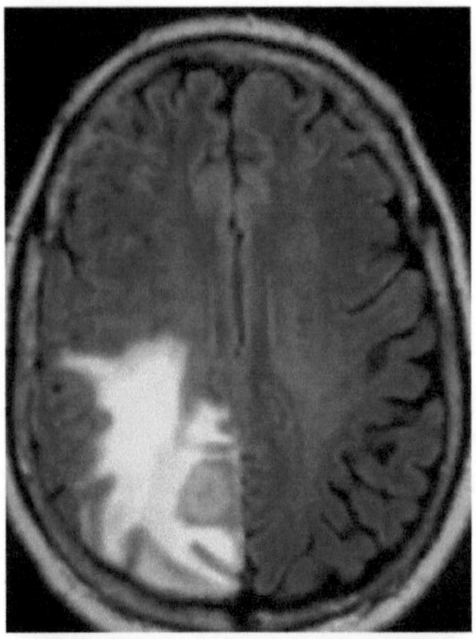

a

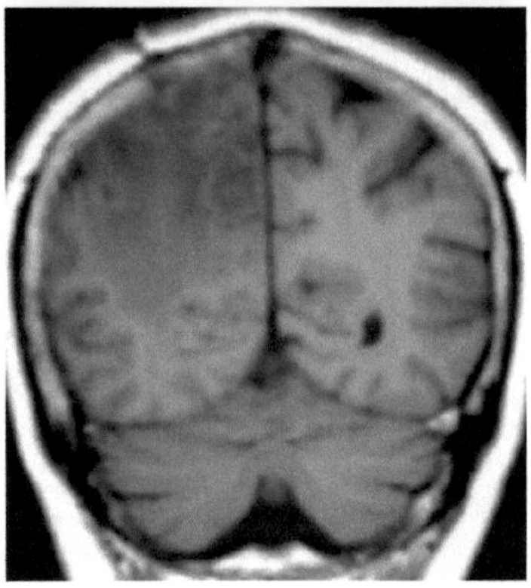

b

Fig. 28.7.3 a,b ▷▷

It is then useful to consider that during the transition from diffuse to anaplastic astrocytoma the Cho signal progressively increases while NAA is decreasing, until the Cho/NAA reaches a plateau at blown anaplastic astrocytoma. Glioblastoma tends to show the highest Cho/NAA levels when they are still well perfused and oxygenated. Then the formation of hypoxic areas within the mass causes a significant drop of Cho signal and the appearance of lipid signals. In this spectrum the creatine signal also has a say. In well-differentiated and oxygenated astrocytomas creatine shows usually normal or slightly elevated levels, then its signal drops significantly. This depletion in creatine usually precedes choline signal drop.

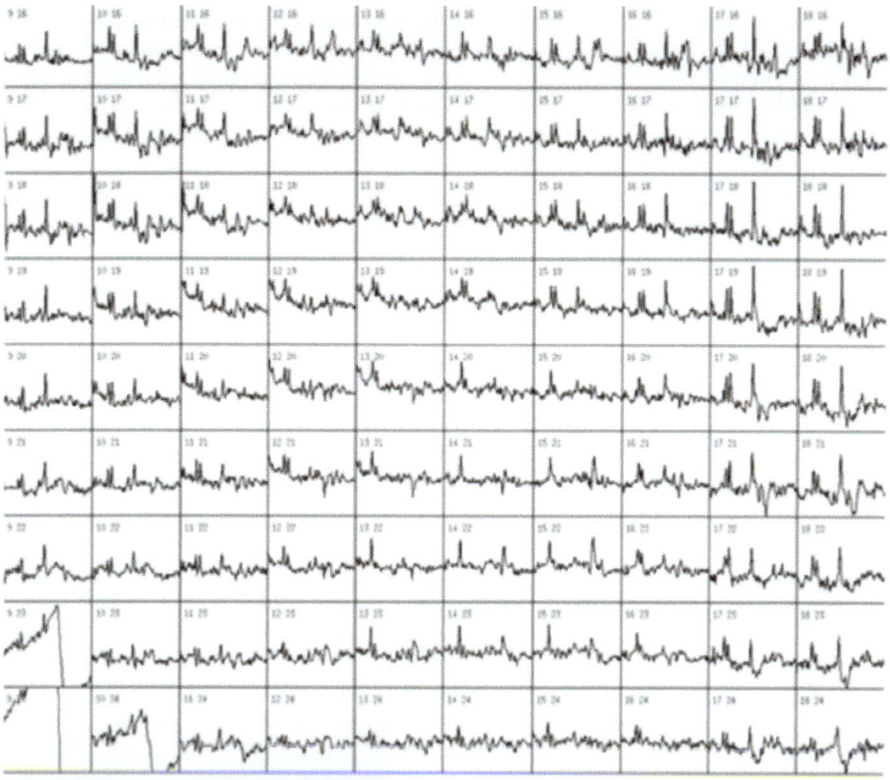

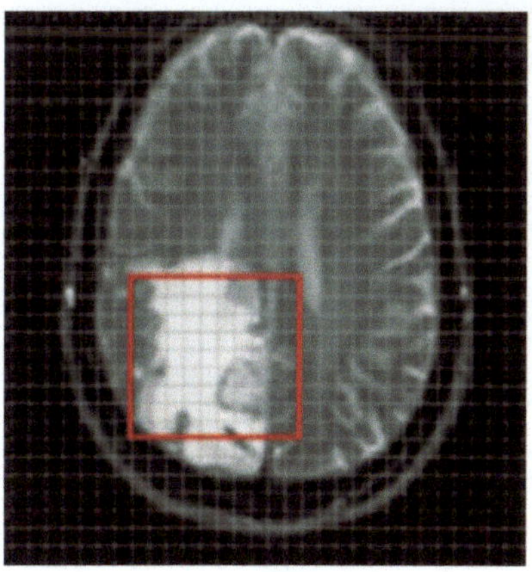

c

Fig. 28.7.4 a–c Axial FLAIR (**a**) and coronal (**b**) SE T1-weighted MR images showing a small mass in the right parasagittal occipital lobe. The mass showed a ring of enhancement on post-contrast T1-weighted SE MR image (picture not shown) with an extensive area of T2-weighted hyperintensity around it in this 41-year-old male. ^{1}H-MRSI (**c**) (multivoxel PRESS sequence; TR/TE=1,500/136 ms; 32×32 matrix; FOV= 200×200×20 cm3) shows a heterogeneous metabolic lesion with elevated choline signal in the voxel corresponding to the ring of enhancement. Note the presence of elevated lipid signal in the core of the lesion corresponding to the necrotic centre of the lesion. In the extensive area with T2-signal abnormality, there is mild NAA signal loss; choline and creatine are within normal. These findings suggest this to be an area of vasogenic oedema. The volume of spectra displayed (**b**) are indicated in the reference T2-weighted SE MR image. The diagnosis of metastasis was confirmed on neuropathologic examination

Spectroscopic imaging is also particularly useful for defining target volumes for radiotherapy and for evaluating heterogeneous tumour response to therapy. Incorporation of MRSI into the treatment-planning process may have the potential to improve control while reducing complications (Pirzkall et al. 2001).

In patients with high-grade gliomas the most common and significant clinical problem is the definitive diagnosis of tumour recurrence as opposed to delayed radiation necrosis (DRN). ^{1}H-MRSI has been shown to be useful for improving diagnostic acumen, when MRI cannot reliably differentiate between these entities (Taylor et al. 1996; Rock et al. 2002; Schlemmer et al. 2002). In cases of suspected recurrent tumours that have recently changed their MRI signal characteristics since the previous examination, the finding of increased choline suggests the diagnosis of recurrent tumour. Conversely, the absence of voxels with elevated choline within the volumes of T2-signal abnormality or contrast enhancement suggests the diagnosis of DRN. The lipid signal tends to be most elevated in areas of DRN or mixed tumour and necrosis than in pure tumour. ^{1}H-MRSI cannot distinguish either pure tumour or pure necrosis from areas of mixed tumour and necrosis.

28.5 Perfusion MR Imaging

At the time of this writing, perfusion MR imaging is increasingly being used as a diagnostic and research tool. However, it is important to remark that it is still relatively new and promising rather than a standard technique for evaluating tumour grading and malignancy. With very short imaging and data processing times and the use of a standard dose of gadolinium chelate, the differential scanning calorimetry (DSC) method can easily be incorporated into the routine clinical evaluation of brain tumours. Cerebral blood volume (CBV) measurements are a relative rather than an absolute quantification of blood volume. Relative CBV maps can be generated after selecting the arterial input function (AIF) in one of the main feeding vessels (i.e., middle cerebral artery).

In the interpretation of rCBV maps it is very important to correlate them with conventional MR images that may show areas of blood–brain barrier (BBB) disruption or T2* signal loss due to susceptibility effects within the tumour. A severe breakdown

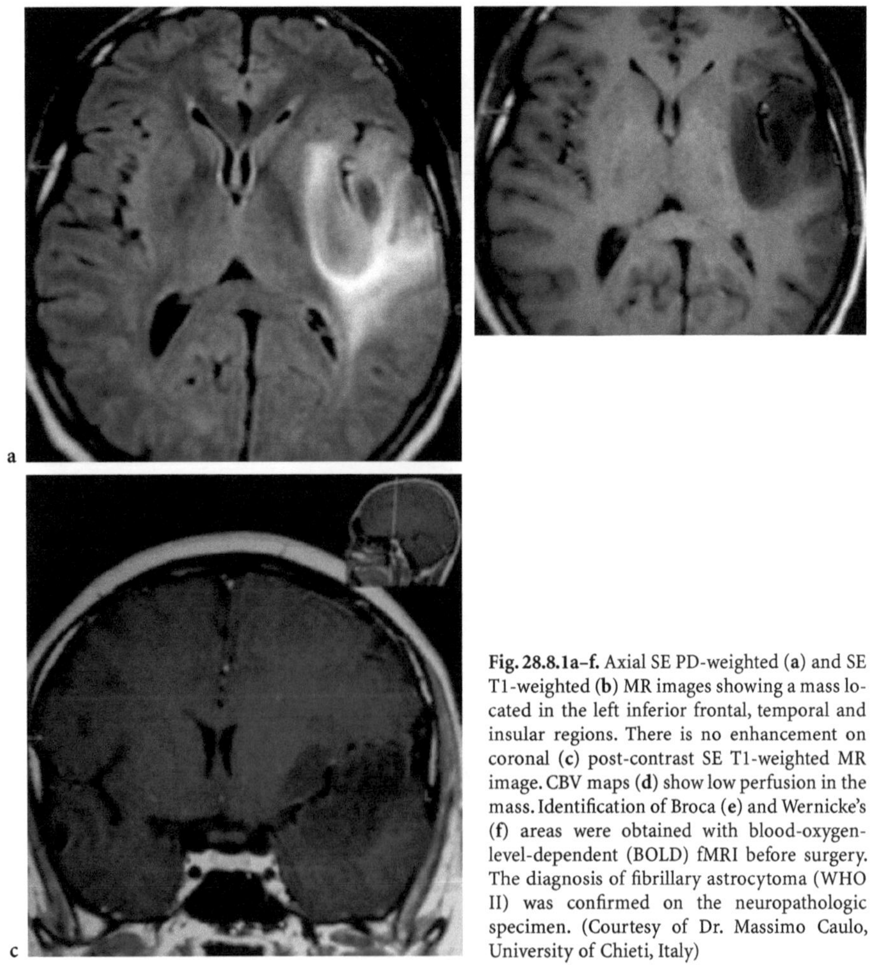

Fig. 28.8.1a–f. Axial SE PD-weighted (**a**) and SE T1-weighted (**b**) MR images showing a mass located in the left inferior frontal, temporal and insular regions. There is no enhancement on coronal (**c**) post-contrast SE T1-weighted MR image. CBV maps (**d**) show low perfusion in the mass. Identification of Broca (**e**) and Wernicke's (**f**) areas were obtained with blood-oxygen-level-dependent (BOLD) fMRI before surgery. The diagnosis of fibrillary astrocytoma (WHO II) was confirmed on the neuropathologic specimen. (Courtesy of Dr. Massimo Caulo, University of Chieti, Italy)

of the BBB may cause inaccurate rCBV estimation in GBM, metastasis, meningioma or lymphoma. In the presence of these lesions it is appropriate to give the patient a small baseline dose of contrast agent before the perfusion study. While conventional T1-weighted MR images show areas of disrupted or absent BBB breakdown, variations in rCBV demonstrate geographic differences within the tumour and are a sign of heterogeneous vascularity.

Several recent studies have found a significant correlation between tumour rCBV and glioma grade (Aronen et al. 1994; Knopp et al. 1999; Roberts et al. 2000; Lev et al. 2004). In a study of 22 patients, all high grade (III and IV) gliomas had normalised CBV values greater than the defined cut-off ratio of 1.5 (Lev et al. 2004). High CBV value was found in a significant number of grade II gliomas that histopathology later showed to be oligodendrogliomas. In the same study correlation with survival was better for CBV than enhancement on T1-weighted MR images. The value of maximum rCBV in a preoperative study of histologically proven GBM may vary over a wide range, but the mean is usually higher than maximum rCBV measured in grade III and II gliomas. This is explained by the larger vascular heterogeneity of GBM with frequent areas of necrosis. The absence of necrosis and the lower vascular heterogeneity explains the lesser variation in maximum rCBV in anaplastic astrocytomas. The finding of low rCBV values in non-enhancing gliomas would add evidence to the preoperative diagnosis of a well-differentiated low-grade II astrocytoma (Fig 28.8.1), while high rCBV values will suggest an undifferentiated anaplastic astrocytoma (Fig. 28.8.2). However,

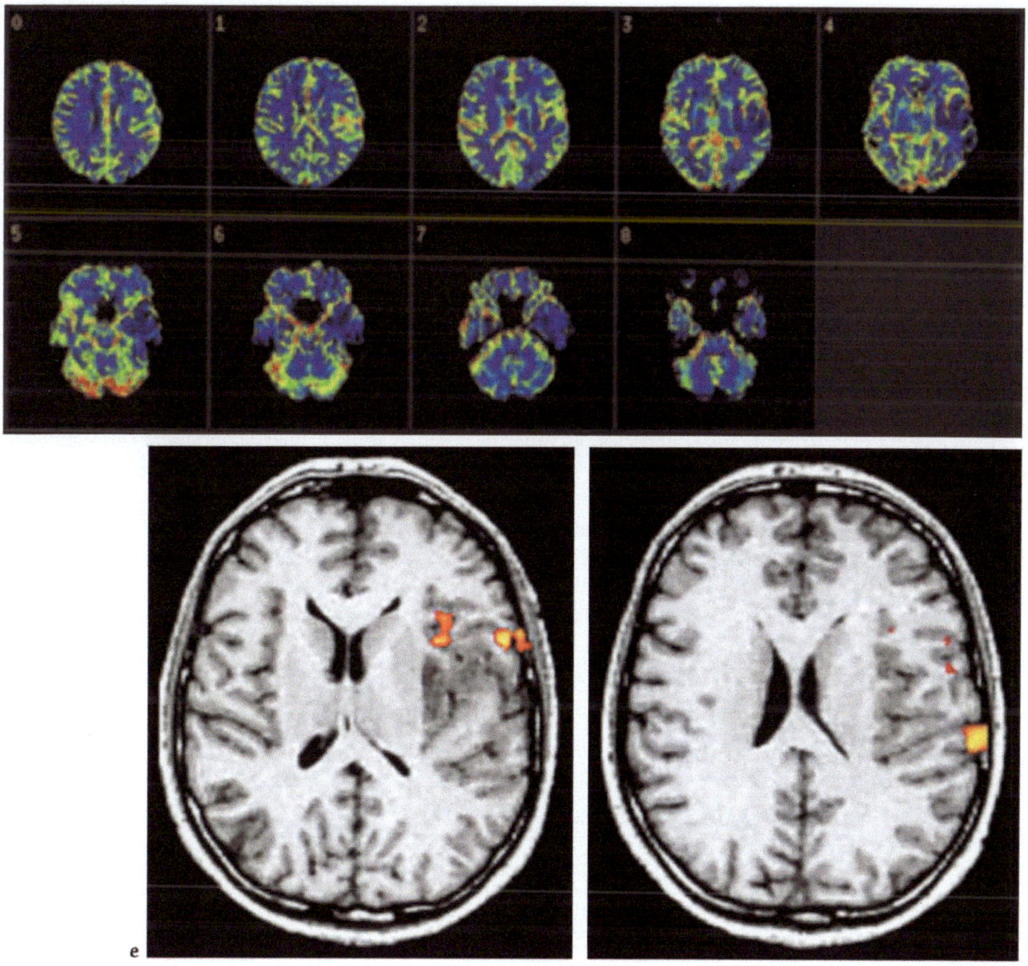

d e f

it is important to emphasize once again that the transition from low-grade to high-grade gliomas is a spectrum without well-established boundaries and that there may be overlap of rCBV values between different glioma grades. In another recent study Law et al. (2003) evaluated sensitivity, specificity and predictive values of perfusion, proton spectroscopic and conventional MR imaging in 106 patients with known histopathologic diagnosis. They showed that rCBV and metabolite ratios (Cho/NAA and Cho/Cr) both individually and in combination can increase the sensitivity and positive predictive values (PPV) in determining grade when compared with conventional MRI alone. The best diagnostic predictor was rCBV. High-grade and low-grade gliomas can be distinguished at the same level of significance also with the arterial spin labelling (ASL) technique (Warmuth et al. 2003). A close linear correlation between DSC-MR and ASL in the tumour region of interest has been demonstrated. Blood flow is underestimated with ASL at low flow rates.

Another application of rCBV maps is guidance of biopsy sampling during stereotactic and open surgery. Foci of increased vascularity within non-enhancing brain glioma can be identified. Zones of higher vascularity are likely to represent the area of the tumour with the highest grade.

Soon et al. have shown that DSC-MRI is a valuable adjunct to conventional imaging also in assessing tumour response during therapy. They have shown that rCBV maps correlate better with clinical follow-up than do gadolinium enhanced T1-weighted MR images, in 18 patients with recurrent GBM receiving an antiangiogenic drug (thalidomide) and carboplatin (Cha et al. 2000).

Preliminary studies have shown that rCBV maps can demonstrate differences in vascularity between delayed radiation necrosis (DRN) and recurrent tumour. These two conditions are easily distinguished by histopathology, but they are often indistinguishable on clinical and conventional imaging grounds. Neovascularity is a distinguished feature of most recurrent GBM and will show as an area of increased rCBV on DSC-MR images. Conversely, the presence of coagulative necrosis mixed with signs of extensive vascular injury is characteristic of DRN that will show up as areas of low rCBV on perfusion images. The ASL method has also shown promising results on the differential diagnosis of DRN vs recurrent GBM, especially in those lesions with areas of T2* magnetic susceptibility due to deposits of hemosiderin or calcium and in lesions near the base of the skull at the air–bone interface.

The contribution of perfusion MRI in the differentiation of GBM, metastasis and lymphoma is still controversial, and additional studies need to be done. As with MR spectroscopic imaging, the finding of increased rCBV in the area around an enhancing mass suggests the diagnosis of glioblastoma rather than a metastasis. In a study of 51 patients (33 gliomas, 18 metastases) the measured rCBV in the peri-tumoral region of high-grade gliomas and metastases was statistically significant: 1.31 ± 0.97 (mean±SD) and 0.39 ± 0.19, respectively (Law et al. 2002). The finding of low rCBV in an enhancing mass suggests the diagnosis of lymphoma, especially when the mass is located in the deep grey matter, subependymal periventricular regions or corpus callosum, which are common locations for primary cerebral lymphoma (Sugahara et al. 1999). On neuropathology lymphoma shows low vascularity despite invasion of the vessel lumina and around endothelial cells of the host. A study of 24 patients demonstrated that rCBV and analysis of the intensity-time curves may be useful in distinguishing primary lymphoma from glioblastoma (Hartmann et al. 2003). The maximum rCBV ratio in lymphoma was significantly lower than that for GBM ($p<0.0001$). Lymphoma showed a characteristic type of curve with a significant increase in signal intensity above the baseline due to massive leakage of contrast media into the interstitial space.

Fig. 28.8.2a–c. Axial FLAIR (**a**) MR images show an infiltrating mass along the left pyramidal tracts in the pons, posterior limb of internal capsule and corona radiata. There is no enhancement on axial (**b**) post-contrast SE T1-weighted MR image. In this patient, high blood volumes on CBV maps (**c**) suggested the diagnosis of anaplastic astrocytoma (WHO III), which was confirmed on the neuropathologic specimen. (Courtesy of Dr. Massimo Caulo, University of Chieti, Italy)

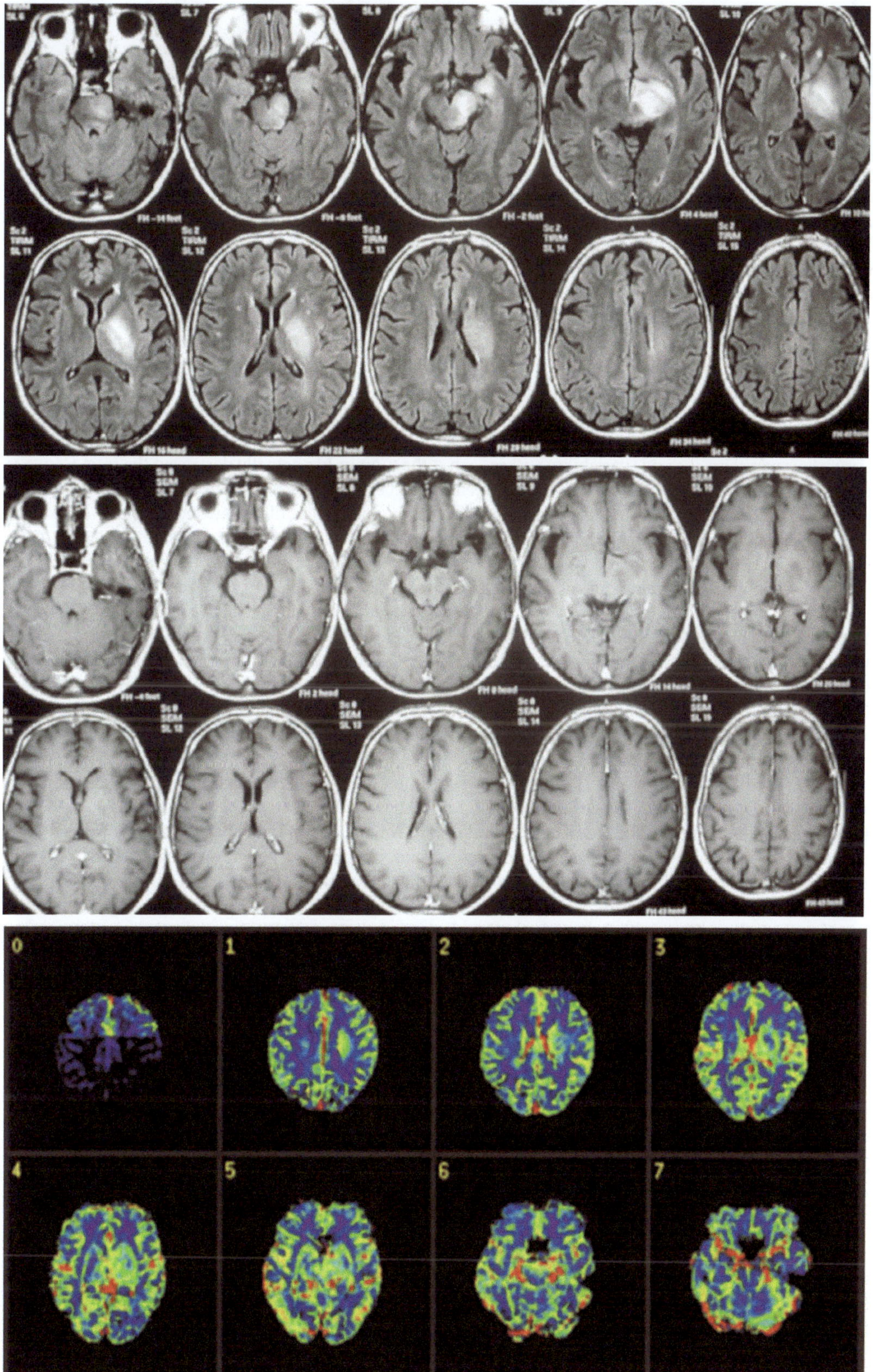

a

b

c

28.6 Diffusion MR and Tractography

Since the pioneering work of the early 1990s, there has been a great interest in the use of diffusion-weighted imaging (DWI) and diffusion-tensor imaging (DTI) to characterise different tumour types and grade. The use of DWI is valuable in the differentiation between epidermoids and arachnoid cysts in the brain (Fig. 28.9.1) and spine. ADC of epidermoid tumours is very low compared to ADC of arachnoid cysts, which is similar to CSF (Tsuruda et al. 1990). Low ADC values are also measured in abscesses due to the viscosity of their contents (Kono et al. 2001). DWI has been much less successful in determining type and grade of a tumour. The majority of brain tumours have higher ADC values than normal brain tissue; however, there is a wide variability within each tumour type and extensive overlap between different types and grades. There is also a large overlap with other brain pathologies. Low-grade astrocytomas have higher ADC values than high-grade gliomas. A steep increase in ADC value may occur when tumour cells start colonising normal tissue, due to extracellular water increase. This change soon becomes visible also on T2-weighted MR images. As cellular density increases the amount of extracellular water diminishes and ADC decreases. In the solid regions of gliomas (Gupta et al. 2000) and meningiomas, a linear correlation between ADC and cellular density has been found. In gliomas Gupta et al. also showed a linear correlation between decreasing ADC and increasing choline values. The highest ADC value within tumours is measured in cystic or necrotic regions (Brunberg et al. 1995). ADC is also quite elevated in areas of vasogenic oedema. In the peri-tumoral region, where T2-weighted signal is abnormal, significantly higher mean diffusivity (MD) and lower fractional anisotropy (FA) than in normal-appearing white matter have been demonstrated. Furthermore, the peri-tumoral MD of metastases measured significantly greater than that of gliomas (Lu et al. 2003). On the other hand peri-tumoral FA measurements showed no significant statistical difference. The higher MD around metastatic lesions may be due to an extracellular water increase greater than in gliomas. The decreasing FA in glioma may be induced by both increased water content and tumour infiltration, which are comparable with the metastasis-related changes caused by increased water content alone. In conclusion, most diffusion studies agree that MD (ADC) is highest in the necrotic tumour core, followed by oedematous brain, non-enhancing tumour component, and enhancing tumour in this order. FA values are reduced in most high-grade tumours. However, in their small series of patients Sinha et al. (2002) have shown that FA added no benefit to tissue differentiation. Conversely, FA may help in understanding the effect of brain tumours on adjacent white matter fibres. A large solitary mass may cause mass effect with distortion of nearby white matter (Fig. 28.9.2). On conventional MR images it might be very difficult to determine whether a prominent and eloquent white matter tract such as the corticospinal tract has been destroyed, infiltrated or simply displaced. Colour-coded DTI and tractography may demonstrate that a large tumour located in the expected position of the pyramidal tract has displaced the tract, changing its orientation (Wieshmann et al. 2000). In a different case, tractography may show that the tumour has actually destroyed the tract (Mori et al. 2002). DTI may indicate that anatomically intact white matter bundles may be present in abnormal-appearing areas of the brain (Witwer et al. 2002). A correlation of this new information with patient clinical deficits before and after tumour surgery will determine the impact of DTI and tractography in surgical planning. It is clear that postoperative preservation of function also depends on identification of white matter tracts that may originate from eloquent cortex and cross a potentially resectable region of the tumour. The potential of delineating white matter pathways serving cortical language sites identified by intraoperative electrocortical language mapping has also been demonstrated (Henry et al. 2004).

Animal and human studies have shown that DWI may be sensitive to monitoring tumour response during radiotherapy and chemotherapy. An early increase in ADC during therapy may suggest therapy-induced necrosis. DWI may also help in differentiating tumour recurrence from delayed radiation injury. Lesions with recurrent tumour showed significantly lower ADC values than lesions without recurrence (Hein et al. 2004).

28.7 Image-Guided Neurosurgery

In neurosurgery it is not always easy to localise a lesion, particularly when it is small, deep seated, and characterised by morphological features similar to the normal brain. As Lars Leksell has said, "No technique in neurosurgery could be too refined, particularly in reference to the ability to localise lesions...".

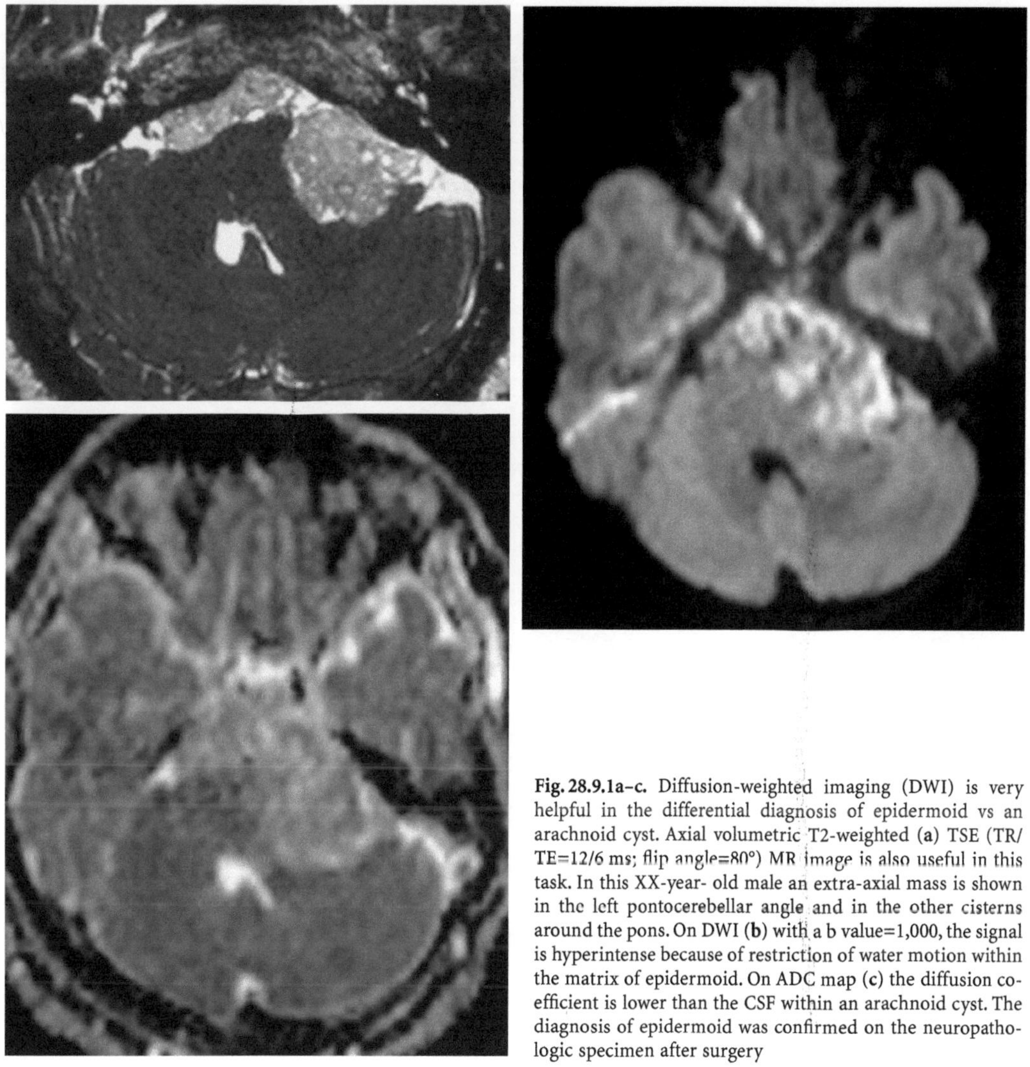

Fig. 28.9.1a–c. Diffusion-weighted imaging (DWI) is very helpful in the differential diagnosis of epidermoid vs an arachnoid cyst. Axial volumetric T2-weighted (a) TSE (TR/TE=12/6 ms; flip angle=80°) MR image is also useful in this task. In this XX-year- old male an extra-axial mass is shown in the left pontocerebellar angle and in the other cisterns around the pons. On DWI (b) with a b value=1,000, the signal is hyperintense because of restriction of water motion within the matrix of epidermoid. On ADC map (c) the diffusion coefficient is lower than the CSF within an arachnoid cyst. The diagnosis of epidermoid was confirmed on the neuropathologic specimen after surgery

Little data substantiate the assertion that "Cytoreductive surgery is essential" in most patients with glioma (Kowalczuk et al. 1997). Whether surgical resection impacts survival is, however, nearly irrelevant to the practising neuro-oncologist. Beginning any protocol of brain tumour treatment after surgical resection whenever possible is in the best interests of the patient, regardless of whether the subsequent survival interval is lengthened. Overall tumour morphology (i.e., heterogeneity) is probably the single-most important feature of patient survival. The optimal characterisation of tumour morphology requires multiple stereotactic sampling of the tumour mass in the centre and at the periphery of the lesion. This crucial histologic information should be correlated with high-resolution MR imaging modalities. A combined neuroimaging, histologic and genetic assessment of the tumour would be the most appropriate to determine prognosis and decide therapeutic protocol.

Since their development 20 years ago, navigational devices have provided the neurosurgeon a high degree of surgical accuracy and precision for planning of multiple procedures. Image-guided neurosurgery represents a substantial improvement in the microsurgical treatment of tumours and other intracranial lesions. With the progressive development of software and hardware, the acceptance of image-guided neurosurgery has increased dramatically.

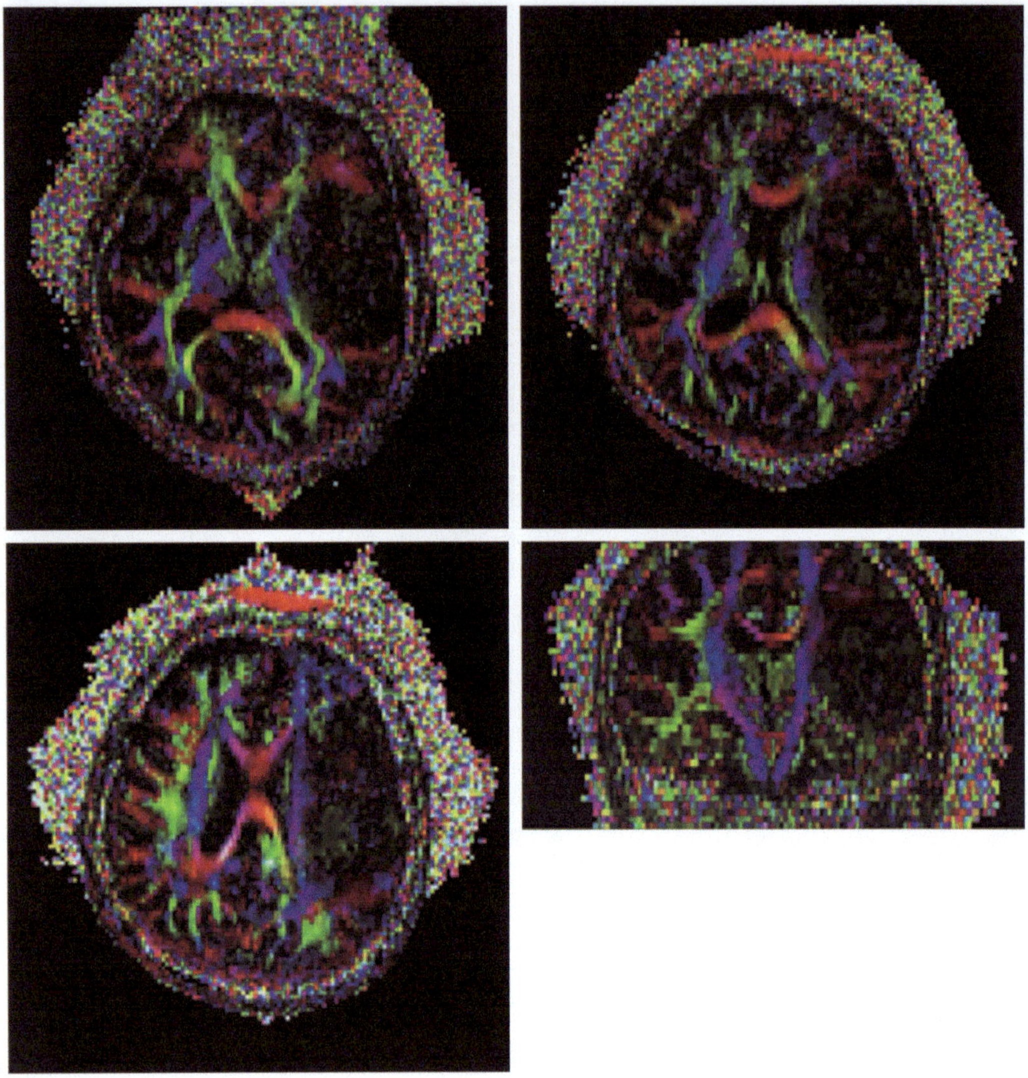

a b c d ▷▷

Additional image data are required to analyze the nature and the dimensions of pathological processes and the surrounding tissue. In this context, functional MRI (fMRI), single photon emission computed tomography (SPECT), and positron emission tomography (PET), as well as special modalities of CT and MR imaging, are routinely used. Multiple modalities are used to detect cerebral lesions as well as adjacent functional eloquent regions preoperatively and intraoperatively. The integration of multiple image information guarantees more accurate planning and realisation of surgical procedures, supports the surgeon to avoid additional intraoperative traumatism and offers a higher level of safety and precision.

Neuronavigation systems are now routinely used in the neurosurgical practice and are quite easy to manage. The day before surgery, adhesive markers are placed on the head skin of the patient, and CT or MR are carried out, so that the images can be transferred into the neuronavigation system and the preoperative surgical plan is feasible. The theoretical basis of neuronavigation is based on the 3D-built reconstruction space through the 3D definition of each marker. A neuronavigation tool is composed of a camera, reference arch, and pointer that allow the lateral, an-

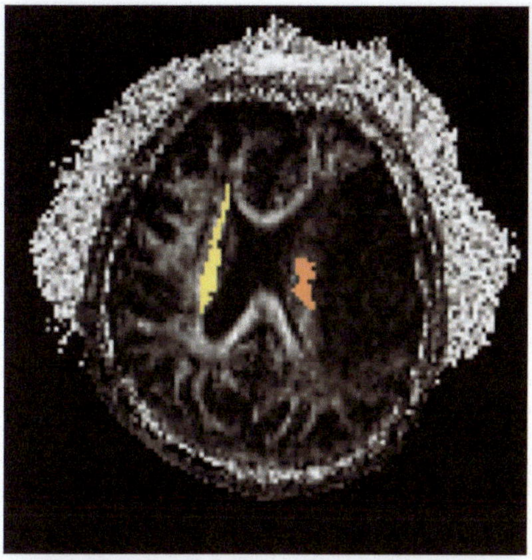
e

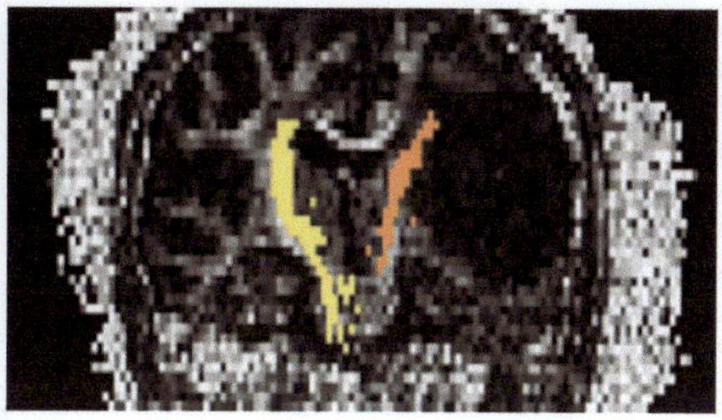
f

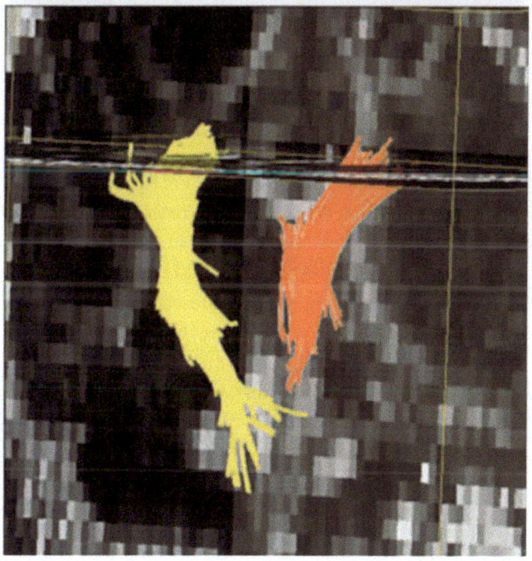
g

Fig. 28.9.2a–g. On conventional MR images it might be very difficult to determine whether a prominent and eloquent white matter tract, such as the corticospinal tract, has been destroyed, infiltrated or simply displaced. Colour-coded DTI and tractography may demonstrate that a large tumour located in the expected position of the pyramidal tract has displaced the tract, changing its orientation. Colour-coded anisotropy axial DTI maps at the level of the posterior limb of the internal capsule (PLIC) (**a**) and corona radiate (**b** and **c**) show displacement of the pyramidal tract toward the midline in a 69-year-old female with a large mass in the left fronto-parietal region. Coronal colour-coded DTI maps (**d**) confirm the displacement of the left pyramidal tract. Tractography (**e, f, g**) of the left (orange) and right (yellow) pyramidal tracts, reconstructed with a single region of interest placed in each PLIC, confirmed thinning and displacement of the pyramidal tract toward the midline on the left side. Tractography was performed with the DTI Studio software developed by Hangyi Hjang, Johns Hopkins University, Baltimore, USA.

teroposterior and vertical coordinates of the markers and subsequently of each point of the brain volume. After this crucial step, the software is able to acquire the head volume in the 3D preoperative CT or MR, and it is possible to define the lesion morphology and its relationship with contiguous areas in all phases of the surgical procedure.

A major technical limitation of neuronavigation systems based on preoperative imaging is represented by dynamic changes of the intracranial contents (brain shift) due to tumour removal and/or CSF leakage that could occur during the surgical procedure. The surgeon then is faced with possible changing of the intraoperative field for which the preoperative imaging data is not accurate, since the information is not updated during the course of surgery. It is clear that intraoperatively acquired images will provide better information. A number of high-tech tools for use during neurosurgical procedures have been developed in recent years, such as intraoperative ultrasound, intraoperative CT and MR, which are considered the superior imaging method for surgery image guidance.

The possibility of detecting, during surgery, eloquent areas allows a reduction of postoperative morbidity. Functional MR and conventional MR data transferred into the navigation device allow recognizing the relation between the eloquent cortical area and the tumour, particularly when a low-grade glioma has to be removed. In this particular situation conventional MR images support the surgeon in tumour boundary definition, while detection of functional areas is suggested by activated fMRI areas. In the past this surgery was performed exclusively by intraoperative electrocortical mapping (ECM), which is still considered the gold standard method. The association of fMRI and ECM has dramatically reduced the length of surgery, an advantage for the patient. Patients with tumours near language-eloquent areas can be treated in asleep–awake anaesthesia.

The possibility of detecting preoperatively the histological features of an intracranial tumour is the common endpoint of neuroradiologists and neurosurgeons. MR spectroscopic imaging could identify areas of tumours with higher density or higher proliferative index, which can become the preferred target of the surgical resection. Unfortunately, the reliability of this technique is not complete, and a surgical specimen collection (biopsy or tumour removal) still represents the procedure allowing the diagnosis. MR spectroscopy could be used in image-guided surgery. The abnormal areas could be easily recognised and surgically collected. This nice interaction between radiologists and surgeons will allow better integration of multiple imaging modalities in the operating room and will lead to more accurate diagnosis and tumour resection for the best care treatment. The surgeon involved in oncology is aware of the importance of a team composed of radiologist, pathologist, oncologist, physicist, and radiotherapist.

28.8 Integrating Multiple Biologic Parameters and Conclusions

Over the past 30 years extraordinary advances in imaging techniques have been made. It is now possible to diagnose readily with CT or conventional MRI the presence of a mass in a few minutes. The type and grade of the tumour is diagnosed accurately in the majority of cases. Unfortunately, none of these technical improvements has made a significant difference in survival of patients with gliomas. Nevertheless, it is mandatory to continue to develop and refine new and less-invasive imaging methods that measure multiple biologic parameters of this complex and relentless disease. The goals of imaging in front of a new presumed glioma should be the following: (1) determine the most likely grade of the mass; (2) determine whether it is a homogeneous or a heterogeneous lesion and identify those areas that will grow faster; (3) define the virtual border that separates volumes of dense tumoral cells with dead normal brain tissue from volumes of functioning brain tissue with scarce and slow growing tumoral cells; (4) identify the areas within or adjacent to the imaging abnormality that cannot be removed (e.g., grey and white matter eloquent structures).

It is well-known that the actual extension of a glioma is indicated neither by CT nor conventional MRI nor any of the more sophisticated imaging techniques. Meticulous neuropathologic studies have demonstrated that tumour cells can be found far from any MR-defined abnormality (Scherer 1940; Burger et al. 1983; Kelly et al. 1987). If "optimal gross resection" is the goal of therapy, we should provide neurosurgeons and other therapists with accurate multiparametric maps of the tumour. The most advanced and necrotic area of the tumour will be defined by post-contrast images. fluorodeoxyglucose (FDG)-PET will outline areas of solid tumour with high glucose consumption. Perfusion MR imaging will outline areas with increased vascularity and elevated angiogenesis. These areas are likely to grow very fast and, therefore, should be taken out. MR spectroscopic imaging will outline zones of increased cellular density and membrane turnover in areas with abnormal T2-weighted signal, distinguishing these from areas of predominant vasogenic oedema. MR spectroscopic imaging will also distinguish areas with severe NAA and neuroaxonal loss and unlikely functioning tissue from areas with abnormal T2-weighted signal but relatively spared NAA signal. In the latter areas it is likely that residual brain tissue is functioning despite evidence of tumour infiltration. Functional MRI and DTI tractography will inform surgeons and therapists of what they cannot remove or treat.

References

Ackerstaff E, Glunde K et al (2003) Choline phospholipid metabolism: a target in cancer cells? J Cell Biochem 90:525–533

Alger JR, Frank JA et al (1990) Metabolism of human gliomas: assessment with H-1 MR spectroscopy and F-18 fluorodeoxyglucose PET. Radiology 177:633–641

Aronen HJ, Gazit IE et al (1994) Cerebral blood volume maps

of gliomas: comparison with tumor grade and histologic findings. Radiology 191:41–51

Balesaria S, Brock C et al (1999) Loss of chromosome 10 is an independent prognostic factor in high-grade gliomas. Br J Cancer 81:1371–1377

Bauman G, Lote K et al (1999) Pretreatment factors predict overall survival for patients with low-grade glioma: a recursive partitioning analysis. Int J Radiat Oncol Biol Phys 45:923–929

Bhakoo KK, Williams SR et al (1996) Immortalization and transformation are associated with specific alterations in choline metabolism. Cancer Res 56:4630–4635

Bizzi A, Movsas B et al (1995) Response of non-Hodgkin lymphoma to radiation therapy: early and long-term assessment with H-1 MR spectroscopic imaging. Radiology 194:271–276

Bruhn H, Frahm J et al (1989) Noninvasive differentiation of tumors with use of localized H-1 MR spectroscopy in vivo: initial experience in patients with cerebral tumors. Radiology 172:541–548

Brunberg JA, Chenevert TL et al (1995) In vivo MR determination of water diffusion coefficients and diffusion anisotropy: correlation with structural alteration in gliomas of the cerebral hemispheres. AJNR Am J Neuroradiol 16:361–371

Burger PC, Dubois PJ et al (1983) Computerized tomographic and pathologic studies of the untreated, quiescent, and recurrent glioblastoma multiforme. J Neurosurg 58:159–169

Cairncross JG, Ueki K et al (1998) Specific genetic predictors of chemotherapeutic response and survival in patients with anaplastic oligodendrogliomas. J Natl Cancer Inst 90:1473–1479

Cha S, Knopp EA et al (2000) Dynamic contrast-enhanced T2-weighted MR imaging of recurrent malignant gliomas treated with thalidomide and carboplatin. AJNR Am J Neuroradiol 21:881–890

Cha S, Knopp EA et al (2002) Intracranial mass lesions: dynamic contrast-enhanced susceptibility-weighted echo-planar perfusion MR imaging. Radiology 223:11–29

Chow KL, Gobin YP et al (2000) Prognostic factors in recurrent glioblastoma multiforme and anaplastic astrocytoma treated with selective intra-arterial chemotherapy. AJNR Am J Neuroradiol 21:471–478

Conturo TE, Lori NF et al (1999) Tracking neuronal fiber pathways in the living human brain. Proc Natl Acad Sci USA 96:10422–10427

DeAngelis LM (2001) Brain tumors. N Engl J Med 344:114–123

De Edelenyi FS, Rubin C et al (2000) A new approach for analyzing proton magnetic resonance spectroscopic images of brain tumors: nosologic images. Nat Med 6:1287–1289

Delbeke D, Meyerowitz C et al (1995) Optimal cutoff levels of F-18 fluorodeoxyglucose uptake in the differentiation of low-grade from high-grade brain tumors with PET. Radiology 195:47–52

Demaerel P, Johannik K et al (1991) Localized 1H NMR spectroscopy in fifty cases of newly diagnosed intracranial tumors. J Comput Assist Tomogr 15:67–76

Fortin D, Cairncross GJ et al (1999) Oligodendroglioma: an appraisal of recent data pertaining to diagnosis and treatment. Neurosurgery 45:1279–1291; discussion 1291

Fujimaki TM, Nakamura MO et al (1991) Correlation between bromodeoxyuridine-labeling indices and patient prognosis in cerebral astrocytic tumors of adults. Cancer 67:1629–1634

Fulham MJ, Bizzi A et al (1992) Mapping of brain tumor metabolites with proton MR spectroscopic imaging: clinical relevance. Radiology 185:675–686

Gupta RK, Cloughesy TF et al (2000) Relationships between choline magnetic resonance spectroscopy, apparent diffusion coefficient and quantitative histopathology in human glioma. J Neurooncol 50:215–226

Hara T, Kondo T et al (2003) Use of 18F-choline and 11C-choline as contrast agents in positron emission tomography imaging-guided stereotactic biopsy sampling of gliomas. J Neurosurg 99:474–479

Harting I, Hartmann M et al (2003) Differentiating primary central nervous system lymphoma from glioma in humans using localised proton magnetic resonance spectroscopy. Neurosci Lett 342:163–166

Hartmann M, Heiland S et al (2003) Distinguishing of primary cerebral lymphoma from high-grade glioma with perfusion-weighted magnetic resonance imaging. Neurosci Lett 338:119–122

Hein PA, Eskey CJ et al (2004) Diffusion-weighted imaging in the follow-up of treated high-grade gliomas: tumor recurrence versus radiation injury. AJNR Am J Neuroradiol 25:201–209

Henry RG, Berman JI et al (2004) Subcortical pathways serving cortical language sites: initial experience with diffusion tensor imaging fiber tracking combined with intraoperative language mapping. Neuroimage 21:616–622

Hoshino TP, Wilson M, CB et al (1989) Prognostic implications of the bromodeoxyuridine labeling index of human gliomas. J Neurosurg 71:335–341

Hoshino TT, Muraoka JJ et al (1980) An autoradiographic study of human gliomas: growth kinetics of anaplastic astrocytoma and glioblastoma multiforme. Brain 103:967–984

Hoshino TW, CB (1979) Cell kinetic analysis of human malignant brain tumors (gliomas). Cancer 44:956–962

Howard AP, SR (1953) Synthesis of deoxyribonucleic acid in normal and irradiated cells and its relation to chromosomal breakage. Heredity 6 [Suppl]:261–273

Kelly PJ, Daumas-Duport C et al (1987) Imaging-based stereotaxic serial biopsies in untreated intracranial glial neoplasms. J Neurosurg 66:865–874

Kim S, Chung JK et al (2004) 11C-methionine PET as a prognostic marker in patients with glioma: comparison with(18)F-FDG PET. Eur J Nucl Med Mol Imaging

Kleihues P, Cavenee WK (eds) (2000) World Health Organization Classification of tumours: pathology and genetics of tumours: pathology and genetics of tumours of the nervous system. IARC Press, Lyon, France pp 6-7

Knopp EA, Cha S et al (1999) Glial neoplasms: dynamic contrast-enhanced T2*-weighted MR imaging. Radiology 211:791–798

Kono K, Inoue Y et al (2001) The role of diffusion-weighted imaging in patients with brain tumors. AJNR Am J Neuroradiol 22:1081–1088

Kowalczuk A, Macdonald RL et al (1997) Quantitative imaging study of extent of surgical resection and prognosis of malignant astrocytomas. Neurosurgery 41:1028–1036; discussion 1036–1038

Kuesel AC, Sutherland GR et al (1994) ^{1}H-MRS of high grade astrocytomas: mobile lipid accumulation in necrotic tissue. NMR Biomed 7:149–155

Law M, Cha S et al (2002) High-grade gliomas and solitary metastases: differentiation by using perfusion and proton spectroscopic MR imaging. Radiology 222:715–721

Law M, Yang S et al (2003) Glioma grading: sensitivity, specificity, and predictive values of perfusion MR imaging and proton MR spectroscopic imaging compared with conventional MR imaging. AJNR Am J Neuroradiol 24:1989–1998

Lee YY, van Tassel P (1989) Intracranial oligodendrogliomas: imaging findings in 35 untreated cases. AJR Am J Roentgenol 152:361–369

Lev MH, Ozsunar Y et al (2004) Glial tumor grading and outcome prediction using dynamic spin-echo MR susceptibility mapping compared with conventional contrast-enhanced MR: confounding effect of elevated rCBV of oligodendrogliomas (corrected). AJNR Am J Neuroradiol 25:214–221

Li X, Lu Y et al (2002) Analysis of the spatial characteristics of metabolic abnormalities in newly diagnosed glioma patients. J Magn Reson Imaging 16:229–237

Lori NF, Akbudak E et al (2002) Diffusion tensor fiber tracking of human brain connectivity: acquisition methods, reliability analysis and biological results. NMR Biomed 15:494–515

Lu S, Ahn D et al (2003) Peritumoral diffusion tensor imaging of high-grade gliomas and metastatic brain tumors. AJNR Am J Neuroradiol 24:937–941

Macara IG (1989) Elevated phosphocholine concentration in ras-transformed NIH 3T3 cells arises from increased choline kinase activity, not from phosphatidylcholine breakdown. Mol Cell Biol 9:325–328

Mendelsohn M (1962) Autoradiographic analysis of cell proliferation in spontaneous breast cancer of C3H mouse III. The growth fraction. J Natl Cancer Inst 28:1015–1029

Mori S, van Zijl PC (2002) Fiber tracking: principles and strategies—a technical review. NMR Biomed 15:468–480

Mori S, Frederiksen K et al (2002) Brain white matter anatomy of tumor patients evaluated with diffusion tensor imaging. Ann Neurol 51:377–380

Negendank W (1992) Studies of human tumors by MRS: a review. NMR Biomed 5:303–324

Nordqvist AC, Smurawa H et al (2001) Expression of matrix metalloproteinases 2 and 9 in meningiomas associated with different degrees of brain invasiveness and edema. J Neurosurg 95:839–844

Ogawa T, Shishido F et al (1993) Cerebral glioma: evaluation with methionine PET. Radiology 186:45–53

Ohtani T, Kurihara H et al (2001) Brain tumour imaging with carbon-11 choline: comparison with FDG PET and gadolinium-enhanced MR imaging. Eur J Nucl Med 28:1664–1670

Olson JD, Riedel E et al (2000) Long-term outcome of low-grade oligodendroglioma and mixed glioma. Neurology 54:1442–1448

Paek SH, Kim CY et al (2002) Correlation of clinical and biological parameters with peritumoral edema in meningioma. J Neurooncol 60:235–245

Patronas NJ, Brooks RA et al (1983) Glycolytic rate (PET) and contrast enhancement (CT) in human cerebral gliomas. AJNR Am J Neuroradiol 4:533–535

Pierpaoli C, Basser PJ (1996) Toward a quantitative assessment of diffusion anisotropy. Magn Reson Med 36:893–906

Pirotte B, Goldman S et al (1995) Use of positron emission tomography (PET) in stereotactic conditions for brain biopsy. Acta Neurochir (Wien) 134:79–82

Pirotte B, Goldman S et al (2004) Comparison of 18F-FDG and 11C-methionine for PET-guided stereotactic brain biopsy of gliomas. J Nucl Med 45:1293–1298

Pirzkall A, McKnight TR et al (2001) MR-spectroscopy guided target delineation for high-grade gliomas. Int J Radiat Oncol Biol Phys 50:915–928

Podo F (1999) Tumour phospholipid metabolism. NMR Biomed 12:413–439

Poptani H, Gupta RK et al (1995) Characterization of intracranial mass lesions with in vivo proton MR spectroscopy. AJNR Am J Neuroradiol 16:1593–1603

Preul MC, Caramanos Z et al (1996) Accurate, noninvasive diagnosis of human brain tumors by using proton magnetic resonance spectroscopy. Nat Med 2:323–325

Reeves GI, Marks JE (1979) Prognostic significance of lesion size for glioblastoma multiforme. Radiology 132:469–471

Roberts HC, Roberts TP et al (2000) Quantitative measurement of microvascular permeability in human brain tumors achieved using dynamic contrast-enhanced MR imaging: correlation with histologic grade. AJNR Am J Neuroradiol 21:891–899

Rock JP, Hearshen D et al (2002) Correlations between magnetic resonance spectroscopy and image-guided histopathology, with special attention to radiation necrosis. Neurosurgery 51:912–919; discussion 919–920

Scherer H (1940) The forms of growth in gliomas and their practical significance. Brain 63:1–35

Schlemmer HP, Bachert P et al (2002) Differentiation of radiation necrosis from tumor progression using proton magnetic resonance spectroscopy. Neuroradiology 44:216–222

Shimizu H, Kumabe T et al (2000) Correlation between choline level measured by proton MR spectroscopy and Ki-67 labeling index in gliomas. AJNR Am J Neuroradiol 21:659–665

Sijens PE, Levendag PC et al (1996) 1H MR spectroscopy detection of lipids and lactate in metastatic brain tumors. NMR Biomed 9:65–71

Sinha S, Bastin ME et al (2002) Diffusion tensor MR imaging of high-grade cerebral gliomas. AJNR Am J Neuroradiol 23:520–527

Smith JS, Perry A et al (2000) Alterations of chromosome arms 1p and 19q as predictors of survival in oligodendrogliomas, astrocytomas, and mixed oligoastrocytomas. J Clin Oncol 18:636–645

Sugahara T, Korogi Y et al (1999) Perfusion-sensitive MRI of cerebral lymphomas: a preliminary report. J Comput Assist Tomogr 23:232–237

Tamiya T, Kinoshita K et al (2000) Proton magnetic resonance spectroscopy reflects cellular proliferative activity in astrocytomas. Neuroradiology 42:333–338

Taylor JS, Langston JW et al (1996) Clinical value of proton magnetic resonance spectroscopy for differentiating recurrent or residual brain tumor from delayed cerebral necrosis. Int J Radiat Oncol Biol Phys 36:1251–1261

Tedeschi G, Lundbom N et al (1997) Increased choline signal coinciding with malignant degeneration of cerebral gliomas: a serial proton magnetic resonance spectroscopy imaging study. J Neurosurg 87:516–524

Tsuruda JS, Chew WM et al (1990) Diffusion-weighted MR imaging of the brain: value of differentiating between extraaxial cysts and epidermoid tumors. AJNR Am J Neuroradiol 11:925–931; discussion 932–934

Usenius JP, Vainio P et al (1994) Choline-containing compounds in human astrocytomas studied by 1H NMR spectroscopy in vivo and in vitro. J Neurochem 63:1538–1543

Van Laere K, Ceyssens S et al (2004) Direct comparison of (18)F-FDG and (11)C-methionine PET in suspected recurrence of glioma: sensitivity, inter-observer variability and prognostic value. Eur J Nucl Med Mol Imaging Aug 10; [Epub ahead of print]

Velema JP, Percy CL (1987) Age curve of central nervous system tumor incidence in adults: variation of shape by histologic type. JNCI 79:623

Villringer A, Rosen BR et al (1988) Dynamic imaging with lanthanide chelates in normal brain: contrast due to magnetic susceptibility effects. Magn Reson Med 6:164–174

Warburg O (1956) On the origin of cancer cells. Science 123:309–314

Warmuth C, Gunther M et al (2003) Quantification of blood flow in brain tumors: comparison of arterial spin labeling and dynamic susceptibility-weighted contrast-enhanced MR imaging. Radiology 228:523–532

Warren KE, Patronas N et al (2001) Comparison of one-, two-, and three-dimensional measurements of childhood brain tumors. J Natl Cancer Inst 93:1401–1405

Wetzel SG, Cha S et al (2002) Relative cerebral blood volume measurements in intracranial mass lesions: interobserver and intraobserver reproducibility study. Radiology 224:797–803

Wieshmann UC, Symms MR et al (2000) Diffusion tensor imaging demonstrates deviation of fibres in normal appearing white matter adjacent to a brain tumour. J Neurol Neurosurg Psychiatry 68:501–503

Witwer BP, Moftakhar R et al (2002) Diffusion-tensor imaging of white matter tracts in patients with cerebral neoplasm. J Neurosurg 97:568–575

Yoshii YM, Tsuboi YK et al (1986) Estimation of growth fraction with bromodeoxyuridine in human central nervous system tumors. J Neurosurg 65:659–663

Zoula S, Herigault G et al (2003) Correlation between the occurrence of ^{1}H-MRS lipid signal, necrosis and lipid droplets during C6 rat glioma development. NMR Biomed 16:199–212

29 Head Trauma

ZEE CHI-SHING, MARCEL MAYA, JOHN L. GO, PAUL E. KIM, and ILHAMI KOVANLIKAYA

CONTENTS

Craniocerebral trauma is the major cause of accidental death in the United States, particularly in the juvenile and young adult groups (CAVENESS 1979; KIM and ZEE 1995; GEAN 1994; GENNARELLI 1985). Severe traumatic brain injury (TBI) accounts for a death rate of 16.9 per 100,000 population per year (SOSIN et al. 1989). Motor vehicles (57%), firearms (14%), and falls (12%) were the most frequent causes. The rate of brain-injury-associated death for males is 3 times that of females. Head injuries are responsible for 200–300 hospital admissions per 100,000 population per year in the United States (BAKAY and GLASSAUER 1980). Most of the admissions last only a few days and the patients are admitted for clinical observation. Head injury is not only a cause of death but also a cause of serious financial burden to the society providing treatment and care to these patients. Loss of labor and reduced productivity to the society further adds to the negative impact. The majority of the patients suffering head injuries are considered as having "mild head injury." Most patients recover fully from mild TBI, but 15–29% may suffer significant neurocognitive problems (HOFMAN et al. 2001). Common symptoms include attention deficit, deficit in working memory and speed of information processing, headaches, dizziness, and irritability.

Severe and moderate head injuries, or even some minor head injuries, can often be associated with rotational forces that produce shear stresses on the brain parenchyma. The brain is soft and malleable. Relatively little force is required to distort the shape of the brain. There are significant differences in density between the cerebrospinal fluid of the ventricles and the surrounding white matter. Differences in density also exist between gray and white matter to a lesser degree. When the skull is rapidly rotated, the superficial gray matter is carried along but the deeper white matter lags behind, causing axial stretching, separation, and disruption of nerve fiber tracts. Shear stresses are most marked at junctions between tissues of different densities. As a result, shear injuries commonly occur at junction of gray and white matter, but they are also found in the deeper white matter of corpus callosum, centrum semiovale, basal ganglia, brainstem (midbrain and rostral pons), and cerebellum.

GENTRY et al. (1988) studied 63 cases of acute head injury and 15 patients with chronic head injury. Corpus callosal injury was found in 47% of the patients. The corpus callosum is prone to injury because of its rigid attachment to the falx and its relationship

Z. CHI-SHING, MD
Professor of Radiology and Neurosurgery, Director of Neuroradiology, Department of Imaging, University of Southern California University Hospital, 1500 San Pablo Street, Los Angeles, CA 90033, USA
M. MAYA, MD
Clinical and Interventional Neuroradiology, Residency Training Program Director, S. Mark Taper Foundation Imaging Center, Cedars-Sinai Medical Center, 8700 Beverly Boulevard, Suite M-335, Los Angeles, CA 90033, USA
J.L. GO, MD
Assistant Professor of Radiology and Otolaryngology, Division of Neuroradiology, Department of Radiology, University of Southern California Keck School of Medicine, 1200 North State Street, Room 3740F, Los Angeles, CA 90033, USA
P.E. KIM, MD; I. KOVANLIKAYA, MD
Assistant Professor of Radiology, Division of Neuroradiology, Department of Radiology, University of Southern California Keck School of Medicine, 1200 North State Street, Room 3740B, Los Angeles, CA 90033, USA

to the independently mobile cerebral hemisphere. Because the falx is broader posteriorly, it effectively prevents transient displacement of the splenium of the corpus callosum, causing greater shear to occur within the fibers of the latter. Gentry et al. also found that diffuse axonal lesions of the lobar white matter and brainstem are usually very small in size and difficult to detect on computed tomography (CT) or magnetic resonance imaging (MRI), while those in the corpus callosum are larger and readily visible on CT or MRI. Pathologically, the diagnosis of diffuse axonal injury depends on the identification of axonal bulbs microscopically. Early injury of axons is best detected immunocytochemically. The most sensitive indicator of injured axons is the presence of beta-amyloid precursor protein in the damaged axons. Injured axons may be seen within 2–3 h of injury and as long as 99 days after trauma (Blumbergs et al. 1994; Hardman and Manoukian 2002).

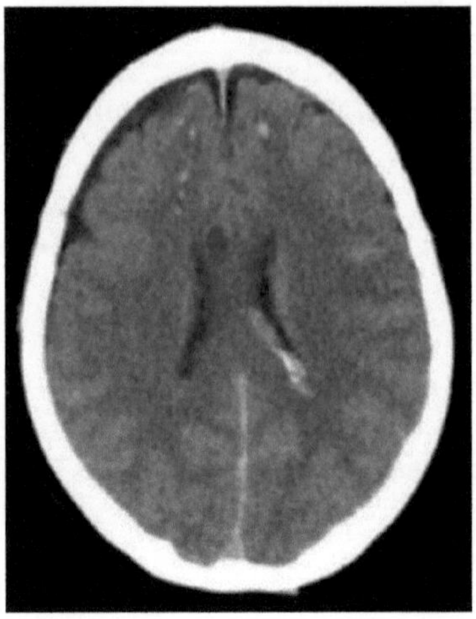

Fig. 29.1 Intraventricular hemorrhage and diffuse axonal Injury. Axial CT scan demonstrate the presence of intraventricular hemorrhage in the left lateral ventricle and a small petechial hemorrhage in the frontal white matter

29.1 Computed Tomography in Traumatic Brain Injury

The advent of CT in the early 1970s revolutionized the diagnosis and management of head trauma patients, and CT remains the most efficient method for evaluating acute head trauma today (Zee and Go 1998). It is widely available, fast, and accurate for detecting acute hemorrhage (Schynoll et al. 1993). High-resolution CT is excellent for evaluating facial and skull fractures. Neurosurgically significant lesions, such as epidural hematomas, subdural hematomas, or depressed skull fractures, are all readily detected by CT. CT is excellent for detecting intraventricular hemorrhage, which is commonly associated with shear injuries of the corpus callosum and white matter (Fig. 29.1) (Gentry et al. 1988).

CT does have a number of pitfalls when used to evaluate head injuries. Isodense or low-density acute hemorrhages are seen in patients who are severely anemic or suffer from disseminated intravascular coagulopathy. A small subdural hematoma or epidural hematoma may not be detected if the appropriate setting for window width and level is not used. CT is also less sensitive than MRI for detecting diffuse axonal injury, cortical contusion, deep cerebral/brainstem injury, and small subdural hematomas (Hans et al. 1984; Kelly et al. 1988; Zee and Go 1998). The early detection of many extra-axial hematomas has been made possible by the increase in the number of CT scans performed in head trauma patients. This results in early surgical interventions in these patients, with a marked improvement in their morbidity and mortality (Jeret et al. 1993; Miller et al. 1988; Servadei et al. 1988; Johnson and Lee 1992).

Diffuse axonal injury (DAI) refers to white matter injury caused by unequal rotation or deceleration of adjacent tissues of differing density and rigidity (Adams et al. 1982; Strich 1961). The most common shearing lesions are seen in the parasagittal white matter. As the shearing force increases, the corpus callosum and dorsolateral brainstem become injured. Internal capsule, cerebellar hemisphere, and sometimes the basal ganglia and thalami may also be involved (Hammound and Wasserman 2002). Clinically, patients may present in a comatose state despite a relatively benign appearance of their CT scans. On CT, DAI involving the white matter may present as multiple, small, focal low-density lesions in the white matter (Cordobes et al. 1986; Zimmerman et al. 1978). These tend to be ovoid or elliptical with the long axis oriented in the direction of the injured axons (Gentry et al. 1989). Hemorrhage may or may not be seen in these low-density areas (Sasiadek et al. 1991). They are typically less than 1 cm in size and spare the adjacent cortical surface of the brain. Lesions are usually located entirely within the white matter or at the gray-white matter junction and are seen in both hemispheres (Gentry et al. 1988). Cerebral swelling with obliteration of the basal cisterns and compression of the lateral ventricles and third ventricle can be an early finding. After about 3 weeks, enlargement of the cerebral sulci and basal cisterns and dilatation of the ventricles can be seen with well-defined foci of hypointensity in the white matter (ZIMMERMAN et al. 1978). SASIADEK et al. (1991) reported that the typical CT findings of DAI were small hemorrhagic lesions, most often in the cerebral white matter and internal capsule. Hemorrhagic lesions resulting from shearing injury in the cerebral white matter and gray-white matter junction are easily identified on CT in the acute stage. However, CT is limited in the evaluation of DAI. MITTL et al. (1994) found abnormalities compatible with DAI on MRI (spin-echo T2-weighted and T2*-weighted gradient echo images) in 30% of patients with normal head CT scans following minor head trauma (Fig. 29.2).

29.2 Magnetic Resonance Imaging in Traumatic Brain Injury

MRI has rapidly become the imaging modality of choice for most neurological disease. In the arena of TBI, MRI has become an important adjunct to CT in the evaluation of patients with DAI, cortical contusion, subcortical gray matter injury, and primary brainstem injury (GENTRY et al. 1988). DAI most frequently involves the white matter of the frontal and temporal lobes, the corpus callosum, and corona radiata (Figs. 29.3, 29.4). Cortical contusions most commonly involve the inferior, lateral, and anterior portions of the frontal and temporal lobes where they are exposed to the rough bony surface of the frontal and temporal fossa. Primary brainstem injury occurs in the dorsolateral aspects of the midbrain.

Several different MR sequences have been studied in the evaluation of head trauma. The utility of fluid-attenuated inversion-recovery sequences in the evaluation of head trauma has been reported by several authors, who found the sensitivity of FLAIR images to be equal or superior to conventional T2-weighted spin-echo images. MRI is indicated when there is a significant discrepancy between the patient's clinical condition and the CT findings, which could be unremarkable in some instances. Gradient echo images further enhance the sensitivity in detecting hemorrhagic shearing injury in the acute phase (deoxyhemoglobin) and chronic phase (hemosiderin) of the injury (Fig. 29.5). This is due to the shortening of T2* by the heterogeneous local magnetic field arising from paramagnetic blood breakdown products. These changes can persist for months to years after the head trauma. T2*-weighted images are critical in the evaluation of patients with chronic head injury. YANAGAWA et al. (1978) found that there is a correlation between the lesions seen on gradient echo images and the Glasgow Coma Score and the duration of unconsciousness. They also found the number of hemorrhagic lesions detected by gradient echo sequences per patient was significantly higher than those seen by T2-FSE.

Magnetization transfer (MT) imaging is based on the principle that protons bound in macromolecules exhibit T1 relaxation coupling with protons in the aqueous phase. Application of an off-resonance saturation pulse can effectively saturate bound protons selectively. Subsequent exchange of longitudinal magnetization with free water protons reduces the signal

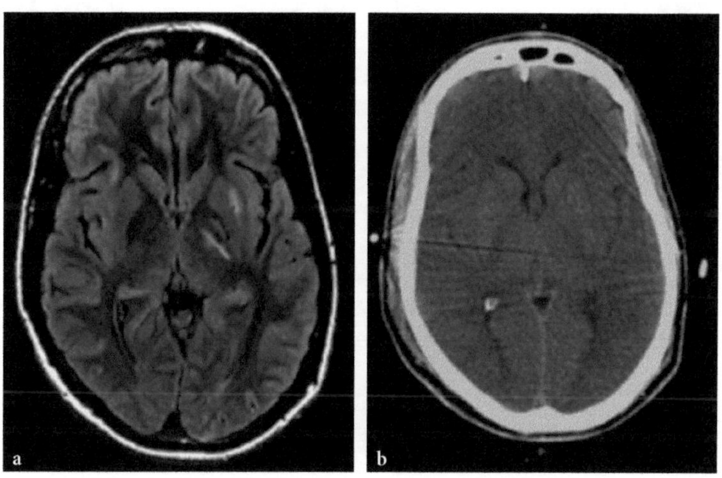

Fig. 29.2a,b. Diffuse axonal injury detected by MRI with a normal-appearing CT scan. **a** Axial FLAIR sequence demonstrates shearing injury involving the left internal capsule and external capsule. **b** Axial CT scan at the same level reveals no abnormality in the left internal capsule or external capsule

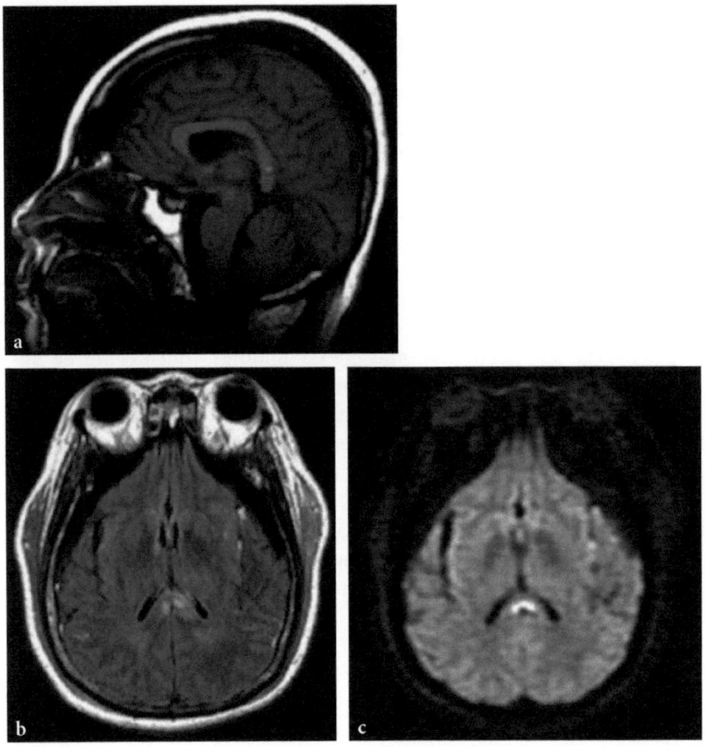

Fig. 29.3a–c. Diffuse axonal injury involving the corpus callosum. **a** Sagittal T1-weighted image demonstrates a focal hyperintense hemorrhage in the splenium of the corpus callosum. **b** Axial FLAIR sequence reveals abnormal signal in the splenium of the corpus callosum. In addition, high-signal material is seen in the left sylvian fissure and cortical sulci, consistent with subarachnoid hemorrhage. **c** Axial diffusion-weighted image demonstrate high signal intensity in the splenium of the corpus callosum, consistent with restricted diffusion

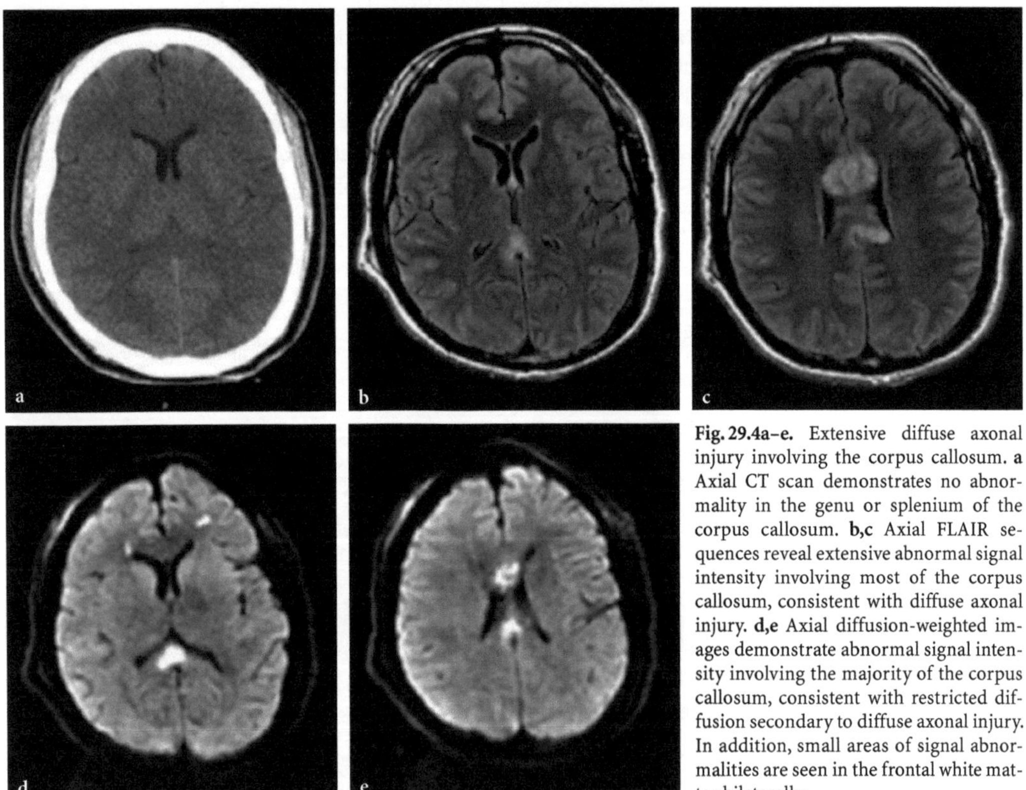

Fig. 29.4a–e. Extensive diffuse axonal injury involving the corpus callosum. **a** Axial CT scan demonstrates no abnormality in the genu or splenium of the corpus callosum. **b,c** Axial FLAIR sequences reveal extensive abnormal signal intensity involving most of the corpus callosum, consistent with diffuse axonal injury. **d,e** Axial diffusion-weighted images demonstrate abnormal signal intensity involving the majority of the corpus callosum, consistent with restricted diffusion secondary to diffuse axonal injury. In addition, small areas of signal abnormalities are seen in the frontal white matter bilaterally

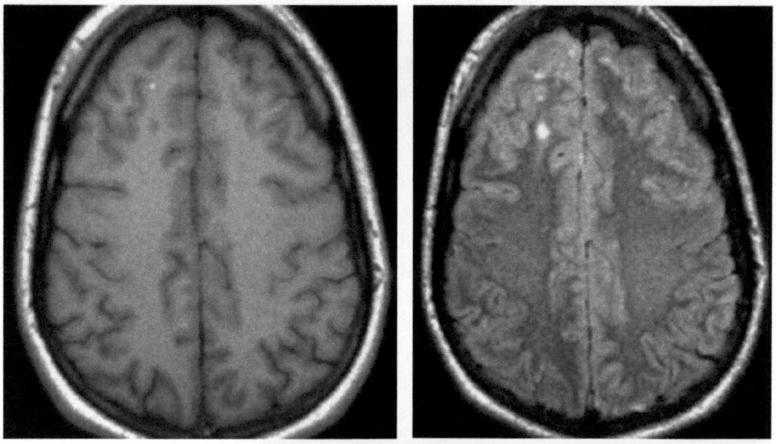

a b

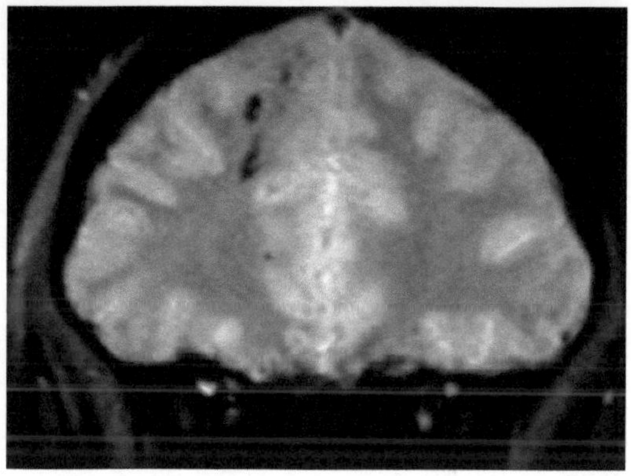

c

Fig. 29.5a–c. Diffuse axonal injury demonstrated by gradient echo images. **a** Axial T1-weighted sequence reveals a tiny hyperintense petechial hemorrhage in the right frontal white matter. **b** Axial FLAIR sequence demonstrates small hyperintense areas in the right frontal white matter. **c** Coronal gradient echo sequence clearly shows several hypointense areas of petechial hemorrhage, consistent with diffuse axonal injury

intensity detected from these free protons. The magnetization transfer ratio (MTR) provides a quantitative index of this MT effect and may be a quantitative measure of the structural integrity of the tissue (Bagley et al. 2000). Experimental models of DAI in pigs showed reduced MTR values in regions of histologically proven axonal injury. McGowen et al. (2000) found that the MTR in the splenium of the corpus callosum was lower in patients who suffered minor head injury compared with a control group, but no significant reduction in MTR was found in the pons. All the patients demonstrated impairment of at least three measures on neuropsychological tests, and in two cases a significant correlation was found between regional MTR values and neuropsychological performance. McGowen et al. also found that quantitative MT can be used to detect lesions of DAI even when conventional T2-weighted MRI is negative. Bagley et al. (2000) found that average MTR values were higher in all areas of white matter in patients without persistent neurological deficit than in patients with deficits. They concluded that detection of an abnormal MTR in normal-appearing white matter may suggest a poor prognosis.

Magnetic resonance spectroscopy (MRS) provides a noninvasive method of evaluating microscopic injury of the white matter in patients with DAI and may help to predict outcome. MRS is a sensitive tool in detecting DAI and may be particularly useful in evaluating patients with mild TBI with unexplained neurological and cognitive deficits. Since DAI disturbs the balance of chemicals that exist in the brain, such as N-acetyl aspartate (NAA), lactate, choline and high-energy phosphates, MRS can provide an index of neuronal and axonal viability by measuring levels of NAA. A majority of mildly brain injured patients, as well as those severely injured, showed a reduction in NAA levels and NAA/creatine ratio in the splenium of the corpus callosum compared with normal controls. Reduced NAA levels, corresponding to neuronal injury, were observed in patients with elevated lactate up to 24 h following the TBI. Marked reduction of NAA in the white matter continues into the subacute phase. However, in some patients normal NAA levels may be detected 6 months following the trauma (Brooks et al. 2001). Elevated lactate levels on MRS in normal-appearing tissues on MRI correlates with poor clinical outcome (Condon et al. 1998).

Animal studies of diffusion-weighted imaging demonstrated conflicting results in the change of apparent diffusion coefficient (ADC) due to DAI (Alsop et al. 1996; Hanstock et al. 1994; Ito et al. 1996). Liu et al. (1999) reported the first clinical study of diffusion-weighted imaging in DAI. They performed diffusion-weighted imaging in patients with acute and subacute DAI and demonstrated that a significant decrease in ADC values can be seen in areas of DAI up to 18 days following head injury. This probably reflects cellular swelling or cytotoxic edema in the acute stage. The authors hypothesize that very low ADC values, compared with acute ischemia, might be due to the presence of blood products and ruptured axons with membrane fragmentation, which restrict the free movement of water molecules. In the first few hours following traumatic brain injury, DAI is characterized by disruption of the cytoskeletal network and axonal membranes. Histological abnormalities seen in association with DAI decrease the diffusion along axons and increase the diffusion in directions perpendicular to them. White matter structures with reduced diffusion anisotropy are detected in the first 24 h in patients suffering from DAI after TBI. A follow-up study revealed several regions that might have recovered from the injury 1 month later (Fig. 29.6).

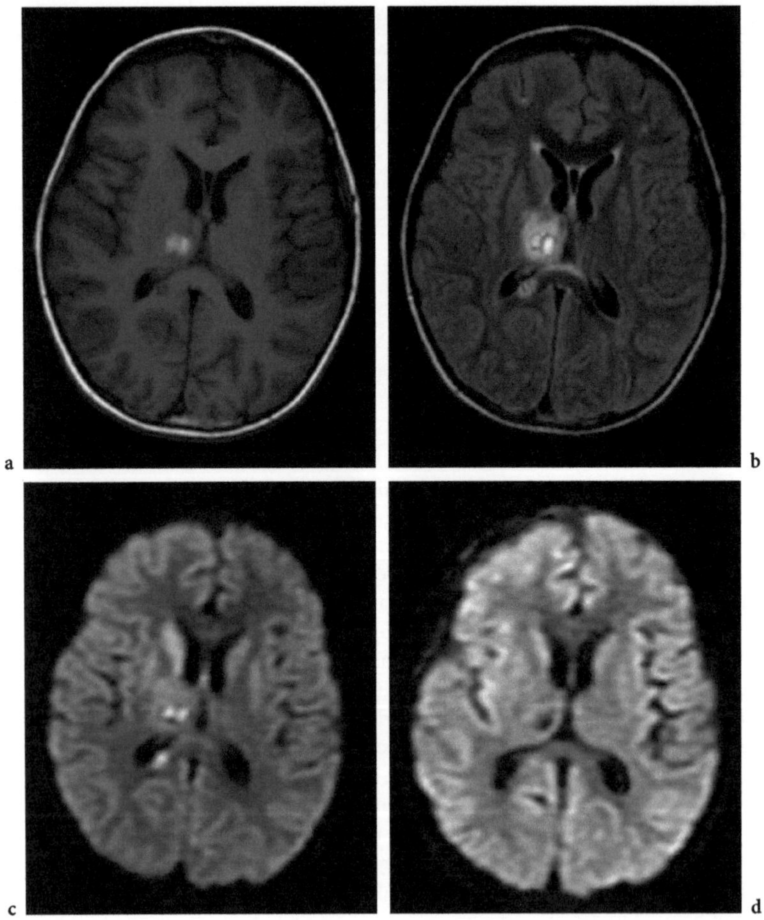

Fig. 29.6a–d. Diffuse axonal injury in the right thalamus. **a** Axial T1-weighted image demonstrates a focal high signal intensity area in the right thalamus, consistent with hemorrhage. **b** Axial FLAIR sequence demonstrates abnormal signal intensity in the right thalamus as well as in the right side of the splenium of the corpus callosum. **c** Axial diffusion-weighted image reveals restricted diffusion in the right thalamus and right side of the splenium of the corpus callosum. **d** Axial diffusion-weighted image obtained 1 month later demonstrates no evidence of restricted diffusion. A hypointense area is seen in the right thalamus, consistent with encephalomalacia

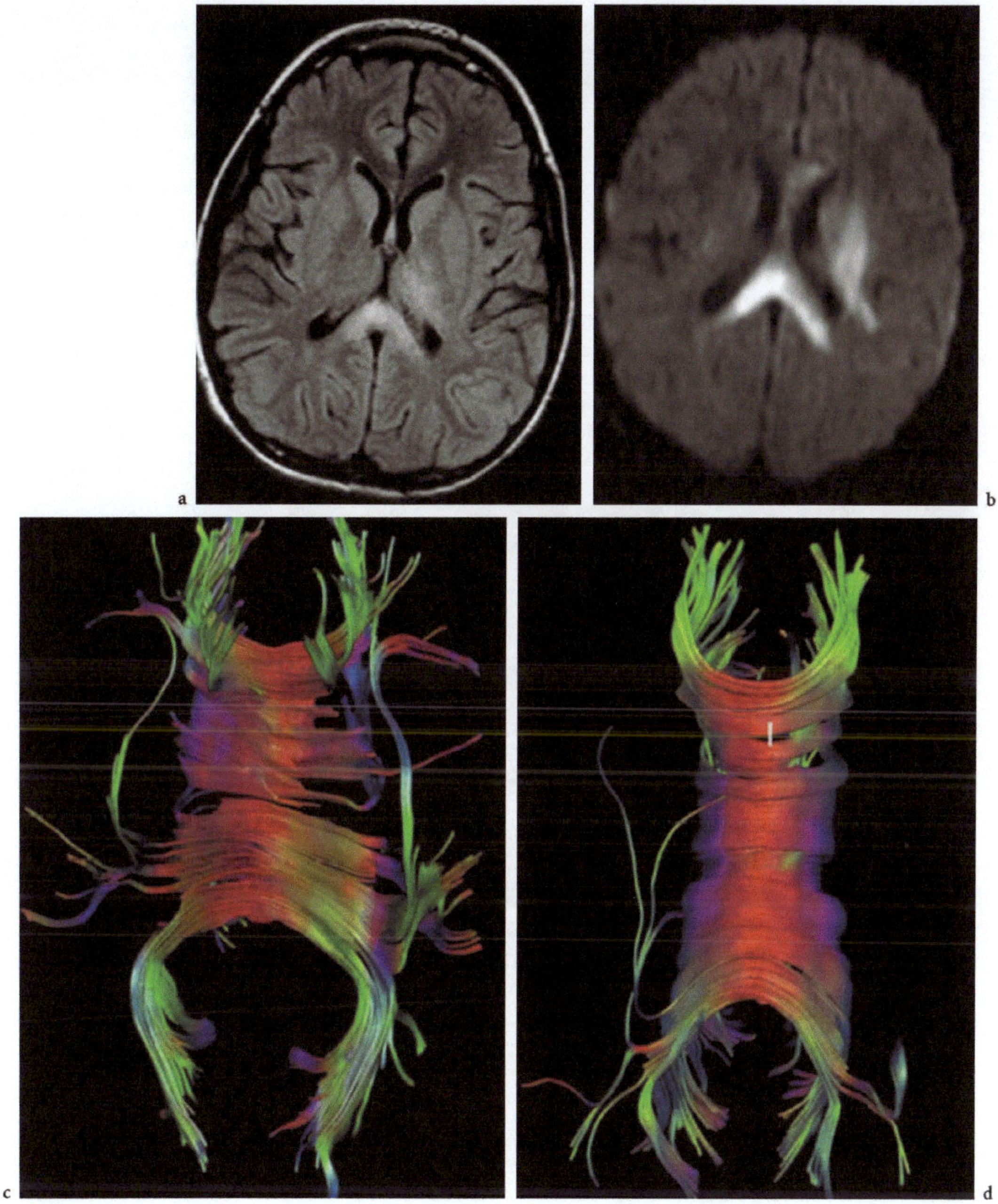

Fig. 29.7a–d. Traumatic swelling of the splenium of the corpus callosum. **a** Axial FLAIR sequence demonstrates abnormal signal intensity in the splenium of the corpus callosum. **b** Axial diffusion-weighted image reveals abnormal signal in the splenium, consistent with restricted diffusion secondary to diffuse axonal injury. Some abnormal signal is also seen in the genu of the corpus callosum and left basal ganglia. **c** Three-dimensional diffusion tensor white matter tractography demonstrating alteration and irregularity of the callosal tracts, most likely indicating cytoskeletal alterations in the white matter. **d** Three-dimensional diffusion tensor white matter tractography of a normal subject for comparison

The diffusion tensor imaging technique might provide a tool for early detection of DAI in patients with minor traumatic head injury (Fig. 29.7) (ARFANAKIS et al. 2002).

29.3 Brainstem Injury

Traumatic brainstem injuries may be classified as primary or secondary, depending on whether the lesion occurred at the time of impact or subsequent to it. Primary lesions include brainstem contusion, shearing injury, and pontomedullary rest (COOPER et al. 1979). Secondary lesions include hypoxic/ischemic injury and Duret hemorrhage (FRIEDE and ROESSMAN 1966). Duret hemorrhage is always seen in association with transtentorial herniation and is thought to result from damage to the medial pontine perforating branches of the basilar artery. Therefore, Duret hemorrhage is seen anterior to the pons. CT is somewhat limited in detecting brainstem lesions, and MRI is the preferred imaging modality for evaluating these lesions. DAI of the brainstem usually produces lesions that are small to microscopic in size and are frequently located in the midbrain and rostral pons (Fig. 29.8). GENTRY et al. (1989) reported that MRI demonstrated a significantly higher number of lesions in traumatic brainstem injury than CT. Patients with traumatic brainstem injury had a significantly higher frequency of corpus callosum and white matter shearing lesions. GENTRY et al. also found the mean Glasgow Coma Score at admission was significantly lower in patients with evi-

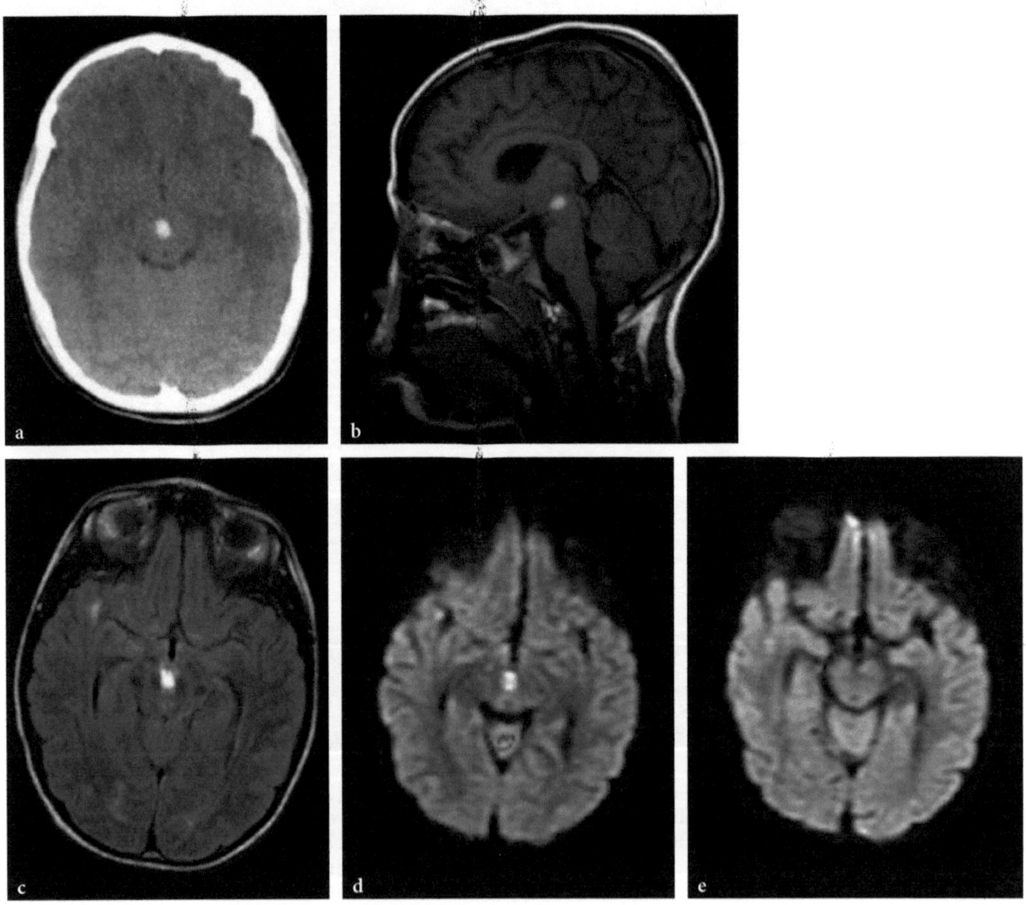

Fig. 29.8a–e. Brainstem hemorrhage. **a** Axial CT scan shows high-density hemorrhage in the midbrain. **b** Sagittal T1-weighted image shows focal hyperintense hemorrhage in the midbrain. **c** Axial FLAIR sequence demonstrates abnormal high signal intensity in the midbrain. **d** Axial diffusion-weighted image demonstrate focal hyperintensity in the midbrain, consistent with restricted diffusion. **e** Axial diffusion-weighted image obtained 3 weeks following the trauma demonstrates no abnormality

dence of brainstem injury on MRI. Traumatic injury to the brainstem involving the dentato-rubro-olivary pathway can result in unilateral or bilateral olivary hypertrophy, which is readily detected by MRI as a focal area of enlargement with high signal intensity on T2-weighted images in the region of the inferior olivary nucleus (Birbamer et al. 1993).

29.4 Cerebral Swelling

Traumatic cerebral swelling can occur secondary to cerebral hyperemia or cerebral edema. Cerebral hyperemia results from a loss of normal autoregulation of cerebral blood flow, which is secondary to elevation of systemic blood pressure. The cerebral blood flow then passively follows systemic blood pressure. Loss of autoregulation of cerebral blood flow is more common in children. Cerebral edema results from an increase in water content. Diffuse brain injury can cause generalized cerebral swelling (Yoshino et al. 1985). Infarction, secondary to intracranial and extracranial vascular injury, is seen with edema. On CT, the edematous brain is hypodense due to increased water content and there is subsequent loss of the normal differentiation between gray and white matter. Ventricular compression and sulcal effacement are also seen. In children, diffuse cerebral edema and subarachnoid hemorrhage are frequently seen as a result of closed head trauma (Segall et al. 1980). When diffuse cerebral swelling is predominantly due to cerebral hyperemia, initial CT scans may show a slight increase in overall density of the brain. This is particularly common in children. Unilateral cerebral swelling is seen frequently with ipsilateral subdural hematoma, less frequently in ipsilateral epidural hematoma, and occasionally as an isolated finding (Lobato et al. 1980).

29.5 Post-traumatic Atrophy of Cerebrum, Cerebellum, and Corpus Callosum

Atrophy of the cerebrum may occur focally or diffusely in patients with previous head trauma (Bakay and Glassauer 1980; Tsai et al. 1978). In such cases, both CT and MRI will show both widening of the cortical sulci and concordant ventriculomegaly in the affected areas. Cerebellar atrophy is demonstrated by the prominence of subarachnoid and cisternal space in the posterior fossa. Time-dependent atrophic changes occurring after TBI can be quantified using MR volumetric studies and, in the chronic stages, these studies may be predictive of eventual cognitive outcome (Bakay and Glassauer 1980). Focal atrophy may present as focal areas of encephalomalacia or porencephalic cyst. Sometimes, it may be difficult to differentiate encephalomalacia from porencephalic cyst on CT as both entities show low density. Since porencephalic cyst contains cerebrospinal fluid, it is generally of lower density than areas of encephalomalacia. On MRI, they can easily be differentiated from each other on the FLAIR sequence, as porencephalic cyst shows low signal intensity whereas encephalomalacia demonstrates high signal intensity.

In patients with long-standing, severe closed head injury and diffuse white matter injury, atrophy of the corpus callosum can occur. The degree of corpus callosal atrophy correlates significantly with the chronicity of the injury. MRI provides an in vivo determination of corpus callosal atrophy which may reflect the severity of DAI. The MRI findings of corpus callosal atrophy following closed head trauma appear to correlate clinically with post-traumatic hemispheric disconnection effects (Benavidez et al. 1999). Reduction in fornix size and hippocampal volume has also been reported in patients with TBI (Tate and Bigler 2000). We have recently observed a case of post-traumatic seizure in a patient with previous temporal lobe injury. MRI of the temporal lobe demonstrated temporal lobe encephalomalacia and bilateral mesial temporal sclerosis.

29.6 Correlation of Neuroimaging and Neurotraumatic Outcome

The role of advanced neuroimaging techniques in TBI management is undergoing a fundamental change. Historically, the radiographic findings in neurotrauma have focused on the descriptive anatomy of lesions with little regard to correlation with clinical outcomes of patients. Given the wide spectrum of traumatic mechanisms coupled with the complexity of neurophysiological autoregulation, prognostication based solely on location, number, and size of lesions has been poor at best. However, recent advances in neuroimaging have opened new opportunities to understanding the biology of neurotrauma as well as stratifying the clinical outcomes based on physiological, functional, and anatomical imaging correlates. With the growing widespread use of MRI, single-photon emission CT, and positron emission tomography (PET) scanning, new techniques are being applied to trauma situations which aim to improve clinical diagnosis and prognosis.

With the widespread adoption of advanced neuroimaging studies, neuroradiologists have gained the ability to correlate subtle changes in neurophysiology and map them anatomically. MRI can detect punctate areas of hemorrhage, differentiate between vasogenic and cytotoxic edema, and demonstrate areas of ischemia/infarct with much greater precision and speed than earlier-generation neuroimaging modalities. While several studies have examined the link between TBI and routine MRI findings, these investigations have focused primarily on lesional anatomy (Hofman et al. 2001; Tate and Bigler 2000; Udstuen and Claar 2001). However, with the development of MRS, MT, diffusion/perfusion imaging, and functional imaging, our understanding of the neurophysiology of TBI has been greatly enhanced (Hammound and Wasserman 2002).) For example, both MRS and MT imaging have been shown to quantify damage after TBI, as reported by Sinson et al. (2001). Post-traumatic differences in NAA/Cr ratios between patients with good and poor outcomes were observed but were not statistically significant. Furthermore, McGowan et al. (2000) have reported that quantitative MT imaging can be utilized to detect abnormalities associated with mild TBI which are not detected on routine CT or MRI. Although there was only a weak correlation between the MRI and neurophysiological data, refinements in the technique may allow development of a grading system to predict extent of injury (Zee et al. 2002). In fact, mild TBI is becoming an intense area of focus given its high prevalence in the population and the greater sensitivity of advanced MRI techniques. Hofman et al. (2001) recently reported the largest prospective study to date correlating neuroimaging findings and neurocognitive tests in patients with mild TBI. Their results suggest that even mild trauma to the brain results in abnormalities identified on single-photon emission CT (SPECT) and MRI which were previously not apparent. Unfortunately, the correlation between the two imaging techniques and neurocognitive tests was poor. Nevertheless, the data would support the further application of MRI and SPECT imaging to patients with head trauma given the sensitivity of these techniques to post-traumatic brain lesions.

The future of TBI research and neuroimaging is bright. We are no longer limited to simple anatomical descriptive analysis but can extend our involvement into the arena of microscopic imaging and the sphere of outcomes research. The role of the neuroradiologist as prognosticator is becoming more important as the tools at our disposal allow better understanding of the link between what we see and what clinicians observe.

References

Adams JH et al (1982) Diffuse axonal injury due to non-missile head injury in humans: an analysis of 45 cases. Ann Neurol 12:557-563

Alsop D et al (1996) Detection of acute pathologic changes following experimental traumatic brain injury using diffusion weighted magnetic resonance imaging. J Neurotrauma 13:515-521

Arfanakis K et al (2002) Diffusion tensor MR imaging in diffuse axonal injury. AJNR 23:794-802

Ashikaga R et al (1997) MRI of head injury using FLAIR. Neuroradiology 39:239-242

Bagley IJ et al (2000) Magnetization transfer imaging of traumatic brain injury. J Magn Reson Imaging 1-8

Bakay L, Glassauer FE (1980) Head injury. Boston, Little Brown

Benavidez DA, Fletcher JM, Hannay HJ et al (1999) Corpus callosum damage and interhemispheric transfer of information following closed head injury in children. Cortex 35:315-336

Birbamer G et al (1993) Post-traumatic segmental myoclonus associated with bilateral olivary hypertrophy. Acta Neurol Scand 87:505-509

Blumbergs PC et al (1994) Staining of amyloid precursor protein to study axonal damage in mild head injury. Lancet 344:1055-1056

Brooks WM et al (2001) Magnetic resonance spectroscopy in traumatic brain injury. J Head Trauma Rehabil 16:149-164

Caveness WF (1979) Incidence of cranio-cerebral trauma in 1976 with trend from 1970 to 1975. In: Thompson RA, Green JRG (eds) Advances in neurology, vol 22. Raven, New York, pp 1-3

Condon B et al (1998) Early 1H magnetic resonance spectroscopy of acute head injury: four cases. J Neurotrauma 15:563-571

Cooper PR, Maravilla K, Kirkpatrick J et al (1979) Traumatically-induced brain stem hemorrhage and the computerized tomographic scan: clinical, pathological, and experimental observations. Neurosurgery 4:115-124

Cordobes F, Lobato RD, Rivas JJ et al (1986) Post-traumatic diffuse axonal brain injury: analysis of 78 patients studied with computed tomography. Acta Neurochir 81:27-35

Friede RL, Roessman U (1966) The pathogenesis of secondary midbrain hemorrhages. Neurology 16:1210-1216

Gean AD (1994) Imaging of head trauma. Raven, New York

Gennarelli TA (1985) Emergency department management of head injuries. Emerg Med Clin North Am 2:749-760

Gentry LR, Godersky JC, Thompson BH (1988) MR imaging of head trauma: review of the distribution and radiopathologic features of traumatic lesions. AJR 150:663-672
Gentry LR et al (1988) Prospective comparative study of intermediate field MR and CT in the evaluation of closed head trauma. AJNR 9:91-100
Gentry LR, Godersky JC, Thompson BH (1989) Traumatic brain stem injury: MR imaging. Radiology 171:177-178
Hammound DA, Wasserman BA (2002) Diffuse axonal injuries: pathophysiology and imaging. Neuroimag Clin North Am 12:205-216
Hans JS, Kaufman B, Alfidi RJ et al (1984) Head trauma evaluated by magnetic resonance and computed tomography: a comparison. Radiology 150:71-77
Hanstock C et al (1994) Diffusion weighted imaging differentiates ischemic tissue from traumatic tissue. Stroke 25:843-848
Hardman JM, Manoukian A (2002) Neuroimag Clin North Am 12:175-187
Hofman P et al (2001) MR imaging, single-photon emission CT, and neurocognitive performance after mild traumatic brain injury. AJNR 22:441-449
Ito J et al (1996) Characterization of edema by diffusion weighted imaging in experimental traumatic brain injury. J Neurosurg 84:97-103
Jeret JS, Mandell M, Anziska B et al (1993) Clinical predictors of abnormality disclosed by computed tomography after mild head trauma. Neurosurgery 32:9-15
Johnson MH, Lee SH (1992) Computed tomography of acute cerebral trauma. RCNA 30:325-352
Kelly AB, Zimmerman RD, Snow RB et al (1988) Head trauma: comparison of MR and CT-experience in 100 patients. AJNR 9:699-708
Kim PE, Zee CS (1995) The radiologic evaluation of craniocerebral missile injuries. Neurosurg Clin North Am 6:669-687
Liu AY et al (1999) Traumatic brain injury: diffusion weighted MR imaging findings. AJNR 20:1636-1641
Lobato RD, Sarabia R, Cordobes F et al (1980) Post traumatic cerebral hemispheric swelling. J Neurosurg 68:417-423
McGowen J et al (2000) Magnetization transfer imaging in the detection of injury associated with mild head trauma. AJNR 21:875-880
Miller JD, Tocher JL, Jones PA (1988) Extradural hematoma: earlier detection, better results (editorial). Brain Inj 2:83-86
Mittl RL et al (1994) Prevalence of MR evidence of diffuse axonal injury in patients with mild head injury and normal CT findings. AJNR 15:1583-1589
Sasiadek M, Marciniak R, Bem Z (1991) CT appearance of shearing injuries of the brain. Bildgebung 58:148-149
Sinson G et al (2001) Magnetization transfer imaging and proton MR spectroscopy in the evaluation of axonal injury: correlation with clinical outcome after traumatic brain injury. AJNR 22:143-151
Schynoll W, Overton D, Krome R et al (1993) A prospective study to identify high-yield criteria associated with acute intracranial computed tomography findings in head injury patients. Am J Emerg Med 11:321-326
Segall HD, McComb JG, Tsai FY, Miller JH (1980) Neuroradiology in head trauma. In: Gwinn JL, Stanley P (eds) Diagnostic imaging in pediatric trauma, chap 3. Springer, Berlin Heidelberg New York
Servadei F, Piazzi G, Seracchioli A et al (1988) Extradural hematomas: an analysis of the changing characteristics of patients admitted from 1980 to 1986. Diagnostic and therapeutic implication in 158 cases. Brain Inj 2:87-100
Sosin DM et al (1989) Head injury-associated deaths in the United States from 1979 to 1986. JAMA 262:2251
Strich SJ (1961) Shearing of nerve fibers as a cause of brain damage due to head injury: a pathological study of twenty cases. Lancet I:2443-2448
Tsai FY, Huprich JE, Gardner FC et al (1978) Diagnostic and prognostic implications of computed tomography of head trauma. J Comput Assist Tomogr 2:323-331
Tate DF, Bigler ED (2000) Fornix and hippocampal atrophy in traumatic brain injury. Learn Mem 7:442-446
Udstuen GJ, Claar JM (2001) Imaging of acute head injury in the adult. Neuroimag Clin North Am 11:433-445
Yanagawa Y et al (1978) A quantitative analysis of head injury using T2-weighted gradient-echo imaging. J Trauma 49:272-277
Yoshino E, Yamaki T, Higuchi T et al (1985) Acute brain edema in fatal head injury: analysis by dynamic CT scanning. J Neurosurg 63:830-839
Zee CS, Go JL (1998) CT of head trauma. Neuroimag Clin North Am 8:525-539
Zee CS et al (2002) Imaging of sequelae of head trauma. Neuroimag Clin North Am 12:325-338
Zee CS, Segall HD, Destian S, Ahmadi J (1996) Radiologic evaluation of head trauma. In: Wilkins R, Rengachary S (eds) Neurosurgery. McGraw-Hills, New York, pp 2675-2687
Zimmerman RA, Bilaniuk LT, Gennarelli T (1978) Computed tomography of shearing injuries of the cerebral white matter. Radiology 127:393-396

30 Psychiatric Disorders

Fabio Sambataro and Alessandro Bertolino

CONTENTS

Magnetic resonance imaging applications to evaluate white matter physiology and pathology in psychiatric disorders include: structural magnetic resonance imaging (MRI), proton magnetic resonance spectroscopy (^{1}H-MRS), diffusion tensor imaging (DTI), and magnetization transfer imaging (MTI).

30.1. Diffusion Tensor Imaging

Diffusion tensor imaging (DTI) is an MRI application providing a means to examine the microstructure of brain tissues, particularly of white matter. The tensor is a mathematical construct useful for describing multidimensional vectorial systems. This construct (the "diffusion tensor") has been applied to diffusion (Basser et al. 1994), and it describes information about the three-dimensional geometry, orientation, and shape of diffusion. The shape of the ellipsoid tensor is linearly dependent on the strength of diffusion along the three main directions (the eigenvalues) of space; therefore, the tensor in white matter will describe an ellipsoid with the longest axis parallel to the axonal direction, as the other two directions are restricted. The tensor fully characterizes the diffusion system providing different measures of diffusion: the apparent diffusion coefficient (ADC) of a certain direction, the degree of anisotropy (fractional anisotropy, FA; relative anisotropy, RA) and primary fiber tract orientation. ADC is calculated by dividing the trace of the tensor by 3 and it is an invariant, thus providing a measure independent of head rotation; it is sensitive to flow in blood vessels and in cerebrospinal fluid (CSF), extracellular and intracellular restrictions of movements, fiber packing and orientation. FA is an invariant measure of the fraction of the magnitude of tensor that can be ascribed to anisotropic diffusion and it can be considered a measure of how elongated the ellipsoid in each voxel is. RA is an invariant normalized standard deviation representing the ratio of the anisotropic part to its isotropic part. Volume ratio (VR) is a measure of the sphericity of the tensor, calculated by dividing the ellipsoid volume by the volume of a sphere with a radius of 1. Minimum/maximum ratio (A) is the ratio between the minimum and the maximum of the eigenvalues, thus dependent on sorting based on size order. There are also some measures that reflect the intervoxel diffusion coherence between tensors and can be used to study fiber orientation and organization at a macroscopic level: correlation measure of organization (Basser and Pierpaoli 1996), geometric measures of weighted average tensor (Westin et al. 1997), intervoxel coherence (Pfefferbaum et al. 2000), and lattice index of anisotropy (Pierpaoli and Basser 1996).

The MR pulse sequences used to acquire diffusion-weighted MR images can be divided in echo-planar imaging and navigator methods, that allow respectively a single and a multiple shot for acquisition of one image, the latter employing navigator MR signals to detect and correct bulk motion. However, DTI sequences still suffer from some problems. The echo-planar imaging techniques are very fast, but

F. Sambataro, MD
Department of Neurology and Psychiatry, Policlinico, University of Bari, Piazza Giulio Cesare, 11, 70124 Bari, Italy
A. Bertolino, MD, PhD
Department of Neurology and Psychiatry, Policlinico, University of Bari, Piazza Giulio Cesare, 11, 70124 Bari, Italy

being very sensitive to magnetic field inhomogeneities (e.g., interfaces between brain, bone and air; Taber et al. 2002) this method can result in artifacts in areas exhibiting large variation of magnetic susceptibility; moreover they are also susceptible to chemical shift artifacts caused by the different properties of fat and water. Spatial resolution is limited (the imaging matrix acquired is rather coarse, thus making the voxel dimension larger than some white matter structures, resulting in partial volume artifacts), and signal averaging may be necessary, leading to a high sensitivity to motion artifacts. Navigator methods have an excellent spatial resolution and smaller artifacts, but more than 10 min is needed to acquire an image along with synchronization with the heart rate, thus limiting routine use of this technique in the clinical setting.

DTI data can be analyzed with two different approaches: region of interest (ROI) and voxelwise analyses. In the first, the study is performed in specific ROIs identified in relevant white matter regions, with limited anatomical reproducibility, fewer statistical tests and the possibility of false negative results. With the latter approach, brains are normalized into a standard space and then tested for group differences in FA, thus studying the entire volume; this method may have increased risk of type I errors.

Several research groups have already used DTI in a variety of conditions. For example, diffusivity is usually increased in elderly people (Gideon et al. 1994; Engelter et al. 2000; Abe et al. 2002) while FA is decreased (Pfefferbaum et al. 2000; Sullivan et al. 2001; Abe et al. 2002), even though these results are not unequivocal (Helenius et al. 2002) and not all brain regions undergo these changes in the same way. Decreased anisotropy can be found in demyelinating diseases, including leukodystrophies (Ito et al. 2002), multiple sclerosis (Filippi et al. 2002), and human immunodeficiency virus-1 (HIV-1) infection (Filippi et al. 2001; Pomara et al. 2001), suggesting that DTI can be considered as a measure of myelin integrity.

30.1.2 Future Applications

Diffusion tensor tractography is an imaging technique that uses the principal diffusion direction measured with DTI to compute the underlying tissue fiber pathways or "tracts" (Basser et al. 2000), thus allowing a three-dimensional visualization of white matter fiber tracts and the identification of specific physical connections between different brain regions. After segmentation of the white matter and identification of specific ROIs, the tracing process starts with selection of starting pixels or "seed points" within these regions. The direction of maximum diffusion is then interpolated between the neighboring voxels, thus defining a path of fibers. The iterative repetition of this process can define a fiber tract. Unfortunately use of this technique is limited by quality of the data (DTI images have a low signal-to-noise ratio) and the diffusion model (the tensor formalism) used for the analysis.

30.2 Magnetization Transfer Imaging and T_2 Relaxographic Imaging

Some other MR applications might be helpful along with DTI studies (Lim and Helpern 2002): Magnetization transfer imaging (MTI) is a relatively new imaging technique that uses off-resonance radiofrequency irradiation to transfer energy between bound and mobile pools of water. The magnetization transfer ratio (MTR) depends on protein concentration, exchange kinetics and relaxation rates of bound water. MTR data are stable and show only small changes across brain development in healthy individuals (Silver et al. 1997). Studies in multiple sclerosis have confirmed that this technique is more sensitive to subtle changes of the white matter than conventional MRI (Filippi et al. 1995).

T_2 relaxographic imaging (T_2RI) can be used to quantify the amount of myelin by examining T_2 relaxation distributions believed to be due to water confined within myelin bilayers. A reduction in these components would indicate lower quantities of myelin. These studies use long echo trains and nonlinear fitting methods (MacKay et al. 1994).

30.3 Psychiatric Disorders

White matter changes have been found in various psychiatric disorders. Most work has been done on schizophrenia, but there are also some studies on alcoholism, HIV-1 infection, mood disorders, and Alzheimer disease.

30.3.1 Schizophrenia

A popular theory about the pathophysiology of schizophrenia hypothesizes that this condition is associated with altered brain development (WEINBERGER et al. 1987). Moreover, if a node of a brain network is damaged early in development, other nodes in the network may be affected. Therefore, disrupted connectivity of cortico-cortical and cortico-subcortical circuitry might be a logical consequence of altered brain development (FRISTON 1998). A large series of clinical and cognitive phenomena are consistent with these contentions (WEINBERGER et al. 2003). Moreover, post-mortem studies in schizophrenia have produced robust evidence consistent with altered brain development and altered connectivity in this disorder. For example, several studies have reported increased neuronal density, decreased neuropil, and abnormalities in the neurons of layer III of the prefrontal cortex (PFC), the neurons responsible for cortico-cortical projections (BUXHOEVEDEN et al. 2000; SELEMON and GOLDMAN-RAKIC 1999). Other studies in PFC have reported reductions in the size of the soma of neurons (RAJKOWSKA et al. 1998), also correlating with the extent of dendritic arborization, and with the number of dendritic spines – a measure of synaptic contacts– (ROBERTS et al. 1996). Signs of apoptotic or necrotic cell death or of gliosis (a marker of degenerative disorders) have never been reported, further corroborating the evidence for altered brain development and connectivity. Similar results have also been reported for the hippocampus (for review see WEINBERGER 1999), further suggesting that altered development of the latter and of its connectivity with the PFC might be instrumental in the pathophysiology of schizophrenia.

These post-mortem findings are also consistent with in vivo studies performed with structural MRI indicating reduced volume of the hippocampus (NELSON et al. 1998), of the PFC (including prefrontal white matter; BREIER et al. 1992; BUCHANAN et al. 1998), and alteration of the connectivity between these two brain regions (WRIGHT et al. 1999). Similar MRI studies on global brain volume have also revealed small decreases in global white matter volume calculated from the associated measure of ventricular ratios (CANNON et al. 1998; WRIGHT et al. 2000), even though these results have not been universally confirmed (LIM et al. 1998). Some authors have reported reduced prefrontal lobe white matter volume (BREIER et al. 1992). Other structural MRI studies have reported alterations in the white matter of schizophrenic patients in the adhesio interthalamica (SNYDER et al. 1998), corpus callosum (CASANOVA et al. 1990; DELISI et al. 1997; DEQUARDO 1999; DEQUARDO et al. 1996; DOWNHILL et al. 2000; GUNTHER et al. 1991; HOFF et al. 1994; LEWINE et al. 1990; NARR et al. 2000; NASRALLAH et al. 1986; ROSSI et al. 1989; STRATTA et al. 1989; TIBBO et al. 1998; UEMATSU and KAIYA 1988; WOODRUFF et al. 1993), and cavum septi pellucidi (DEGREEF et al. 1992; KWON et al. 1998; NOPOULOS et al. 1996, 1997), even though there have also been negative reports.

Consistent with all these studies and with their indications, studies in animal models of schizophrenia have suggested that altered development of the hippocampus, of the PFC, and of their connectivity may be plausibly involved in the pathophysiology of this disorder. More specifically, developmental lesions of the hippocampus in nonhuman primates and in rodents selectively disrupt development of prefrontal neurons (BERTOLINO et al. 1997, 2002), and of their function for cognition (LIPSKA et al. 2002) and for regulation of dopamine release (LIPSKA et al. 1995; BERTOLINO et al. 1999).

Molecular studies in post-mortem tissue and in animal models also suggest that white matter might be associated with altered connectivity in schizophrenia. Studies of genome-wide expression analysis using DNA microarray and RT-PCR (based on a reverse transcriptase-polymerase chain reaction of a messenger RNA) (COPLAND et al. 2002; TKACHEV et al. 2003) have examined the dorsolateral PFC of patients with chronic schizophrenia. More than 6500 genes were examined and a significant (up to 50%) downregulation of the expression (HAKAK et al. 2001) of seven genes was found, these being responsible for oligodendrocyte cell differentiation and maturation, myelination, and glutamate excitotoxicity response (myelin-associated glycoprotein; CNP; myelin and lymphocyte protein, MAL; gelsolin, GSN; ErbB3, and transferrin). Other studies in knock-out mice suggest a possible role for some myelin-related genes in the pathogenesis of schizophrenia (BARTSCH et al. 1997; BARTSCH 1996; FURUKAWA et al. 1997; LASSMANN et al. 1997; MONTAG et al. 1994).

If altered connectivity of brain regions is implicated in the pathophysiology of schizophrenia, it is logical to expect that the interconnecting white matter fibers might be affected. In a ^{1}H-MRS study LIM et al. (1998) have reported selective reductions of N-acetyl aspartate (NAA) in prefrontal and parietal white matter. Although extremely useful in accounting for partial volume effects of gray and white matter, their sophisticated technique did not allow for more detailed regional analysis. This is important especially for gray matter, since one of the assumptions of their work is that NAA concentration is stable across functionally distinct cortical areas (e.g., dorsolateral and medial prefrontal cortices). Other ^{1}H-MRS studies have reported no neurochemical differences in prefrontal white matter and in centrum semiovale in patients with schizophrenia (Bertolino et al. 1996, 1998a,b, 2001; Callicott et al. 1998), schizophreniform disorder (Bertolino et al. 2003), and bipolar disorder (Bertolino et al. 2003).

DTI is the most suitable technique to evaluate the integrity of white matter fiber tracts. The first DTI study in patients with schizophrenia was performed by Buchsbaum et al. (1998) in five chronic patients and six controls who also underwent ^{18}F-fluorodeoxyglucose positron emission tomography (PET-FDG) scans. After spatial normalization, these authors reported significantly reduced prefrontal white matter RA. There were no correlations between the glucose metabolic rates of frontal cortex and the striatum assessed by PET-FDG. The authors have interpreted these results as suggestive of impairment of frontostriatal connectivity. Lim et al. (1999) studied 10 men with schizophrenia and 10 healthy controls with a pulsed gradient spin-echo echo-planar imaging DTI. For data analysis, they used a ROI approach identifying three lobar regions: prefrontal, temporo-parietal, and parieto-occipital. After using tissue segmentation contours to minimize the echo-planar warping effect, they reported widespread lower bilateral FA in the white matter of the patients from frontal to occipital regions. These widespread bilateral diffusion deficits have been also found by Agartz et al. (2001) and by Minami et al. (2003). No differences in the anisotropy of gray matter were found in these studies.

Other authors have focused their attention on specific regions: Foong et al. (2000a) studied 20 patients and 25 controls, identifying ROIs in the genu and splenium of the corpus callosum. They found significantly increased mean diffusivity and a significant reduction in FA in the splenium, but not in the genu. These results have been confirmed by Agartz et al. (2001) and Ardekani et al. (2003), who reported reduced FA also in forceps major. Ardekani et al. (2003) also found bilateral reduction in FA in the white matter of the anterior parahippocampal gyrus (PHG). Sun et al. (2003) have reported increased FA values in the anterior cingulate bundle. Some studies have focused on specific fiber tracts, reporting decreased FA in the left uncinate fasciculus, the most prominent tract of temporal-frontal connections (Burns et al. 2003; Kubicki et al. 2002a), and in the left arcuate fasciculus, one of the white matter tracts of parietal-frontal connections (Burns et al. 2003). Some of these results have not been confirmed in a recent study in patients with early-onset schizophrenia by Kumra et al. (2004). These authors demonstrated reduced FA in bilateral frontal lobes (at +5, +10 and +20 mm above the anterior-posterior commissure plane, AC-PC) and in the right occipital region; no statistical difference between patients and healthy controls was found in the genu and splenium of the corpus callosum.

Kalus et al. (2004), co-registering a high-resolution 3D-MPRAGE T1-weighted sequence with DTI, measured the intervoxel coherence (COH; an index of the degree to which the vectors point in the same direction) in the hippocampus of patients with schizophrenia. Despite lack of statistical difference in the volume of the hippocampus compared with normals, the DTI data showed that COH was reduced in patients in the bilateral posterior hippocampus and left total hippocampus. The limitations of this study include the small sample size and the potential confounding effect of pharmacotherapy.

Clinical symptomatology of the patients studied has been found to correlate with anisotropy indexes: decreased FA in inferior prefrontal white matter regions was associated with impulsivity (measured by the Motor Impulsiveness factor of the Barratt Impulsiveness Scale), and higher trace correlated with Aggressiveness (measured with the Assaultiveness scale of the Buss Durkee Hostility Inventory and with the Aggression scale of the Life History of Aggression; Hoptman et al. 2002) or with greater severity of the negative symptoms of schizophrenia, measured by the Schedule for the Assessment of Negative Symptoms (Wolkin et al. 2003).

Other studies have reported negative results. Steel et al. (2001) studied 10 patients and 10 controls with ^{1}H-MRS and DTI, examining frontal and occipital white matter. In patient they found nonsignificant reductions (of about 10–15%) in prefrontal white matter NAA levels, and no differences in white matter anisotropy. Also Foong et al. (2002) did not find any difference between patients and control groups.

MTR has also been used in schizophrenia: with a ROI approach, Foong et al. (2000b) have shown significant bilateral alterations in the temporal lobe white matter in 25 patients with schizophrenia, and a similar statistical trend in left and frontal lobes; using a voxelwise controlled approach in the same data, the authors showed a significant reduction in MTR in the inferior and middle frontal, inferior and middle temporal, and superior parietal gyri, particularly in the frontal and temporal regions (Foong et al. 2001). Negative symptom scores on the Positive And Negative Syndrome Scale (PANSS) were correlated with decreased MTR in left parietal and temporo-occipital regions. The limitations of this study include the small sample size and the gender distribution (19 men, 6 women).

T_2RI is likely to be used to corroborate the disconnection hypothesis of schizophrenia, looking to the disruptions of white matter.

30.3.2 Alcoholism

Application of these techniques to alcoholism has been limited. Pfefferbaum et al. (2000) performed a controlled DTI study of the genu and splenium of the corpus callosum and the centrum semiovale of 15 detoxified chronic patients with alcohol addiction, measuring the correlation between white matter microstructure changes and performance on neuropsychological tests assessing working memory and attention. They measured the FA and COH using a voxelwise approach. A brief neurocognitive battery based on the Dementia Rating Scale, and Backward Digit, Block Spans and Trail Making B for the assessment of attention and working memory, were administered. FA was lower in the patient group compared with control subjects in the genu and centrum semiovale; the COH was lower only in the splenium. Patients had lower neuropsychological performance, and working memory accuracy correlated positively with the splenium FA, whereas attention correlated positively with the COH. Consistent with post-mortem studies (de la Monte 1988), these results have suggested disruption of white matter microstructure in these patients and have also suggested that disruption of connectivity can be associated with impairment of working memory and attention. In another study, Pfefferbaum and Sullivan (2002) also found that FA and COH in the above-mentioned regions correlated with lifetime alcohol consumption.

Lower anisotropy in frontal white matter can be found also in individuals with cocaine dependence, confirming that the alterations in orbitofrontal connectivity might be involved in the pathogenesis of this disorder (Lim et al. 2002). These results are consistent with findings of white matter hyperintensities reported in cocaine abusers, probably associated with the vasoconstrictive effects of this drug.

30.3.3 HIV-1 Infection

Two studies have used DTI to examine the white matter in patients with HIV-1 infection. Filippi et al. (2001) studied 10 patients with a wide range of viral loads (from undetectable to greater than 400,000 HIV messenger RNA copies/mm^3). They used a ROI approach identifying regions in the genu and splenium of corpus callosum as well as bilaterally in frontal and parietal-occipital subcortical white matter and centrum semiovale. Patients were divided into three groups according to viral load level: undetectable, intermediate, and high levels. Clinical MRI scans showed only mild brain atrophy. Patients in the first group did not show any changes in diffusivity compared with healthy controls. Anisotropy index was significantly decreased in the genu and splenium of the corpus callosum in the other two groups; mean diffusivity was reduced in these regions only in the patients with high viral loads. Pomara et al. (2001) studied six non-demented HIV-1 patients and nine controls. They used a ROI approach identifying regions in the genu, splenium of the corpus callosum and bilaterally in the internal capsule, frontal, parietal, and temporal white matter. MRI scans did not show any alteration in white matter and mean diffusivity did not differ in any of these regions, while FA was decreased in frontal white matter and increased in the internal capsule. These studies show that very subtle alterations of white matter that are invisible on conventional MRI scans could be detected by DTI. Further studies with larger patient samples and neuropsychological assessments are needed.

30.3.4 Mood Disorders

White matter hyperintensities (WMH) are focal white matter abnormalities that appear as high MR signal intensity areas on T2-weighted images. The findings of WMH have been consistently replicated in patients with bipolar disorder (Deicken et al. 1991; Dupont et al. 1987, 1990, 1995). These lesions can be classified into two broad categories according to criteria established by Fazekas et al. (1987): periventricular, ranging from pencil-thin lining to irregular broad shapes extending to the deep white matter; and deep white matter lesions, ranging from punctate foci to large confluent areas. The presence of WMH might be associated with increased risk for bipolar disorder and for unipolar depression

(Coffey et al. 1990), but there are also some negative studies (Breeze et al. 2003). The etiology of WMH is unclear, but chronically reduced cerebral perfusion, cardiovascular risk factors (Claus et al. 1996; Liao et al. 1997), hypertension (Dufouil et al. 2001; Veldink et al. 1998), atherosclerosis, tobacco smoking (Gonzalez-Pinto et al. 1998), decreased serum cholesterol (Glueck et al. 1994; Swartz 1990), arteriolar hyalinization and lacunar infarcts and diabetes mellitus (Manolio et al. 1994), nutritional deficiency, demyelination, gliosis, and spongiosis (Drayer 1988; Grafton et al. 1991) might play an important role. However, WMH can be seen occasionally in healthy individuals (Katzman et al. 1999), especially in elderly subjects (Austrom et al. 1990), in whom WMH are associated with lower performances on tests of frontal lobe function (Baum et al. 1996; Boone et al. 1992; DeCarli et al. 1995).

Etiopathogenesis of late-life depression is at present uncertain. Some reports of WMH have induced researchers to focus their attention on white matter and subcortical vascular changes (Krishnan et al. 1997), particularly in medial orbital prefrontal regions (MacFall et al. 2001). In frontal cortex neuropathological studies have found altered neuronal and glial cell morphology and density (Rajkowska et al. 1999). Some imaging studies have shown that prefrontal cortex, anterior cingulate, amygdala, and striatum are involved (Drevets et al. 1997; Mayberg 1994). Neuropsychological functions (e.g., attention, speed of processing, and executive functions, which rely upon the integrity of fronto-striatal system that is located in frontal white matter) are impaired in geriatric depressed patients (Lockwood et al. 2000). One DTI study, by Alexopoulos et al. (2000), was performed in 13 geriatric patients with major depression during an open-label treatment with citalopram as an antidepressant. An ROI approach was used and five regions were identified in the frontal white matter along the AC-PC plane. After 12 weeks eight subjects achieved remission, defined as not having depressive symptoms for at least two consecutive weeks. Using survival analysis with proportional risk factors to study the correlation between FA and remission covarying for age, they found that FA of the ROI drawn at 10 and 15 mm from the AC-PC plane, lateral to the anterior cingulate, including fibers of the cortico-striatal pathways, was associated with the remission of depressive symptoms. Reduced FA in that region was associated with poor outcome.

MR studies on white matter integrity of patients with bipolar disorder (BP) suggest consistent frontal white matter changes measured with different techniques such as T1 proton relaxation times (Dolan et al. 1990) and morphometric analysis on T1-weighted images (Lopez-Larson et al. 2002). Recently, Adler et al. (2004) performed a controlled study with DTI in nine patients with BP-I treated with standard pharmacotherapy. Four ROIs were identified in prefrontal white matter along the AC-PC plane. After covarying for age and education, FA was significantly reduced in patients in the ROIs identified at 25 and 30 mm above the AC-PC plane. No significant difference in ADC values was found in any of the ROIs. The limitations of the study include the small sample size and the anisotropic nature of the voxels that can cause partial volume effects.

30.3.5 Alzheimer Disease

Alzheimer disease (AD) is mainly due to alterations affecting gray matter, but there are some post-mortem studies that have also shown loss of axons and death of oligodendrocytes (Brun and Englund 1986; Englund 1998). Diffusion-weighted imaging (DWI) studies have shown reduced diffusion within the splenium and body of the corpus callosum (Hanyu et al. 1999). DTI studies performed in the early stages of the disease have found increased mean diffusivity and decreased FA in the splenium of the corpus callosum, superior longitudinal fasciculus, and left cingulum, but also in the frontal, temporal, and parietal white matter (Bozzali et al. 2001, 2002; Rose et al. 2000; Sandson et al. 1999; Takahashi et al. 2002). These changes (mean diffusivity and eigenvalues) in the posterior cingulate may be associated with the degree of cognitive impairment measured by Mini Mental State Examination (Yoshiura et al. 2002); Bozzali et al. (2002) found that FA and mean diffusivity of the overall white matter were associated with lower scores on this cognitive assessment scale.

30.3.6 Other Conditions

White matter abnormalities have been reported with MRI also in obsessive compulsive disorder (OCD). Rosenberg et al. (1997) found a larger corpus callosum in treatment-naïve OCD pediatric patients. Jenike et al. (1996) showed a significant decrease in total white matter in adult patients with OCD.

BREITER et al. (1994) found decreased posterior white matter levels, particularly in the retrocallosal region. All these studies suggest impaired corticocortical and subcortical connectivity.

O'SULLIVAN et al. (2001) found that diffusion anisotropy was reduced in the white matter of older subjects and negatively correlated with age in this group. Moreover, executive dysfunction measured by the Trail Making Test was associated with an increase in mean diffusivity, especially in anterior white matter.

30.3.7 Conclusions

From the various studies reviewed here, it possible to draw the following conclusions:

- Most of the DTI studies performed to date in patients with schizophrenia show widespread bilateral anisotropic diffusion deficits in white matter in comparison with healthy controls. The regions most frequently studied have been the frontal, parietal, and occipital lobes, and specific fiber tracts such as the corpus callosum, uncinate and arcuate fasciculi, and cingulate bundle. The consistency of these findings is rather limited, although some agreement has been reached on decreased anisotropy in the splenium of the corpus callosum in adult-onset schizophrenia.
- ^{1}H-MRS and MR structural findings in the white matter of patients with schizophrenia are controversial. The involvement of prefrontal white matter needs to be clarified with more suitable methods.
- The lack of univocal findings in all the MRI studies may be associated with the small sample sizes, differences in MRI methodology, and clinical confounding factors (treatment, chronicity, etc.).
- As for the data on white matter lesions in patients with alcoholism, HIV-1 infection, mood disorders, and AD, the scarcity of the studies does not allow evaluation of the consistency of the results.

Integrity of white matter provides coordinated communication of specific brain regions in complex domains, such as higher cognitive function or mood regulation (DAVIDSON et al. 2000). Post-mortem, genetic, MRI, ^{1}H-MRS, and DTI studies provide some support for the involvement of white matter abnormalities in the pathogenesis of some psychiatric disorders, especially schizophrenia and mood disorders.

However, the role played by white matter in the pathophysiology of such psychiatric disorders may be secondary to cortical alterations.

In schizophrenia, abnormalities of both white and gray matters have been described. The former may be related to genetic susceptibility to develop the disease, whereas the latter may be secondary to the disease process. In fact, gray matter volume is usually reduced in the neocortex as well as in subcortical structures such as the thalamus (O'LEARY et al. 1994), amygdala, and hippocampus (WRIGHT et al. 2000).

Better understanding of white matter alterations will probably be achieved with an extensive use of MRI and DTI, although further improvements in resolution and analysis methods are desirable. DTI can yield more powerful results using other techniques (MTI, T2-RI, tractography), in association with measures of functionality (fMRI and neuropsychological testing) and genetic analyses, as well as with clinical symptomatology and treatment outcomes.

Even with the limitations detailed above, at present DTI seems the only approach that can be used to noninvasively track white matter fibers and to assess "in vivo" their integrity at the microstructural level.

References

Adler CM, Holland SK, Schmithorst V, Wilke M, Weiss KL, Pan H, Strakowski SM (2004) Abnormal frontal white matter tracts in bipolar disorder: a diffusion tensor imaging study. Bipolar Disord 6:197-203

Agartz I, Andersson JL, Skare S (2001) Abnormal brain white matter in schizophrenia: a diffusion tensor imaging study. Neuroreport 12:2251-2254

Akbarian S, Bunney WE Jr, Potkin SG et al (1993a) Altered distribution of nicotinamide-adenine dinucleotide phosphate-diaphorase cells in frontal lobe of schizophrenics implies disturbances of cortical development. Arch Gen Psychiatry 50:169-177

Akbarian S, Vinuela A, Kim JJ, Potkin SG, Bunney WE Jr, Jones EG (1993b) Distorted distribution of nicotinamide-adenine dinucleotide phosphate-diaphorase neurons in temporal lobe of schizophrenics implies anomalous cortical development. Arch Gen Psychiatry 50:178-187

Akbarian S, Kim JJ, Potkin SG, Hetrick WP, Bunney WE Jr, Jones EG (1996) Maldistribution of interstitial neurons in prefrontal white matter of the brains of schizophrenic patients. Arch Gen Psychiatry 53:425-436

Alexopoulos GS, Meyers BS, Young RC et al (2000) Executive dysfunction and long-term outcomes of geriatric depression. Arch Gen Psychiatry 57:285-290

Anderson SA, Volk DW, Lewis DA (1996) Increased density of microtubule associated protein 2-immunoreactive neurons in the prefrontal white matter of schizophrenic subjects. Schizophr Res 19:111-119

Andreasen NC, Arndt S, Swayze V II, Cizadlo T, Flaum M, O'Leary D, Ehrhardt JC, Yuh WTC (1994) Thalamic abnormalities in schizophrenia visualized through magnetic resonance image averaging. Science 266:294-298

Ardekani BA, Nierenberg J, Hoptman MJ, Javitt DC, Lim KO (2003) MRI study of white matter diffusion anisotropy in schizophrenia. Neuroreport 14:2025-2029

Austrom MG, Thompson RF Jr, Hendrie HC et al (1990) Foci of increased T2 signal intensity in MR images of healthy elderly subjects. A follow-up study. J Am Geriatr Soc 38:1133-1138

Bailer U, Leisch F, Meszaros K et al (2000) Genome scan for susceptibility loci for schizophrenia. Neuropsychobiology 42:175-182

Ballmaier M, Sowell ER, Thompson PM, Kumar A, Narr KL, Lavretsky H, Welcome SE, DeLuca H, Toga AW (2004) Mapping brain size and cortical gray matter changes in elderly depression. Biol Psychiatry 55:382-389

Bartsch S, Montag D, Schachner M, Bartsch U (1997) Increased number of unmyelinated axons in optic nerves of adult mice deficient in the myelin-associated glycoprotein (MAG). Brain Res 762:231-234

Bartsch U (1996) Myelination and axonal regeneration in the central nervous system of mice deficient in the myelin-associated glycoprotein. J Neurocytol 25:303-313

Basser PJ, Mattiello J, LeBihan D (1994) Estimation of the effective self-diffusion tensor from the NMR spin echo. J Magn Reson B 103:247-254

Basser PJ, Pierpaoli C (1996) Microstructural and physiological features of tissues elucidated by quantitative-diffusion-tensor MRI. J Magn Reson B 111:209-219

Baum KA, Schulte C, Girke W, Reischies FM, Felix R (1996) Incidental white-matter foci on MRI in "healthy" subjects: evidence of subtle cognitive dysfunction. Neuroradiology 38:755-760

Bertolino A, Nawroz S, Mattay VS, Barnett AS, Duyn JH, Moonen CT, Frank JA, Tedeschi G, Weinberger DR (1996) Regionally specific pattern of neurochemical pathology in schizophrenia as assessed by multislice proton magnetic resonance spectroscopic imaging. Am J Psychiatry 153:1554-1563

Bertolino A, Saunders RC, Mattay VS, Bachevalier J, Frank JA, Weinberger DR (1997) Altered development of prefrontal neurons in rhesus monkeys with neonatal mesial temporo-limbic lesions: a proton magnetic resonance spectroscopic imaging study. Cereb Cortex 7:740-748

Bertolino A, Callicott JH, Elman I, Mattay VS, Tedeschi G, Frank JA, Breier A, Weinberger DR (1998a) Regionally specific neuronal pathology in untreated patients with schizophrenia: a proton magnetic resonance spectroscopic imaging study. Biol Psychiatry 43:641-648

Bertolino A, Knable MB, Saunders RC, Callicott JH, Kolachana B, Mattay VS, Bachevalier J, Frank JA, Egan M, Weinberger DR (1999) The relationship between dorsolateral prefrontal N-acetylaspartate measures and striatal dopamine activity in schizophrenia. Biol Psychiatry 45:660-667

Bertolino A, Callicott JH, Mattay VS, Weidenhammer KM, Rakow R, Egan MF, Weinberger DR (2001) The effect of treatment with antipsychotic drugs on brain N-acetylaspartate measures in patients with schizophrenia. Biol Psychiatry 49:39-46

Bertolino A, Roffman JL, Lipska BK, van Gelderen P, Olson A, Weinberger DR (2002) Reduced N-acetylaspartate in prefrontal cortex of adult rats with neonatal hippocampal damage. Cereb Cortex 12:983-990

Bertolino A, Frye M, Callicott JH, Mattay VS, Rakow R, Shelton-Repella J, Post R, Weinberger DR (2003a) Neuronal pathology in the hippocampal area of patients with bipolar disorder: a study with proton magnetic resonance spectroscopic imaging. Biol Psychiatry 53:906-913

Bertolino A, Sciota D, Brudaglio F, Altamura M, Blasi G, Bellomo A, Antonucci N, Callicott JH, Goldberg TE, Scarabino T, Weinberger DR, Nardini M (2003b) Working memory deficits and levels of N-acetylaspartate in patients with schizophreniform disorder. Am J Psychiatry 160:483-489

Boone KB, Miller BL, Lesser IM et al (1992) Neuropsychological correlates of white-matter lesions in healthy elderly subjects. A threshold effect. Arch Neurol 49:549-554

Bozzali M, Franceschi M, Falini A et al (2001) Quantification of tissue damage in AD using diffusion tensor and magnetization transfer MRI. Neurology 57:1135-1137

Bozzali M, Falini A, Franceschi M et al (2002) White matter damage in Alzheimer's disease assessed in vivo using diffusion tensor magnetic resonance imaging. J Neurol Neurosurg Psychiatry 72:742-746

Breeze JL, Hesdorffer DC, Hong X, Frazier JA, Renshaw PF (2003) Clinical significance of brain white matter hyperintensities in young adults with psychiatric illness. Harv Rev Psychiatry 11:269-283

Breier A, Buchanan RW, Elkashef A, Munson RC, Kirkpatrick B, Gellad F (1992) Brain morphology and schizophrenia. A magnetic resonance imaging study of limbic, prefrontal cortex, and caudate structures. Arch Gen Psychiatry 49:921-926

Breiter HC, Filipek PA, Kennedy DN et al (1994) Retrocallosal white matter abnormalities in patients with obsessive-compulsive disorder. Arch Gen Psychiatry 51:663-664

Brun A, Englund E (1986) A white matter disorder in dementia of the Alzheimer type: a pathoanatomical study. Ann Neurol 19:253-262

Brzustowicz LM, Hodgkinson KA, Chow EW, Honer WG, Bassett AS (2000) Location of a major susceptibility locus for familial schizophrenia on chromosome 1q21-q22. Science 288:678-682

Buchanan RW, Vladar K, Barta PE, Pearlson GD (1998) Structural evaluation of the prefrontal cortex in schizophrenia. Am J Psychiatry 155:1049-1055

Buchsbaum MS, Tang CY, Peled S et al (1998) MRI white matter diffusion anisotropy and PET metabolic rate in schizophrenia. Neuroreport 9:425-430

Burnashev N (1996) Calcium permeability of glutamate-gated channels in the central nervous system. Curr Opin Neurobiol 6:311-317

Burns J, Job D, Bastin ME et al (2003) Structural disconnectivity in schizophrenia: a diffusion tensor magnetic resonance imaging study. Br J Psychiatry 182:439-443

Buxhoeveden D, Roy E, Switala A, Casanova MF (2000) Reduced interneuronal space in schizophernia. Biol Psychiatry 47:681-683

Cahn W, Hulshoff Pol HE, Lems EBTE, van Haren NEM, Schnack HG, Van der Linden JA et al (2002) Brain volume changes in first-episode schizophrenia: a one-year follow-up study. Arch Gen Psychiatry 59:1002-1010

Callicott JH, Egan MF, Bertolino A, Mattay VS, Langheim FJ, Frank JA, Weinberger DR (1998) Hippocampal N-acetyl aspartate in unaffected siblings of patients with schizo-

phrenia: a possible intermediate neurobiological phenotype. Biol Psychiatry 44:941-950
Cannon TD, van Erp TG, Huttunen M et al (1998) Regional gray matter, white matter, and cerebrospinal fluid distributions in schizophrenic patients, their siblings, and controls. Arch Gen Psychiatry 55:1084-1091
Casanova MF, Zito M, Goldberg T et al (1990) Shape distortion of the corpus callosum of monozygotic twins discordant for schizophrenia. Schizophr Res 3:155-156
Claus JJ, Breteler MM, Hasan D et al (1996) Vascular risk factors, atherosclerosis, cerebral white matter lesions and cerebral perfusion in a population-based study. Eur J Nucl Med 23:675-682
Coffey CE, Figiel GS, Djang WT, Weiner RD (1990) Subcortical hyperintensity on magnetic resonance imaging: a comparison of normal and depressed elderly subjects. Am J Psychiatry 147:187-189
Connor JR (1994) Iron acquisition and expression of iron regulatory proteins in the developing brain: manipulation by ethanol exposure, iron deprivation and cellular dysfunction. Dev Neurosci 16:233-247
Copland C, Dracheva S, Davis KL, Haroutunian V (2002) mRNA expression of three isoforms of myelin associated glycoprotein (MAG) in patients with schizophrenia (abstract). Abstr Soc Neurosci 28:494.4
Davis KL, Stewart DG, Friedman JI, Buchsbaum M, Harvey PD, Hof PR, Buxbaum J, Haroutunian V (2003) White matter changes in schizophrenia: evidence for myelin-related dysfunction. Arch Gen Psychiatry 60:443-456
de la Monte SM (1988) Disproportionate atrophy of cerebral white matter in chronic alcoholics. Arch Neurol 45:990-992
DeCarli C, Murphy DG, Tranh M et al (1995) The effect of white matter hyperintensity volume on brain structure, cognitive performance, and cerebral metabolism of glucose in 51 healthy adults. Neurology 45:2077-2084
Degreef G, Lantos G, Bogerts B, Ashtari M, Lieberman J (1992) Abnormalities of the septum pellucidum on MR scans in first-episode schizophrenic patients. AJNR Am J Neuroradiol 13:835-840
Deicken RF, Reus VI, Manfredi L, Wolkowitz OM (1991) MRI deep white matter hyperintensity in a psychiatric population. Biol Psychiatry 29:918-922
DeLisi LE, Sakuma M, Tew W, Kushner M, Hoff AL, Grimson R (1997) Schizophrenia as a chronic active brain process: a study of progressive brain structural change subsequent to the onset of schizophrenia. Psychiatry Res 74:129-140
DeQuardo JR (1999) Landmark analysis of corpus callosum shape in schizophrenia. Biol Psychiatry 46:1712-1714
DeQuardo JR, Bookstein FL, Green WD, Brunberg JA, Tandon R (1996) Spatial relationships of neuroanatomic landmarks in schizophrenia. Psychiatry Res 67:81-95
Dolan RJ, Poynton AM, Bridges PK, Trimble MR (1990) Altered magnetic resonance white-matter T1 values in patients with affective disorder Br J Psychiatry 157:107-110
Downhill JE Jr, Buchsbaum MS, Wei T et al (2000) Shape and size of the corpus callosum in schizophrenia and schizotypal personality disorder. Schizophr Res 42:193-208
Drayer BP (1988) Imaging of the aging brain. I. Normal findings. Radiology 166:785-796
Drevets WC, Price JL, Simpson JR Jr et al (1997) Subgenual prefrontal cortex abnormalities in mood disorders. Nature 386:824-827
Dufouil C, de Kersaint-Gilly A, Besancon V et al (2001) Longitudinal study of blood pressure and white matter hyperintensities: the EVA MRI Cohort. Neurology 56:921-926
Dupont RM, Jernigan TL, Gillin JC, Butters N, Delis DC, Hesselink JR (1987) Subcortical signal hyperintensities in bipolar patients detected by MRI. Psychiatry Res 21:357-358
Dupont RM, Jernigan TL, Butters N et al (1990) Subcortical abnormalities detected in bipolar affective disorder using magnetic resonance imaging. Clinical and neuropsychological significance. Arch Gen Psychiatry 47:55-59
Dupont RM, Butters N, Schafer K, Wilson T, Hesselink J, Gillin JC (1995) Diagnostic specificity of focal white matter abnormalities in bipolar and unipolar mood disorder. Biol Psychiatry 38:482-486
Ekelund J, Lichtermann D, Hovatta I et al (2000) Genome-wide scan for schizophrenia in the Finnish population: evidence for a locus on chromosome 7q22. Hum Mol Genet 9:1049-1057
Englund E (1998) Neuropathology of white matter changes in Alzheimer's disease and vascular dementia. Dement Geriatr Cogn Disord 9 [Suppl 1]:6-12
Faraone SV, Matise T, Svrakic D et al (1998) Genome scan of European-American schizophrenia pedigrees: results of the NIMH Genetics Initiative and Millennium Consortium. Am J Med Genet 81:290-295
Fazekas F, Chawluk JB, Alavi A, Hurtig HI, Zimmerman RA (1987) MR signal abnormalities at 1.5 T in Alzheimer's dementia and normal aging. AJR Am J Roentgenol 149:351-356
Filippi CG, Ulug AM, Ryan E, Ferrando SJ, van Gorp W (2001) Diffusion tensor imaging of patients with HIV and normal-appearing white matter on MR images of the brain. AJNR Am J Neuroradiol 22:277-283
Filippi M, Campi A, Dousset V et al (1995) A magnetization transfer imaging study of normal-appearing white matter in multiple sclerosis. Neurology 45:478-482
Filippi M, Tortorella C, Rovaris M (2002) Magnetic resonance imaging of multiple sclerosis. J Neuroimaging 12:289-301
Foong J, Maier M, Clark CA, Barker GJ, Miller DH, Ron MA (2000a) Neuropathological abnormalities of the corpus callosum in schizophrenia: a diffusion tensor imaging study. J Neurol Neurosurg Psychiatry 68:242-244
Foong J, Maier M, Barker GJ, Brocklehurst S, Miller DH, Ron MA (2000b) In vivo investigation of white matter pathology in schizophrenia with magnetisation transfer imaging. J Neurol Neurosurg Psychiatry 68:70-74
Foong J, Symms MR, Barker GJ, Maier M, Miller DH, Ron MA (2002) Investigating regional white matter in schizophrenia using diffusion tensor imaging. Neuroreport 13:333-336
Foong J, Symms MR, Barker GJ, Maier M, Woermann FG, Miller DH, Ron MA (2001) Neuropathological abnormalities in schizophrenia: evidence from magnetization transfer imaging. Brain 124:882-892
Friston KJ (1998) The disconnection hypothesis. Schizophr Res 30:115-125
Furukawa K, Fu W, Li Y, Witke W, Kwiatkowski DJ, Mattson MP (1997) The actin-severing protein gelsolin modulates calcium channel and NMDA receptor activities and vulnerability to excitotoxicity in hippocampal neurons. J Neurosci 17:8178-8186
Glueck CJ, Tieger M, Kunkel R, Hamer T, Tracy T, Speirs J (1994) Hypocholesterolemia and affective disorders. Am J Med Sci 308:218-225

Gonzalez-Pinto A, Gutierrez M, Ezcurra J et al (1998) Tobacco smoking and bipolar disorder. J Clin Psychiatry 59:225-228

Grafton ST, Sumi SM, Stimac GK, Alvord EC Jr, Shaw CM, Nochlin D (1991) Comparison of postmortem magnetic resonance imaging and neuropathologic findings in the cerebral white matter. Arch Neurol 48:293-298

Gunther W, Petsch R, Steinberg R et al (1991) Brain dysfunction during motor activation and corpus callosum alterations in schizophrenia measured by cerebral blood flow and magnetic resonance imaging. Biol Psychiatry 29:535-555

Gurling HM, Kalsi G, Brynjolfson J et al (2001) Genomewide genetic linkage analysis confirms the presence of susceptibility loci for schizophrenia, on chromosomes 1q32.2, 5q33.2, and 8p21-22 and provides support for linkage to schizophrenia, on chromosomes 11q23.3-24 and 20q12.1-11.23. Am J Hum Genet 68:661-673

Hakak Y, Walker JR, Li C et al (2001) Genome-wide expression analysis reveals dysregulation of myelination-related genes in chronic schizophrenia. Proc Natl Acad Sci USA 98:4746-4751

Hanyu H, Asano T, Sakurai H et al (1999) Diffusion-weighted and magnetization transfer imaging of the corpus callosum in Alzheimer's disease. J Neurol Sci 167:37-44

Hirsch SR, Weinberger DR (2003) Schizophrenia, 2nd edn. Blackwell, Oxford

Hoff AL, Neal C, Kushner M, DeLisi LE (1994) Gender differences in corpus callosum size in first-episode schizophrenics. Biol Psychiatry 35:913-919

Hoffman RE, Dobscha SK (1989) Cortical pruning and the development of schizophrenia: a computer model. Schizophr Bull 15:477-490

Hoptman MJ, Volavka J, Johnson G, Weiss E, Bilder RM, Lim KO (2002) Frontal white matter microstructure, aggression, and impulsivity in men with schizophrenia: a preliminary study. Biol Psychiatry 52:9-14

Hulshoff Pol HE, Brans RG, van Haren NE, Schnack HG, Langen M, Baare WF, van Oel CJ, Kahn RS (2004) Gray and white matter volume abnormalities in monozygotic and same-gender dizygotic twins discordant for schizophrenia. Biol Psychiatry 55:126-130

Ito R, Mori S, Melhem ER (2002) Diffusion tensor brain imaging and tractography. Neuroimaging Clin North Am 12:1-19

Jenike MA, Breiter HC, Baer L et al (1996) Cerebral structural abnormalities in obsessive-compulsive disorder. A quantitative morphometric magnetic resonance imaging study. Arch Gen Psychiatry 53:625-632

Karas GB, Burton EJ, Rombouts SA, van Schijndel RA, O'Brien JT, Scheltens P, McKeith IG, Williams D, Ballard C, Barkhof F (2003) A comprehensive study of gray matter loss in patients with Alzheimer's disease using optimized voxel-based morphometry. Neuroimage 18:895-907

Katzman GL, Dagher AP, Patronas NJ (1999) Incidental findings on brain magnetic resonance imaging from 1000 asymptomatic volunteers. JAMA 282:36-39

Kaufmann CA, Suarez B, Malaspina D et al (1998) NIMH Genetics Initiative Millennium Schizophrenia Consortium: linkage analysis of African-American pedigrees. Am J Med Genet 81:282-289

Keshavan MS, Anderson S, Pettegrew JW (1994) Is schizophrenia due to excessive synaptic pruning in the prefrontal cortex? The Feinberg hypothesis revisited. J Psychiatr Res 28:239-265

Krishnan KR, Hays JC, Blazer DG (1997) MRI-defined vascular depression. Am J Psychiatry 154:497-501

Kubicki M, Westin CF, Maier SE et al (2002a) Uncinate fasciculus findings in schizophrenia: a magnetic resonance diffusion tensor imaging study. Am J Psychiatry 159:813-820

Kubicki M, Westin CF, Maier SE, Mamata H, Frumin M, Ersner-Hershfield H, Kikinis R, Jolesz FA, McCarley R, Shenton ME (2002b) Diffusion tensor imaging and its application to neuropsychiatric disorders. Harv Rev Psychiatry 10:324-336

Kumra S, Ashtari M, McMeniman M, Vogel J, Augustin R, Becker DE, Nakayama E, Gyato K, Kane JM, Lim K, Szeszko P (2004) Reduced frontal white matter integrity in early-onset schizophrenia: a preliminary study. Biol Psychiatry 55:1138-1145

Kwon JS, Shenton ME, Hirayasu Y et al (1998) MRI study of cavum septi pellucidi in schizophrenia, affective disorder, and schizotypal personality disorder. Am J Psychiatry 155:509-515

Lassmann H, Bartsch U, Montag D, Schachner M (1997) Dying-back oligodendrogliopathy: a late sequel of myelin-associated glycoprotein deficiency. Glia 19:104-110

Le Bihan D, Breton E, Lallemand D, Grenier P, Cabanis E, Laval-Jeantet M (1986) MR imaging of intravoxel incoherent motions: application to diffusion and perfusion in neurologic disorders. Radiology 161:401-417

Le Bihan D, Mangin JF, Poupon C, Clark CA, Pappata S, Molko N, Chabriat H (2001) Diffusion tensor imaging: concepts and applications. J Magn Reson Imaging 13:534-546

Levinson DF, Mahtani MM, Nancarrow DJ et al (1998) Genome scan of schizophrenia. Am J Psychiatry 155:741-750

Lewine RR, Gulley LR, Risch SC, Jewart R, Houpt JL (1990) Sexual dimorphism, brain morphology, and schizophrenia. Schizophr Bull 16:195-203

Liao D, Cooper L, Cai J et al (1997) The prevalence and severity of white matter lesions, their relationship with age, ethnicity, gender, and cardiovascular disease risk factors: the ARIC Study. Neuroepidemiology 16:149-162

Lieberman J, Chakos M, Wu H, Alvir J, Hoffman E, Robinson D, Bilder R (2001) Longitudinal study of brain morphology in first episode schizophrenia. Biol Psychiatry 49:487-499

Lim KO, Helpern JA (2002) Neuropsychiatric applications of DTI - a review. NMR Biomed 15:587-593

Lim KO, Adalsteinsson E, Spielman D, Sullivan EV, Rosenbloom MJ, Pfefferbaum A (1998) Proton magnetic resonance spectroscopic imaging of cortical gray and white matter in schizophrenia. Arch Gen Psychiatry 55:346-352

Lim KO, Hedehus M, Moseley M, de Crespigny A, Sullivan EV, Pfefferbaum A (1999) Compromised white matter tract integrity in schizophrenia inferred from diffusion tensor imaging. Arch Gen Psychiatry 56:367

Lim KO, Choi SJ, Pomara N, Wolkin A, Rotrosen JP (2002) Reduced frontal white matter integrity in cocaine dependence: a controlled diffusion tensor imaging study. Biol Psychiatry 51:890-895

Lipska BK, Aultman JM, Verma A, Weinberger DR, Moghaddam B (2002) Neonatal damage of the ventral hippocampus impairs working memory in the rat. Neuropsychopharmacology 27:47-54

Lipska BK, Weinberger DR (1995) Genetic variation in vulnerability to the behavioral effects of neonatal hippocampal damage in rats. Proc Natl Acad Sci USA 92:8906-8910

Lockwood KA, Alexopoulos GS, Kakuma T, Van Gorp WG

(2000) Subtypes of cognitive impairment in depressed older adults. Am J Geriatr Psychiatry 8:201-208
Lopez-Larson MP, DelBello MP, Zimmerman ME, Schwiers ML, Strakowski SM (2002) Regional prefrontal gray and white matter abnormalities in bipolar disorder. Biol Psychiatry 52:93-100
MacFall JR, Payne ME, Provenzale JE, Krishnan KR (2001) Medial orbital frontal lesions in late-onset depression. Biol Psychiatry 49:803-806
Manolio TA, Kronmal RA, Burke GL et al (1994) Magnetic resonance abnormalities and cardiovascular disease in older adults. The Cardiovascular Health Study. Stroke 25:318-327
Mayberg HS (1994) Frontal lobe dysfunction in secondary depression. J Neuropsychiatry Clin Neurosci 6:428-442
Michael D. Nelson MD, Andrew J, Saykin AJ, Laura A. Flashman LA, Riordan HJ, Henry J (1998) Riordan hippocampal volume reduction in schizophrenia as assessed by magnetic resonance imaging: a meta-analytic study. Arch Gen Psychiatry 55:433-440
Minami T, Nobuhara K, Okugawa G et al (2003) Diffusion tensor magnetic resonance imaging of disruption of regional white matter in schizophrenia. Neuropsychobiology 47:141-145
Montag D, Giese KP, Bartsch U et al (1994) Mice deficient for the myelin-associated glycoprotein show subtle abnormalities in myelin. Neuron 13:229-246
Mowry BJ, Ewen KR, Nancarrow DJ et al (2000) Second stage of a genome scan of schizophrenia: study of five positive regions in an expanded sample. Am J Med Genet 96:864-869
Narr KL, Thompson PM, Sharma T, Moussai J, Cannestra AF, Toga AW (2000) Mapping morphology of the corpus callosum in schizophrenia. Cereb Cortex 10:40-49
Nasrallah HA, Andreasen NC, Coffman JA et al (1986) A controlled magnetic resonance imaging study of corpus callosum thickness in schizophrenia. Biol Psychiatry 21:274-282
Nopoulos P, Swayze V, Andreasen NC (1996) Pattern of brain morphology in patients with schizophrenia and large cavum septi pellucidi. J Neuropsychiatry Clin Neurosci 8:147-152
Nopoulos P, Swayze V, Flaum M, Ehrhardt JC, Yuh WT, Andreasen NC (1997) Cavum septi pellucidi in normals and patients with schizophrenia as detected by magnetic resonance imaging. Biol Psychiatry 41:1102-1108
O'Sullivan M, Jones DK, Summers PE, Morris RG, Williams SC, Markus HS (2001) Evidence for cortical "disconnection" as a mechanism of age-related cognitive decline. Neurology 57:632-638
Park JP, Moeschler JB, Berg SZ, Wurster-Hill DH (1991) Schizophrenia and mental retardation in an adult male with a de novo interstitial deletion 9(q32q34.1). J Med Genet 28:282-283
Persaud R, Russow H, Harvey I et al (1997) Focal signal hyperintensities in schizophrenia. Schizophr Res 27:55-64
Pfefferbaum A, Sullivan EV (2002) Microstructural but not macrostructural disruption of white matter in women with chronic alcoholism. Neuroimage 15:708-718
Pfefferbaum A, Sullivan EV, Hedehus M, Adalsteinsson E, Lim KO, Moseley M (2000) In vivo detection and functional correlates of white matter microstructural disruption in chronic alcoholism. Alcohol Clin Exp Res 24:1214-1221
Pierpaoli C, Basser PJ (1996) Toward a quantitative assessment of diffusion anisotropy. Magn Reson Med 36:893-906
Pitman RK, Shin LM, Rauch SL (2001) Investigating the pathogenesis of posttraumatic stress disorder with neuroimaging. J Clin Psychiatry 62 [Suppl 17]:47-54
Pomara N, Crandall DT, Choi SJ, Johnson G, Lim KO (2001) White matter abnormalities in HIV-1 infection: a diffusion tensor imaging study. Psychiatry Res 106:15-24
Rajkowska G, Selemon LD, Goldman-Rakic PS (1998) Neuronal and glial somal size in the prefrontal cortex: a postmortem morphometric study of schizophrenia and Huntington disease. Arch Gen Psychiatry 55:215-224
Rajkowska G, Miguel-Hidalgo JJ, Wei J et al (1999) Morphometric evidence for neuronal and glial prefrontal cell pathology in major depression. Biol Psychiatry 45:1085-1098
Riley BP, Tahir E, Rajagopalan S et al (1997) A linkage study of the N-methyl-D-aspartate receptor subunit gene loci and schizophrenia in southern African Bantu-speaking families. Psychiatr Genet 7:57-74
Roberts RC, Conley R, Kung L, Peretti FJ, Chute DJ (1996) Reduced striatal spine size in schizophrenia: a postmortem ultrastructural study. Neuroreport 7:1214-1218
Rose SE, Chen F, Chalk JB et al (2000) Loss of connectivity in Alzheimer's disease: an evaluation of white matter tract integrity with colour coded MR diffusion tensor imaging. J Neurol Neurosurg Psychiatry 69:528-530
Rosenberg DR, Keshavan MS, Dick EL, Bagwell WW, MacMaster FP, Birmaher B (1997) Corpus callosal morphology in treatment-naive pediatric obsessive compulsive disorder. Prog Neuropsychopharmacol Biol Psychiatry 21:1269-1283
Rossi A, Stratta P, Gallucci M, Passariello R, Casacchia M (1989) Quantification of corpus callosum and ventricles in schizophrenia with nuclear magnetic resonance imaging: a pilot study. Am J Psychiatry 146:99-101
Sachdev P, Brodaty H (1999) Quantitative study of signal hyperintensities on T2-weighted magnetic resonance imaging in late-onset schizophrenia. Am J Psychiatry 156:1958-1967
Sandson TA, Felician O, Edelman RR, Warach S (1999) Diffusion-weighted magnetic resonance imaging in Alzheimer's disease. Dement Geriatr Cogn Disord 10:166-171
Selemon LD, Goldman-Rakic PS (1999) The reduced neuropil hypothesis: a circuit based model of schizophrenia. Biol Psychiatry 45:17-25
Silver NC, Barker GJ, MacManus DG, Tofts PS, Miller DH (1997) Magnetisation transfer ratio of normal brain white matter: a normative database spanning four decades of life. J Neurol Neurosurg Psychiatry 62:223-228
Snyder PJ, Bogerts B, Wu H, Bilder RM, Deoras KS, Lieberman JA (1998) Absence of the adhesio interthalamica as a marker of early developmental neuropathology in schizophrenia: an MRI and postmortem histologic study. J Neuroimaging 8:159-163
Staal WG, Hulshoff Pol HE, Schnack HG, van Haren NE, Seifert N, Kahn RS (2001) Structural brain abnormalities in chronic schizophrenia at the extremes of the outcome spectrum. Am J Psychiatry 158:1140-1142
Steel RM, Bastin ME, McConnell S et al (2001) Diffusion tensor imaging (DTI) and proton magnetic resonance spectroscopy (^{1}H MRS) in schizophrenic subjects and normal controls. Psychiatry Res 106:161-170
Stober G, Saar K, Ruschendorf F et al (2000) Splitting schizophrenia: periodic catatonia-susceptibility locus on chromosome 15q15. Am J Hum Genet 67:1201-1207

Stratta P, Rossi A, Gallucci M, Amicarelli I, Passariello R, Casacchia M (1989) Hemispheric asymmetries and schizophrenia: a preliminary magnetic resonance imaging study. Biol Psychiatry 25:275-284

Sun Z, Wang F, Cui L, Breeze J, Du X, Wang X, Cong Z, Zhang H, Li B, Hong N, Zhang D (2003) Abnormal anterior cingulum in patients with schizophrenia: a diffusion tensor imaging study. Neuroreport 14:1833-1836

Swartz CM (1990) Albumin decrement in depression and cholesterol decrement in mania. J Affect Disord 19:173-176

Taber KH, Pierpaoli C, Rose SE, Rugg-Gunn FJ, Chalk JB, Jones DK, Hurley RA (2002) The future for diffusion tensor imaging in neuropsychiatry. J Neuropsychiatry Clin Neurosci 14:1-5

Takahashi S, Yonezawa H, Takahashi J, Kudo M, Inoue T, Tohgi H (2002) Selective reduction of diffusion anisotropy in white matter of Alzheimer disease brains measured by 3.0 Tesla magnetic resonance imaging. Neurosci Lett 332:45-48

Taylor WD, Hsu E, Krishnan KR, MacFall JR (2004) Diffusion tensor imaging: background, potential, and utility in psychiatric research. Biol Psychiatry 55:201-207

Tibbo P, Nopoulos P, Arndt S, Andreasen NC (1998) Corpus callosum shape and size in male patients with schizophrenia. Biol Psychiatry 44:405-412

Tkachev D, Mimmack ML, Ryan MM et al (2003) Oligodendrocyte dysfunction in schizophrenia and bipolar disorder. Lancet 362:798-805

Uematsu M, Kaiya H (1988) The morphology of the corpus callosum in schizophrenia. An MRI study. Schizophr Res 1:391-398

Uranova N, Orlovskaya D, Vikhreva O et al (2001) Electron microscopy of oligodendroglia in severe mental illness. Brain Res Bull 55:597-610

Veldink JH, Scheltens P, Jonker C, Launer LJ (1998) Progression of cerebral white matter hyperintensities on MRI is related to diastolic blood pressure. Neurology 51:319-320

Weinberger D (1999) Cell biology of the hippocampal formation in schizophrenia. Biol Psychiatry 45:395-402

Westin CF, Peled S, Gudbjartsson H, Kikinis R, Jolesz FA (1997) Geometrical diffusion measures from tensor basis analysis (abstract). Proceedings of the 5th scientific meeting of the International Society of Magnetic Resonance in Medicine, Vancouver, British Columbia, p 1742

Williams NM, Rees MI, Holmans P et al (1999) A two-stage genome scan for schizophrenia susceptibility genes in 196 affected sibling pairs. Hum Mol Genet 8:1729-1739

Wolkin A, Choi SJ, Szilagyi S, Sanfilipo M, Rotrosen JP, Lim KO (2003) Inferior frontal white matter anisotropy and negative symptoms of schizophrenia: a diffusion tensor imaging study. Am J Psychiatry 160:572-574

Woodruff PW, Pearlson GD, Geer MJ, Barta PE, Chilcoat HD (1993) A computerized magnetic resonance imaging study of corpus callosum morphology in schizophrenia. Psychol Med 23:45-56

Wright IC, Sharma T, Ellison ZR, McGuire PK, Friston KJ, Brammer MJ, Murray RM, Bullmore ET (1999) Supra-regional brain systems and the neuropathology of schizophrenia. Cereb Cortex 9:366-378

Wright IC, Rabe-Hesketh S, Woodruff PW, David AS, Murray RM, Bullmore ET (2000) Meta-analysis of regional brain volumes in schizophrenia. Am J Psychiatry 157:16-25

Yoshiura T, Mihara F, Ogomori K, Tanaka A, Kaneko K, Masuda K (2002) Diffusion tensor in posterior cingulate gyrus: correlation with cognitive decline in Alzheimer's disease. Neuroreport 13:2299-2302

Subject Index

N

O

List of Contributors

ROLAND BAMMER, PhD
Lucas Center for MR Spectroscopy and Imaging
Department of Radiology
Mail Code 5488, Route 8
Stanford, CA 94305-5488
USA

ALESSANDRO BERTOLINO, MD, PhD
Department of Neurology and Psychiatry
University of Bari
Piazza Giulio Cesare, 11
70124 Bari
Italy

ALBERTO BIZZI, MD
Department of Neuroradiology
Istituto Nazionale Neurologico "Carlo Besta"
Via Celoria, 11
20133 Milano
Italy

LOUIS R. CAPLAN, MD
Beth Israel Deaconess Medical Center
Harvard Medical School
330 Brookline Ave
Boston, MA 02215
USA

MAURICIO CASTILLO, MD, FACR
Professor and Chief of Neuroradiology
Department of Radiology
University of North Carolina
School of Medicne
101 Manning Drive
Campus Box 7510
Chapel Hill, NC 27599-7510
USA

NICOLA DE STEFANO, MD, PhD
Associate Professor
Department of Neurology & Behavioral Sciences
University of Siena
Viale Bracci 2
53100 Siena
Italy

VINCENT DOUSSET, MD, PhD
Professor of Radiology
Service de Neuroradiologie Diagnostique et Thérapeutique
CHU Bordeaux Pellegrin and
Laboratoire de Neurobiologie des Affections de la Myéline
Université Victor Segalen Bourdeaux 2
Place Amélie-Raba Léon
33076 Bordeaux
France

BART J. EMMER, MD, PhD
Department of Radiology
Leiden University Medical Center
Albinusdreef 2
Postbus 9600
2300 RC Leiden
The Netherlands

FRANZ FAZEKAS, MD
Professor, Department of Neurology
and Department of Neuroradiology
Medical University Graz
Auenbruggerplatz 22
8036 Graz
Austria

MASSIMO FILIPPI, MD
Director, Neuroimaging Research Unit
Department of Neurology
Scientific Institute and University Ospedale San Raffaele
Via Olgettina, 60
20132 Milan
Italy

KENNETH W. FISHBEIN, PhD
Nuclear Magnetic Resonance Unit
National Institutes of Health
National Institute of Aging
Intramural Research Program
GRC 4D-08
5600 Nathan Shock Drive
Baltimore, MD 21224
USA

GIOVANNI B. FRISONI, MD
Head, LENITEM – Laboratory of Epidemiology
Neuroimaging & Telemedicine
IRCCS San Giovanni di Dio FBF
The National Center for Research and
Care of Alzheimer's Disease
Via Pilastroni 4
25125 Brescia
Italy

John L. Go, MD
Assistant Professor of Radiology and Otolaryngology
Division of Neuroradiology
Department of Radiology
University of Southern California Keck School of Medicine
1200 North State Street, Room 3740F
Los Angeles, CA 90033
USA

Joao A Gomes, MD
Johns Hopkins Hospital
Neurocritical Care Division, Meyer 8-140
600 N Wolfe St
Baltimore, MD
USA

Simon J. Hickman, MB, BChir, MRCP
NMR Research Unit
Department of Neuroinflammation
Institute of Neurology
University College London
The National Hospital for Neurology and Neurosurgery
Queen Square
London WC1N 3BG
UK

Mark A. Horsfield, PhD
Department of Cardiovascular Sciences
University of Leicester
Faculty of Medicine
Leicester LE1 5WW
UK

Tom W.J. Huizinga, MD
Department of Radiology
Leiden University Medical Center
Albinusdreef 2
Postbus 9600
2300 RC Leiden
The Netherlands

Peter Jezzard, PhD
Professor of Neuroimaging
FMRIB Centre
John Radcliffe Hospital
Department of Clinical Neurology
University of Oxford
Headington, Oxford, OX3 9DU
UK

Alayar Kangarlu, MD
Head of MRI Physics and
Assistant Professor of Clinical Neuroscience
Columbia University College of Physicians
and Surgeons and New York State Psychiatric Institute
1051 Riverside Drive, Unit 74
New York, NY 10032
USA

Paul E. Kim, MD
Assistant Professor of Radiology
Division of Neuroradiology
Department of Radiology
University of Southern California Keck School of Medicine
1200 North State Street, Room 3740B
Los Angeles, CA 90033
USA

Bette K. Kleinschmidt-DeMasters, MD
Departments of Pathology, Neurology, Neurosurgery
University of Colorado
Health Sciences Center, Campus box A-034
4200 East Ninth Avenue
Denver, CO 80262
USA

Michael Knauth, MD
Professor, Department of Neuroradiology
Zentrum Radiologie
Georg-August-Universität Göttingen
Robert-Koch-Straße 40, TL 183
37075 Göttingen
Germany

Ilhami Kovanlikaya, MD
Assistant Professor of Radiology
Division of Neuroradiology, Department of Radiology
University of Southern California Keck School of Medicine
1200 North State Street, Room 3740B
Los Angeles, CA 90033
USA

Dara L. Kraitchman, VMD, PhD
Associate Professor
Johns Hopkins University, School of Medicine
Department of Radiology
Division of Magnetic Resonance Research
601 N. Caroline Street, Office 4231
Baltimore, MD 21287-0845
USA

Robert E. Lenkinski, PhD
Associate Chief for Academic Affairs
Director of Experimental Radiology
and the 3T Magnetic Resonance Imaging/Spectroscopy Program
Beth Israel Deaconess Medical Center
Professor of Radiology, Harvard Medical School
330 Brookline Avenue
Boston, Massachusetts 02215
USA

David K.B. Li, MD, FRCPC
Professor, Department of Radiology
The University of British Columbia
Main Floor
2211 Wesbrook Mall
Vancouver, British Columbia, V6T 2B5
Canada

Carlo Marras, MD
Department of Neurosurgery
Istituto Nazionale Neurologico "Carlo Besta"
Via Celoria, 11
20133 Milano
Italy

Mario Mascalchi, MD
Professor, Sezione di Radiodiagnostica
Dipartimento di Fisiopatologia Clinica
Università di Firenze
Viale Morgagni, 85
50134 Firenze
Italy

MARCEL MAYA, MD
Clinical and Interventional Neuroradiology
Residency Training Program Director
S. Mark Taper Foundation Imaging Center
Cedars-Sinai Medical Center
8700 Beverly Boulevard, Suite M-335
Los Angeles, CA 90033
USA

JOSEPH C. MCGOWAN, PhD
Associate Professor of Electrical Engineering
Department of Electrical Engineering
Maury Hall 227
United States Naval Academy
Annapolis, MD 21402-5025
USA

DAVID H. MILLER, MD, FRCP
NMR Research Unit, Department of Neuroinflammation
Institute of Neurology
The National Hospital for Neurology and Neurosurgery
Queen Square
London WC1N 3BG London
UK

SUSUMU MORI, MD
Department of Radiology and Radiological Science
Johns Hopkins Hospital University Medical School
217 Traylor Bldg.
720 Rutland Ave.
Baltimore, MD 21205
USA
and
F.M. Kirby Research Center for Functional Brain Imaging
Kennedy Krieger Institute, 707 N. Broadway
Baltimore, MD 21205
USA

MARZIA MORTILLA, MD
Department of Radiology
Childrens Hospital Anna Meyer
Florence
Italy

LIDIA NAGAE-POETSCHER, MD
Department of Radiology and Radiological Science
Johns Hopkins Hospital University Medical School
217 Traylor Bldg.
720 Rutland Ave.
Baltimore, MD 21205
USA
and
F.M. Kirby Research Center for Functional Brain Imaging
Kennedy Krieger Institute, 707 N. Broadway
Baltimore, MD 21205
USA

DARIN T. OKUDA, MD
St. Joseph's Hospital & Medical Center
Barrow Neurological Institute
Division of Neurology
350 W. Thomas Road
Phoenix, AZ 85013
USA

DONALD W. PATY, MD, FRCPC
Professor Emeritus, Division of Neurology
The University of British Columbia
Main Floor
2211 Wesbrook Mall
Vancouver BC V6T 2B5
Canada

BIANCA POLLO, MD
Department of Neuropathology
Istituto Nazionale Neurologico "Carlo Besta"
Via Celoria, 11
20133 Milano
Italy

CHARLES RAYBAUD, MD, FRCPC
Division Head of Neuroradiology
Department of Diagnostic Imaging
The Hospital for Sick Children
555 University Avenue
Toronto, Ontario M5G 1X8
Canada

MARIA A. ROCCA, MD
Neuroimaging Research Unit
Department of Neurology
Scientific Institute and University Ospedale San Raffaele
Via Olgettina, 60
20132 Milan
Italy

MARCO ROVARIS, MD
Neuroimaging Research Unit
Department of Neurology
Scientific Institute and University Ospedale San Raffaele
Via Olgettina, 60
20132 Milan
Italy

FABRIZIO SALVI, MD
Sezione di Radiodiagnostica
Dipartimento di Fisiopatologia Clinica
Università di Firenze
Viale Morgagni, 85
50134 Firenze
Italy

FABIO SAMBATARO, MD
Department of Neurology and Psychiatry
University of Bari
Piazza Giulio Cesare, 11
70124 Bari
Italy

STEFAN SCHWARZ, MD
Assistant Professor
Department of Neurology
Klinikum Mannheim
University of Heidelberg
Theodor-Kutzer-Ufer 1-3
68167 Mannheim
Germany

Jack H. Simon, MD, PhD
Departments of Radiology, Neurology, Neurosurgery
University of Colorado
Health Sciences Center
Campus box A-034
4200 East Ninth Avenue
Denver, CO 80262
USA

Richard G. Spencer, PhD, MD
Chief, Nuclear Magnetic Resonance Unit
National Institutes of Health
National Institute of Aging
Intramural Research Program
GRC 4D-08
5600 Nathan Shock Drive
Baltimore, MD 21224
USA

Siegrid Strasser-Fuchs, MD
Professor, Department of Neurology
Medical University Graz
Auenbruggerplatz 22
8036 Graz
Austria

Scott D. Swanson, PhD
Research Assistant Professor
Department of Radiology
University of Michigan
200 Zina Pitcher Place
Ann Arbor, MI 48109-0553
USA

Ahmed Toosy, MD
Department of Headache
Brain Injury and Rehabilitation
Institute of Neurology
Queen Square
London, WC1N 3BG
UK

Anthony Traboulsee, MD, FRCPC
Instructor, Division of Neurology
Department of Medicine
The University of British Columbia
S195-2211 Wesbrook Mall
Vancouver, British Columbia, V6T 2B5
Canada

Mark A. van Buchem, MD, PhD
Professor and Head Neuroradiology
Department of Radiology
Leiden University Medical Center
Albinusdreef 2
Postbus 9600
2300 RC Leiden
The Netherlands

Peter C.M. van Zijl, PhD
Department of Radiology and Radiological Science
Johns Hopkins Hospital University Medical School
217 Traylor Bldg.
720 Rutland Ave.
Baltimore, MD 21205
USA
and
F.M. Kirby Research Center for Functional Brain Imaging
Kennedy Krieger Institute
707 N. Broadway
Baltimore, MD 21205
USA

Timothy L. Vollmer, MD
Chairman, Division of Neurology, 8 BNI
Barrow Neurological Institute
St. Joseph's Hospital and Medical Center
350 West Thomas Road
Phoenix, AZ 85013
USA

Chi Shing Zee, MD
Professor of Radiology and Neurosurgery
Director of Neuroradiology
University of Southern California University Hospital
Department of Imaging
1500 San Pablo Street
Los Angeles, CA 90033
USA

Guojun Zhao, MD
Research Associate, Division of Neurology
Department of Medicine
The University of British Columbia
Gerald McGavin Building
2386 East Mall
Vancouver, British Columbia, V6T 1Z4
Canada

MEDICAL RADIOLOGY Diagnostic Imaging and Radiation Oncology

Titles in the series already published

DIAGNOSTIC IMAGING

Innovations in Diagnostic Imaging
Edited by J. H. Anderson

Radiology of the Upper Urinary Tract
Edited by E. K. Lang

The Thymus - Diagnostic Imaging, Functions, and Pathologic Anatomy
Edited by E. Walter, E. Willich, and W. R. Webb

Interventional Neuroradiology
Edited by A. Valavanis

Radiology of the Pancreas
Edited by A. L. Baert, co-edited by G. Delorme

Radiology of the Lower Urinary Tract
Edited by E. K. Lang

Magnetic Resonance Angiography
Edited by I. P. Arlart, G. M. Bongartz, and G. Marchal

Contrast-Enhanced MRI of the Breast
S. Heywang-Köbrunner and R. Beck

Spiral CT of the Chest
Edited by M. Rémy-Jardin and J. Rémy

Radiological Diagnosis of Breast Diseases
Edited by M. Friedrich and E.A. Sickles

Radiology of the Trauma
Edited by M. Heller and A. Fink

Biliary Tract Radiology
Edited by P. Rossi, co-edited by M. Brezi

Radiological Imaging of Sports Injuries
Edited by C. Masciocchi

Modern Imaging of the Alimentary Tube
Edited by A. R. Margulis

Diagnosis and Therapy of Spinal Tumors
Edited by P. R. Algra, J. Valk, and J. J. Heimans

Interventional Magnetic Resonance Imaging
Edited by J.F. Debatin and G. Adam

Abdominal and Pelvic MRI
Edited by A. Heuck and M. Reiser

Orthopedic Imaging
Techniques and Applications
Edited by A. M. Davies and H. Pettersson

Radiology of the Female Pelvic Organs
Edited by E. K.Lang

Magnetic Resonance of the Heart and Great Vessels
Clinical Applications
Edited by J. Bogaert, A.J. Duerinckx, and F. E. Rademakers

Modern Head and Neck Imaging
Edited by S. K. Mukherji and J. A. Castelijns

Radiological Imaging of Endocrine Diseases
Edited by J. N. Bruneton in collaboration with B. Padovani and M.-Y. Mourou

Trends in Contrast Media
Edited by H. S. Thomsen, R. N. Muller, and R. F. Mattrey

Functional MRI
Edited by C. T. W. Moonen and P. A. Bandettini

Radiology of the Pancreas
2nd Revised Edition
Edited by A. L. Baert
Co-edited by G. Delorme and L. Van Hoe

Emergency Pediatric Radiology
Edited by H. Carty

Spiral CT of the Abdomen
Edited by F. Terrier, M. Grossholz, and C. D. Becker

Liver Malignancies
Diagnostic and Interventional Radiology
Edited by C. Bartolozzi and R. Lencioni

Medical Imaging of the Spleen
Edited by A. M. De Schepper and F. Vanhoenacker

Radiology of Peripheral Vascular Diseases
Edited by E. Zeitler

Diagnostic Nuclear Medicine
Edited by C. Schiepers

Radiology of Blunt Trauma of the Chest
P. Schnyder and M. Wintermark

Portal Hypertension
Diagnostic Imaging-Guided Therapy
Edited by P. Rossi
Co-edited by P. Ricci and L. Broglia

Recent Advances in Diagnostic Neuroradiology
Edited by Ph. Demaerel

Virtual Endoscopy and Related 3D Techniques
Edited by P. Rogalla, J. Terwisscha Van Scheltinga, and B. Hamm

Multislice CT
Edited by M. F. Reiser, M. Takahashi, M. Modic, and R. Bruening

Pediatric Uroradiology
Edited by R. Fotter

Transfontanellar Doppler Imaging in Neonates
A. Couture and C. Veyrac

Radiology of AIDS
A Practical Approach
Edited by J.W.A.J. Reeders and P.C. Goodman

CT of the Peritoneum
Armando Rossi and Giorgio Rossi

Magnetic Resonance Angiography
2nd Revised Edition
Edited by I. P. Arlart, G. M. Bongratz, and G. Marchal

MEDICAL RADIOLOGY Diagnostic Imaging and Radiation Oncology

Titles in the series already published

Pediatric Chest Imaging
Edited by Javier Lucaya
and Janet L. Strife

Applications of Sonography in Head and Neck Pathology
Edited by J. N. Bruneton
in collaboration with C. Raffaelli
and O. Dassonville

Imaging of the Larynx
Edited by R. Hermans

3D Image Processing
Techniques and Clinical Applications
Edited by D. Caramella
and C. Bartolozzi

Imaging of Orbital and Visual Pathway Pathology
Edited by W. S. Müller-Forell

Pediatric ENT Radiology
Edited by S. J. King
and A. E. Boothroyd

Radiological Imaging of the Small Intestine
Edited by N. C. Gourtsoyiannis

Imaging of the Knee
Techniques and Applications
Edited by A. M. Davies
and V. N. Cassar-Pullicino

Perinatal Imaging
From Ultrasound to MR Imaging
Edited by Fred E. Avni

Radiological Imaging of the Neonatal Chest
Edited by V. Donoghue

Diagnostic and Interventional Radiology in Liver Transplantation
Edited by E. Bücheler, V. Nicolas,
C. E. Broelsch, X. Rogiers,
and G. Krupski

Radiology of Osteoporosis
Edited by S. Grampp

Imaging Pelvic Floor Disorders
Edited by C. I. Bartram
and J. O. L. DeLancey
Associate Editors: S. Halligan,
F. M. Kelvin, and J. Stoker

Imaging of the Pancreas
Cystic and Rare Tumors
Edited by C. Procacci
and A. J. Megibow

High Resolution Sonography of the Peripheral Nervous System
Edited by S. Peer and G. Bodner

Imaging of the Foot and Ankle
Techniques and Applications
Edited by A. M. Davies,
R. W. Whitehouse,
and J. P. R. Jenkins

Radiology Imaging of the Ureter
Edited by F. Joffre, Ph. Otal,
and M. Soulie

Imaging of the Shoulder
Techniques and Applications
Edited by A. M. Davies and J. Hodler

Radiology of the Petrous Bone
Edited by M. Lemmerling
and S. S. Kollias

Interventional Radiology in Cancer
Edited by A. Adam, R. F. Dondelinger,
and P. R. Mueller

Duplex and Color Doppler Imaging of the Venous System
Edited by G. H. Mostbeck

Multidetector-Row CT of the Thorax
Edited by U. J. Schoepf

Functional Imaging of the Chest
Edited by H.-U. Kauczor

Radiology of the Pharynx and the Esophagus
Edited by O. Ekberg

Radiological Imaging in Hematological Malignancies
Edited by A. Guermazi

Imaging and Intervention in Abdominal Trauma
Edited by R. F. Dondelinger

Multislice CT
2nd Revised Edition
Edited by M. F. Reiser, M. Takahashi,
M. Modic, and C. R. Becker

Intracranial Vascular Malformations and Aneurysms
From Diagnostic Work-Up
to Endovascular Therapy
Edited by M. Forsting

Radiology and Imaing of the Colon
Edited by A. H. Chapman

Coronary Radiology
Edited by M. Oudkerk

Dynamic Contrast-Enhanced Magnetic Resonance Imaging in Oncology
Edited by A. Jackson, D. L. Buckley,
and G. J. M. Parker

Imaging in Treatment Planning for Sinonasal Diseases
Edited by R. Maroldi and P. Nicolai

Clinical Cardiac MRI
With Interactive CD-ROM
Edited by J. Bogaert,
S. Dymarkowski, and A. M. Taylor

Focal Liver Lesions
Detection, Characterization,
Ablation
Edited by R. Lencioni, D. Cioni,
and C. Bartolozzi

Multidetector-Row CT Angiography
Edited by C. Catalano
and R. Passariello

MR Imaging in White Matter Diseases of the Brain and Spinal Cord
Edited by M. Filippi, N. De Stefano,
V. Dousset, and J. C. McGowan

Paediatric Musculoskeletal Diseases
With an Emphasis on Ultrasound
Edited by D. Wilson

Contrast Media in Ultrasonography
Basic Principles and
Clinical Applications
Edited by Emilio Quaia

Springer

Medical Radiology Diagnostic Imaging and Radiation Oncology

Titles in the series already published

Radiation Oncology

Lung Cancer
Edited by C.W. Scarantino

Innovations in Radiation Oncology
Edited by H. R. Withers and L. J. Peters

Radiation Therapy of Head and Neck Cancer
Edited by G. E. Laramore

Gastrointestinal Cancer – Radiation Therapy
Edited by R.R. Dobelbower, Jr.

Radiation Exposure and Occupational Risks
Edited by E. Scherer, C. Streffer, and K.-R. Trott

Radiation Therapy of Benign Diseases
A Clinical Guide
S. E. Order and S. S. Donaldson

Interventional Radiation Therapy Techniques – Brachytherapy
Edited by R. Sauer

Radiopathology of Organs and Tissues
Edited by E. Scherer, C. Streffer, and K.-R. Trott

Concomitant Continuous Infusion Chemotherapy and Radiation
Edited by M. Rotman and C. J. Rosenthal

Intraoperative Radiotherapy – Clinical Experiences and Results
Edited by F. A. Calvo, M. Santos, and L.W. Brady

Radiotherapy of Intraocular and Orbital Tumors
Edited by W. E. Alberti and R. H. Sagerman

Interstitial and Intracavitary Thermoradiotherapy
Edited by M. H. Seegenschmiedt and R. Sauer

Non-Disseminated Breast Cancer
Controversial Issues in Management
Edited by G. H. Fletcher and S.H. Levitt

Current Topics in Clinical Radiobiology of Tumors
Edited by H.-P. Beck-Bornholdt

Practical Approaches to Cancer Invasion and Metastases
A Compendium of Radiation Oncologists' Responses to 40 Histories
Edited by A. R. Kagan with the Assistance of R. J. Steckel

Radiation Therapy in Pediatric Oncology
Edited by J. R. Cassady

Radiation Therapy Physics
Edited by A. R. Smith

Late Sequelae in Oncology
Edited by J. Dunst and R. Sauer

Mediastinal Tumors. Update 1995
Edited by D. E. Wood and C. R. Thomas, Jr.

Thermoradiotherapy and Thermochemotherapy

Volume 1:
Biology, Physiology, and Physics

Volume 2:
Clinical Applications

Edited by M.H. Seegenschmiedt, P. Fessenden, and C.C. Vernon

Carcinoma of the Prostate
Innovations in Management
Edited by Z. Petrovich, L. Baert, and L.W. Brady

Radiation Oncology of Gynecological Cancers
Edited by H.W. Vahrson

Carcinoma of the Bladder
Innovations in Management
Edited by Z. Petrovich, L. Baert, and L.W. Brady

Blood Perfusion and Microenvironment of Human Tumors
Implications for Clinical Radiooncology
Edited by M. Molls and P. Vaupel

Radiation Therapy of Benign Diseases
A Clinical Guide
2nd Revised Edition
S. E. Order and S. S. Donaldson

Carcinoma of the Kidney and Testis, and Rare Urologic Malignancies
Innovations in Management
Edited by Z. Petrovich, L. Baert, and L.W. Brady

Progress and Perspectives in the Treatment of Lung Cancer
Edited by P. Van Houtte, J. Klastersky, and P. Rocmans

Combined Modality Therapy of Central Nervous System Tumors
Edited by Z. Petrovich, L. W. Brady, M. L. Apuzzo, and M. Bamberg

Age-Related Macular Degeneration
Current Treatment Concepts
Edited by W. A. Alberti, G. Richard, and R. H. Sagerman

Radiotherapy of Intraocular and Orbital Tumors
2nd Revised Edition
Edited by R. H. Sagerman, and W. E. Alberti

Modification of Radiation Response
Cytokines, Growth Factors, and Other Biolgical Targets
Edited by C. Nieder, L. Milas, and K. K. Ang

Radiation Oncology for Cure and Palliation
R. G. Parker, N. A. Janjan, and M. T. Selch

Clinical Target Volumes in Conformal and Intensity Modulated Radiation Therapy
A Clinical Guide to Cancer Treatment
Edited by V. Grégoire, P. Scalliet, and K. K. Ang

Advances in Radiation Oncology in Lung Cancer
Edited by Branislav Jeremić

Springer

MIX
Papier aus verantwortungsvollen Quellen
Paper from responsible sources
FSC® C105338

If you have any concerns about our products,
you can contact us on
ProductSafety@springernature.com

In case Publisher is established outside the EU,
the EU authorized representative is:
Springer Nature Customer Service Center GmbH
Europaplatz 3, 69115 Heidelberg, Germany

Printed by Libri Plureos GmbH
in Hamburg, Germany